Atlas of Thyroid Lesions

Arne Heilo • Eva Sigstad • Krystyna Grøholt
Editors

Atlas of Thyroid Lesions

Springer

Editors
Arne Heilo, MD
Department of Radiology
Oslo University Hospital
Section The Norwegian Radium Hospital
P.Box 4953 Nydalen
0424 Oslo, Norway
AJH@ous-hf.no

Eva Sigstad, MD
Department of Pathology
Oslo University Hospital
Section The Norwegian Radium Hospital
P.Box 4953 Nydalen
0424 Oslo, Norway
ESP@ous-hf.no

Krystyna Grøholt, MD
Department of Pathology
Oslo University Hospital
Section The Norwegian Radium Hospital
P.Box 4953 Nydalen
0424 Oslo, Norway
KKG@ous-hf.no

ISBN 978-1-4939-4081-3 ISBN 978-1-4419-6010-8 (eBook)

DOI 10.1007/978-1-4419-6010-8
Springer New York Dordrecht Heidelberg London

Printed on acid-free paper

Springer is part of Springer Science+Business Media (www.springer.com)

Preface

Thyroid nodules are a common clinical finding in the population, especially in women. The prevalence of palpable nodules is about 5%. At autopsy or ultrasound (US) examination thyroid lesions are found in up to 50% of the adult population. Only about 10% of palpable thyroid nodules are malignant. In Norway there are about 220 new thyroid carcinomas each year. This means that more than 2000 patients have to be examined to find these carcinomas. Due to increased use of computed tomography, magnetic resonance, positron emmision tomography and US examination of the neck for other reasons, more palpable and nonpalpable thyroid lesions, so-called "incidentalomas" are found. Many of these lesions will need further examination.

Until a few years ago, thyroid lesions were resected with no preoperative diagnosis, and as a result, a lot of benign thyroid nodules were removed unnecessarily. In addition, many malignant tumors were not radically removed at primary surgery and the need for regional lymph node resections were not taken into consideration. For many years there has been controversy about the most cost-effective approach in the diagnostic evaluation and treatment of thyroid nodules.

During the past 5 years, the management of patients with thyroid nodules and thyroid carcinoma has changed. In 2006 the American Thyroid Association announced their Management Guidelines for patients with Thyroid Nodules and Differentiated Thyroid Carcinoma [1], and the European Thyroid Association released their European Consensus for the Management of Patients with Differentiated Thyroid Carcinoma of the Follicular Epithelium the same year [2]. In March 2007 the Norwegian guidelines were published [3].

The essential aim of this atlas is to give physicians performing US examinations better knowledge in differentiating between benign, suspicious, and malignant thyroid lesions, and between normal and pathologic neck lymph nodes. There are some features that are typical for one entity, but there are also many overlapping features among the different lesions, which make it impossible to assess the correct diagnosis in every case. The presentation of pathology images may help the cytopathologist/histopathologist in their evaluation of the different specimens, and may also be of interest to the radiologist. A better understanding of the pathology may help the radiologist develop his or her skills. The goal for the patient and the physician should be to prevent surgeries for clinically insignificant benign nodular disease and to perform radical resections of thyroid carcinomas and metastases when needed.

Arne Heilo, MD, Eva Sigstad, MD,
and Krystyna Grøholt, MD

Acknowledgments

I want to thank the whole thyroid team at Rikshospitalet/ Radiumhospitalet for their important contribution and encouragement. I want to thank my closest colleague and best co-operant in ultrasound until 2009, Dr. Kristin Holgersen, who has performed a lot of the ultrasound examinations.

I also want to thank Kaja Heilo, my daughter, for her invaluable help with the layout of the book.

Arne Heilo, MD

Contents

Section I

Introduction

Ultrasound (US) has become a very important tool in the management of thyroid carcinoma, both in primary diagnostics and in the follow-up of patients surgically treated for thyroid carcinoma. According to the Norwegian guidelines [3], "Patients with a palpable thyroid tumor should be referred directly to a center where both US of the whole neck and US-guided cytologic biopsy of the thyroid tumor and of suspicious lymph nodes can be performed. As far as possible, a cytopathologist or a screener should be present to examine the specimen and ensure good quality." In Norway breast screening centers are established in every county. The intention is to implement this work-up model for thyroid nodules in connection with these centers where the radiologists are familiar with the use of US-guided cytologic biopsies in collaboration with cytopathologists.

The most crucial step when evaluating thyroid lesions and cervical lymph nodes is the US examination, along with deciding whether a lesion should be punctured, how many nodules should be punctured, and from what part of the lesion the sample should be collected. This evaluation and decision is based on the experience of the physician performing the examination, but also on the ability of the US equipment to procure the pathology. Many US physicians have limited experience in this field, and the need for a reference atlas is obvious.

Because of the numerous findings of thyroid nodules at different imaging examinations of the neck, it is very important to have a proper policy on how to handle these findings. It is well accepted that nonsuspicious nodules less than 1 cm should be left alone without doing cytologic biopsy or further follow-up, except for patients who have received external radiation to the head or neck during childhood, or in patients with a family history of medullary or papillary thyroid cancer. Any asymptomatic colloid or hypertrophic nodule, thyroiditis, and goiter may, with some exceptions, be included in this policy.

This atlas demonstrates a broad spectrum of US findings in the thyroid gland in patients with benign and malignant thyroid lesions, and also the different features of metastases in the cervical lymph nodes. The diagnoses given in this atlas were principally confirmed by histologic evaluation after surgery. Some cases, however, were confirmed only by cytologic evaluation or histologic evaluation of histologic needle biopsy with clinical follow-up. Lymph node metastases were confirmed by CB and/or thyroglobuline assay in the wash out specimens. In some cases comparable computed tomography or magnetic resonance images are shown, and in most cases the gross pathology and cytologic or histologic findings are presented.

All US images were taken with a Philips HDI 5000 with SonoCT and Xres (Philips Medical Systems, Bothell, WA) using a broadband 12-5-mHz linear transducer. The Doppler images were all taken with a PRF ± 4 cm/s. The CBs were taken with either a 27- or 25-gauge needle, almost always without aspiration. (We only use aspiration if the first attempts give "dry tap".) Histologic needle biopsies were taken with the Bard Magnum reusable biopsy gun (Bard Biopsy Systems,Tempe, AZ) using an 18- or 16-gauge needle with a 22- or 15-mm needle advancement. In very small tumors we used the Bard Monopty disposable gun with an 18-gauge needle and 11-mm needle advancement.

The image presentation starts with an overview of the different features of thyroid lesions described in the literature; one new feature is also presented. The images with comments show our definition of the different features with the terminology we use. Thereafter, images of the different pathologic entities are presented, and US features are described. In each case the reader will have information about the patient's age and sex, a very short clinical history, and the findings on US, cytology, and histology in the cases where either needle biopsy was taken or a resection was performed.

As for US evaluation, the evaluation of the slides with cytologic specimens was based on the experience of the cytopathologist. In almost all cases presented in this atlas there was an immediate on-site evaluation of the smears.

In addition to determining the adequacy of the specimens, on-site evaluation gave the cytopathologist the opportunity to evaluate the specific lesions together with the radiologist. The on-site collaboration between radiologist and cytocytopathologist, made the puncture more focused and accurate, and the cytopathologist was able to achieve a better understanding of the characteristics of the whole lesion, as well as the rest of the thyroid gland. This information in some cases turned out to be of crucial importance to the cytopathologist, and ensured an even better interpretation of the smears.

The cytologic biopsy specimens were prepared fresh, air-dried and stained immediately with Diff-Quick. In cases where the clinical information or morphology indicated the possibility of medullary carcinoma, unstained slides were taken for immunocytochemical staining for calcitonin. In cases suspicious for a lymphocytic lesion (thyroiditis or lymphocytic neoplasm), an additional puncture was performed and the material referred for flow cytometric immunophenotyping. The biopsies were diagnosed according to the World Health Organization classification. Histologic needle biopsy was performed under US guidance in selected cases, mostly in cases with inadequate cytologic biopsy.

The images from the US evaluation were not available for the cytopathologist doing the gross section examination of the resected specimens. For this reason the US images do not precisely show concordance with the images from the gross specimens, the cytology, and histology. The main patterns harmonize, however, to a great extent.

This atlas does not strive to be a complete pathology atlas. The cytologic and histologic images are meant to serve as a cytologic or histologic correspondence to the radiologic images. As such, some of the basic characteristics for each of the entities mentioned are described, some with additional comments due to the experience of the authors.

1 Physical and Technical Essentials

Definitions, Terminology and Abbreviations

There are confusing, and to a certain degree misleading, discrepancies between different countries, different medical centers, and different specialties in the terminology concerning the sampling of specimens for cytology and histology. In the United States, sampling of specimens for cytology and histology are called *biopsy*: fine needle aspiration biopsy (FNAB or FNA biopsy), which gives a specimen for cytology, and coarse or core needle biopsy (CNB), which gives a specimen for histology. In Europe, most often another terminology is used: fine needle aspiration cytology (FNAC or FNAC cytology), cutting biopsy (CB), core needle biopsy (CNB), or just biopsy. Large needle biopsy (LNB) is also used by some authors. Some regard an 18-gauge needle as a fine needle.

The term *histology* is in accordance with cytology, biopsy is not. A biopsy will give a specimen for cytology and histology.

The term *fine needle capillary biopsy* (FNCB) has been used to emphasize sampling without aspiration, a method that is increasingly recognized all over the world. Nevertheless, the terms *FNAC*, *FNAB*, or just *FNA* are still used, although no aspiration has been employed. In this atlas we use the terms *cytologic biopsy* (CB) and *histologic needle biopsy* (HNB) independent of needle size and aspiration.

AP — antero posterior
CB — cytologic biopsy (FNAC, FNAB, FNA, FNCB)
CN — colloid nodule
CT — computed tomography
FA — follicular adenoma
FTC — follicular thyroid carcinoma
FVPTC — follicular variant of PTC
HNB — histologic needle biopsy (CNB, CB, LNB)
LN — lymph node
MR — magnetic resonance
MTC — medullary thyroid carcinoma
PTC — papillary thyroid carcinoma
SD — sagittal diameter
TD — transverse diameter

Evaluation Basics

Ultrasound (US) evaluation in general is uniquely operator dependent. If images from a neck examination are not stored as a lot of parallel slices or as a video uptake, the pathology can only be revealed while examining the area of interest. Still images will sometimes lose important information, *ie,* a malignant infiltration from the tumor into neighboring tissue outside the thyroid gland, which often can be readily revealed in real time.

The evaluation is, however, also highly dependent on the equipment. Using some of the old US machines with low frequency transducers, it is only possible to distinguish between cystic and solid thyroid nodules, while the high-end machines can evaluate very small lesions and lymph nodes [4-7]. Both an experienced physician and premium class equipment is crucial for a good result, *ie* high sensitivity and specificity.

The results are, however, often dependent on cytologic verification of equivocal US findings. It may be difficult to obtain cell material from the most suspicious area. Thus, it is mandatory to have good skill in US-guided free hand puncture technique to achieve a high accuracy [4].

Anatomy

The thyroid gland is composed of a right and a left lobe lying adjacent and lateral to the upper trachea and esophagus, and between the two carotid arteries. The thyroid has a homogeneous echopattern, and is hyperechoic compared with the neighboring strap muscles. An isthmus of variable size connects the two lobes, and in some cases a pyramidal lobe is present, extending upward anterior to the thyroid cartilage. Rarely aberrant thyroid tissue is found in the mediastinum or laterally on the neck. Because of the superficial location of the gland, it is possible to recognize normal anatomic structures less than 1 mm in diameter using a 10- to 15-mHz transducer. When the gland is greatly enlarged, there is a need for transducers with lower frequency, thus giving less resolution with reduced ability to evaluate the findings. The degree of information achieved with ultrasound is reduced when the tumor extends into the mediastinum.

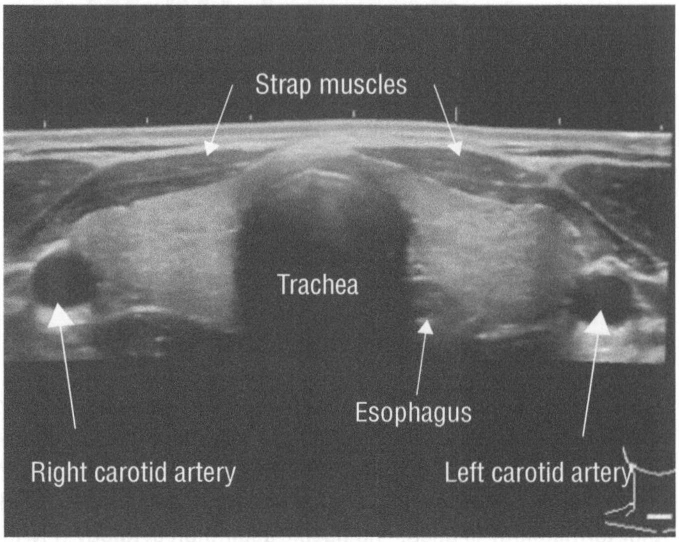

Figure 1-1. Anatomy of the thyroid gland.

Neck lymph nodes are generally superfi dally located, which makes it possible to evaluate them with the same high frequency transducer used for the thyroid gland. Ultrasound may reveal metastatic infi ltration in lymph nodes less than 3 mm in size, which is of utmost importance in efforts to give the patient radical treatment. Because of the great number of neck lymph nodes, it is important to rccord the location of a lymph node metastasis as a guide for the surgeon. There are different international maps available describing neck lymph node localization. In this atlas we refer to the map made by the American Joint Committee on Carcinoma having levels from I-VII.

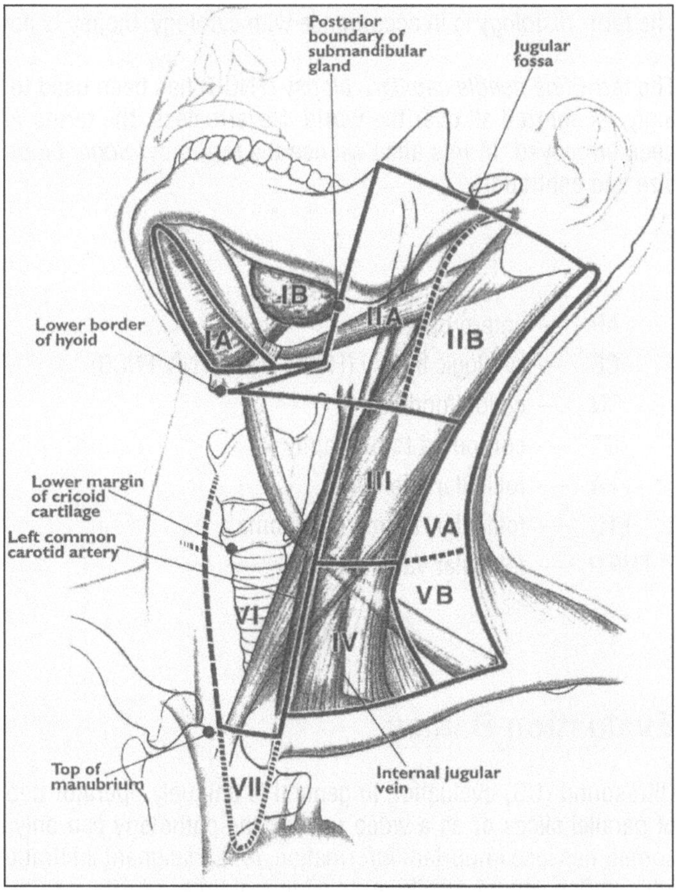

Figure 1-2. Levels of the regonal lymph nodes.

2 Ultrasound Features of Thyroid Lesions

There are many different features indicating a certain benign or malignant tumor type, but many of these are overlapping signs. Combining several features is considered to give the best result. Ultrasound features of benign lesions are often described as a diffusely enlarged gland, a well-circumscribed inhomogeneous hyper- or isoechoic solid lesion, a semi-solid or predominantly cystic lesion, multinodular lesions, and so forth. US features suggestive of malignant thyroid tumors have been described as follows: microcalcifications, hypoechogenicity, a taller than wide lesion, predominantly solid composition, irregular borders, absence of peripheral halo, intranodular hypervascularity, and regional lymphadenopathy [4,8,9]. No single US feature has both a high sensitivity and a high positive predictive value for thyroid carcinoma. The different malignant tumors have to some degree a different appearance on US.

"Comet Tail" Crystals

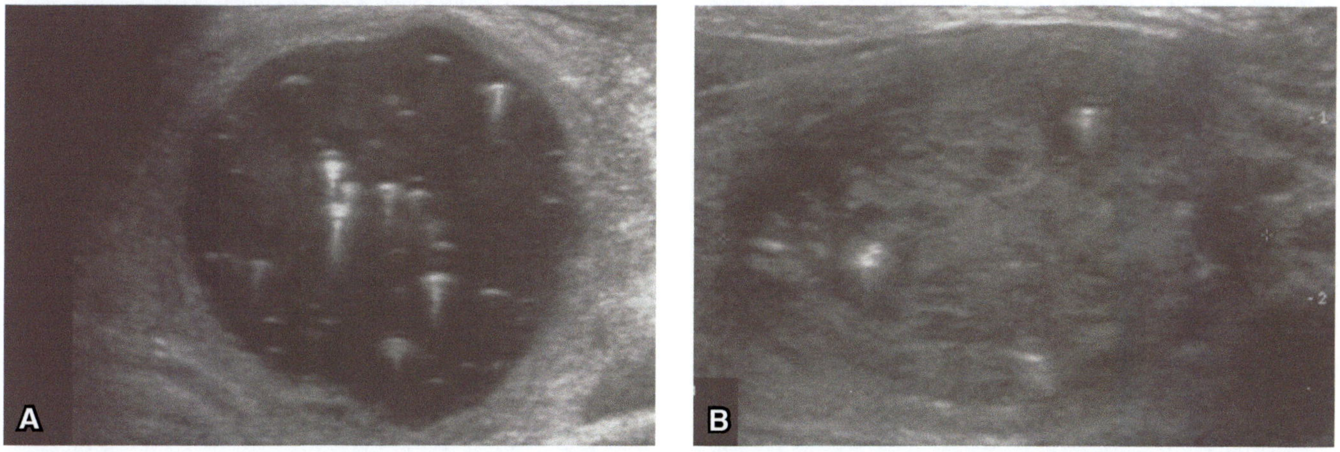

Figure 2-1. "Comet tail" crystals are highly echogenic, tiny, almost shiny foci, often with white tails, seen within both solid and cystic lesions that represent condensed colloid [4,6,7]. The white tail is a result of reverberation artifacts. **A**, Cystic colloid nodule. **B**, Papillary thyroid carcinoma.

Calcifications

Calcifications are described as micro-, coarse, or "eggshell" calcifications.

Microcalcifications

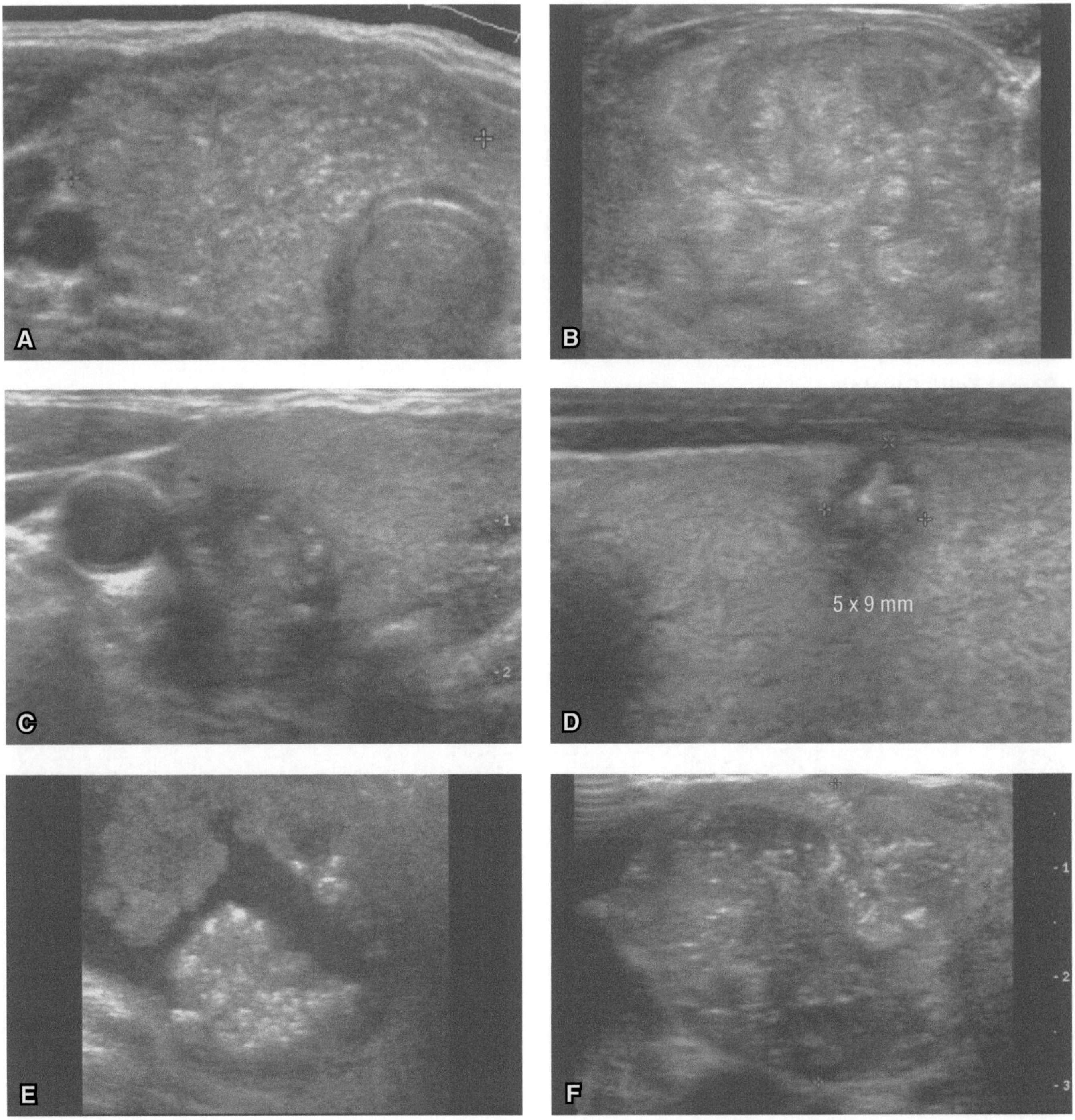

Figure 2-2. Microcalcifications are defined as punctate, highly echogenic, but somewhat pale nonshadowing discrete foci. They are thought to represent calcified psammoma bodies or granular amorphous deposits of calcium [4,10]. If they are innumerable or located in small groups, the tumor is highly suspicious for being a papillary carcinoma. Microcalcifications are also seen in medullary carcinoma, but they tend to be more coarse and with more irregular shape than in papillary carcinoma [6,7,10]. Often a few microcalcifications are also found in other malignant and benign tumors. **A**, Papillary thyroid carcinoma (PTC), innumerable. **B**, PTC, clusters. **C–E**, PTC. **F**, Medullary thyroid carcinoma.

Coarse calcifications

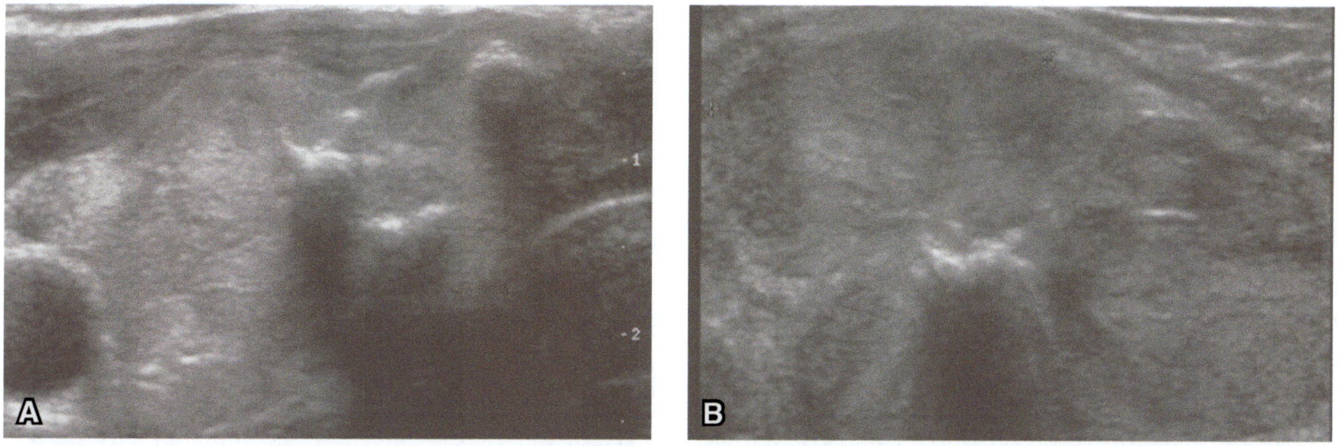

Figure 2-3. Coarse calcifications are defined as large, highly echogenic foci with irregular borders and acoustic shadow. They may appear as one large calcification or a cluster of smaller calcifications. They are suspicious for malignancy, especially if they are located in the central part of the tumor, but they are also often seen in nodular goiter [8,10–13]. There is no exact distinction between the largest microcalcifications and the smallest coarse calcifications. Calcified psammoma bodies will probably always be tiny, but granular amorphous deposits of calcium may vary in size. **A**, Papillary thyroid carcinoma. **B**, Follicular thyroid carcinoma.

"Eggshell" calcifications

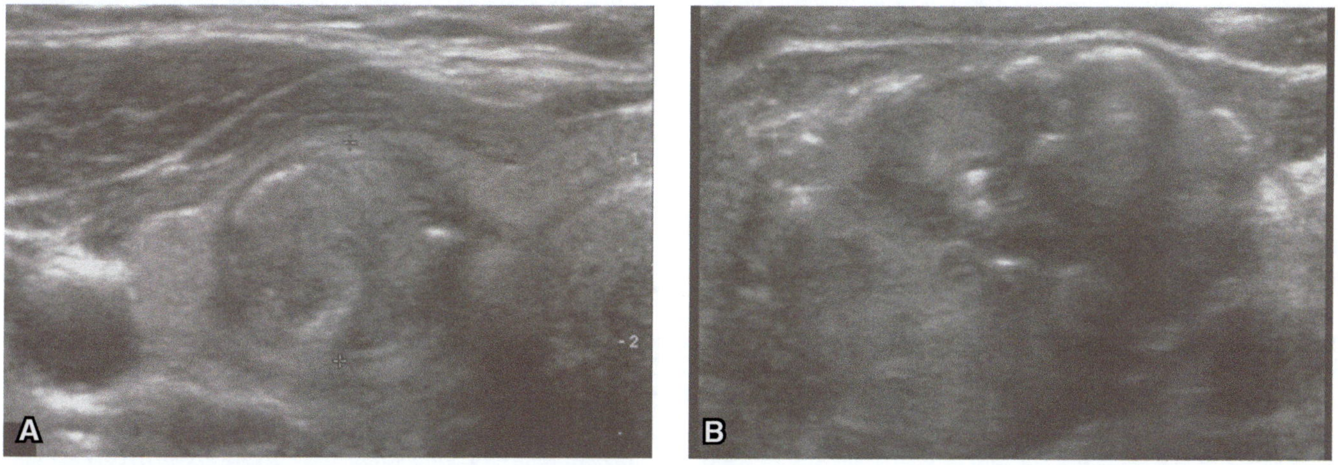

Figure 2-4. "Eggshell" calcifications are thin, peripherally located calcifications that indicate benignity and are usually due to degenerative changes in goiterous nodules [6], but can also be found in malignant tumors. **A**, Papillary thyroid carcinoma. **B**, Colloid nodule.

Histologic morphology

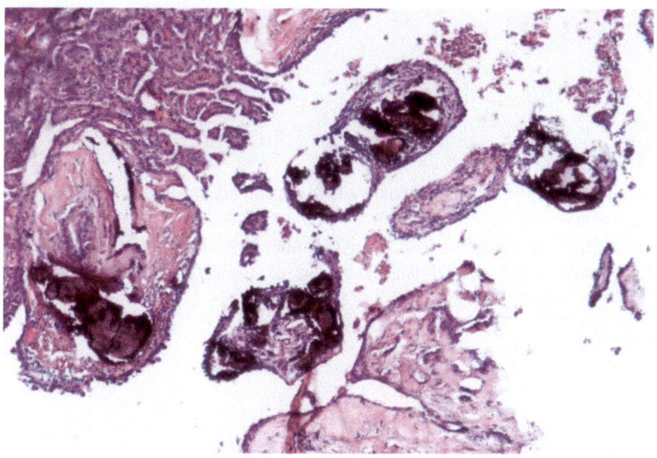

Figure 2-5. From lesions with coarse calcification, "eggshell" calcification, and "comet tail" crystals the histology specimen sometimes contains calcifications irregular in form and shape, in contrast to the true psammomma bodies one may find in specimens from papillary thyroid carcinomas (PTCs) that are circular with concentric rings. Histology: microcalcification bodies in PTC.

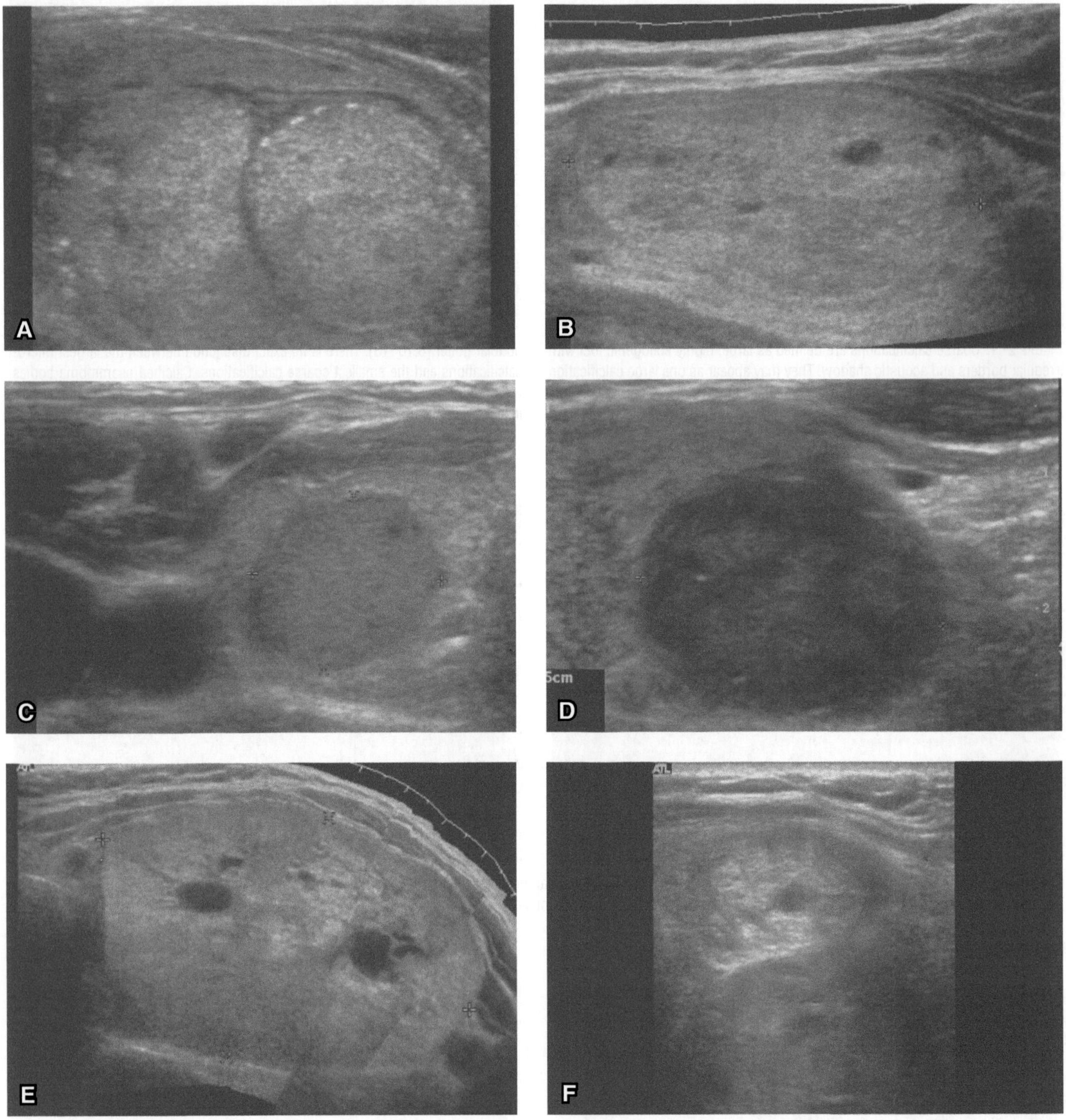

Figure 2-6. Lesions are described as hyperechoic, isoechoic, hypoechoic, anechoic, or with mixed echogenicity. Benign lesions are often hyper- or isoechoic or with mixed echogenicity compared with the echogenicity in the normal tissue of the thyroid gland; malignant tumors are most often hypoechoic [4–7]. A highly hypoechoic lesion is strongly suspicious for malignancy. There is, however, a lot of overlap between benign and malignant lesions. Cystic areas may be either anechoic or hypoechoic depending on the content. **A**, Hyperechoic (colloid nodule [CN]). **B**, Isoechoic (CN). **C**, Hypoechoic (medullary thyroid carcinoma). **D**, Strongly hypoechoic (follicular variant of papillary thyroid carcinoma). **E** and **F**, Mixed echogenicity (CN).

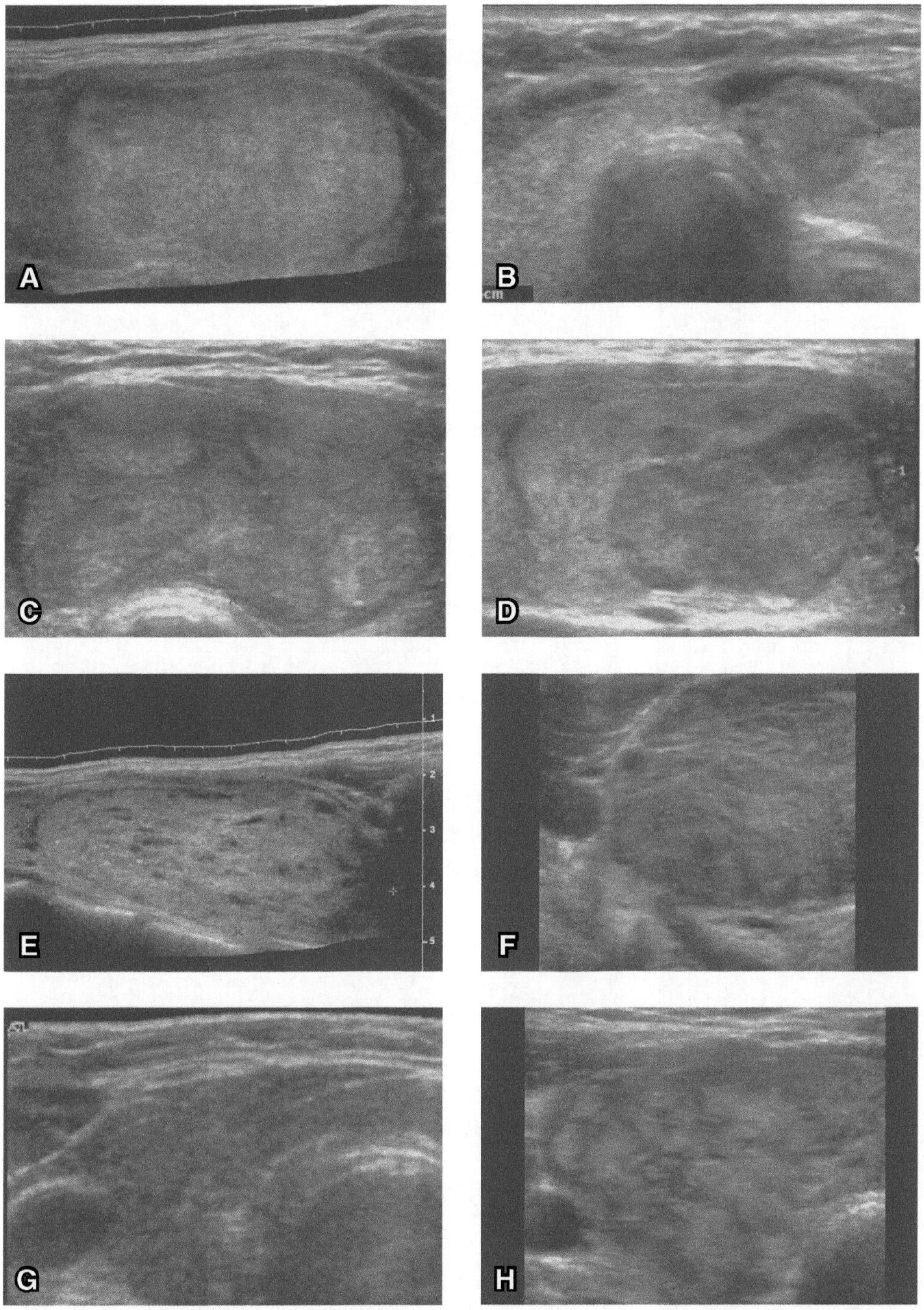

Figure 2-7. Echo pattern or echo texture is described in different ways by different authors. The pattern can be homogeneous or heterogeneous, regular or irregular. It can be lobulated, nodular or granular, spongy or honeycomb-like [6]. A homogeneous echo pattern indicates a benign tumor, and a heterogeneous echo pattern is usually seen in malignant lesions. A lobulated echo pattern may indicate a follicular tumor. Both predominantly large nodular patterns and small nodular patterns are found in goiter, but small nodular and granular patterns are also seen in thyroiditis [6,10]. Linear bright echoes within an enlarged hypoechoic thyroid lobe, so-called "coarse septations", are sometimes found in Hashimoto's thyroiditis. They are caused by fibrous bands [6,10]. Another echo pattern that may be of importance in distinguishing different tumors is geographic echo pattern. This pattern consists of sharply marginated areas of different echogenicity within the tumor. We have found this echo pattern especially in follicular variant of papillary thyroid carcinoma (FVPTC), but also in follicular tumors. **A**, Homogeneous (follicular adenoma [FA]). **B**, Heterogeneous (papillary thyroid carcinoma [PTC]). **C**, Lobulated (FA). **D**, Geographic (FVPTC). **E**, Spongy (colloid nodule). **F**, Coarse septations (lymphoma). **G**, Granular (thyroiditis). **H**, Nodular (thyroiditis).

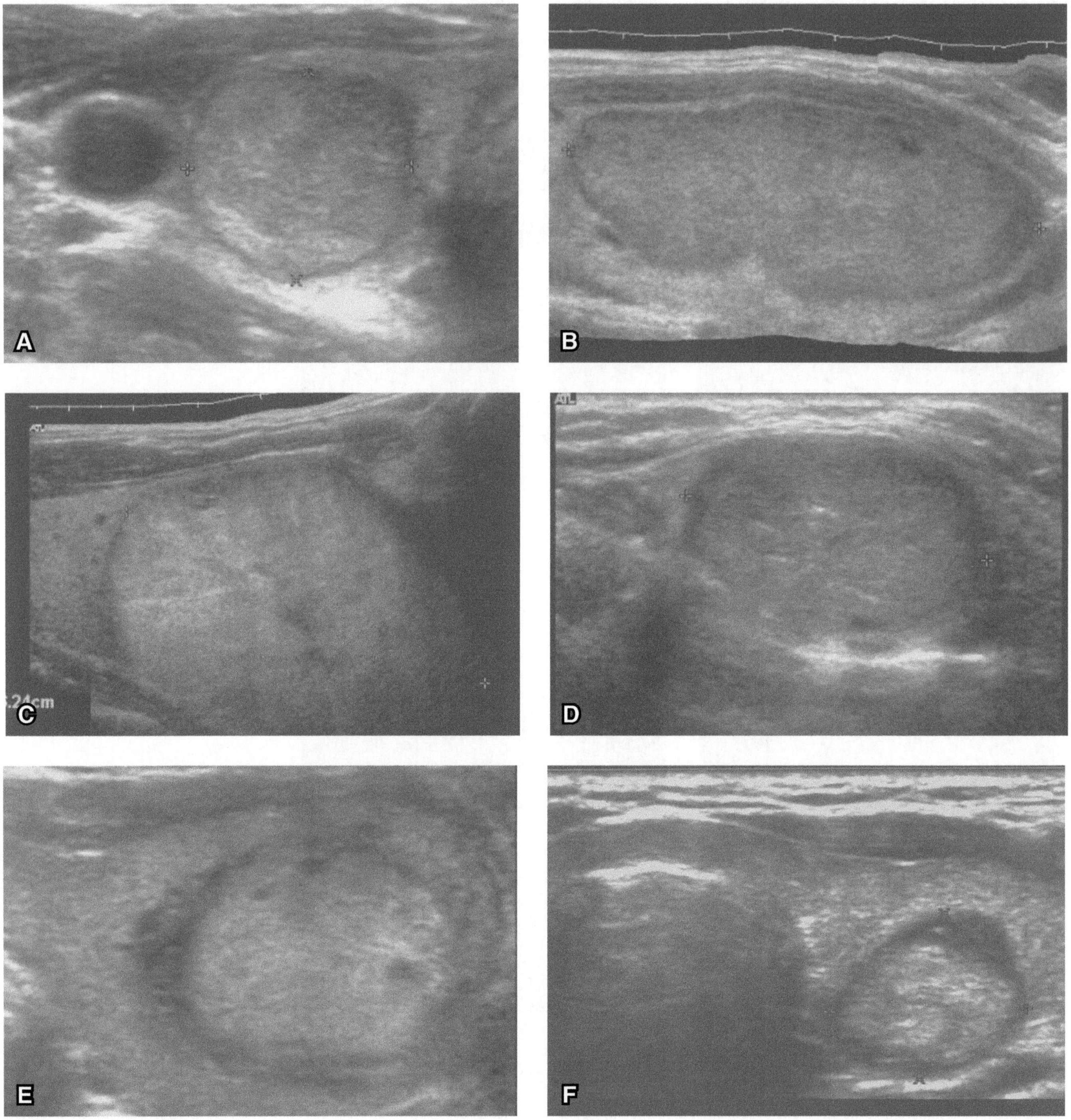

Figure 2-8. Using color Doppler, the peripheral hypoechoic halo especially found in follicular tumors represents peripheral vessels adjacent to the capsule [6,7]. A thin, even halo with a thin vascular rim is strongly indicative of a follicular adenoma (FA). A thick halo usually corresponds with a thick rim of vessels. An even or uneven thick halo is suspicious for follicular carcinoma. A thick halo, however, is sometimes also seen in adenomas, and a segmented thin halo is sometimes found in nodular goiter. **A** and **B**, Thin, even halo (FA). **C**, Thin, uneven halo (follicular thyroid carcinoma [FTC]). **D**, Thick partial halo (FTC). **E** and **F**, Thick, uneven halo (FTC).

Edge Shadow

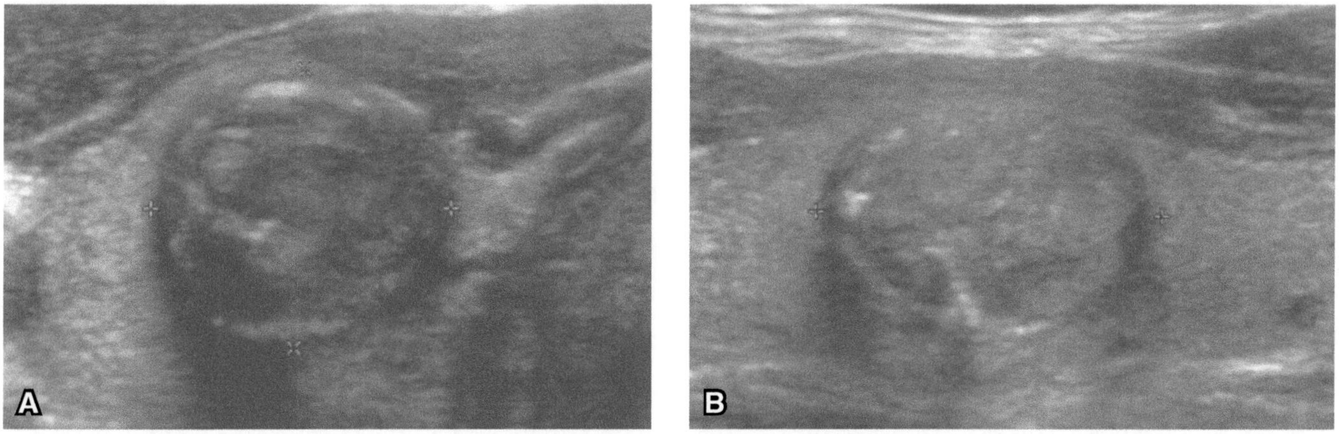

Figure 2-9. Refractive shadows on the side edges of a lesion are probably caused by fibrotic or calcified tissue at the edge of the tumor. Peripheral reactive fibrosis may be prominent in papillary carcinomas [10]. The feature is suspicious for malignancy, but is also seen in benign lesions. This pattern is less prominent in modern ultrasound equipment with cross beam technology. **A**, Colloid nodule. **B**, Papillary thyroid carcinoma.

Infiltration

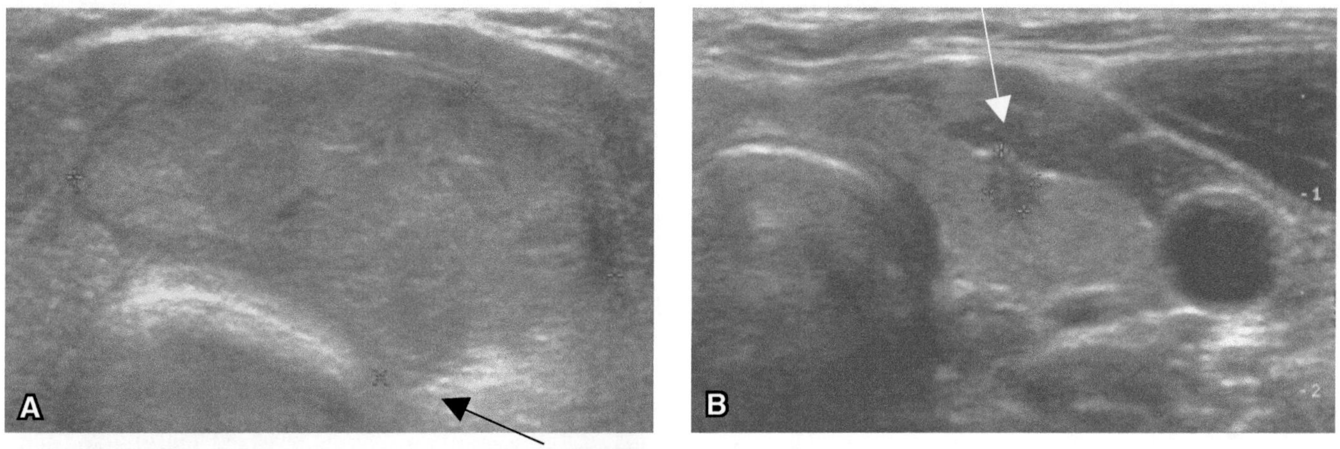

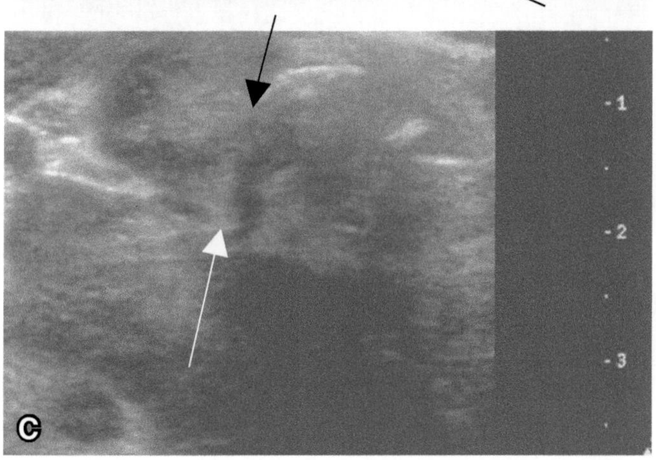

Figure 2-10. A malignant tumor may grow through the thyroid capsule and infiltrate the strap muscles or the trachea, and at a later stage, other adjacent structures. Infiltration is difficult to see on still images, but can more easily be discerned in a real time examination. If the tumor is suspicious for infiltrating the neighborhood, the physician should try to move the tumor or the neighboring structures to verify adhesions or independent movement. **A**, Follicular thyroid carcinoma. **B**, Papillary thyroid carcinoma. **C**, Anaplastic thyroid carcinoma.

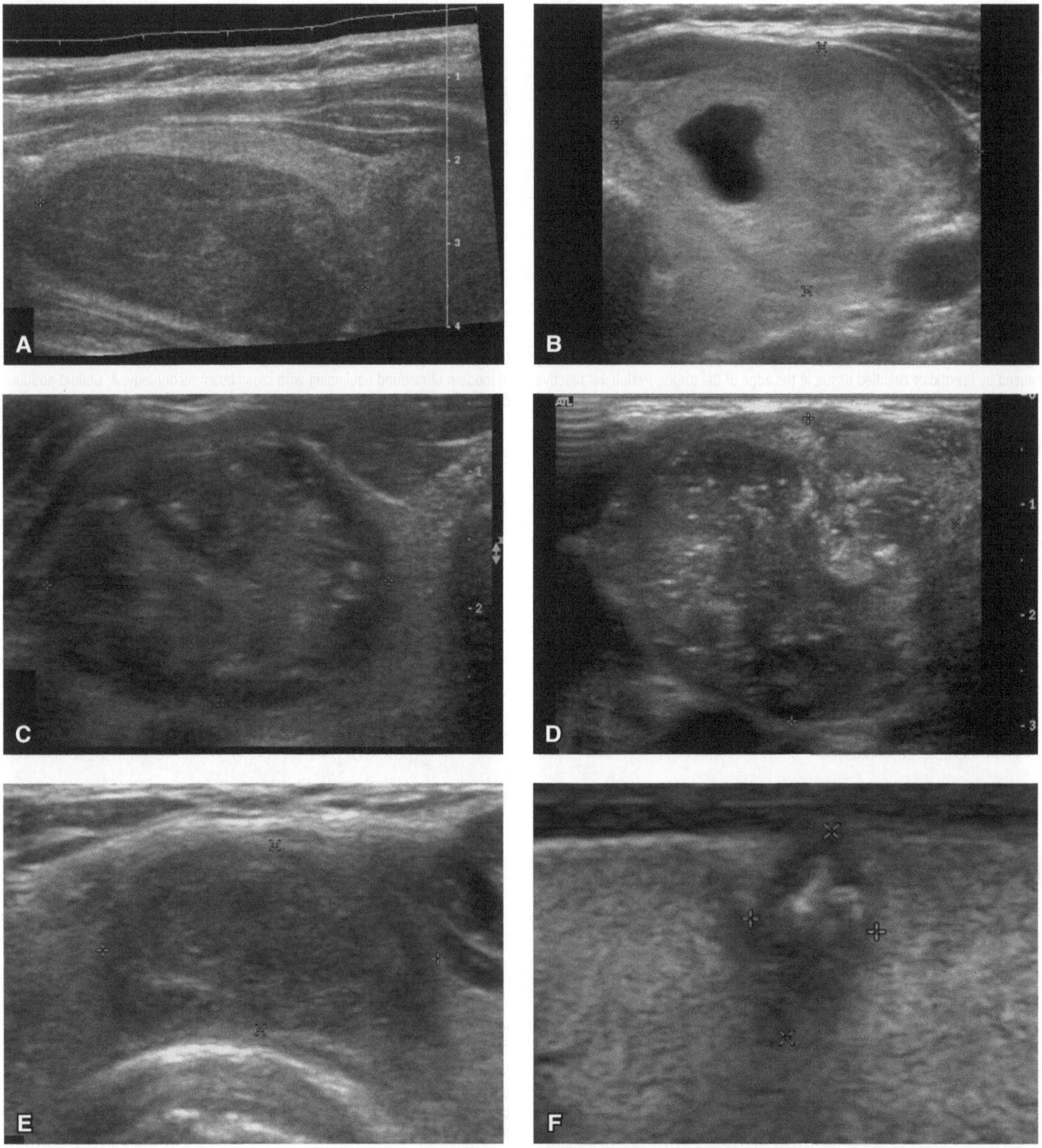

Figure 2-11. The margin of a lesion may be described as well defined or poorly defined, regular or irregular, or the lesion may have a diffuse or blurred margin or be sharply or well circumscribed. A lesion with a well-defined, regular margin is probably benign, and a diffuse or blurred margin is suspicious for malignancy [4,6–10]. **A**, Sharply circumscribed (follicular adenoma). **B**, Well circumscribed (colloid nodule). **C**, Quite well circumscribed (papillary thyroid carcinoma). **D**, Quite well circumscribed (medullary thyroid carcinoma). **E** and **F**, Blurred margin (PTC).

Size and Shape

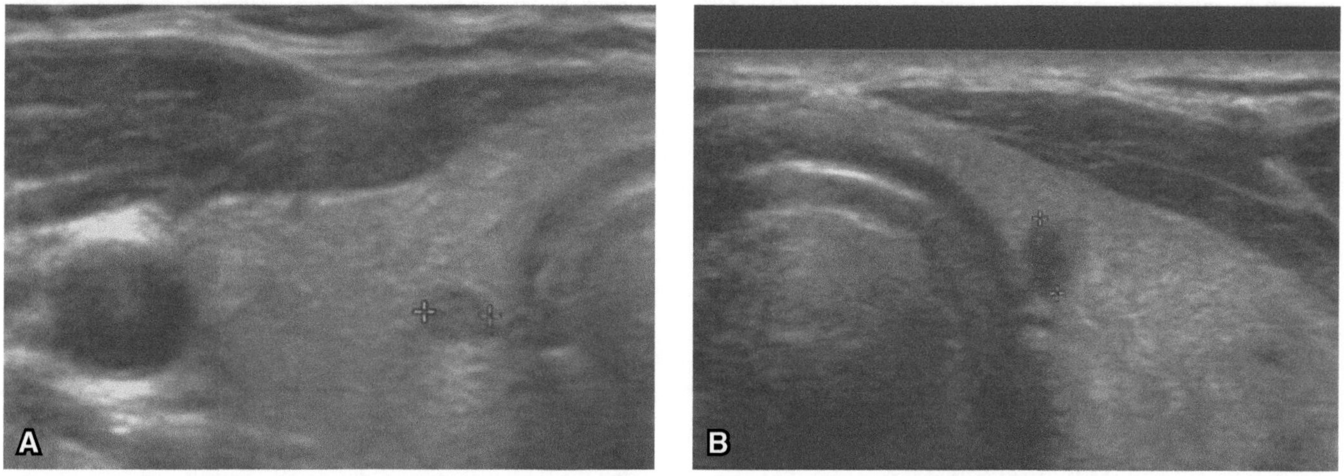

Figure 2-12. A malignant thyroid tumor has no lower size limit. With high resolution ultrasound (US) equipment, papillary carcinomas less than 10 mm in diameter, so-called "microcarcinomas," can also be disclosed [14]. A small, taller than wide nodule, *ie,* with an anteroposterior-to-transverse diameter ≥ 1, is suspicious for malignancy because most benign nodules are wider than tall. However, most malignant tumors also have a taller than wide ratio of less than 1 [8]. Follicular carcinomas often have a diameter of more than 3 cm. Huge, rapidly growing tumors are highly suspicious for anaplastic carcinoma. The description from the US examination has to be precise as to where in the thyroid gland the suspicious lesions are located. This information is of crucial importance, and should be available to the cytopathologist performing the gross examination, and especially in cases where the lesions are small. **A**, Papillary thyroid carcinoma (PTC) 3mm. **B**, PTC 4 mm, taller than wide.

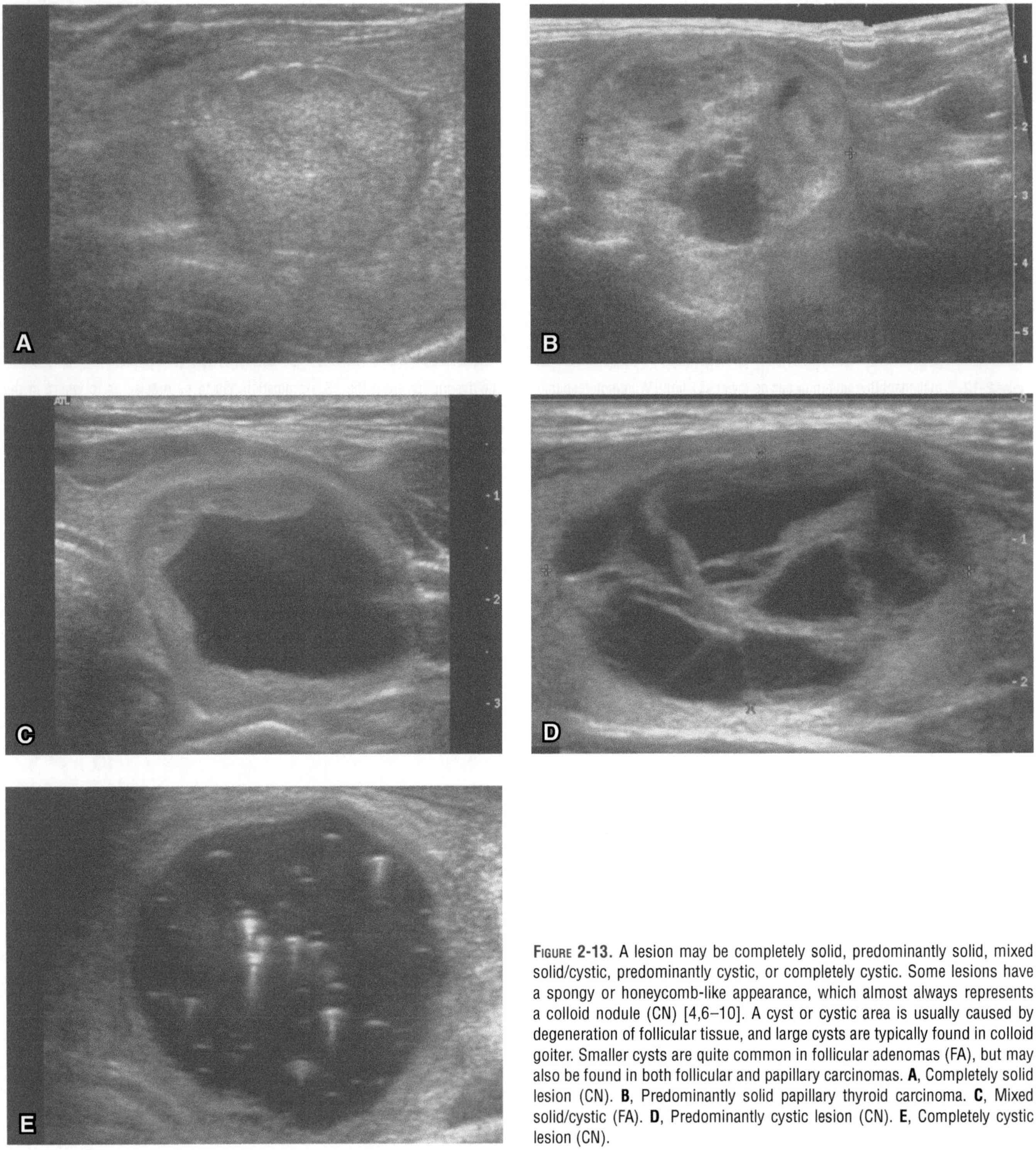

Figure 2-13. A lesion may be completely solid, predominantly solid, mixed solid/cystic, predominantly cystic, or completely cystic. Some lesions have a spongy or honeycomb-like appearance, which almost always represents a colloid nodule (CN) [4,6–10]. A cyst or cystic area is usually caused by degeneration of follicular tissue, and large cysts are typically found in colloid goiter. Smaller cysts are quite common in follicular adenomas (FA), but may also be found in both follicular and papillary carcinomas. **A**, Completely solid lesion (CN). **B**, Predominantly solid papillary thyroid carcinoma. **C**, Mixed solid/cystic (FA). **D**, Predominantly cystic lesion (CN). **E**, Completely cystic lesion (CN).

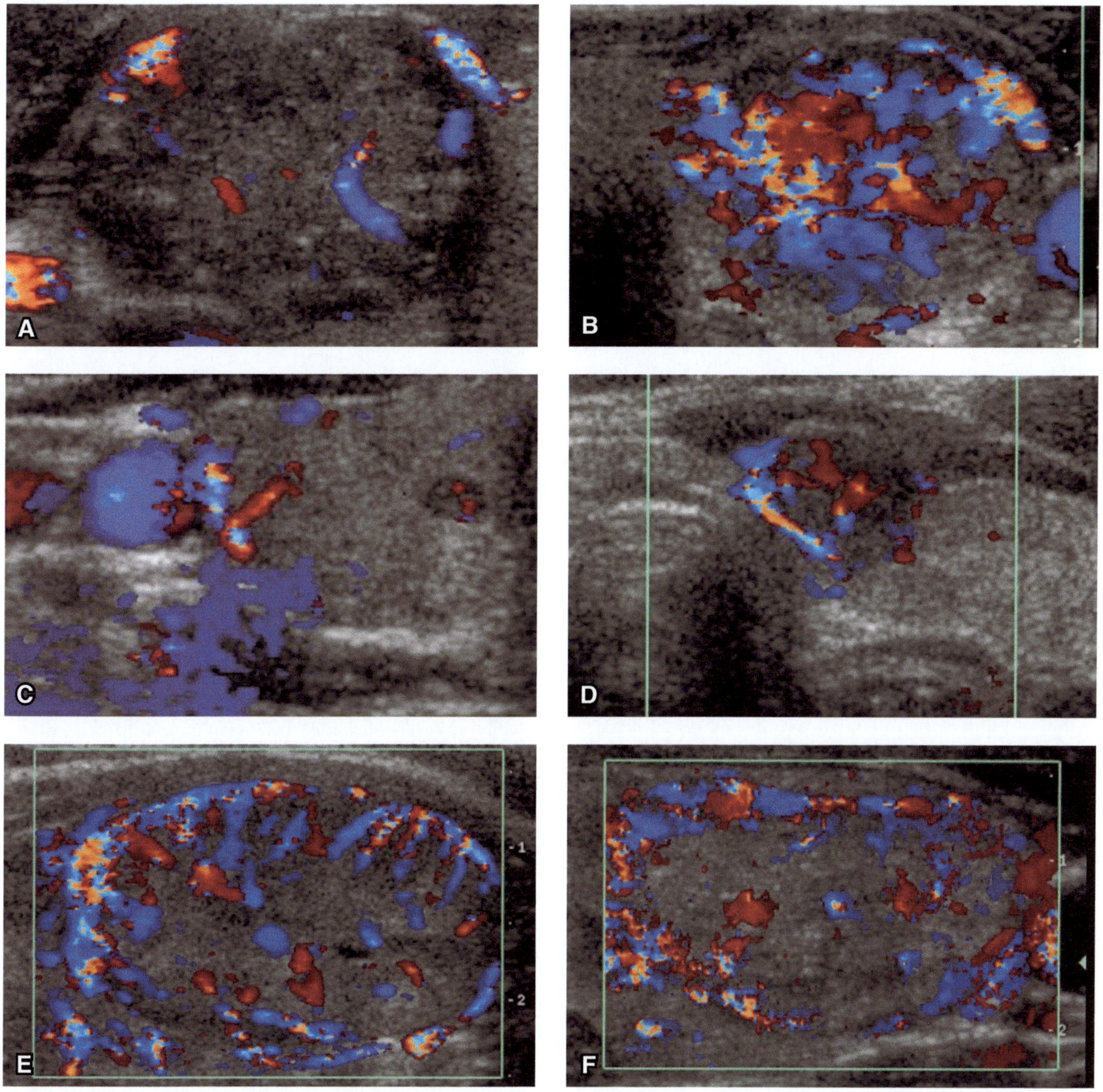

FIGURE 2-14. Normal thyroid tissue is usually richly vascularized. The different degrees of vascularity in a lesion are difficult to evaluate because both benign and malignant lesions and thyroiditis can present with scant, medium, or hypervascularity. The so-called "thyroid inferno," which means excessive flow, can be found in thyroiditis and in solid tumors. Some authors advocate that papillary carcinomas are almost always hypervascular [6], while other authors have found nonhypervascular papillary carcinomas [15,16]. The latter is also our experience. Other authors have classified vascularity in three groups: type 1 — absence of blood flow; type 2 — perinodular blood flow; type 3 — marked intranodular blood flow [4,7,15]. We believe it is more useful to evaluate the different flow patterns. *Disorganized vascularity,* probably due to neovascularity, is highly suspicious for malignancy [7]. In our opinion visible flow within a very small (3–5 mm) hypoechoic lesion is suspicious for malignancy. Follicular adenomas (FAs) and carcinomas often have a typical flow pattern with a more or less rich flow in the peripheral hypoechoic halo with vessels passing from the periphery toward the central part of the tumor, the so-called *spoke-and-wheel-like vascularity* [6]. In our experience it seems that carcinomas may have richer flow in both the periphery and inside the tumor compared with the flow in the adenomas. **A**, Scantly vascularized papillary thyroid carcinoma (PTC). **B**, Hypervascular PTC. **C**, Three-mm PTC with suspicious vascularity. **D**, PTC with pathologic vascularity. **E**, "Spoke-and-wheel-like" vascularity (FA). **F**, Suggestion of "spoke-and-wheel-like" vascularity (colloid nodule).

Section II

Types of Thyroid Lesions

3 Nodular or Colloid Goiter, Hyperplasia, and Cysts

These thyroid nodules are often described as hyperplastic, adenomatous, or colloid. Most cystic thyroid lesions are hyperplastic nodules that have undergone extensive liquefactive degeneration. The common features of a nodular goiter are multinodular, inhomogeneous, well-circumscribed solid, semi-solid or mostly cystic tumors. Some are hyperechoic compared with the echogenicity of the normal thyroid tissue, some are isoechoic, and still others hypoechoic. The hyper- and isoechoic nodules are often partially circumscribed by a thin hypoechoic halo. The nodules may contain coarse calcifications within the tumor, or peripheral "eggshell" calcifications. The cystic areas are often purely anechoic, but they may also be hypoechoic or show fluid-fluid levels due to intracystic bleeding, often with avascular internal debris. Many, even tiny cysts, contain small, strongly hyperechoic foci, often with "comet tail" artifacts. These foci represent crystallized colloid. Some cysts have intracystic avascular septa and/or papillary solid tissue protruding from the wall. Some cystic nodules have a spongy or honeycomb-like appearance. The vascularity varies a lot when evaluated with color Doppler imaging. Sometimes only spreading, faint vascularity is observed throughout the nodule, but often there is strong vascularity inside the nodule combined with a distinct peripheral border flow.

Common Features

Multinodular
Solid, semi-solid, or mostly cystic
Variable internal structure; inhomogeneous; hyper-, iso-, or hypoechoic; cystic or spongyform
Well-circumscribed to poorly encapsulated, merging into normal thyroid tissue
"Eggshell" or coarse calcifications
Strongly hyperechoic foci with "comet tail" artifacts

Cytologic Morphology

Nodular goiter usually presents a picture of thin and/or thick colloid together with some follicular epithelium and macrophages. In old nodes, the colloid may be degenerated. The material from colloid nodules with adenomatous hyperplasia may be very cellular and the amount of colloid scant. Additional punctures in other parts of the lesions may give a more representative specimen that is easier to interpret.

Cystic thyroid lesions are often a challenge to the cytopathologist. This is mainly because papillary thyroid carcinomas may be cystic. The epithelium floating in the fluid is often reactive and irregular, and may be difficult to distinguish from atypical epithelium in a cystic thyroid carcinoma. Many separate air-dried smears from fresh cystic fluid may reveal small papillary cell groups when interpreted immediately.

Colloid Nodules Left Lobe

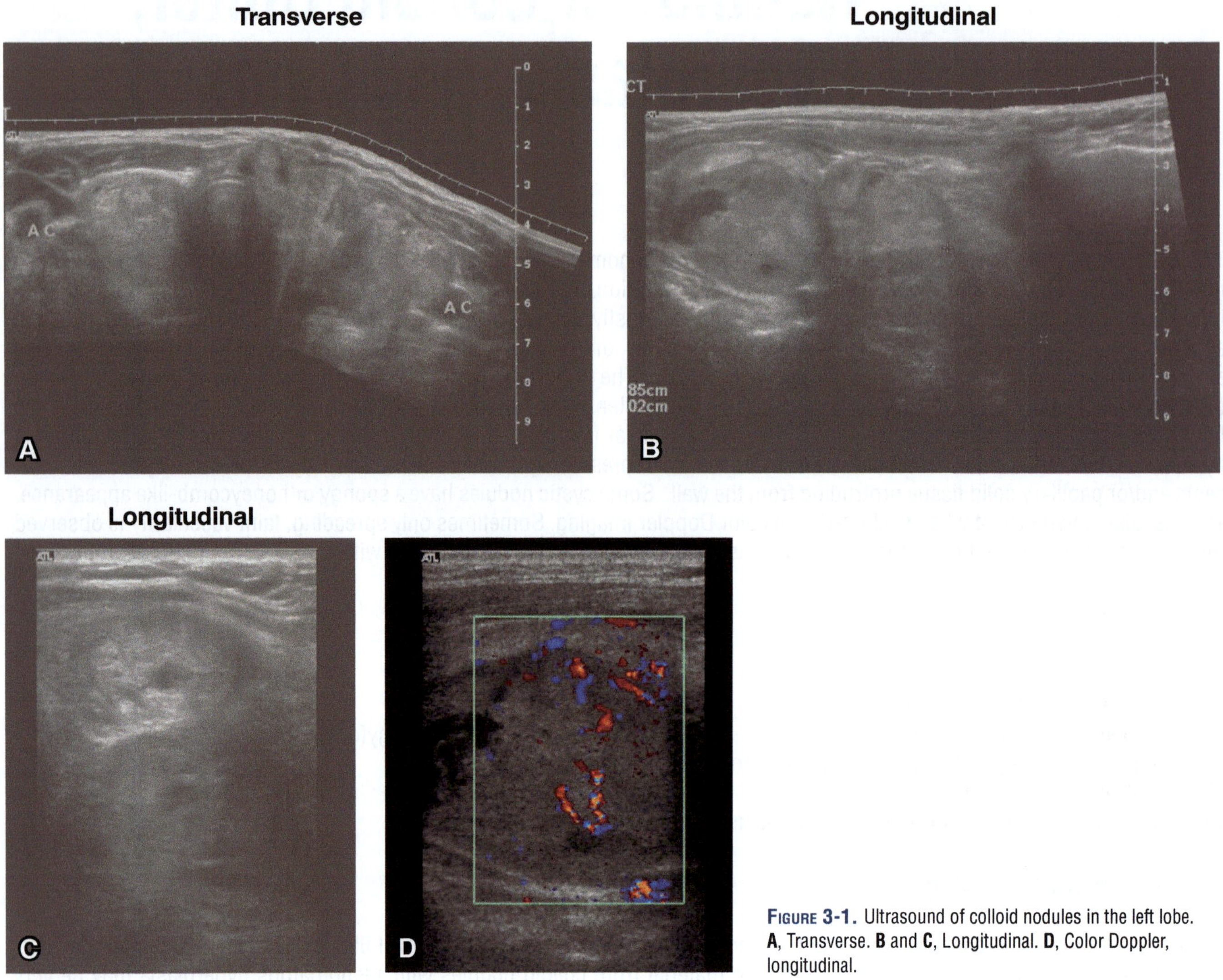

Figure 3-1. Ultrasound of colloid nodules in the left lobe. **A**, Transverse. **B** and **C**, Longitudinal. **D**, Color Doppler, longitudinal.

69-Year-old woman

- **Clinical history:** Surgery for goiter in 1986 and 1998. Now marginal zone B-cell lymphoma in skin. Large thyroid gland on CT. Lymphoma?
- **Ultrasound:** Colloid nodules. Probably follicular tumor posteriorly.
- **Cytology:** Colloid nodules.
- **18-Gauge histologic needle biopsy posteriorly:** Colloid nodule? Follicular tumor?
- **Left hemithyroidectomy:** Colloid nodules.

General features
Multinodular, mixed echogenicity
Inhomogeneous echo pattern
Each lesion quite well circumscribed
Small cysts
A few microcalcifications

Features of tumor posteriorly, left lobe
Hypoechoic
Well circumscribed
Mostly homogeneous echo pattern
Scantly vascularized
Small cysts

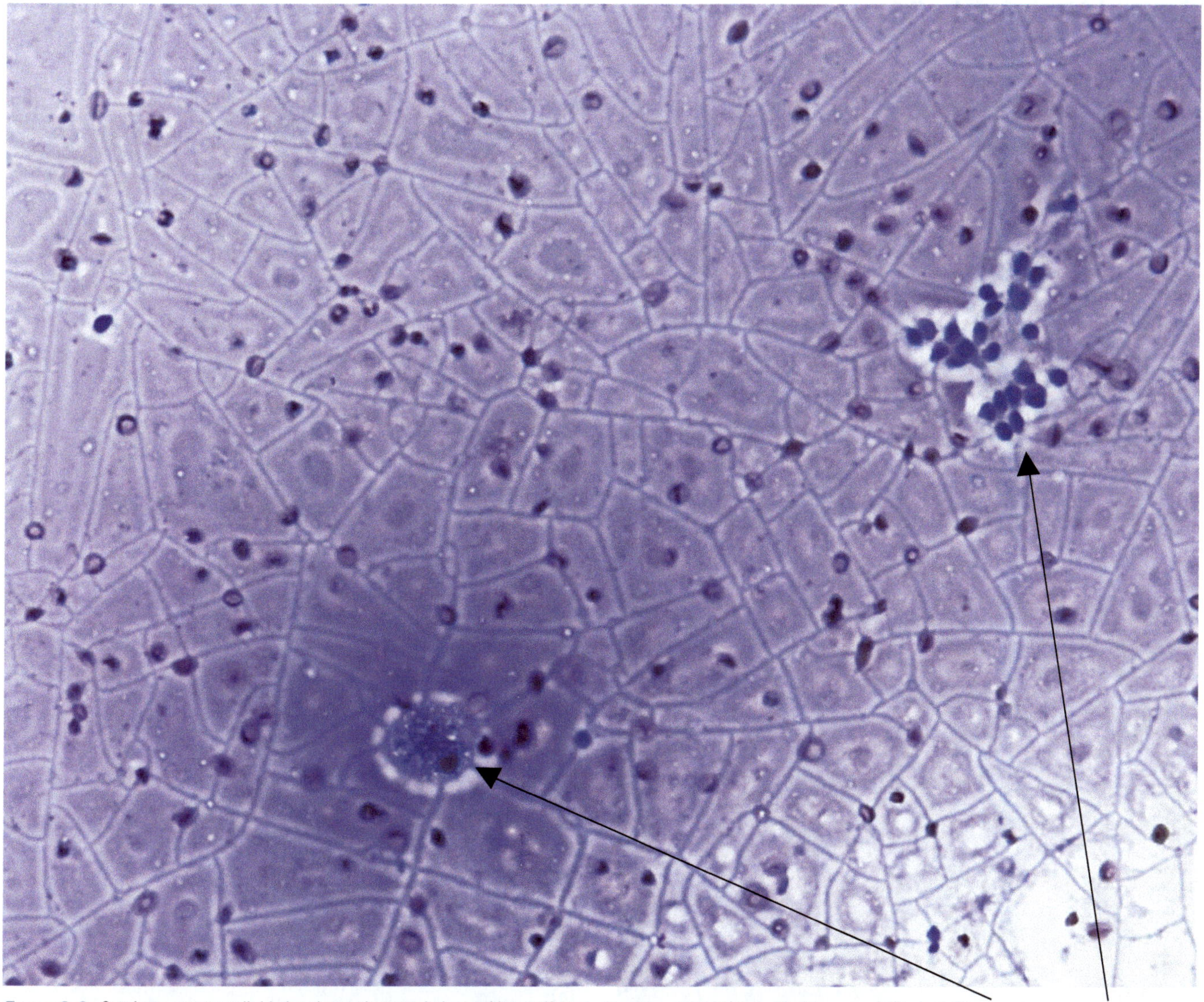

FIGURE 3-2. Cytology: watery colloid showing a characteristic cracking artifact. *Left arrow*, macrophage. *Right arrow*, follicular cells.

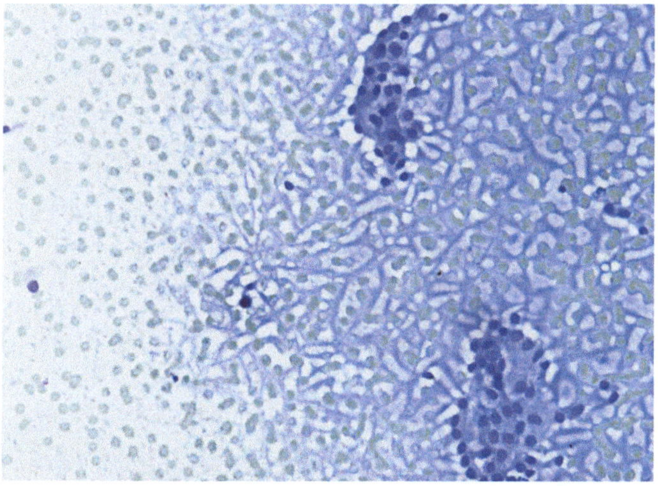

FIGURE 3-3. Colloid and epithelium.

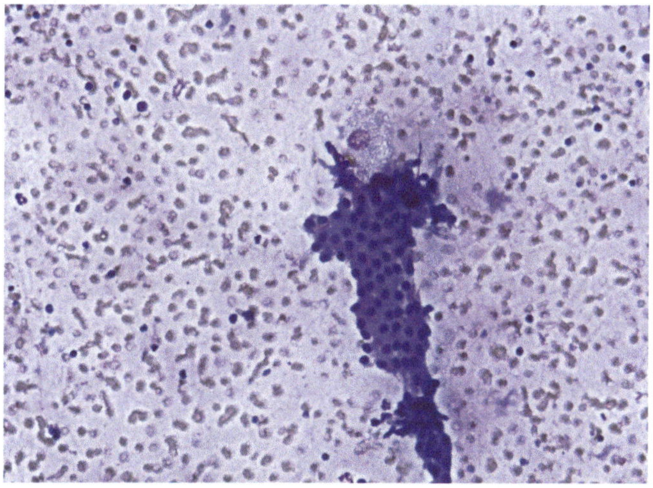

FIGURE 3-4. Colloid, epithelium, and macrophage.

Colloid Nodules Left Lobe

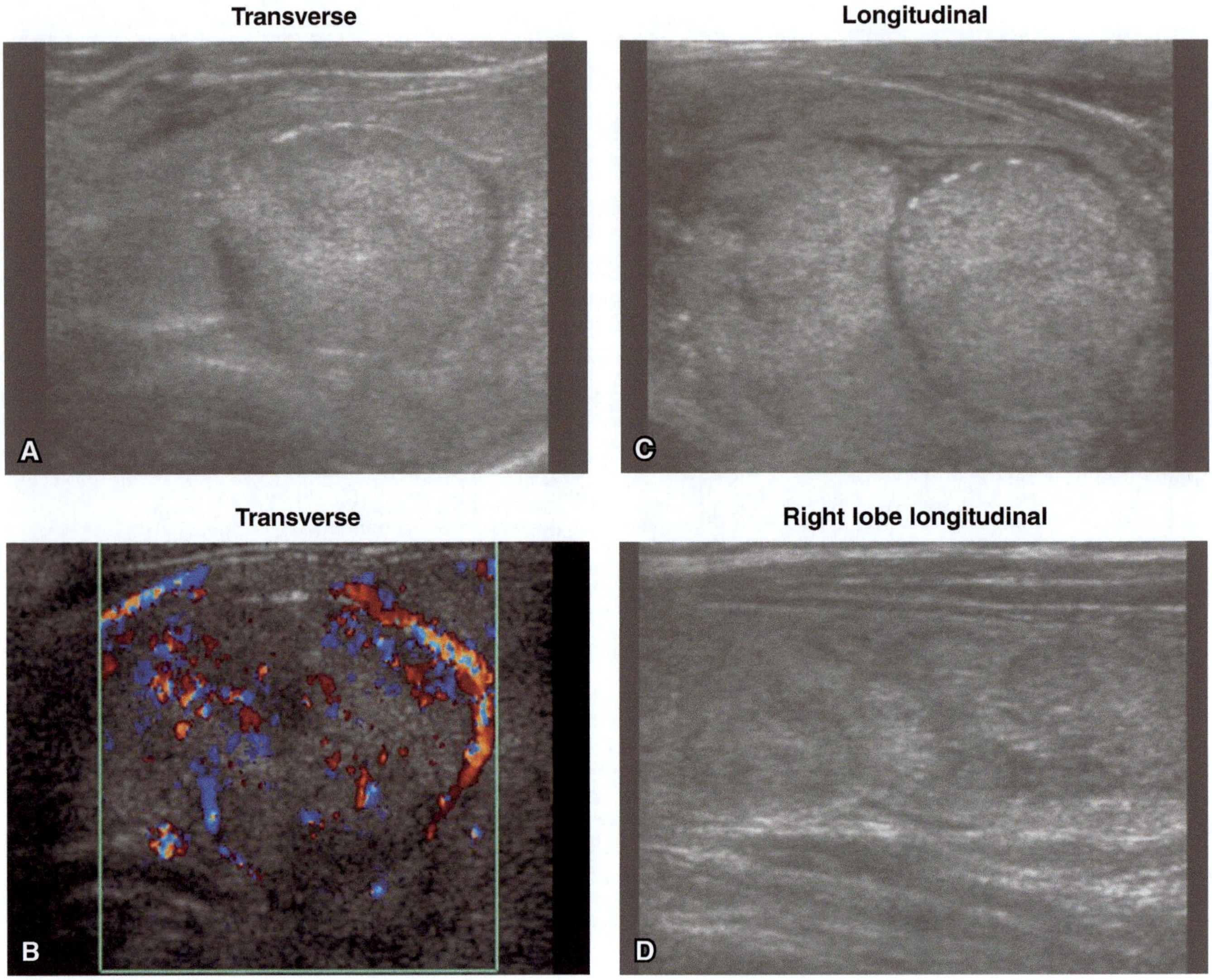

Figure 3-5. Ultrasound of colloid nodules in the left (**A–C**) and right (**D**) lobes. **A**, Transverse, 12 x 21 mm. **B**, Color Doppler, transverse. **C**, Longitudinal, sagittal diameter: 40 mm. **D**, Right lobe longitudinal.

64-Year-old woman

- **Clinical history:** Incidentaloma in left lobe found at CT of the thorax.
- **Ultrasound:** Colloid nodules both lobes.
- **Cytology left lobe:** Colloid nodule.
- **Left hemithyroidectomy:** Colloid nodules.

Features

Multinodular
Iso-/hyperechoic
Inhomogeneous echo pattern
"Eggshell" calcifications
Partially well circumscribed
Partially thin hypoechoic halo
Moderately vascularized

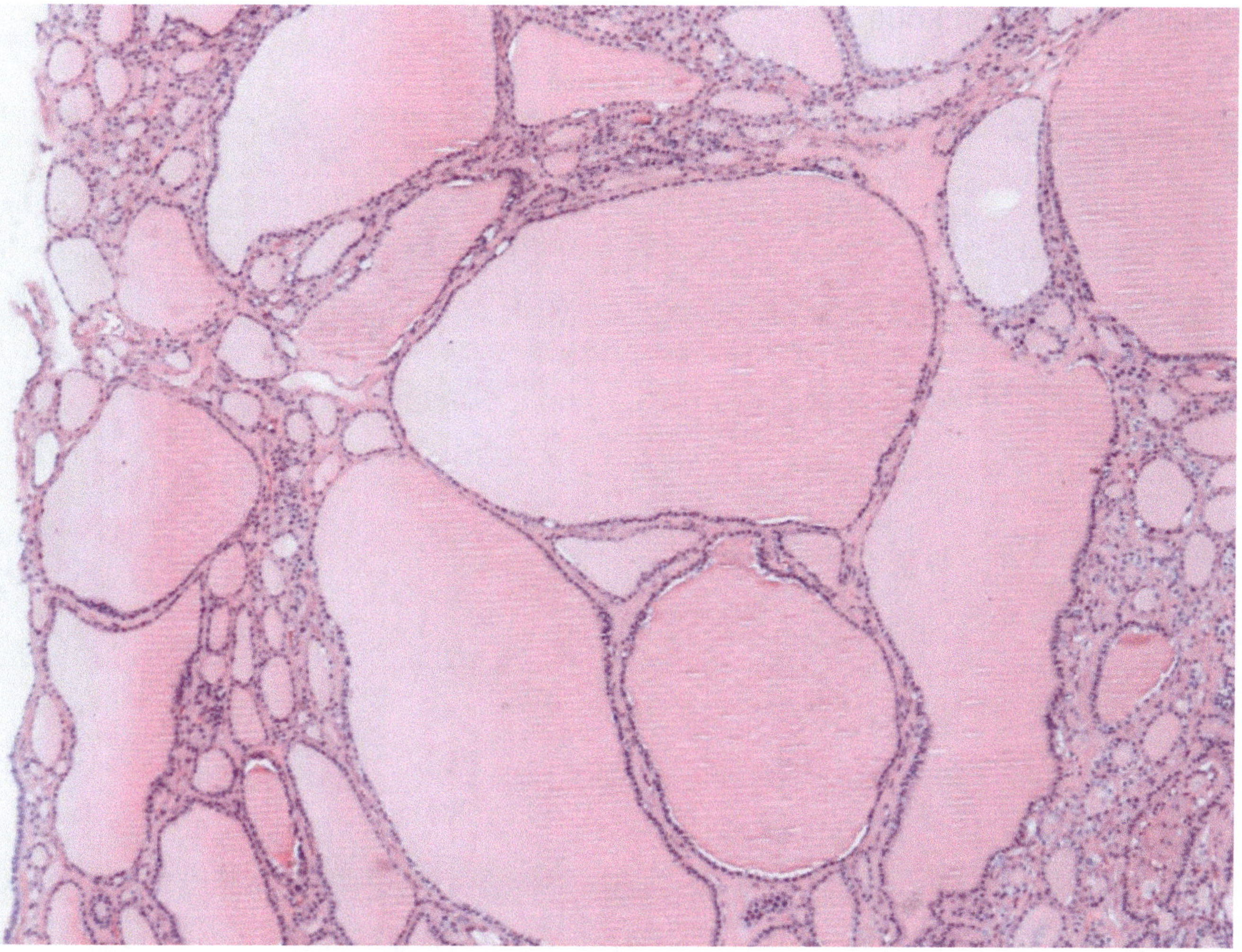

Figure 3-6. Histology: colloid-filled follicles of different size lined by flattened epithelium.

Colloid Nodule Left Lobe

Transverse

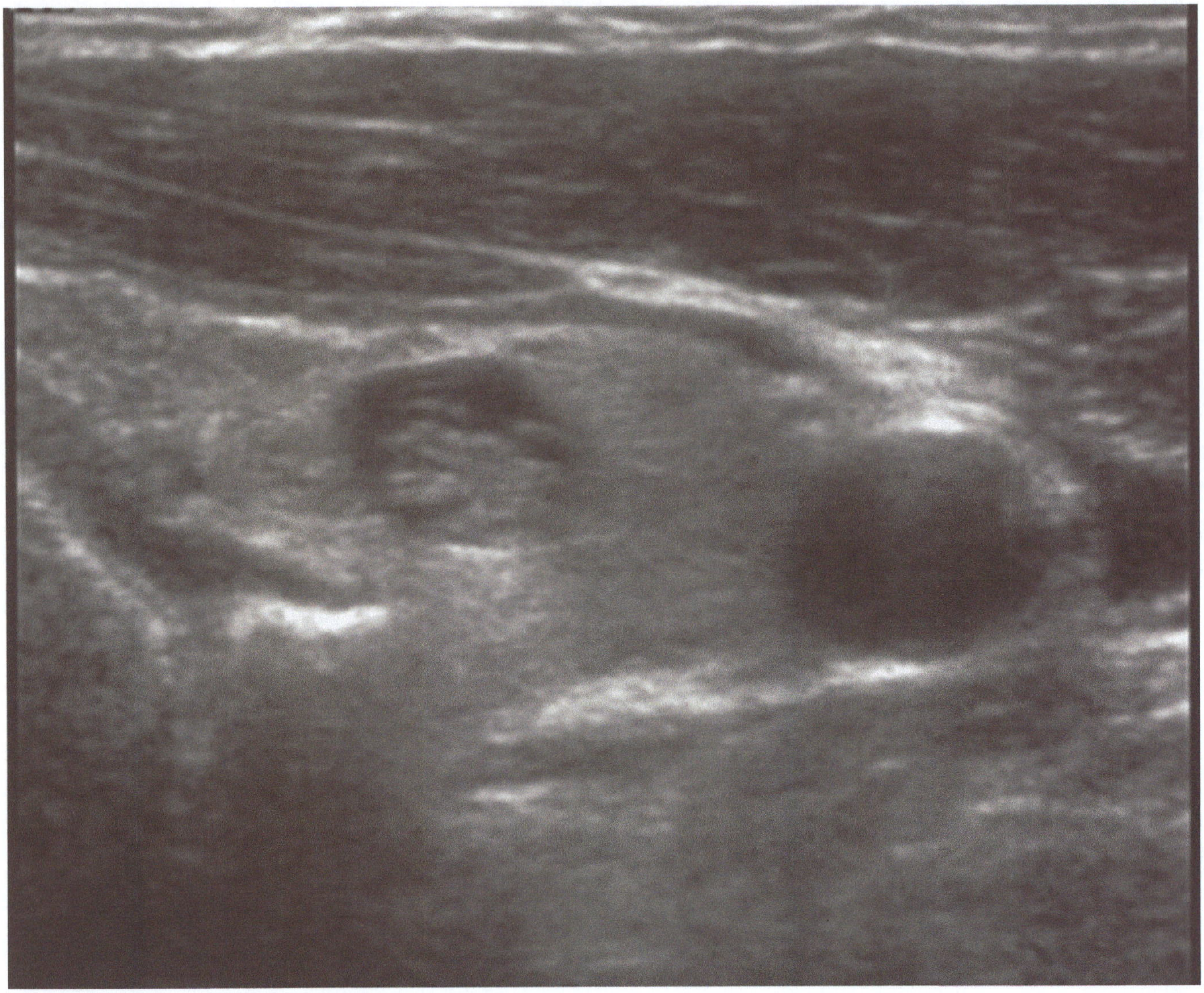

Figure 3-7. Ultrasound of a colloid nodule in the left lobe. Transverse, 7 x 10 mm.

56-Year-old man

- **Clinical history:** Nodular goiter. MR revealed tumor in right lobe. Right hemithyroidectomy revealed follicular carcinoma.
- **Ultrasound left lobe:** Colloid nodule.
- **Cytology:** Insufficient for diagnosis.
- **Left hemithyroidectomy:** Colloid nodule.

Features

Partially iso-and hypoechoic
Inhomogeneous echo pattern
Spongy
Well circumscribed

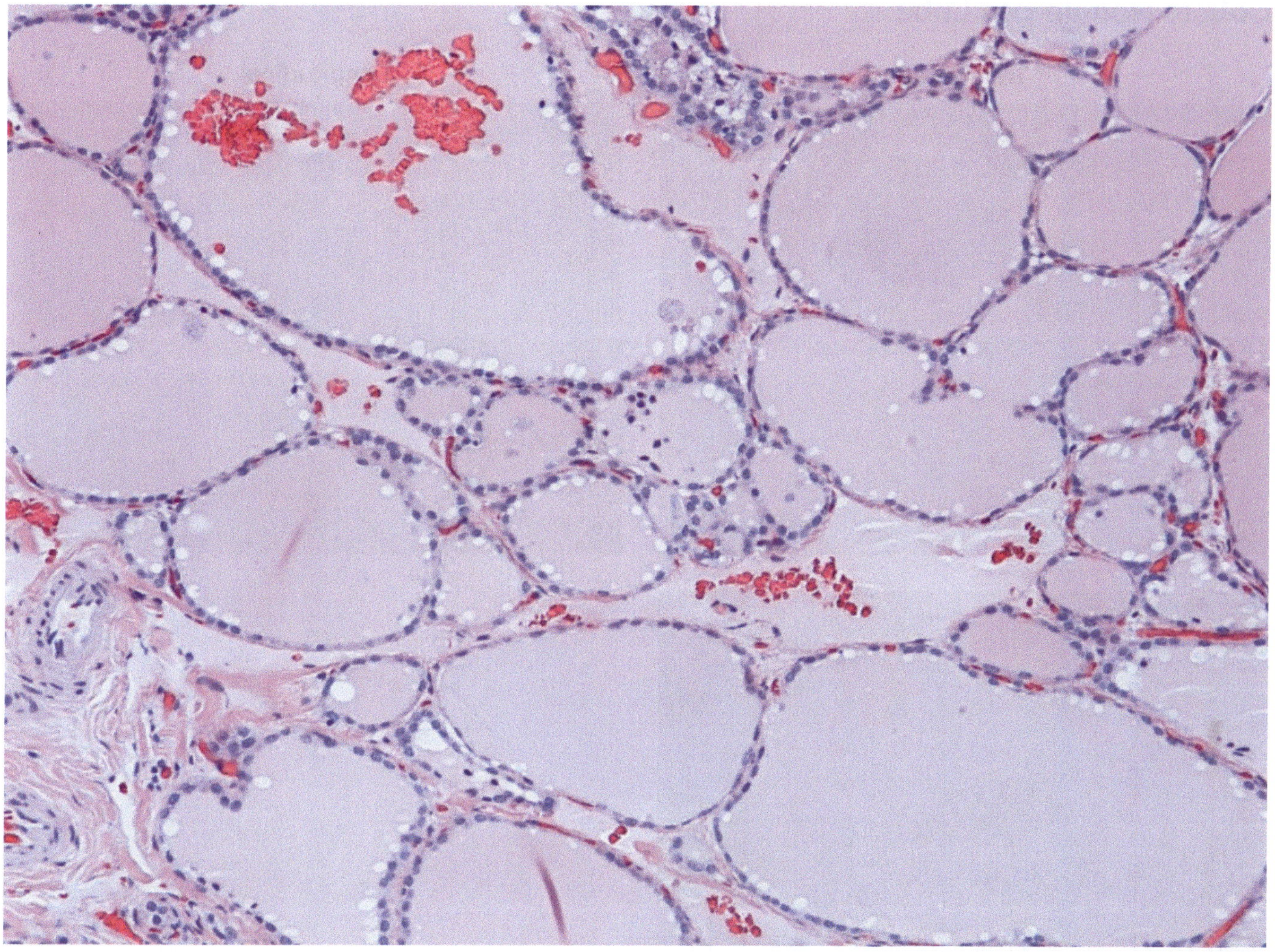

Figure 3-8. Histology: colloid nodule.

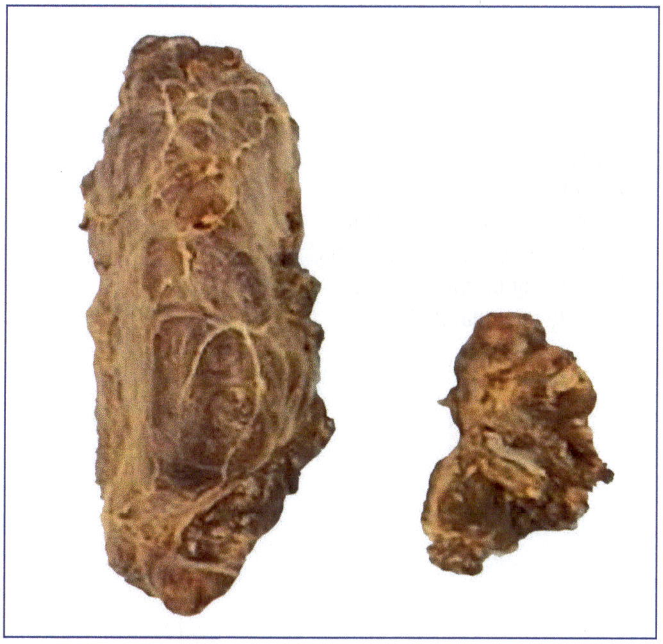

Figure 3-9. Left lobe with colloid nodules.

Colloid Nodule Left Lobe

Transverse	Longitudinal

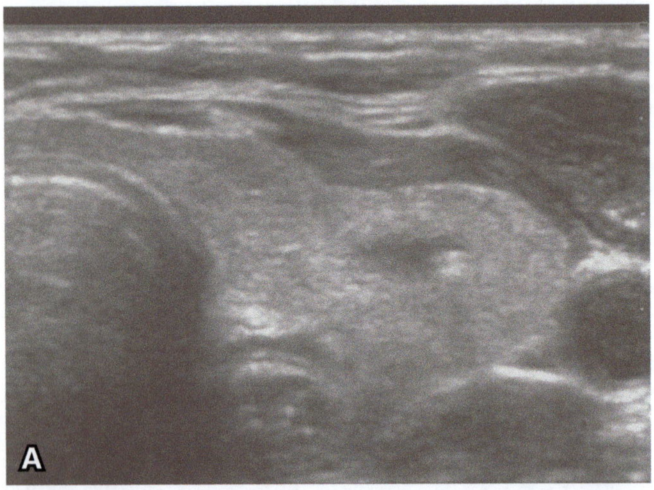

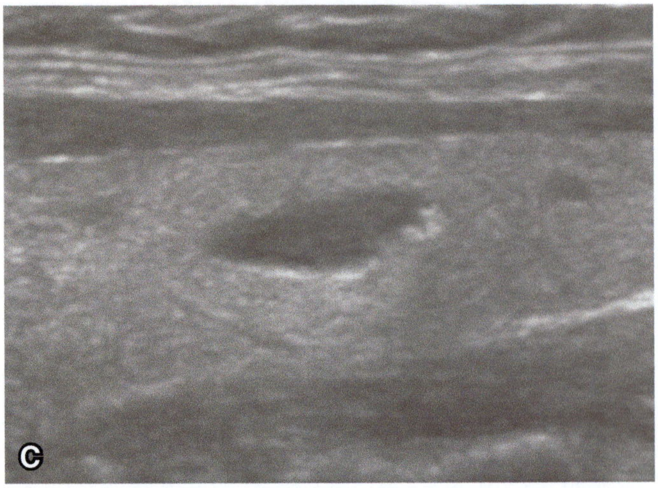

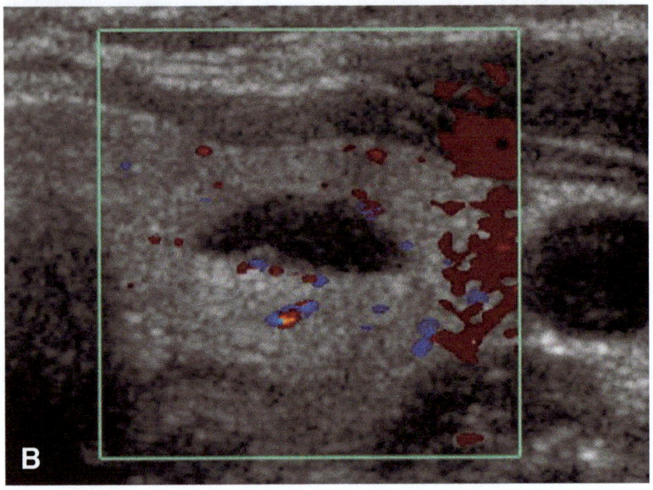

Figure 3-10. Ultrasound of a colloid nodule in the left lobe. **A**, Transverse. **B**, Color Doppler, transverse. **C**, Longitudinal.

37-Year-old woman

- **Clinical history:** Two cold nodules at scintigraphy.
- **Ultrasound:** Papillary thyroid carcinoma (PTC), isthmus/ left lobe. Colloid cyst in left lobe.
- **Cytology:** PTC.
- **Thyroidectomy:** PTC in isthmus. Cystic colloid nodule in left lobe.

See also pages 162–163

Features

Isoechoic
Homogeneous echo pattern
Small cyst with calcifications
Not clearly circumscribed
Scantly vascularized

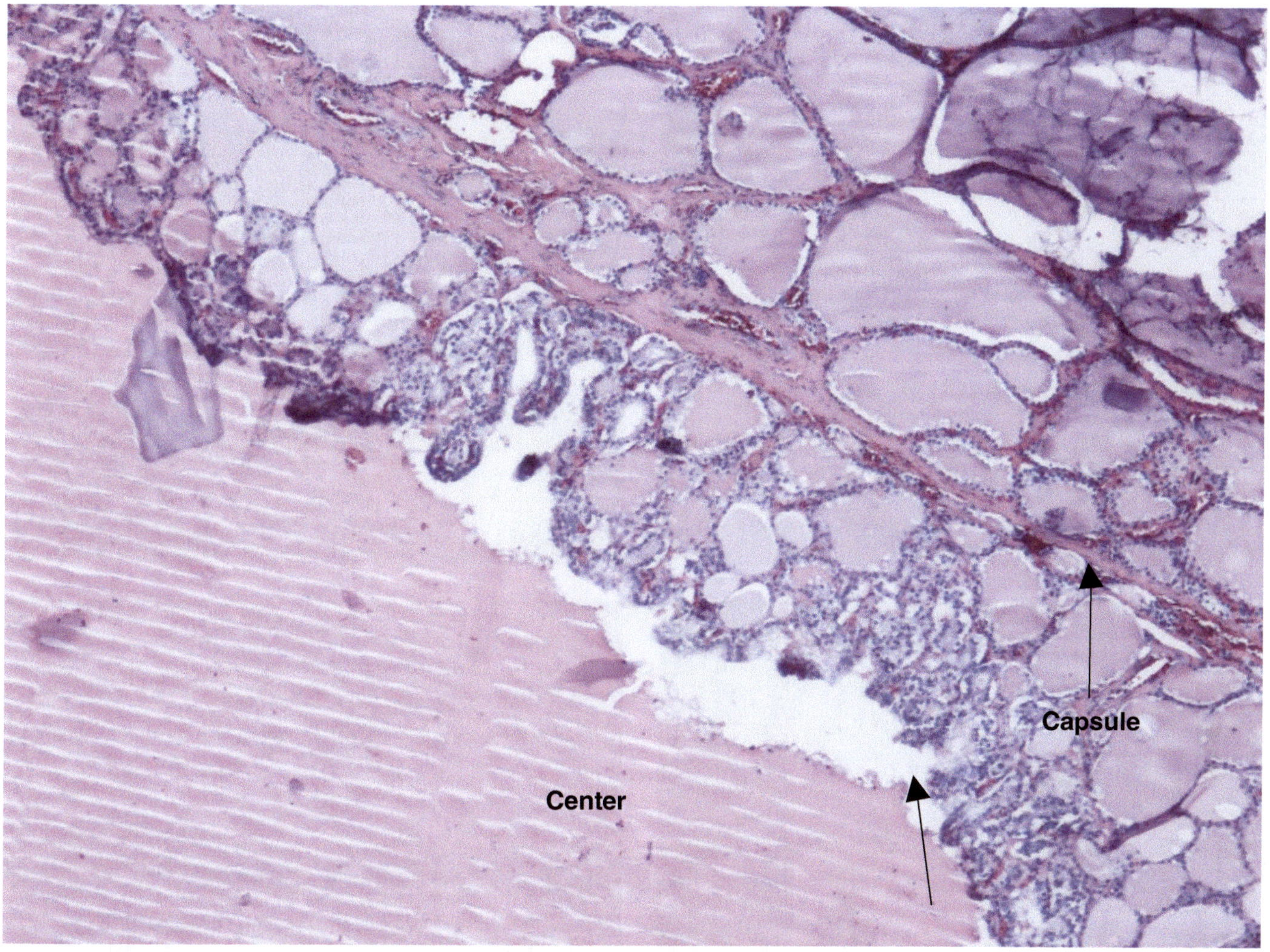

FIGURE 3-11. Histology: nodule rich in colloid in the center. Subcapsular condensation (*arrow*) of small follicles.

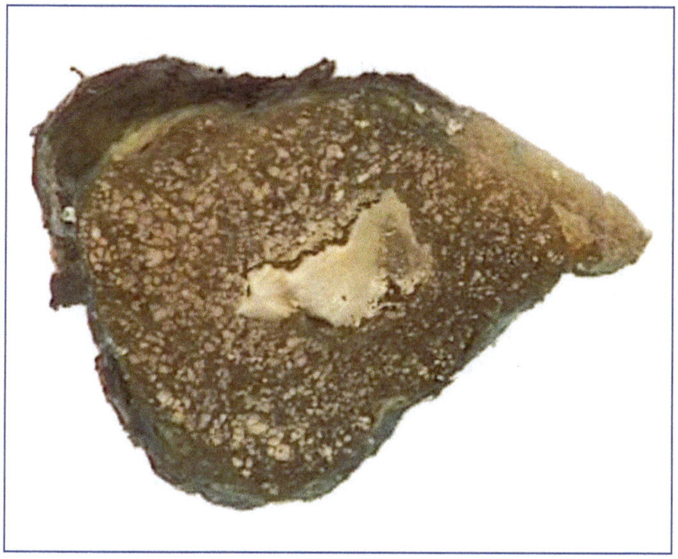

FIGURE 3-12. Gross section: note localized colloid cyst in the center of the nodule.

Colloid Nodule Right Lobe

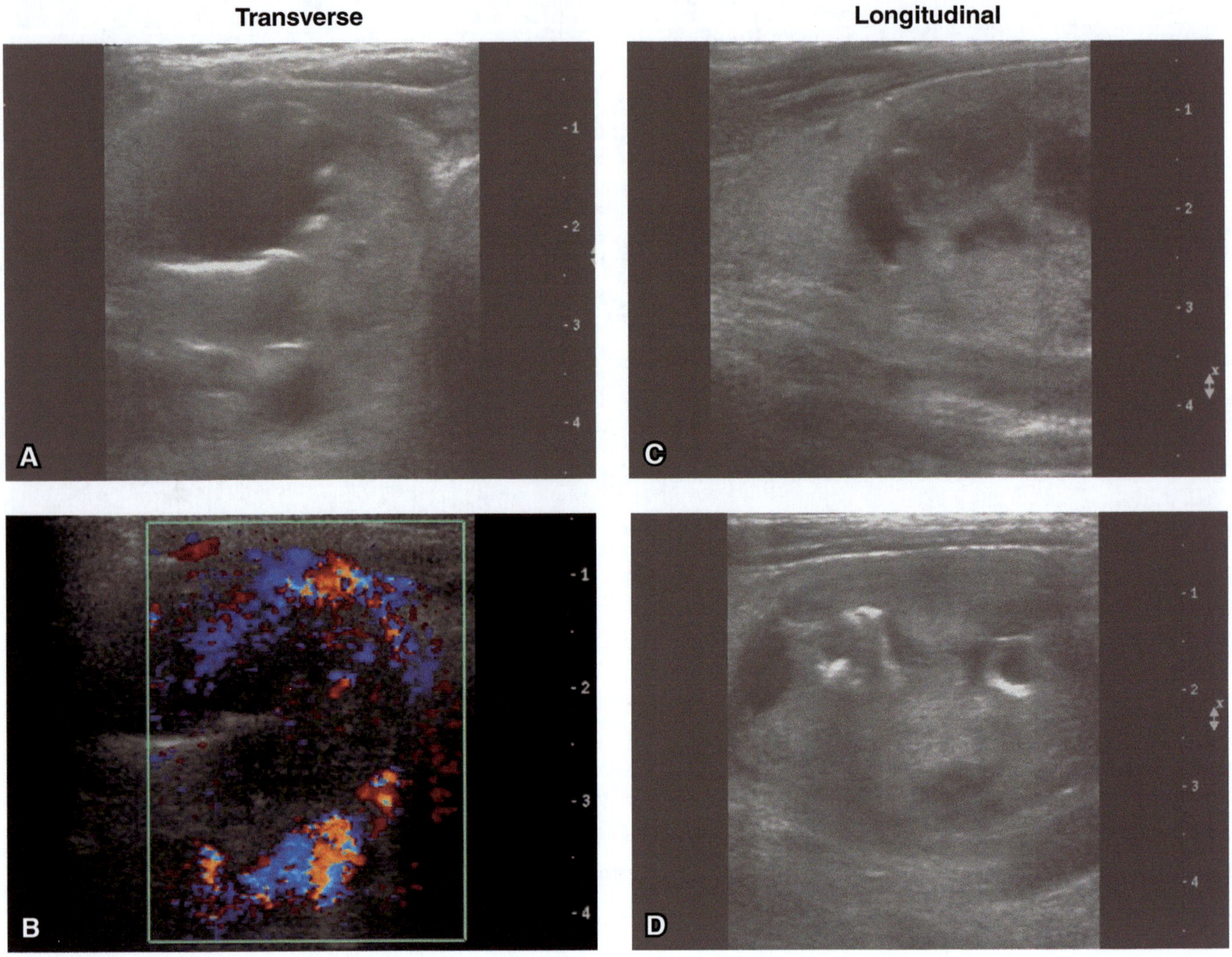

Figure 3-13. Ultrasound of a colloid nodule in the right lobe. **A**, Transverse, **B**, Color Doppler, transverse. **C** and **D**, Longitudinal.

65-Year-old woman

- **Clinical history:** About 10 years ago iodine treatment because of hyperparathyroidism. Nodular goiter present. Metastasis from follicular thyroid carcinoma in left iliac bone revealed 2 weeks before ultrasound examination.
- **Ultrasound:** Tumor consistent with follicular carcinoma in left lobe. Colloid nodule in right lobe.
- **Thyroidectomy:** Widely invasive follicular carcinoma in left lobe. Colloid nodule in right lobe.

See also pages 102–103

Features
Slightly hypoechoic
Inhomogeneous echo pattern
Small cysts
Well circumscribed
Coarse calcifications
Peripheral hypervascularity

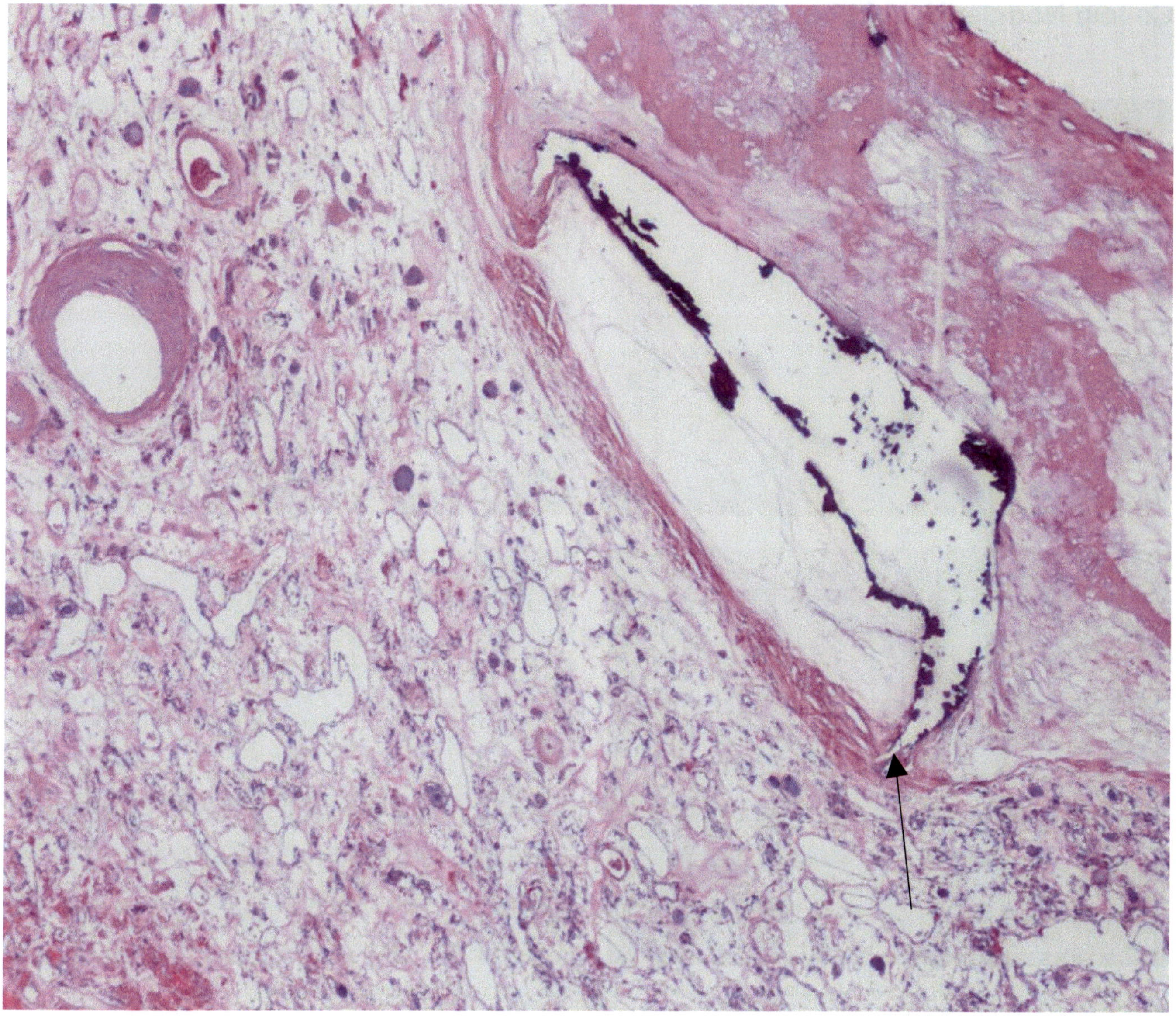

Figure 3-14. Histology: colloid nodule with calcifications in the capsule (*arrow*) and degenerative changes.

Colloid Nodule Right Lobe

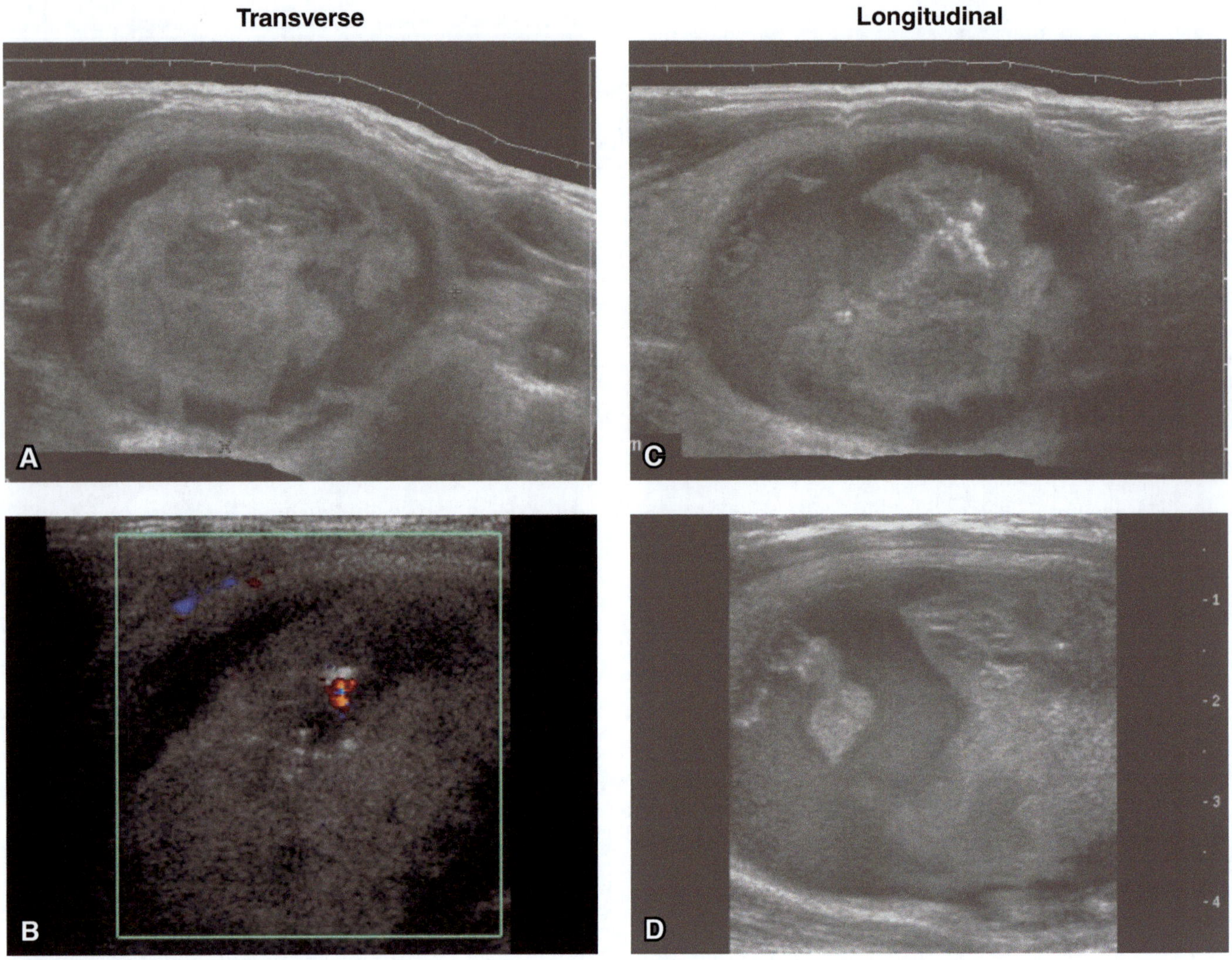

FIGURE 3-15. Ultrasound of a colloid nodule in the right lobe. **A**, Transverse, 37 x 46 mm. **B**, Color Doppler, transverse. **C**, Longitudinal, sagittal diameter: 53 mm. **D**, Longitudinal.

37-Year-old woman

- **Clinical history:** Palpable nodule aspirated for 35 ml of fluid 2 months before ultrasound examination. Rapid refilling.
- **Ultrasound:** Colloid cystic nodules in both lobes.
- **Cytology right lobe:** Cystic fluid.
- **Right hemithyroidectomy:** Cystic colloid nodule.

Features

Isoechoic solid tissue peripherally
Mostly cystic with hemorrhagic fibrinous clots and probably small areas of papillomatous solid tissue
Well circumscribed
Some microcalcifications
Almost avascular

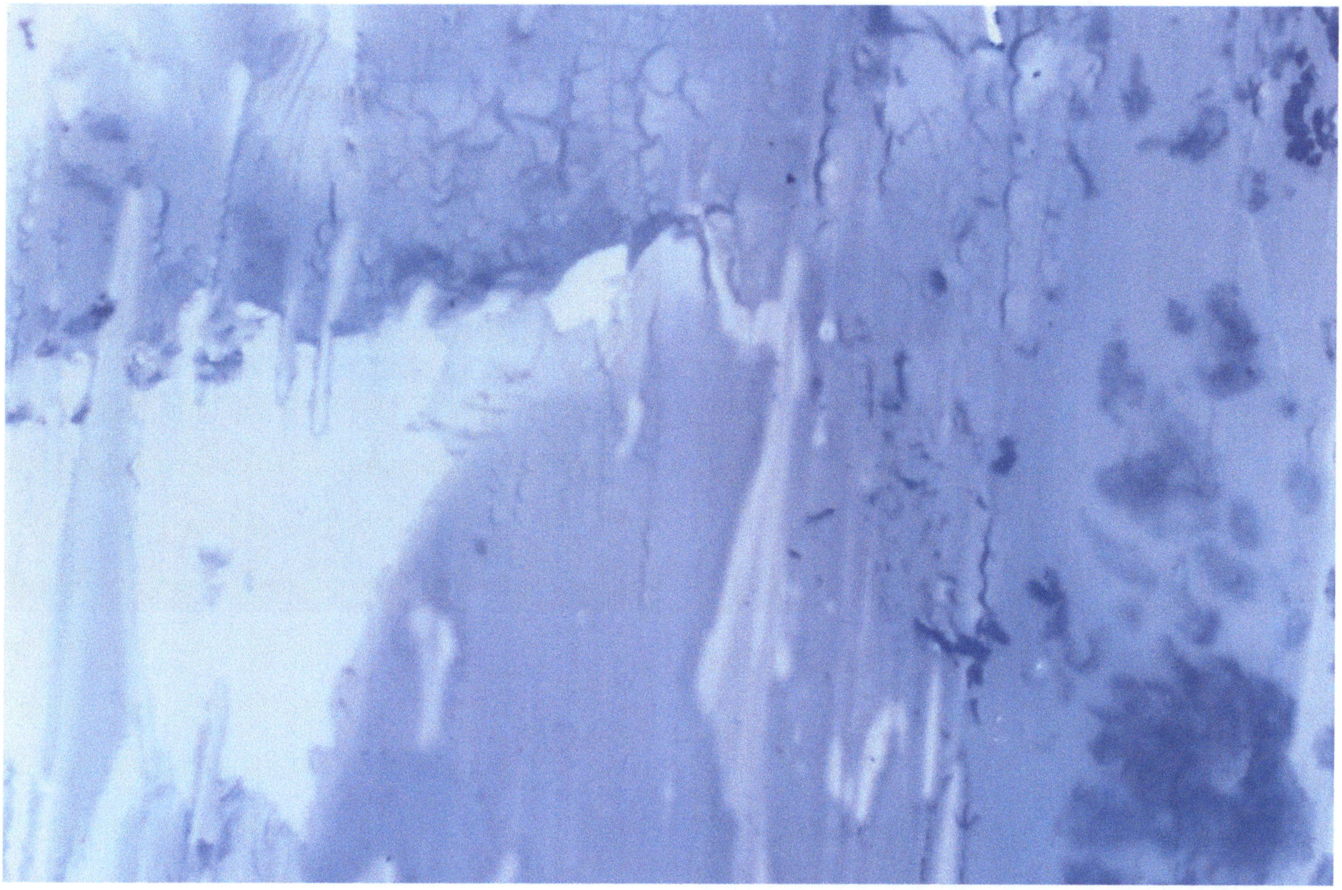

FIGURE 3-16. Cytology: abundant amount of thin colloid.

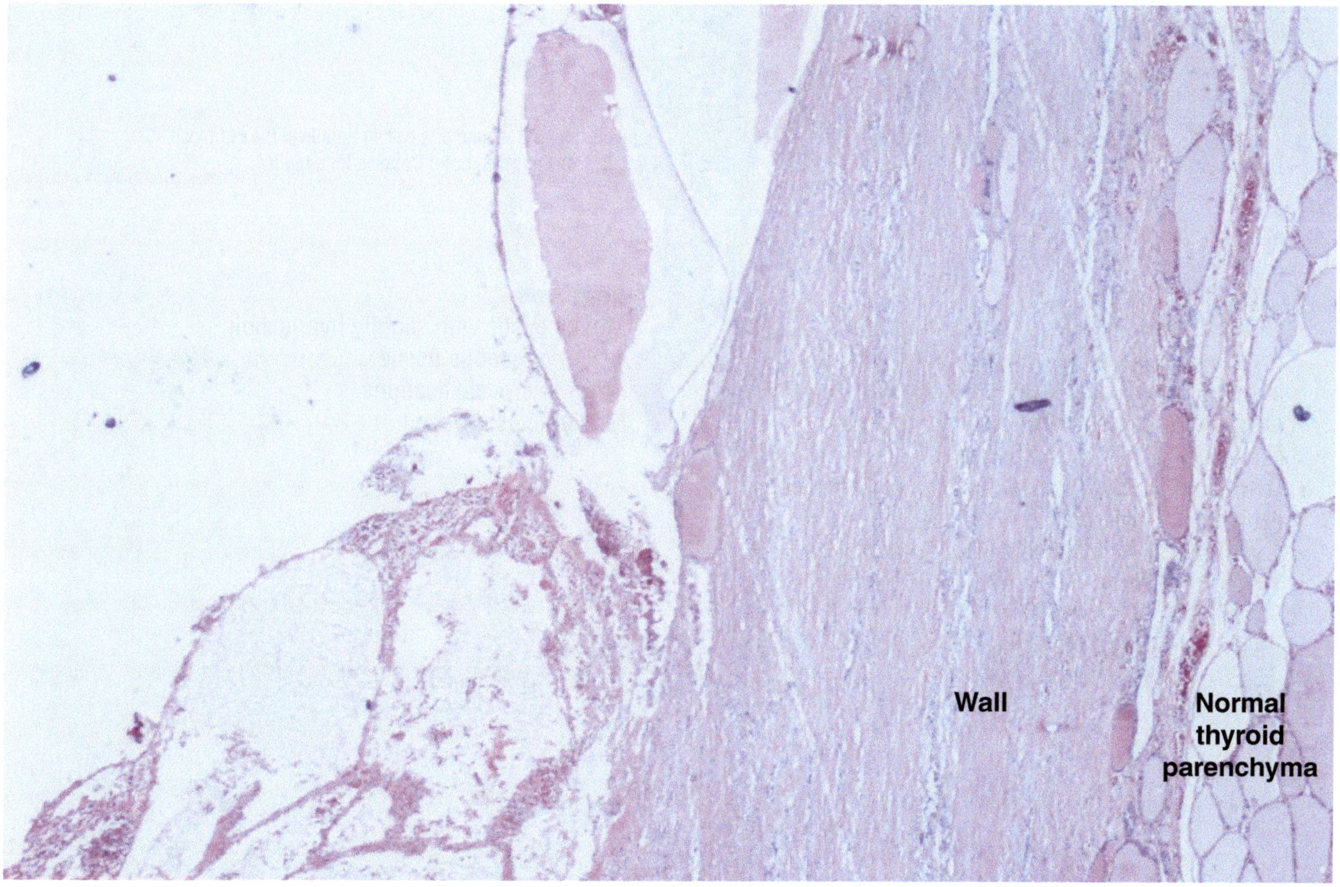

FIGURE 3-17. Histology: from the wall of the cystic colloid nodule.

Colloid Nodule Right Lobe

Transverse

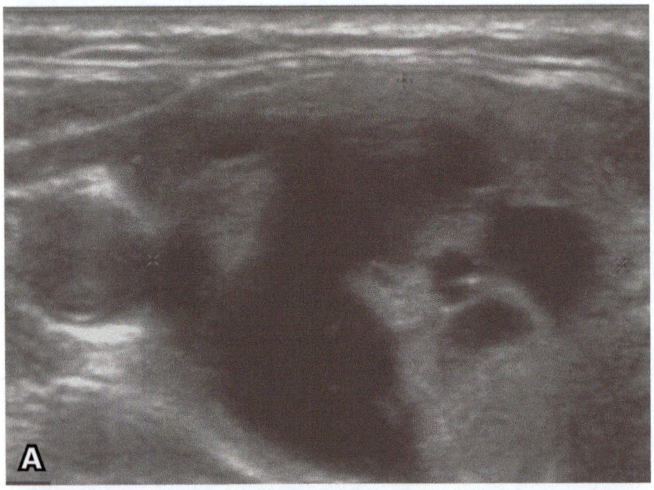

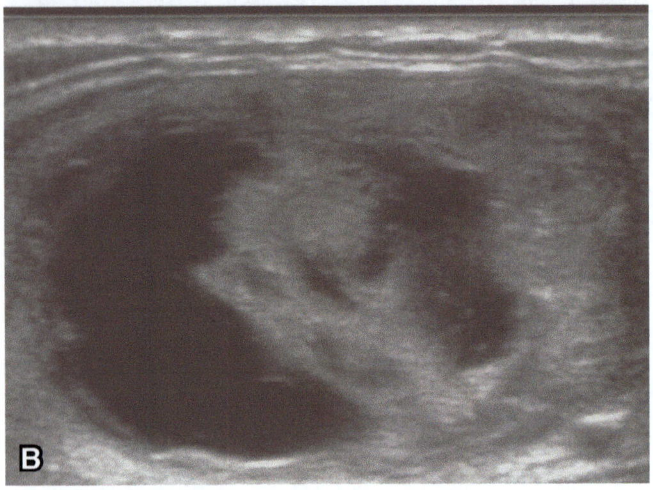

Longitudinal

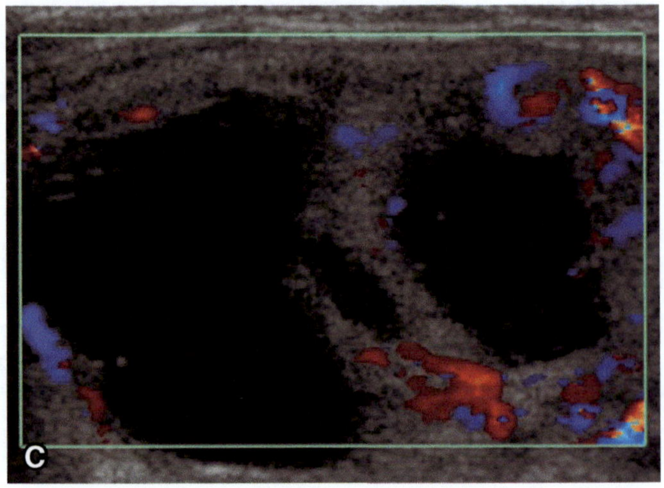

FIGURE 3-18. Ultrasound of a colloid nodule in the right lobe. **A** and **B**, Transverse. **C**, Color Doppler, longitudinal.

49-Year-old woman

- **Clinical history:** Benign tumor in isthmus resected 4 years ago. Examination of two nodules, one in each lobe 1 year ago. Cytology of left lobe suspicious for papillary thyroid carcinoma (PTC). No follow up.
- **Ultrasound:** Cystic colloid nodule in right lobe. Probably colloid nodule in left lobe.
- **Cytology:** PTC in left lobe. Cyst in right lobe.
- **Thyroidectomy:** PTC in left lobe. Cyst in right lobe.

See also pages 174–175

Features

Mostly cystic with slightly hypoechoic homogeneous tissue
A few microcalcifications
Medium vascularized

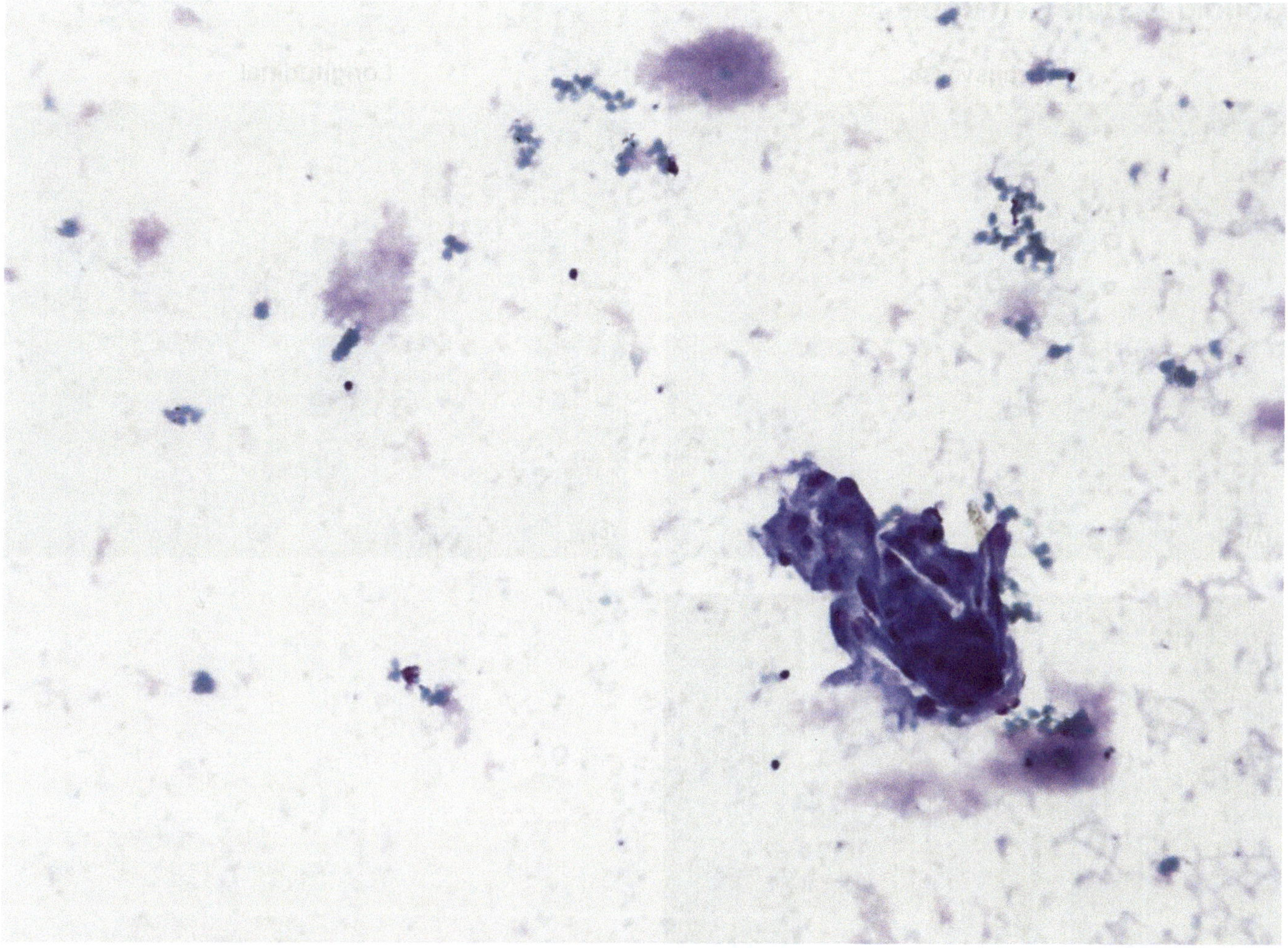

Figure 3-19. Cytology from the right lobe: cystic material with macrophages and metaplastic/reactive epithelium.

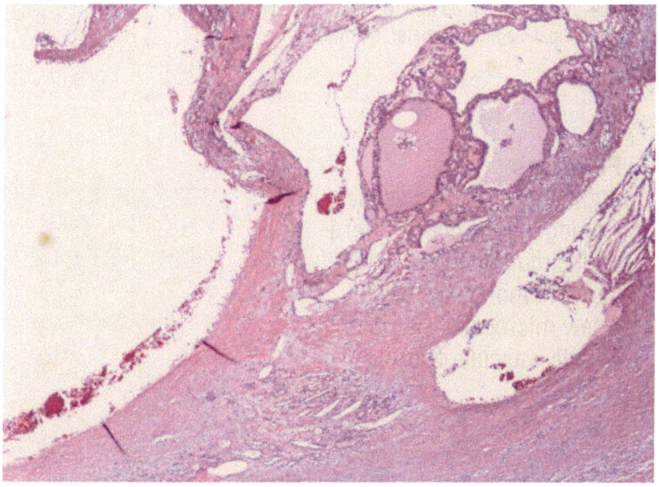

Figure 3-20. Histology: from the wall of the cystic colloid nodule.

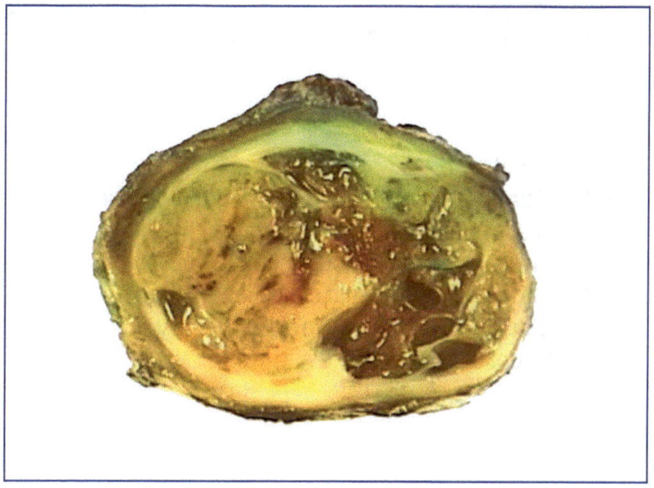

Figure 3-21. Gross examination: cystic colloid nodule.

Colloid Nodule Left Lobe

Transverse

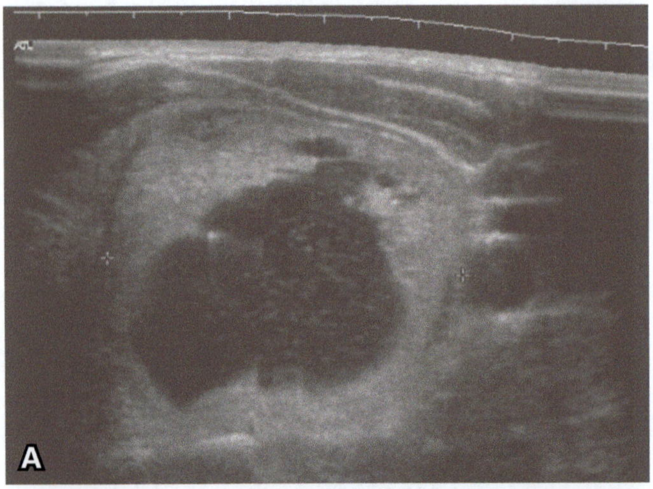

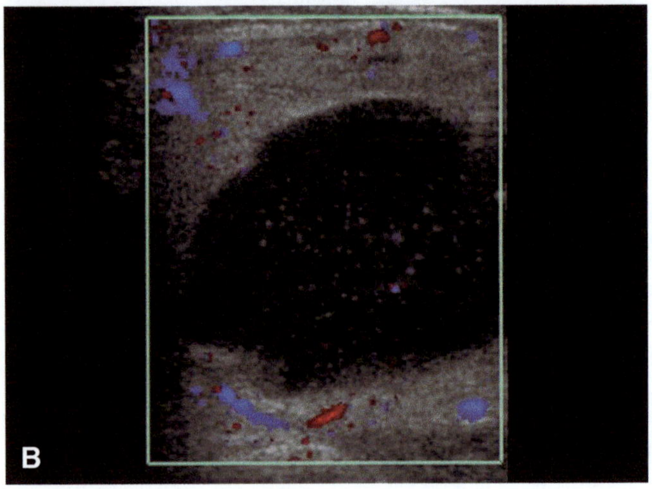

Longitudinal

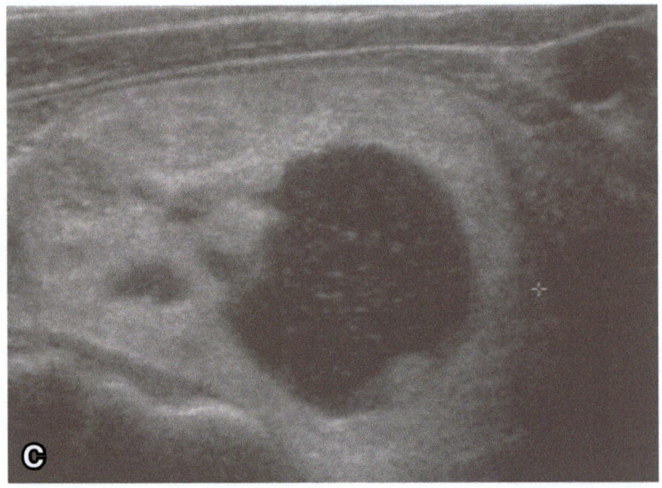

Figure 3-22. Ultrasound of a colloid nodule in the left lobe. **A**, Transverse diameter: 38 mm. **B**, Color Doppler, transverse. **C**, Longitudinal, sagittal diameter: 54 mm.

50-Year-old man

- **Clinical history:** Rapidly growing tumor in left lobe past 2 months.
- **Ultrasound:** Colloid nodule in left lobe.
- **Cytology:** Hemorrhagic cystic fluid.
- **18-Gauge histologic needle biopsy:** Cystic colloid nodule.

Features

Slightly hypoechoic tissue
Homogeneous echo pattern
Well circumscribed
Large hemorrhagic cyst
A few microcalcifications
Scantly vascularized

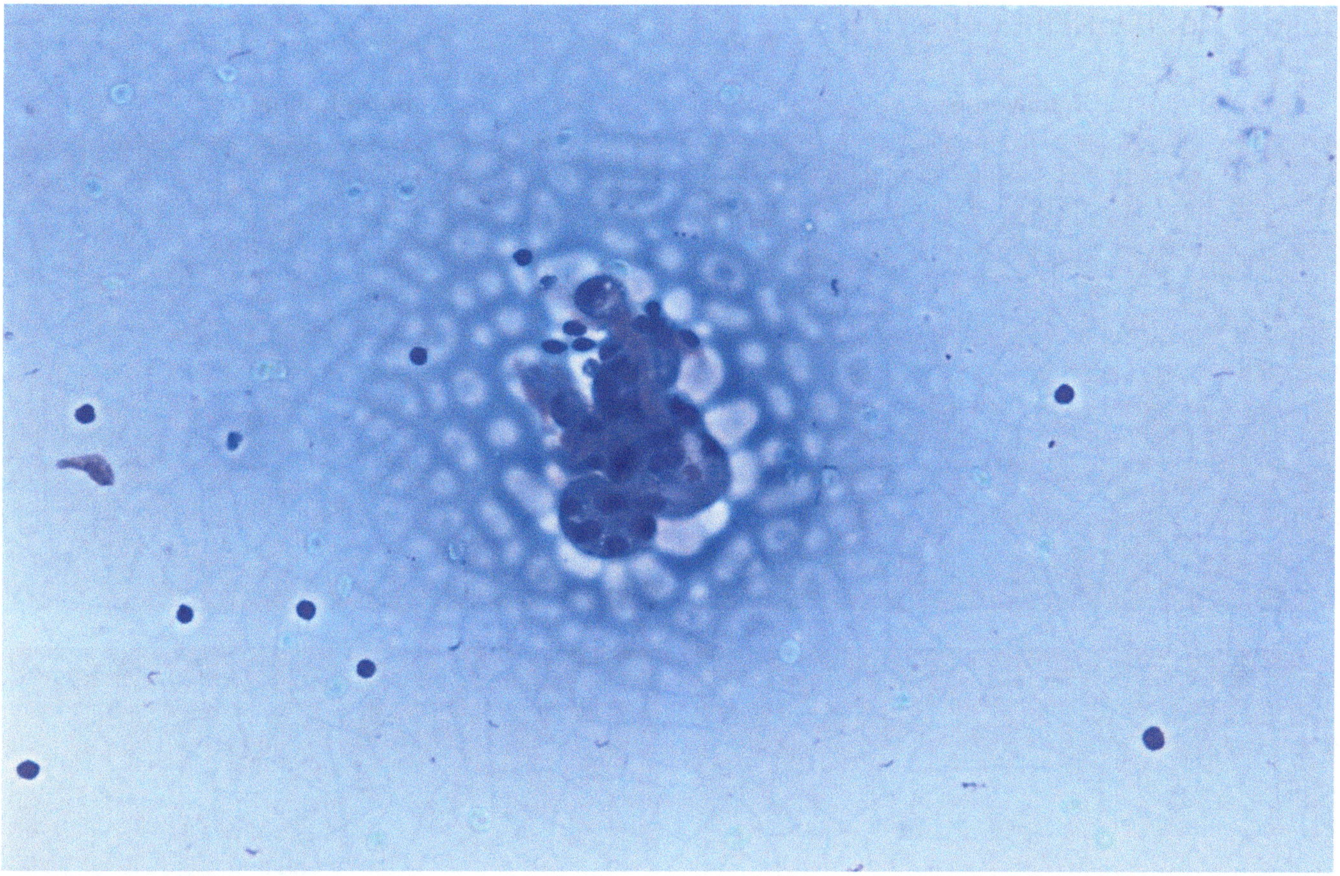

Figure 3-23. Cytology: thin colloid and one group of benign follicular epithelium.

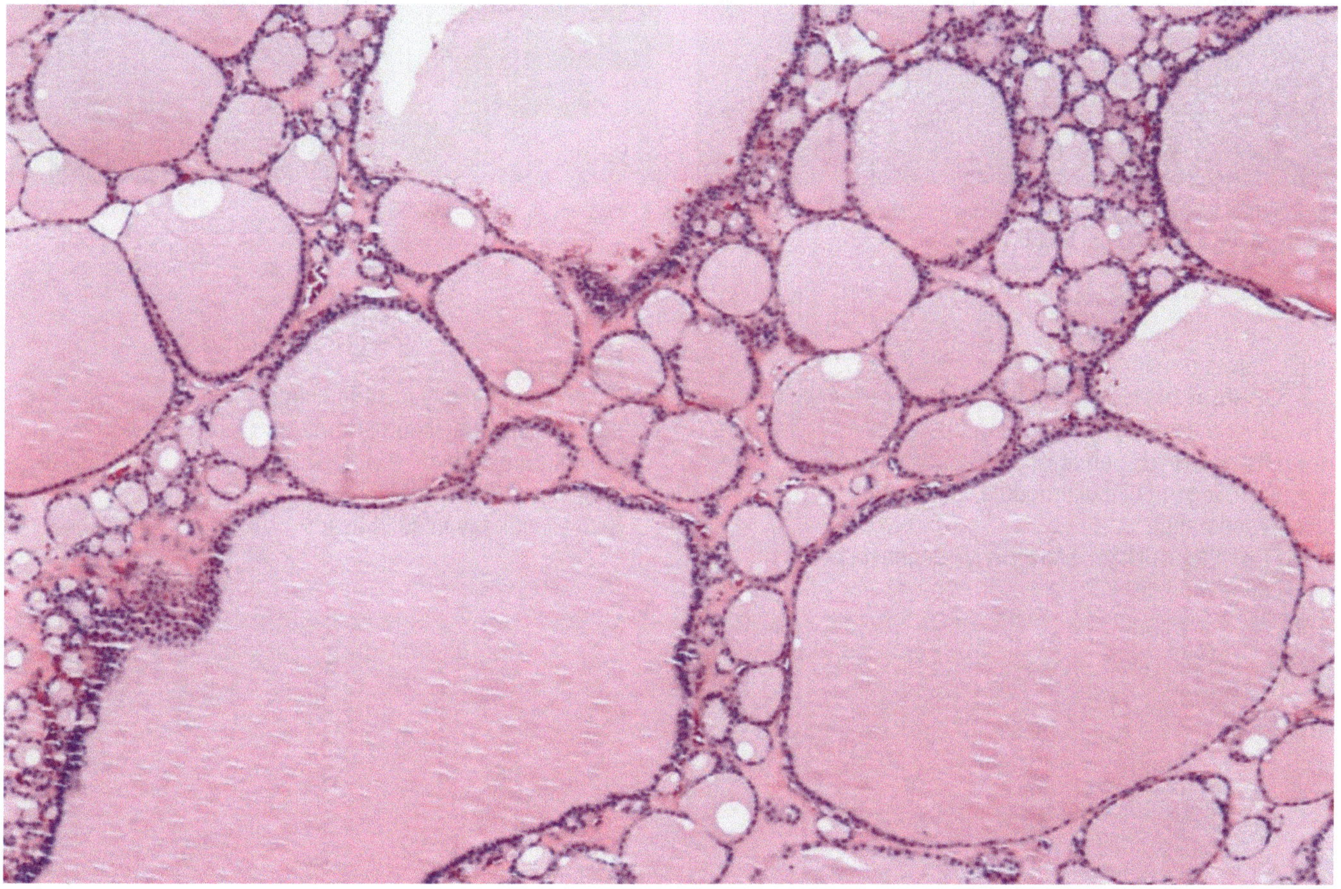

Figure 3-24. Histology: colloid nodule.

Colloid Nodule Right Lobe

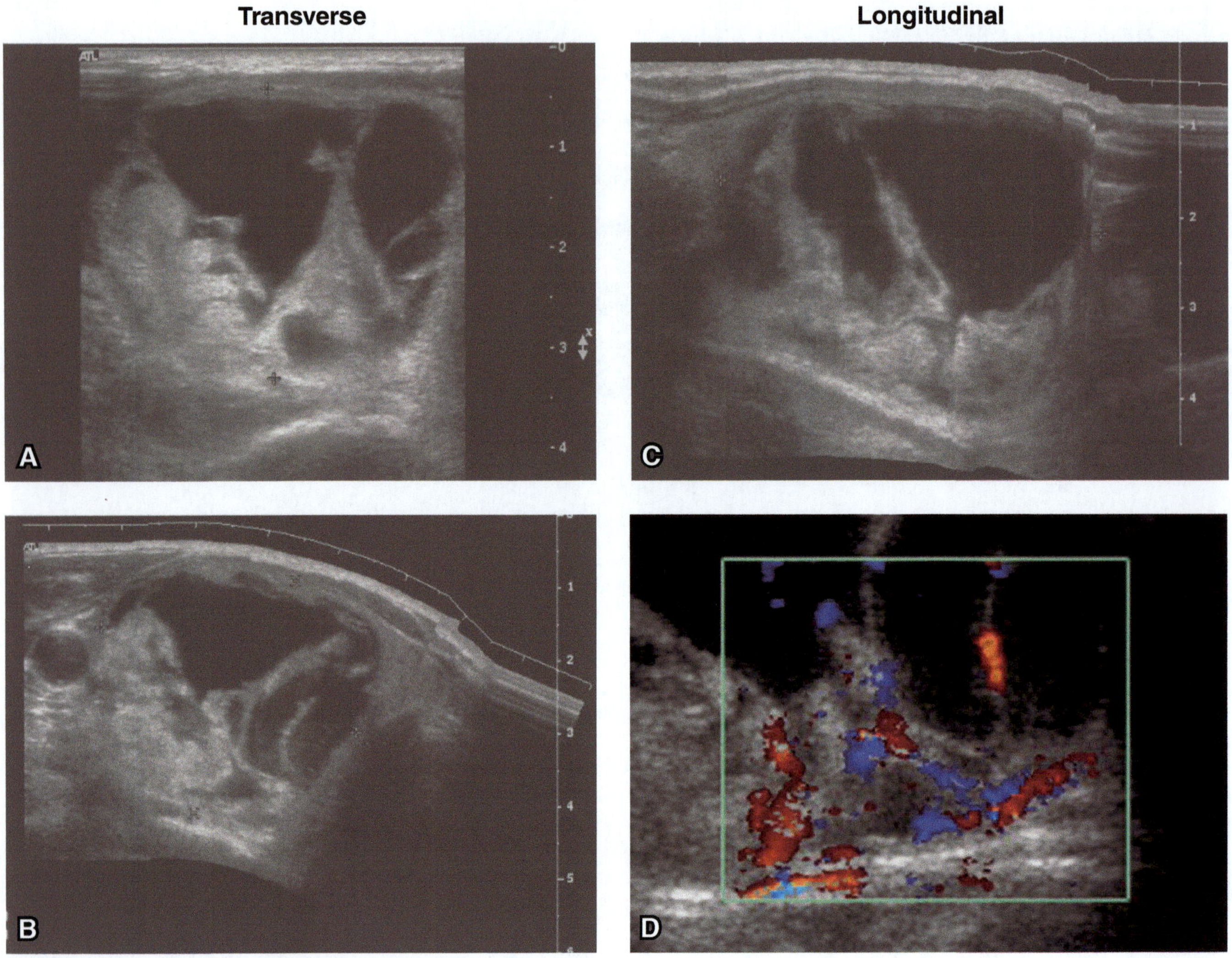

FIGURE 3-25. Ultrasound of a colloid nodule in the right lobe. **A**, Transverse, 35 x 38 mm. **B**, Transverse. **C**, Longitudinal, sagittal diameter: 40 mm. **D**, Color Doppler, longitudinal.

61-Year-old man

- **Clinical history:** Cyst in right lobe past 4 years. Several aspirations.
- **Ultrasound:** Semicystic tumor. Malignant?
- **Cytology:** Follicular nodule with cystic degeneration.
- **Right hemithyroidectomy:** Degenerated colloid nodule.

Features

Mixed echogenicity in solid tissue
Inhomogeneous echo pattern
Well circumscribed
Large cyst with septa
Rich vascularity in solid tissue

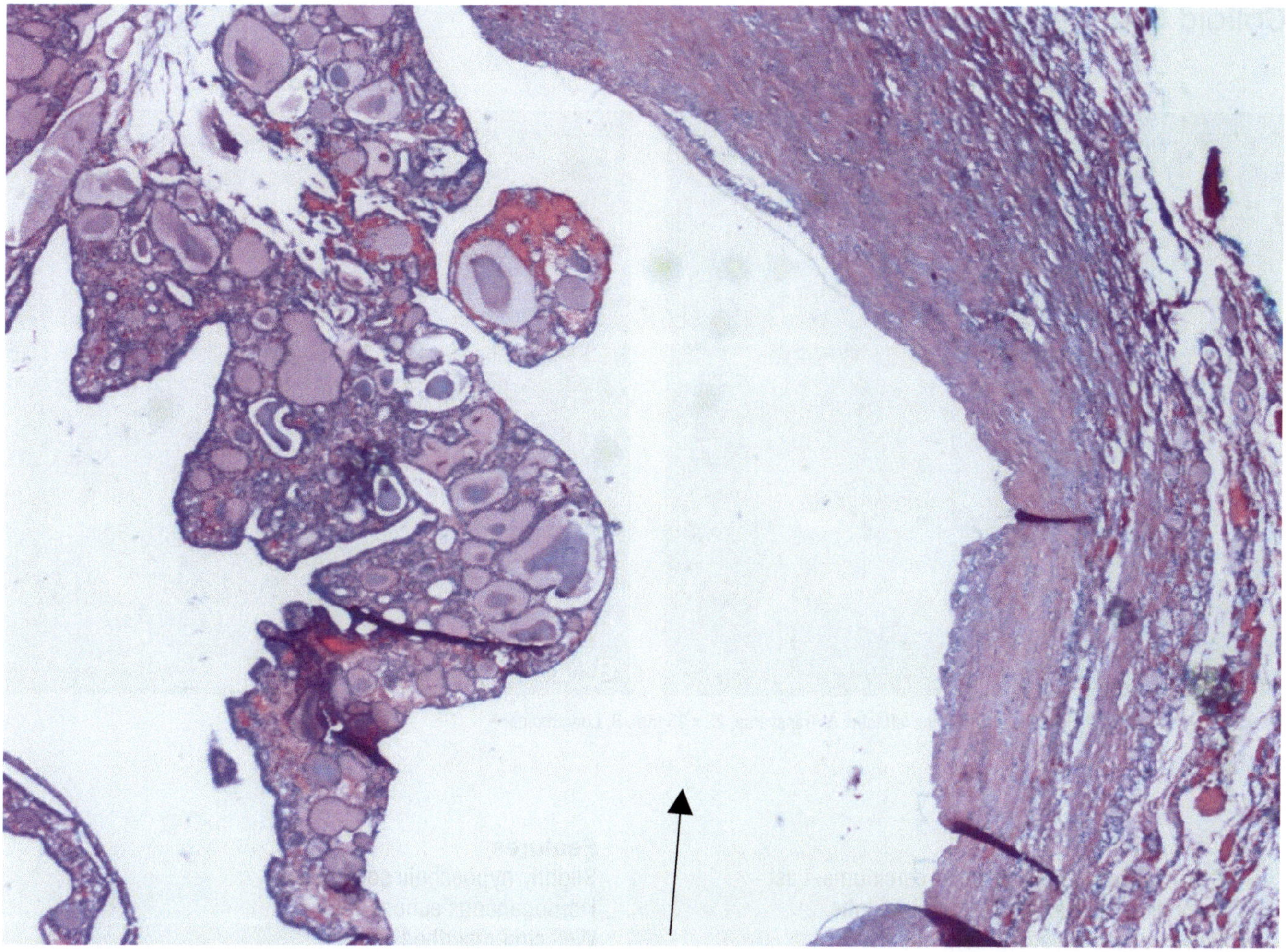

Figure 3-26. Histology: cystic space (*arrow*) within the colloid nodule

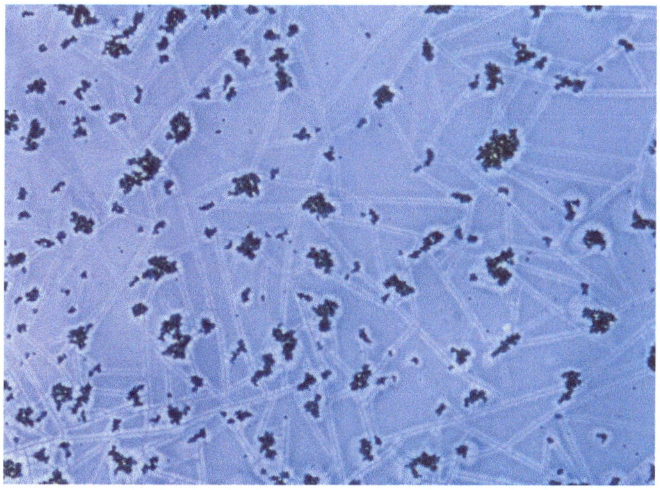

Figure 3-27. Cytology: watery colloid showing a characteristic cracking artifact with erythrocyte aggregates.

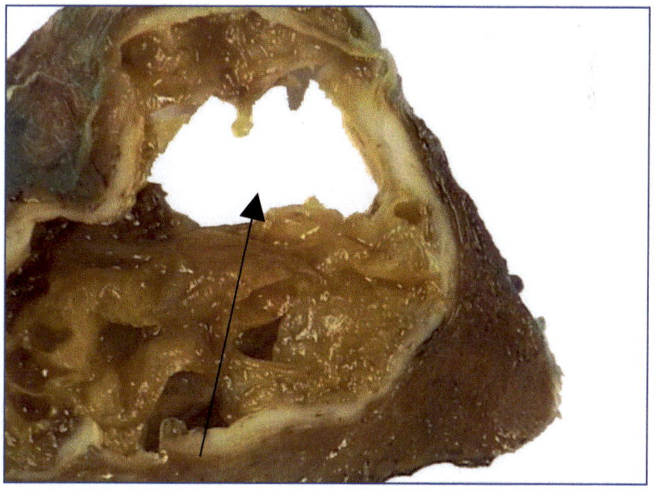

Figure 3-28. Gross section: partially cystic lesion.

Colloid Cyst Left Lobe

Transverse **Longitudinal**

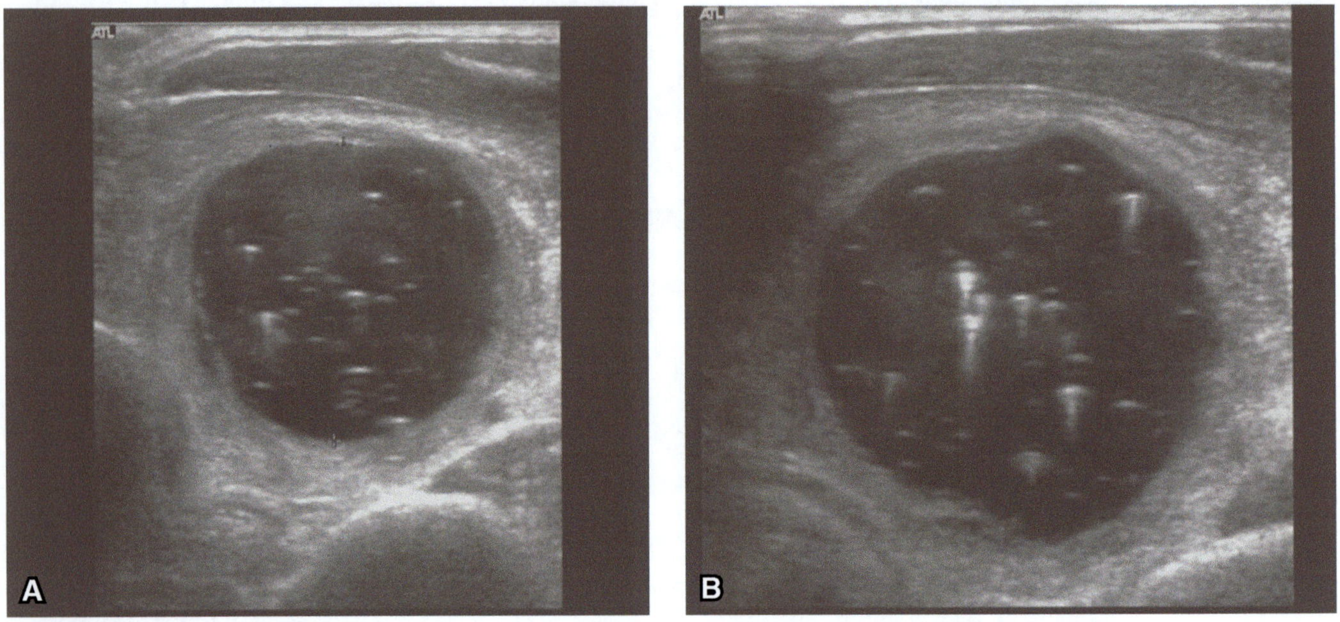

Figure 3-29. Ultrasound of a colloid cyst in the left lobe. **A**, Transverse, 22 x 25 mm. **B**, Longitudinal.

35-Year-old man

- **Clinical history:** Testicular carcinoma. Last week growing tumor in left thyroid lobe.
- **Ultrasound:** Cystic colloid nodule.
- **Cytology:** Cystic colloid nodule.

Features

Slightly hypoechoic solid tissue
Homogeneous echo pattern
Well circumscribed
Large cyst with colloid crystals

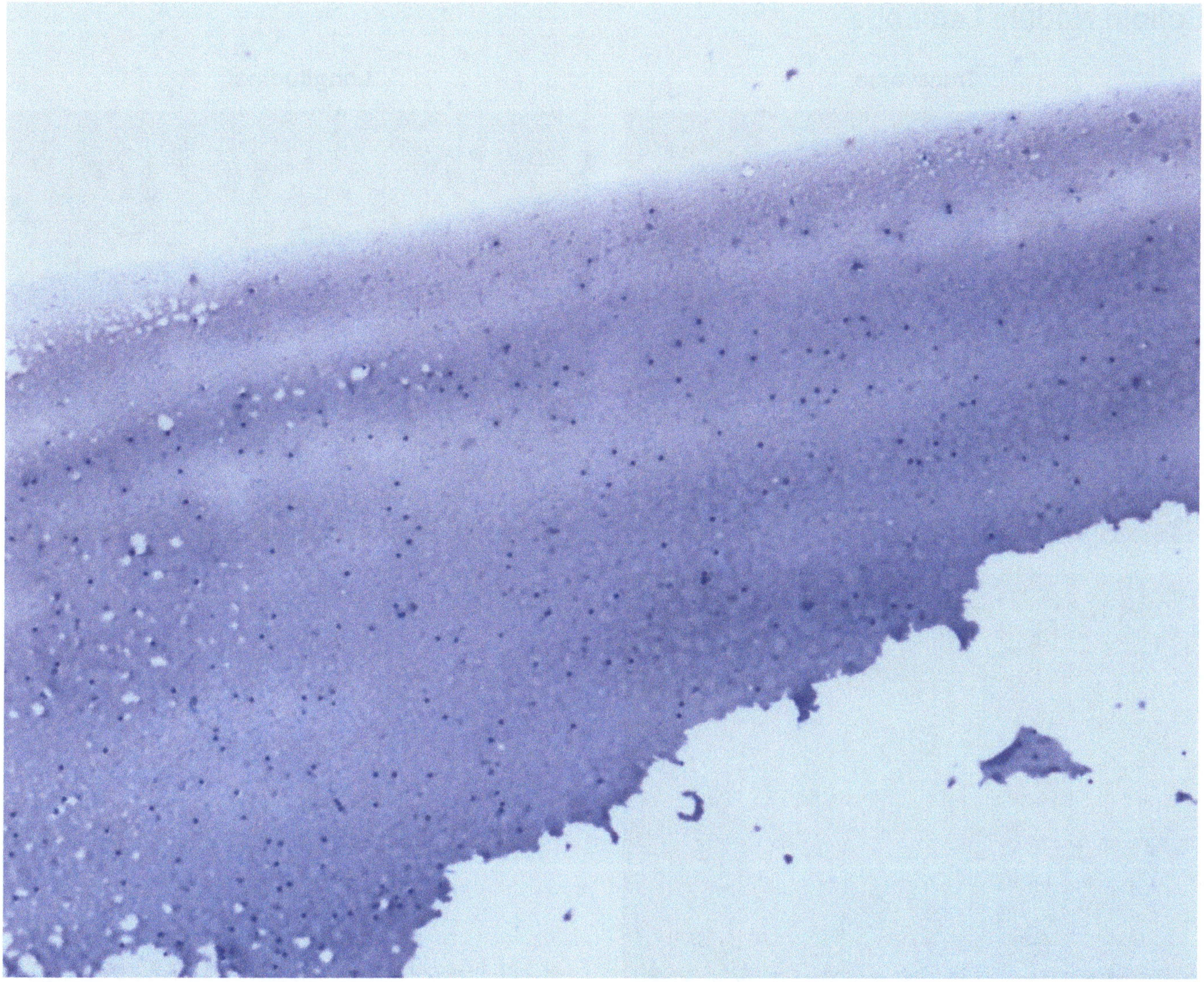

Figure 3-30. Cytology: rich in thin colloid.

Colloid Nodule Left Lobe

Transverse | **Longitudinal**

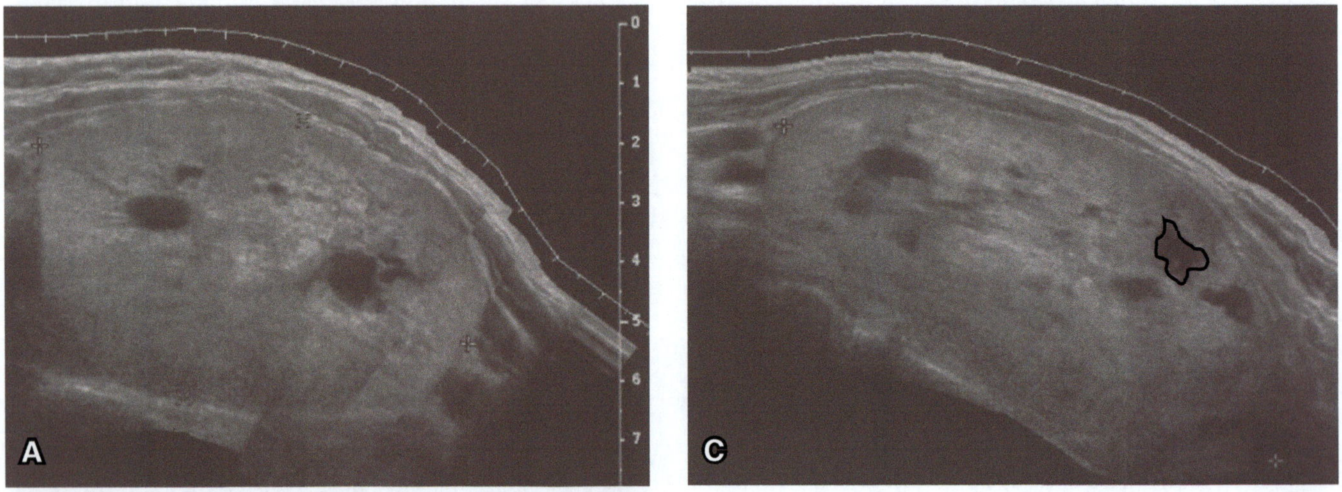

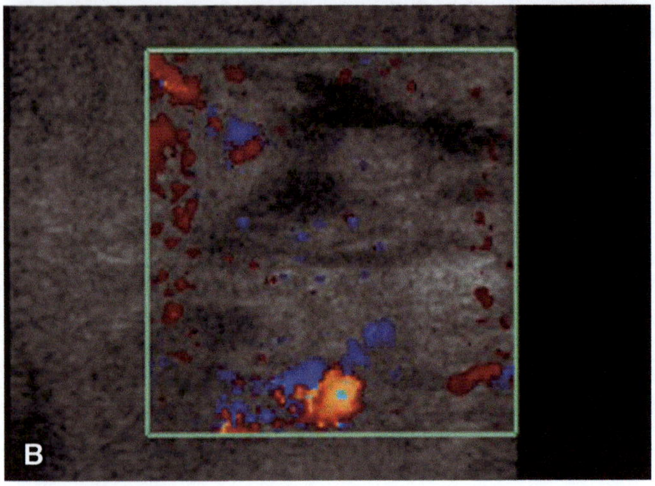

FIGURE 3-31. Ultrasound of a colloid nodule in the left lobe. **A**, transverse, 50 x 80 mm. **B**, Color Doppler, transverse. **C**, Longitudinal, sagittal diameter: 110 mm.

60-Year-old man

- **Clinical history:** Palpable nodule in left lobe past 10 months. Increased size past 2 months.
- **Ultrasound:** Probably colloid nodule.
- **Cytology:** Follicular lesion.
- **16-Gauge histologic needle biopsy:** Colloid nodule.
- **Left hemithyroidectomy:** Colloid nodule.

Features

Hyper-, iso-, and hypoechoic tissue
Small cysts
A few microcalcifications
Well circumscribed
Scantly vascularized

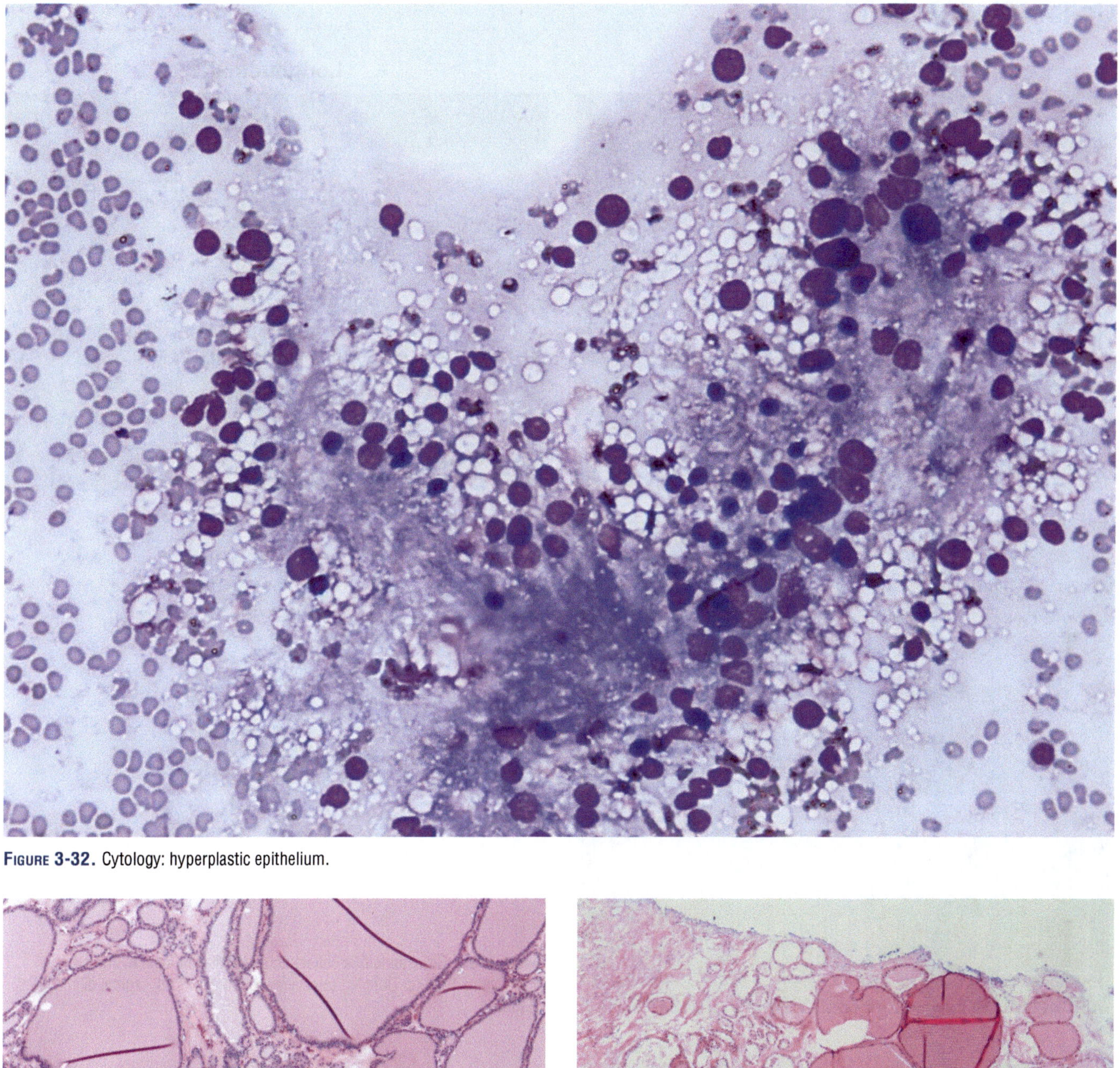

FIGURE 3-32. Cytology: hyperplastic epithelium.

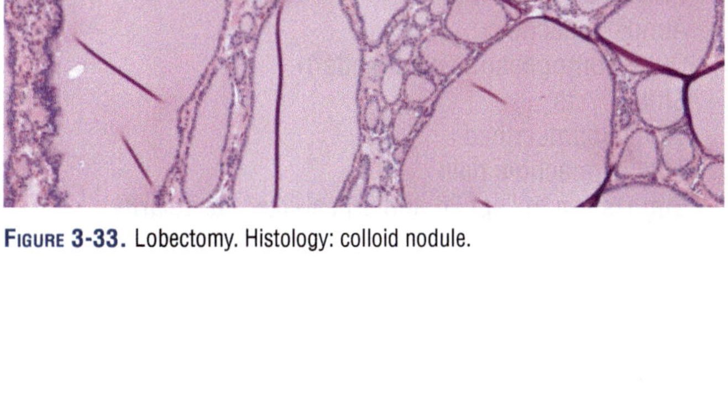

FIGURE 3-33. Lobectomy. Histology: colloid nodule.

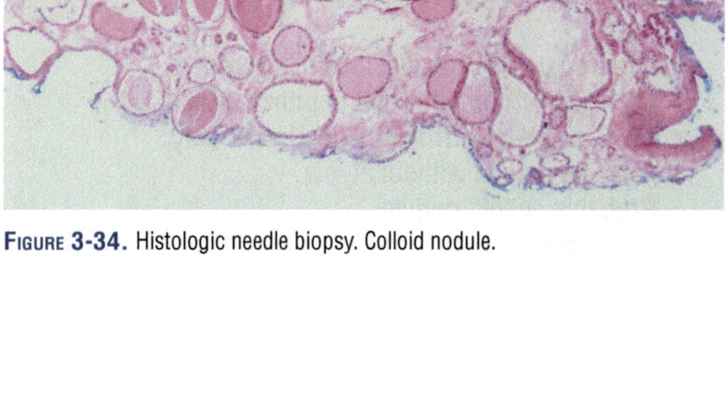

FIGURE 3-34. Histologic needle biopsy. Colloid nodule.

Colloid Nodule Left Lobe

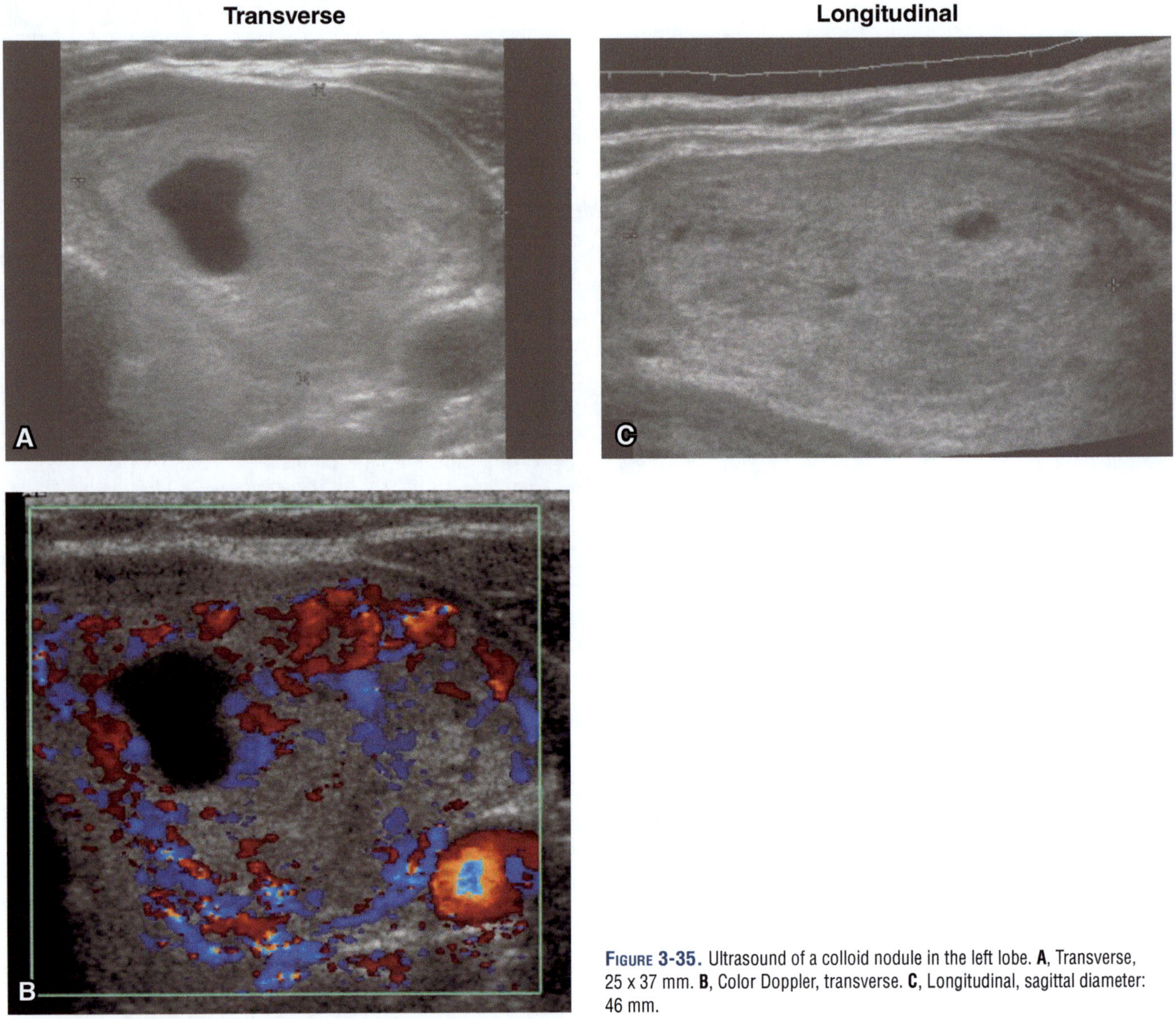

Figure 3-35. Ultrasound of a colloid nodule in the left lobe. **A**, Transverse, 25 x 37 mm. **B**, Color Doppler, transverse. **C**, Longitudinal, sagittal diameter: 46 mm.

51-Year-old woman

- **Clinical history:** Palpable nodule for about 1 year.
- **Ultrasound:** Probably follicular tumor.
- **Cytology:** Some follicular epithelial cells.
- **18-Gauge histologic needle biopsy:** Follicular tissue without atypia. Probably colloid nodule.
- **Left hemithyroidectomy:** Colloid nodule.

Features

Almost isoechoic
Quite homogeneous echo pattern
Small cysts
Well circumscribed
Thin hypoechoic halo
Suggestion of “spoke-and-wheel-like” vascularity

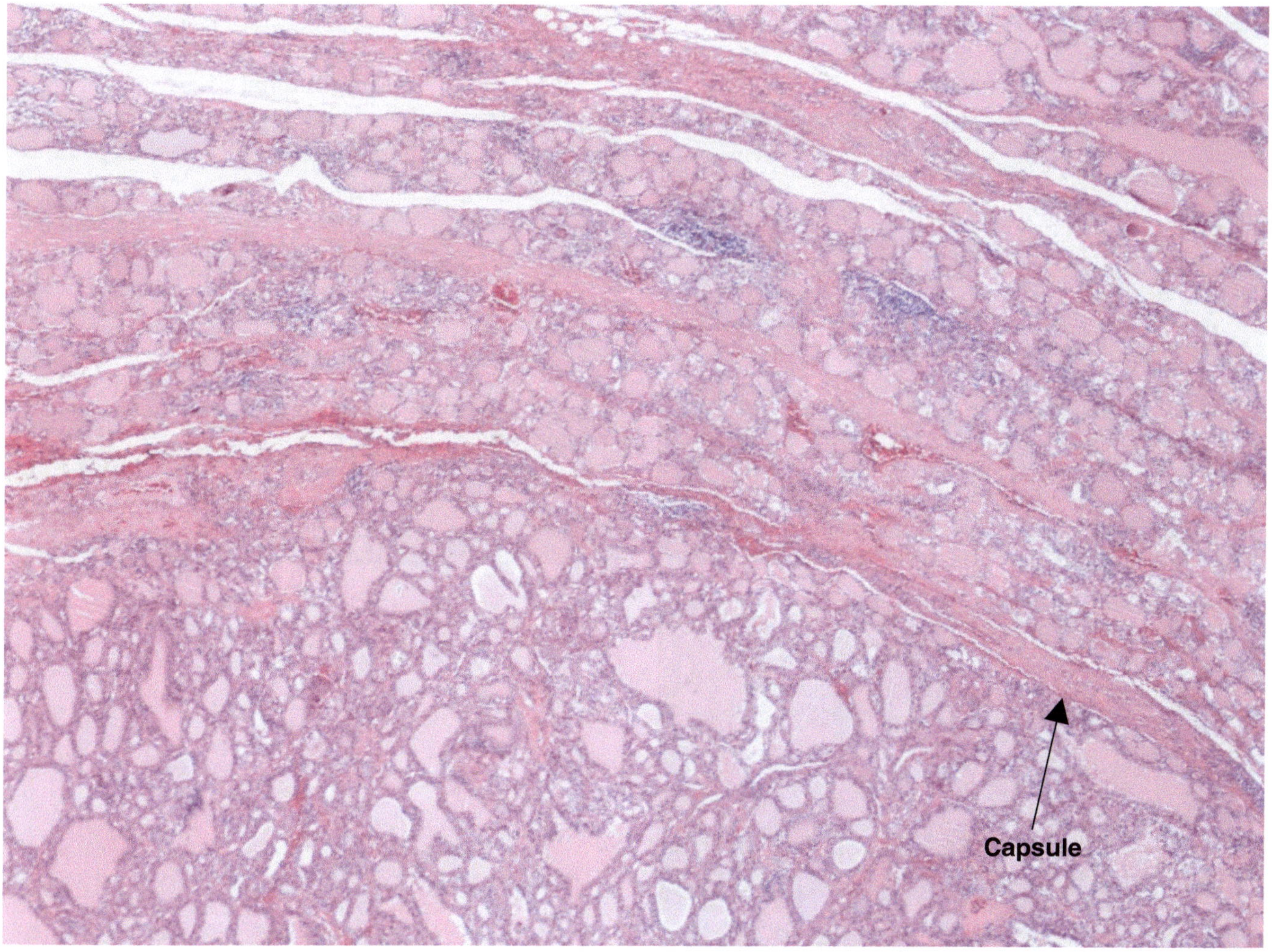

Figure 3-36. Histology: adenomatous colloid nodule.

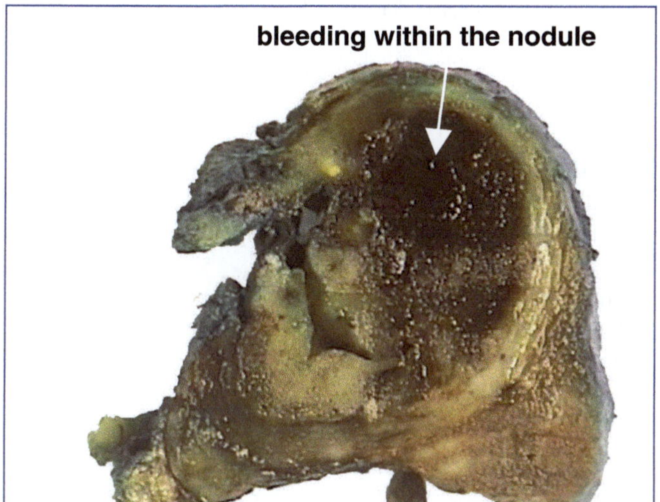

Figure 3-37. Gross section showing bleeding within the nodule (*arrow*).

Colloid Nodule Left Lobe

Transverse | **Longitudinal**

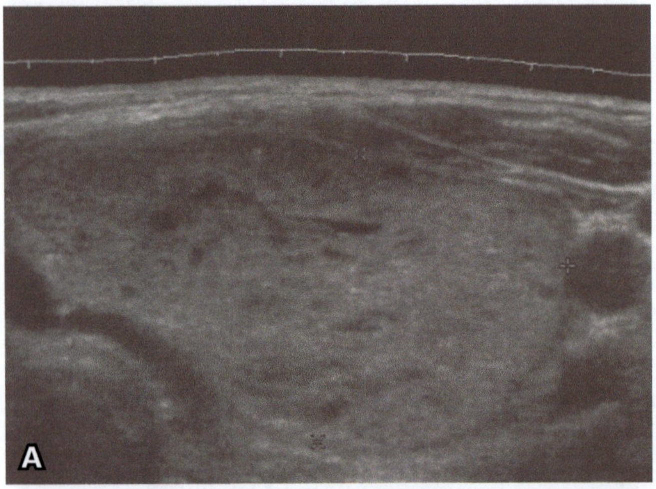

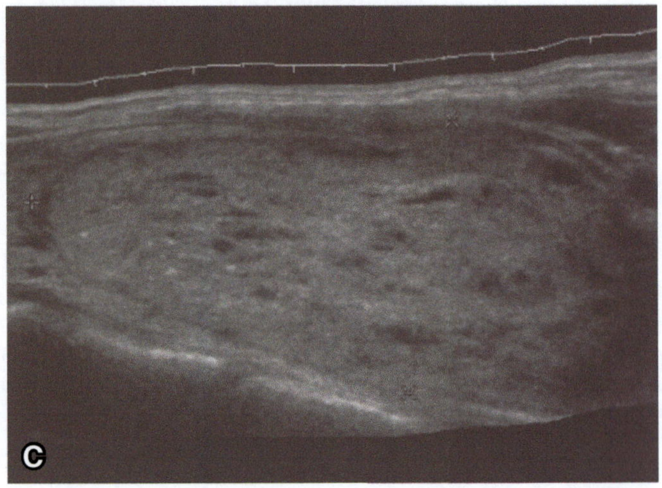

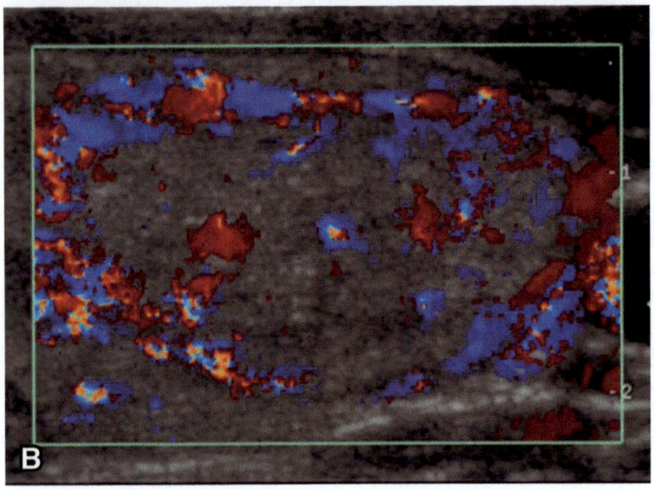

Figure 3-38. Ultrasound of a colloid nodule in the left lobe. **A**, Transverse, 23 x 45 mm. **B**, Color Doppler, Transverse. **C**, Longitudinal, sagittal diameter: 66 mm.

39-Year-old woman

- **Clinical history:** Palpable tumor in left lobe unchanged for more than 1 year.
- **Ultrasound:** Colloid nodule? Follicular adenoma?
- **Cytology:** No diagnostic material.
- **18-Gauge histologic needle biopsy:** Follicular tissue without atypia.
- **Left hemithyroidectomy:** Colloid nodule.

Features

Slightly hypoechoic
Inhomogeneous spongy echo pattern
Well circumscribed
Thin partial hypoechoic halo
A few microcalcifications
Suggestion of "spoke-and-wheel-like" vascularity

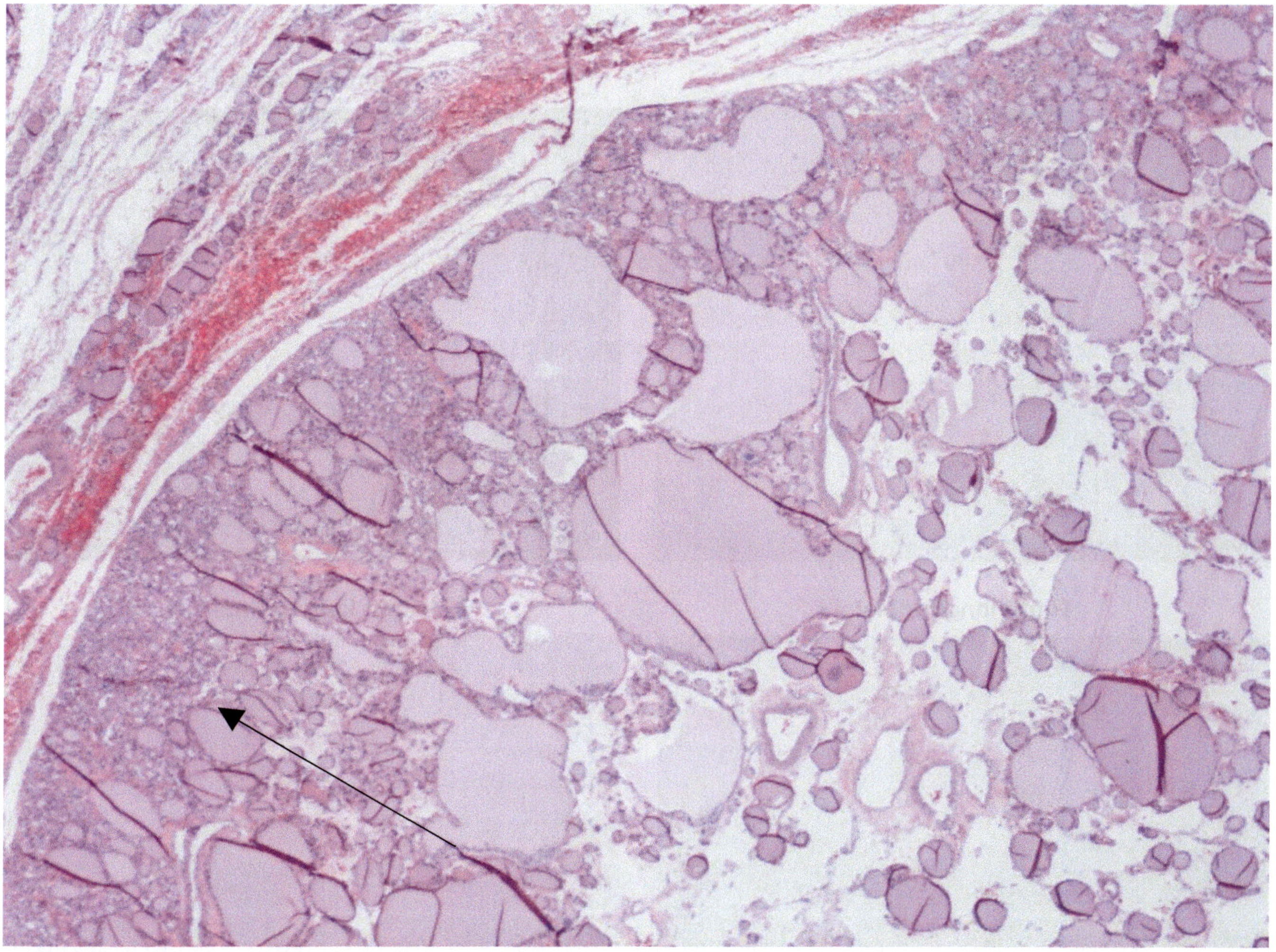

Figure 3-39. Histology: colloid nodule. Subcapsular areas with follicular hyperplasia (*arrow*).

Colloid Nodules Both Lobes

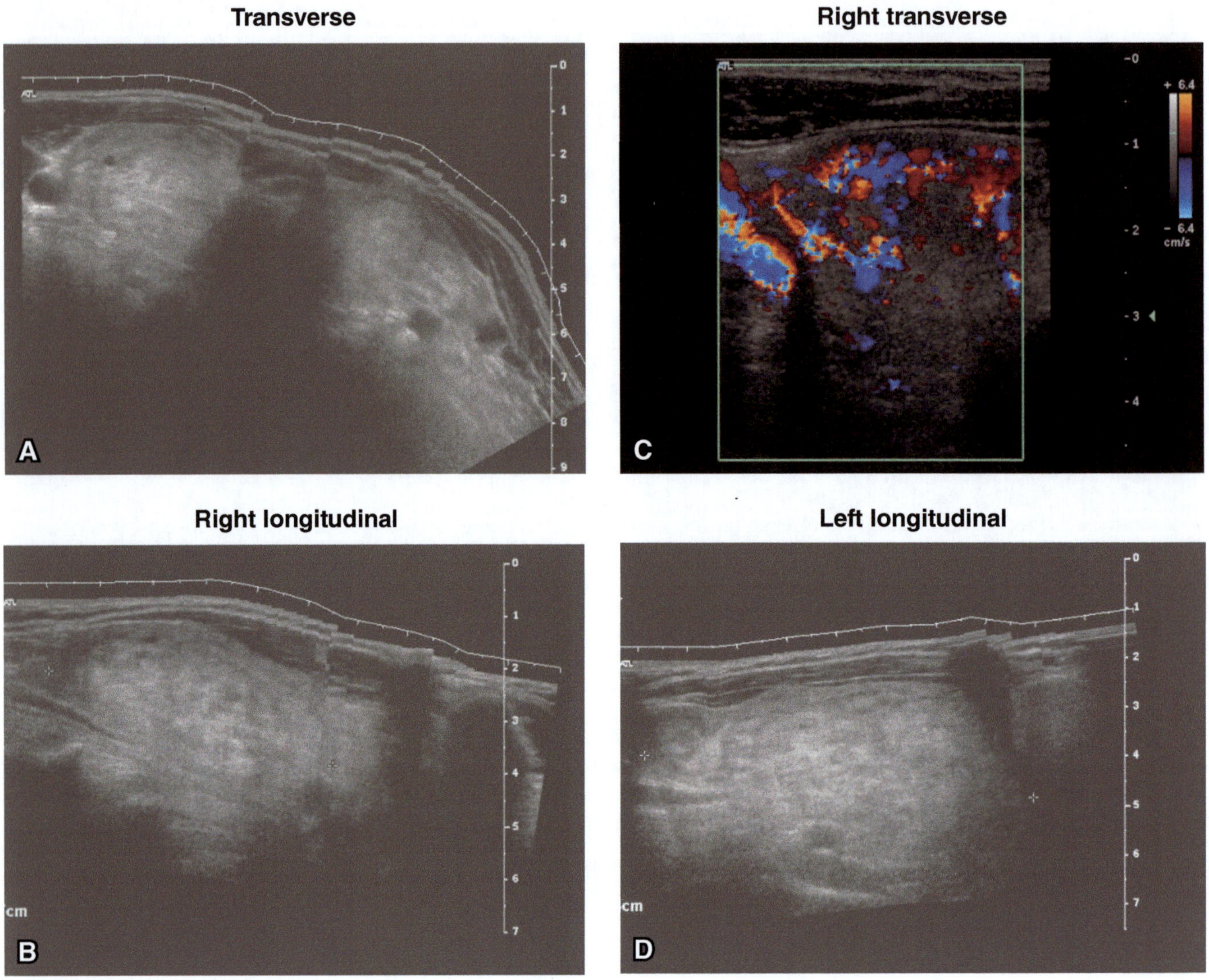

FIGURE 3-40. Ultrasound of colloid nodules in both lobes. **A**, Transverse. **B**, Right lobe longitudinal, sagittal diameter: 57 mm. **C**, Color Doppler. **D**, Left lobe longitudinal, SD: 78 mm.

72-Year-old man

- **Clinical history:** Large goiter for many years with intrathoracic extention. Now increased in size.
- **Ultrasound:** Diffuse goiter? Colloid nodules?
- **Cytology:** Colloid nodules.
- **Thyroidectomy:** Colloid nodules.

General features

Hypoechoic
Inhomogeneous granular echo pattern both lobes
No well defined nodules
A few microcalcifications
Partially well vascularized

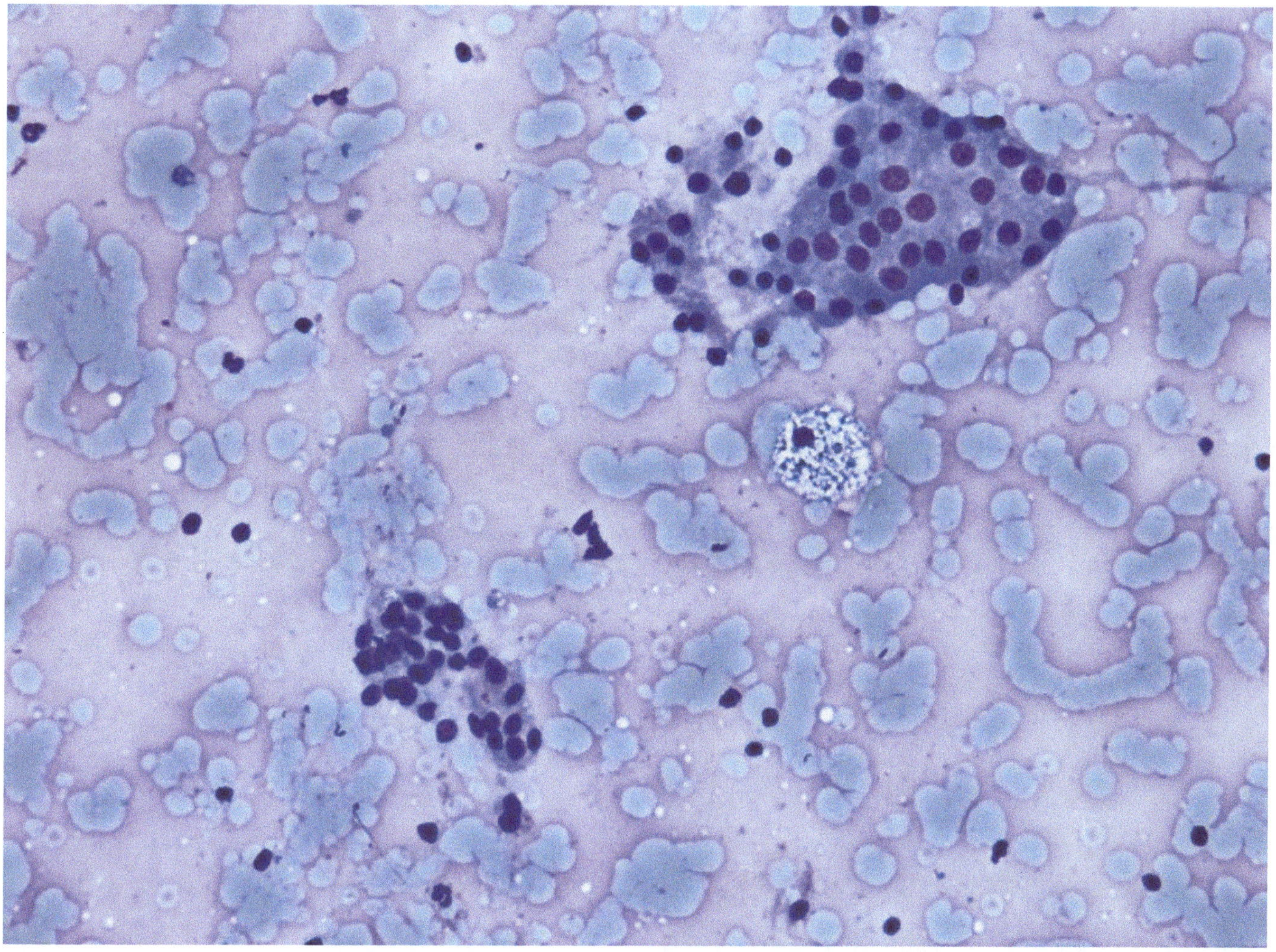

Figure 3-41. Cytology: thin colloid, epithelium, and macrophages.

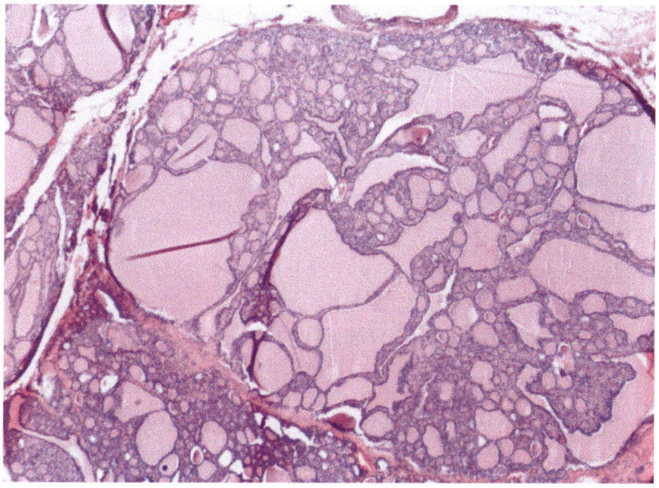

Figure 3-42. Histology: colloid nodule with follicular hyperplasia.

Colloid Nodule Left Lobe

Transverse

Longitudinal

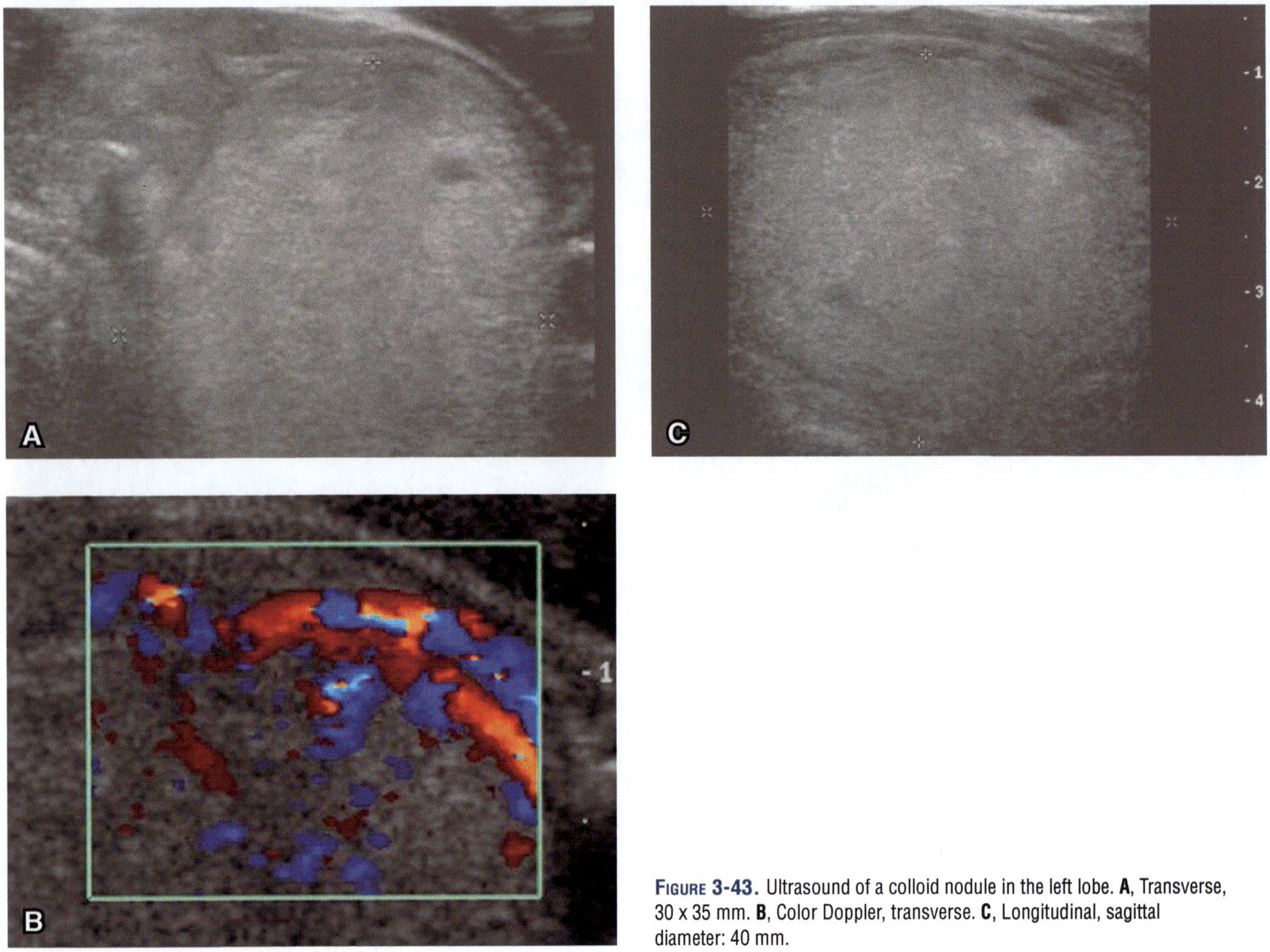

FIGURE 3-43. Ultrasound of a colloid nodule in the left lobe. **A**, Transverse, 30 x 35 mm. **B**, Color Doppler, transverse. **C**, Longitudinal, sagittal diameter: 40 mm.

50-Year-old woman

- **Clinical history:** Incidentaloma found at general clinical examination.
- **Ultrasound:** Probably follicular adenoma.
- **Cytology:** Rich follicular epithelium.
- **18-Gauge histologic needle biopsy:** Follicular tissue.
- **Left hemithyroidectomy:** Colloid nodule.

Features

Isoechoic
Homogeneous echo pattern
Some very small cysts
Well circumscribed
Partial thin hypoechoic halo
Peripheral vascularity

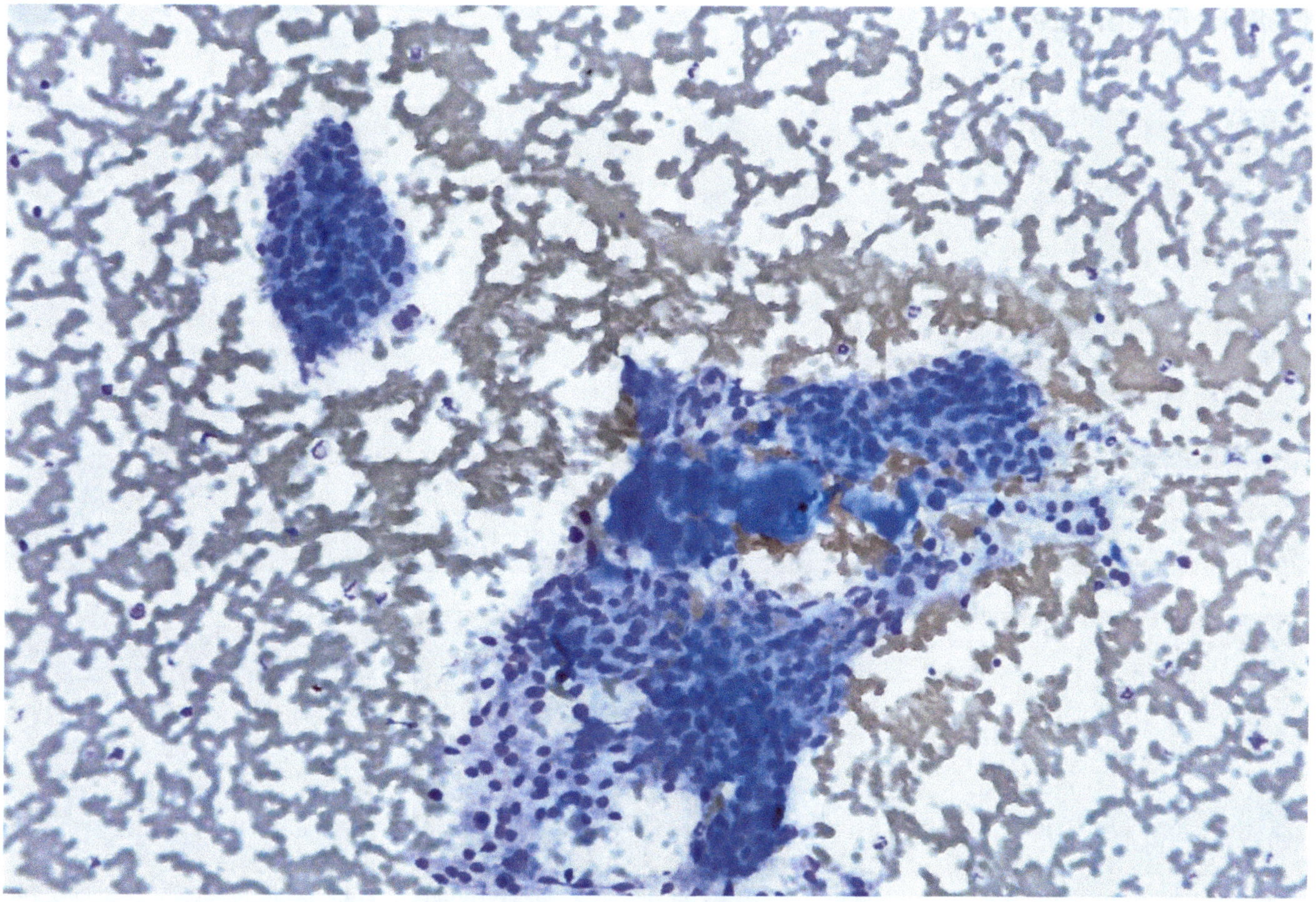

Figure 3-44. Cytology: abundant amount of epithelium on a background rich in blood. The amount of colloid is sparse.

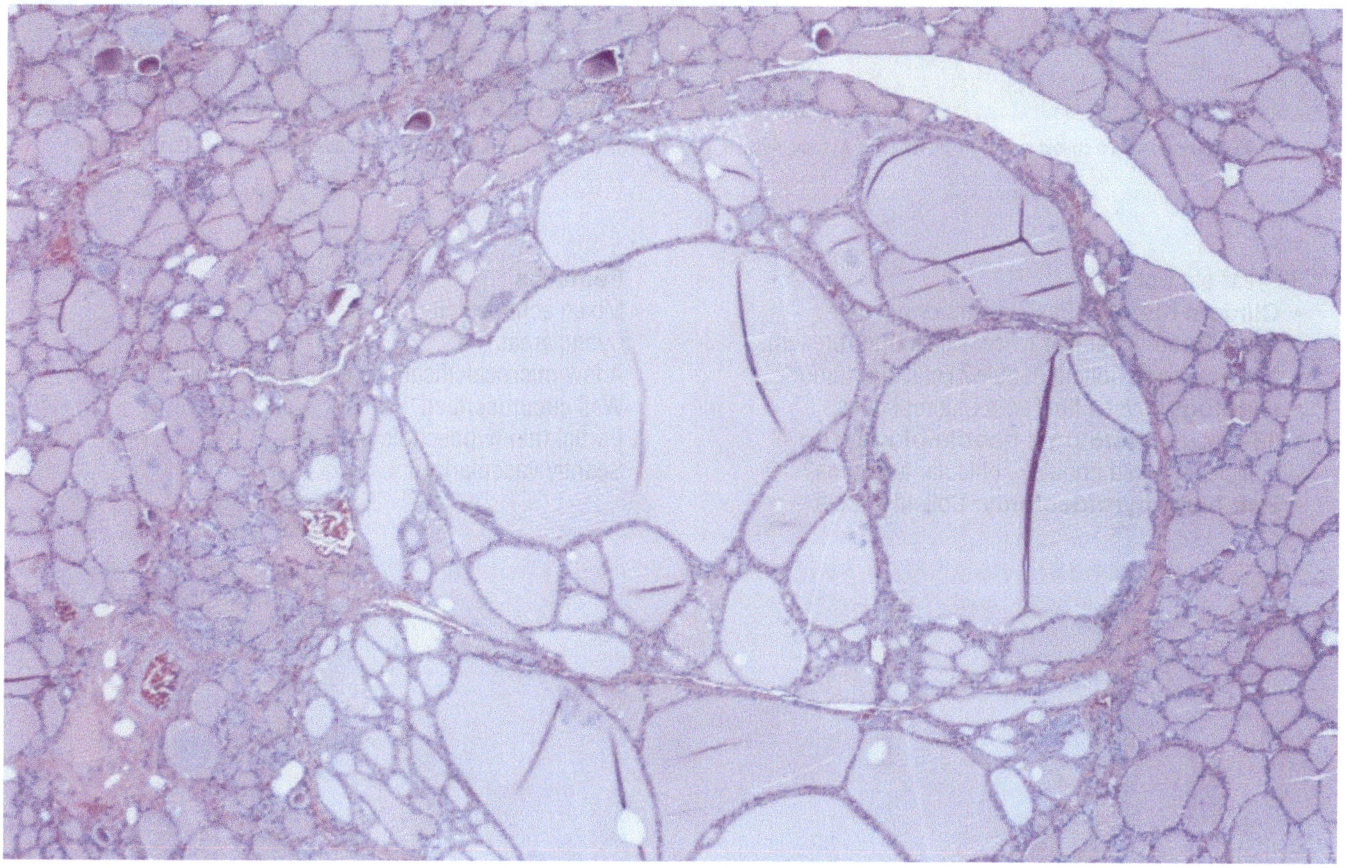

Figure 3-45. Histology: macro- and microfollicular colloid nodules.

Colloid Nodule Left Lobe

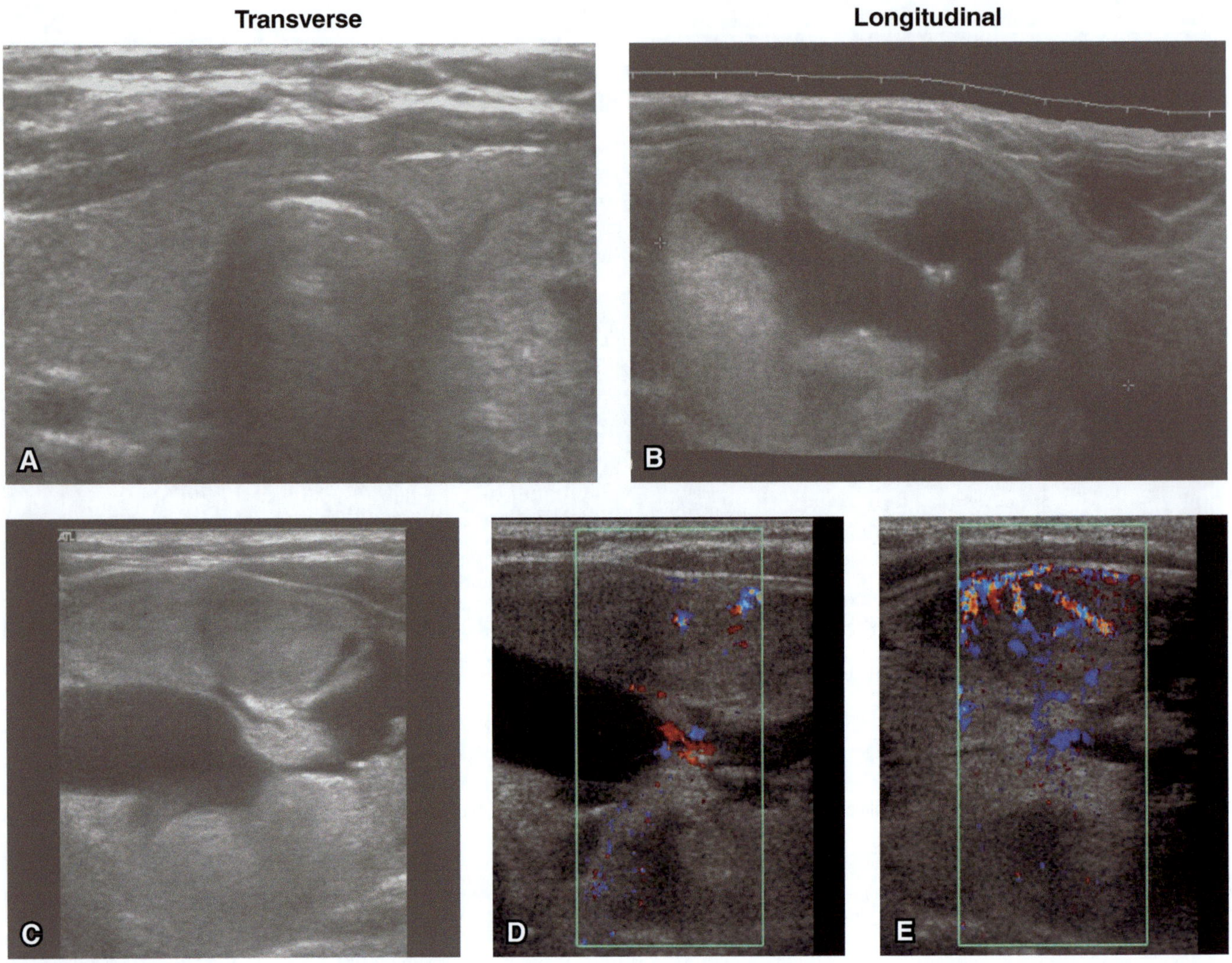

Figure 3-46. Ultrasound of a colloid nodule in the left lobe. **A**, Transverse. **B**, Longitudinal: Sagittal diameter: 60 mm. **C**, Transverse. **D** and **E**, Color Doppler.

33-Year-old woman

- **Clinical history:** Past 2 years cyst in left thyroid lobe. Aspirated twice. New tumor present.
- **Ultrasound:** Colloid nodule? Follicular tumor?
- **Cytology:** Cystic fluid with macrophages.
- **16-Gauge histologic needle biopsy:** Follicles. Colloid nodule? Follicular adenoma?
- **Left hemithyroidectomy:** Colloid nodule.

Features

Mixed echogenicity
Cystic areas
A few microcalcifications or crystallic colloid
Well circumscribed
Partial thin hypoechoic halo
Scantly vascularized

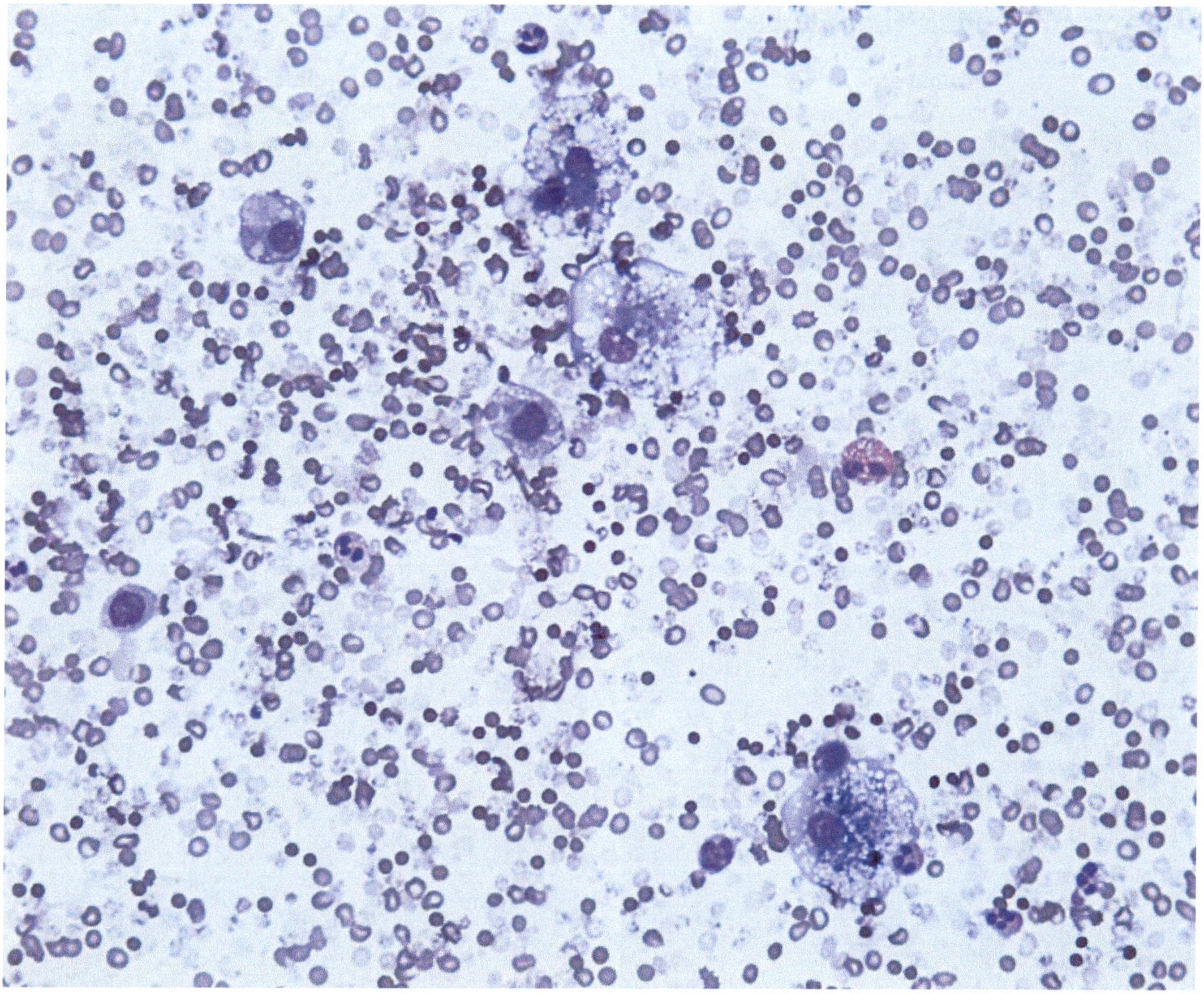

Figure 3-47. Cytology: cystic fluid with several macrophages and rich in erythrocytes.

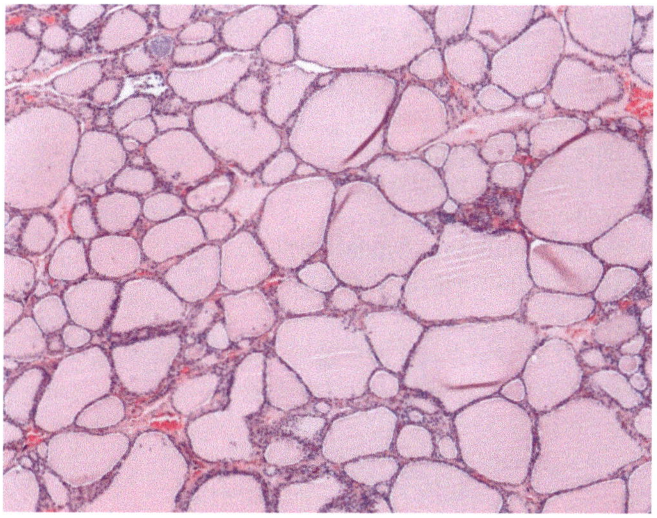

Figure 3-48. Histology: classical colloid nodule.

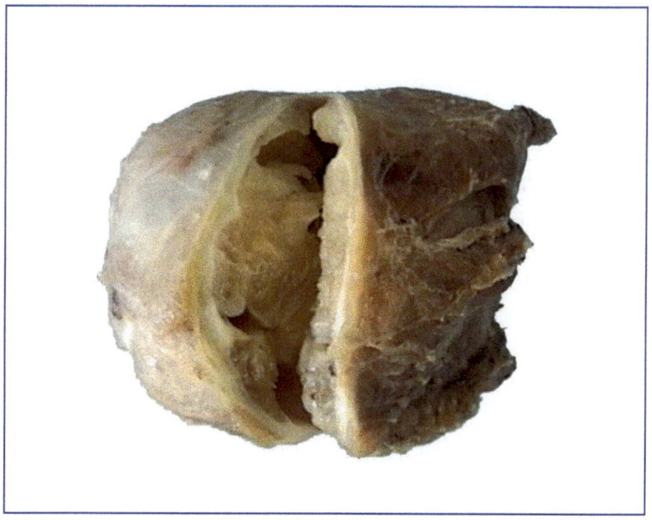

Figure 3-49. Gross section.

Hyperplastic Nodule Right Lobe

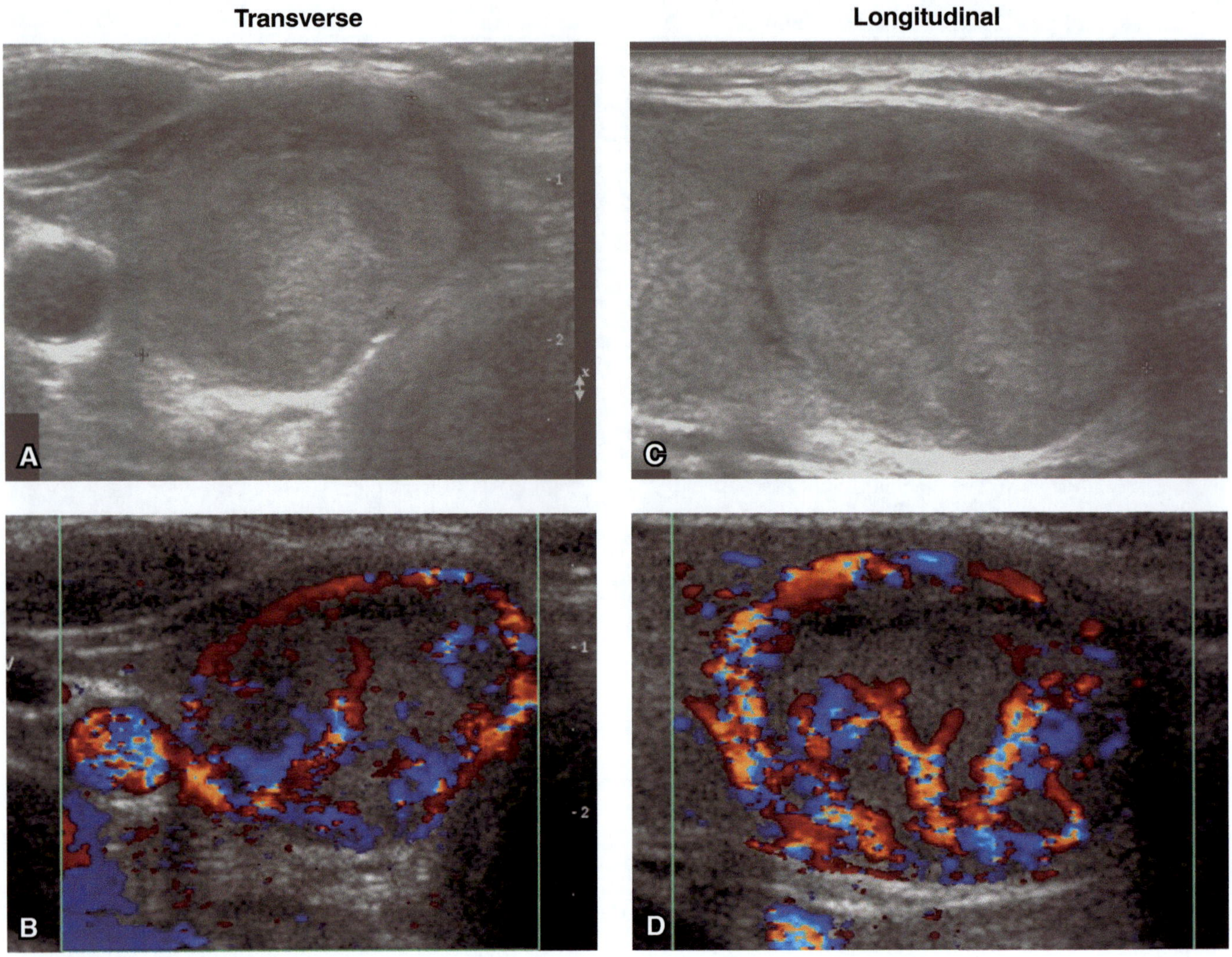

FIGURE 3-50. Ultrasound of a hyperplastic nodule in the right lobe. **A**, Transverse, 17 x 23 mm. **B**, Color Doppler, transverse. **C**, Longitudinal, sagittal diameter: 24 mm. **D**, Color Doppler, longitudinal.

40-Year-old woman

- **Clinical history:** Unknown.
- **Ultrasound:** Probably follicular tumor. Benign? Malignant?
- **Cytology:** Follicular lesion.
- **16-Gauge histologic needle biopsy:** Probably colloid nodule.
- **Right hemithyroidectomy:** Hyperplastic nodule.

Features

Slightly hypoechoic
Inhomogeneous echo pattern
Well circumscribed
Partial thin, uneven hypoechoic halo
"Spoke-and-wheel-like" vascularity

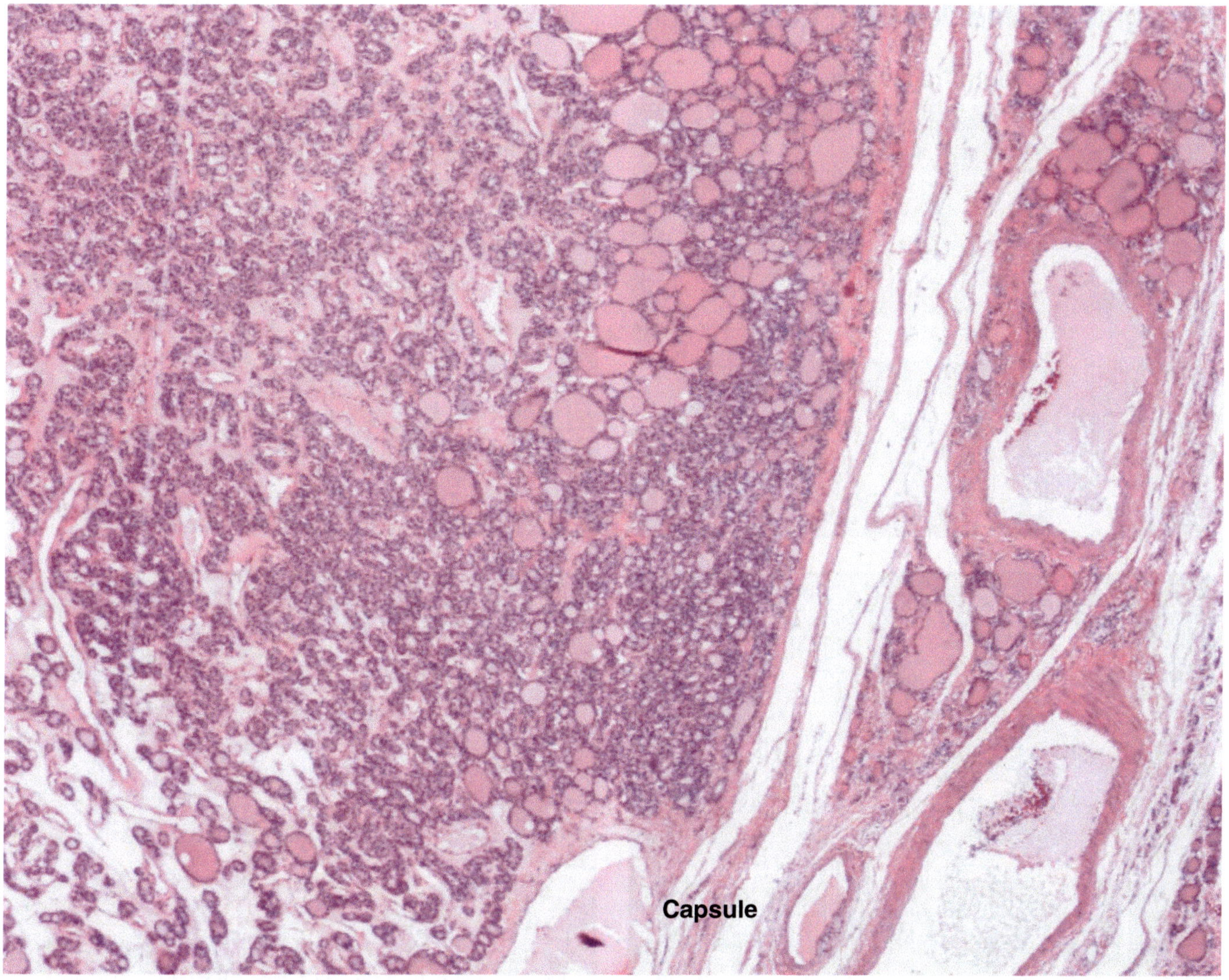

Figure 3-51. Histology: adenomatous colloid nodule.

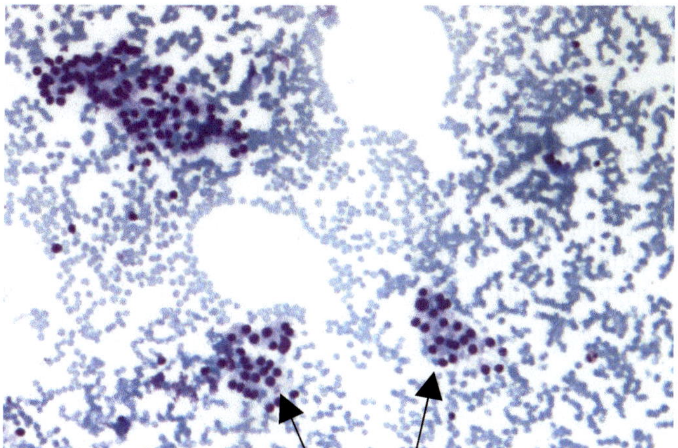

Figure 3-52. Cytology: follicular epithelium (*arrows*) on a background rich in blood.

Hyperplastic Nodules Both Lobes

Right Transverse | **Left Transverse**

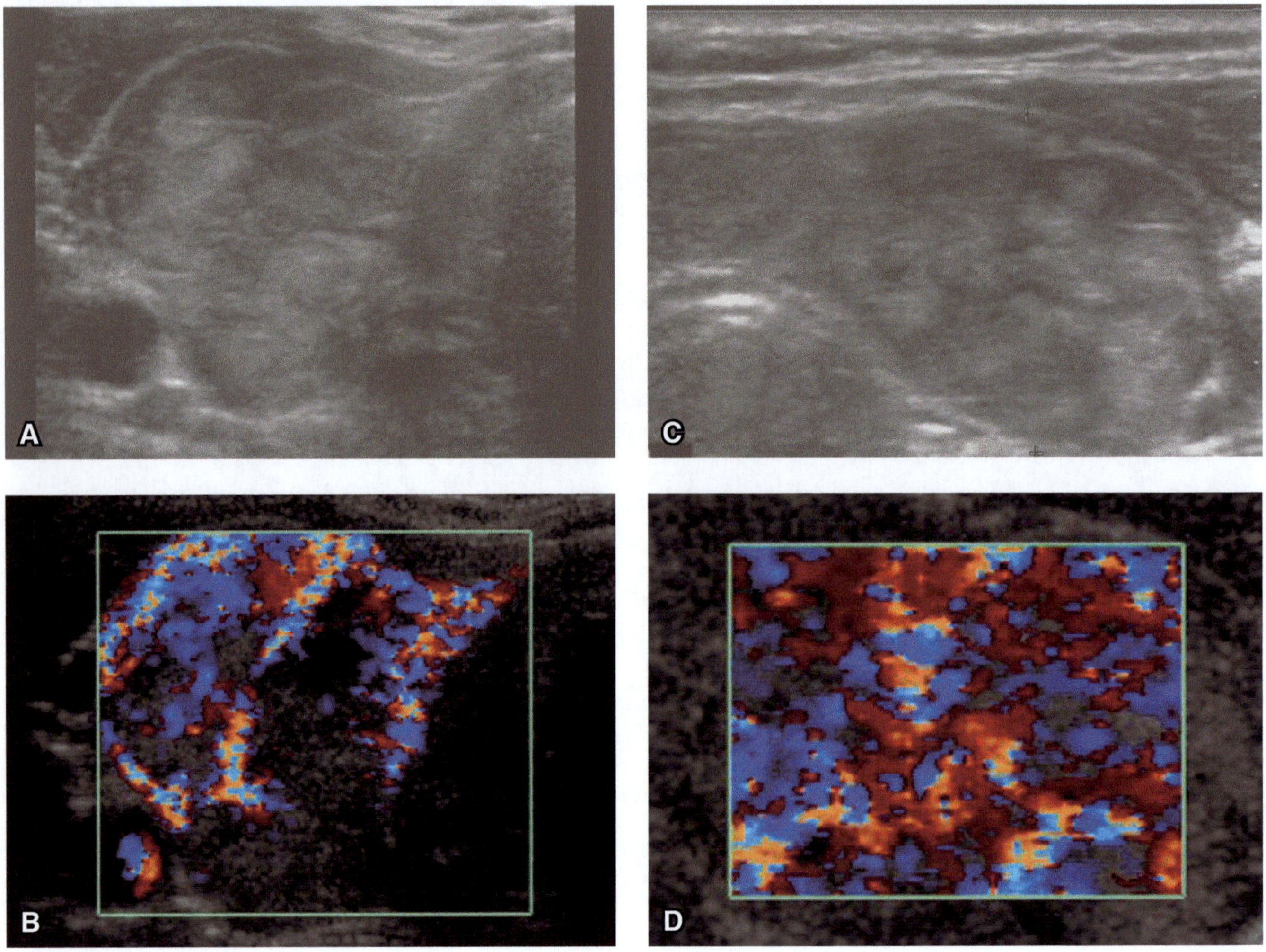

Figure 3-53. Ultrasound of hyperplastic nodules in both lobes. **A**, Right transverse. **B**, Color Doppler, right transverse. **C**, Left transverse. **D**, Color Doppler, left transverse.

42-Year-old woman

- **Clinical history:** Enlarged thyroid for some months with somewhat tender palpable nodules in both lobes.
- **Scintigraphy:** Hyperactivity.
- **Ultrasound:** Nodular irregular tissue. Thyroiditis?
- **Cytology:** Hyperplastic epithelial cells. Thyroiditis? Graves disease?
- **18-Gauge histologic needle biopsy:** Follicular somewhat hyperplastic tissue.
- **Thyroidectomy:** Hyperplastic nodular tissue consistent with hyperthyroidism.

Features
Mixed echogenicity
Nodular echo pattern
Whole gland affected
Hypervascular

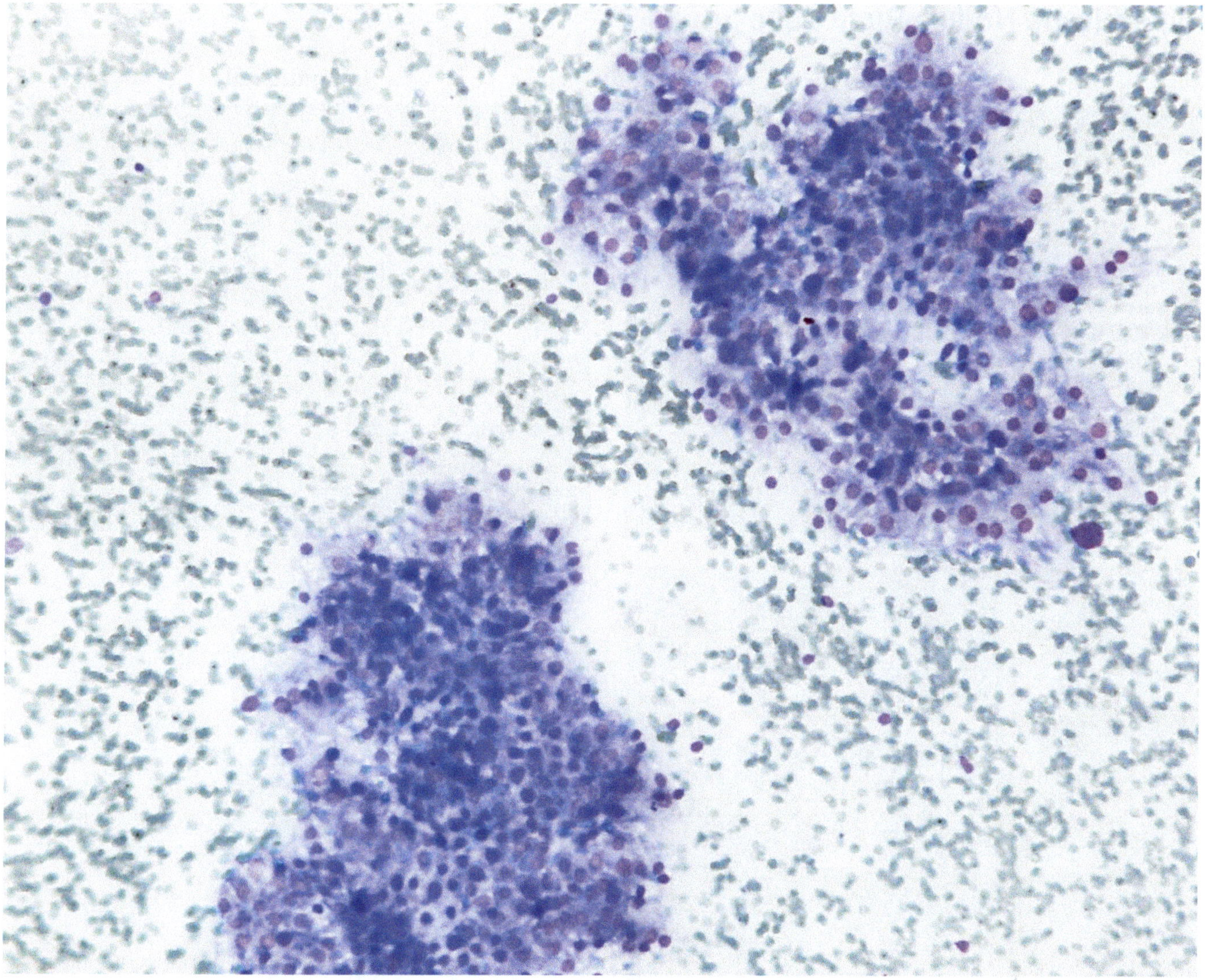

Figure 3-54. Cytology: rich in hyperplastic follicular epithelium.

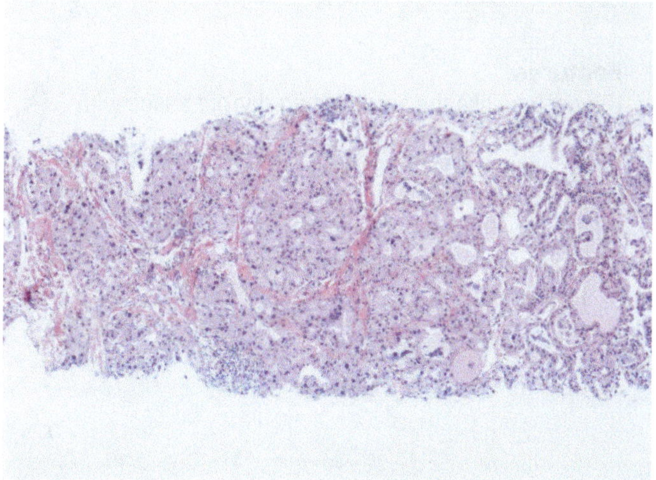

Figure 3-55. Histologic needle biopsy: hyperplastic nodule.

Hyperplastic Nodule Right Lobe

Transverse

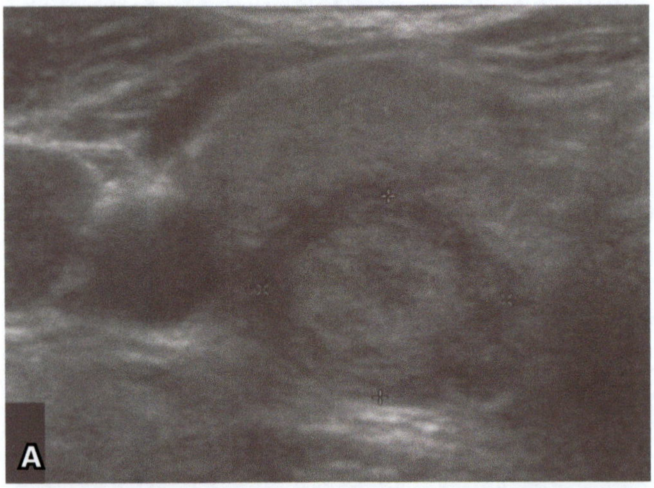

Longitudinal

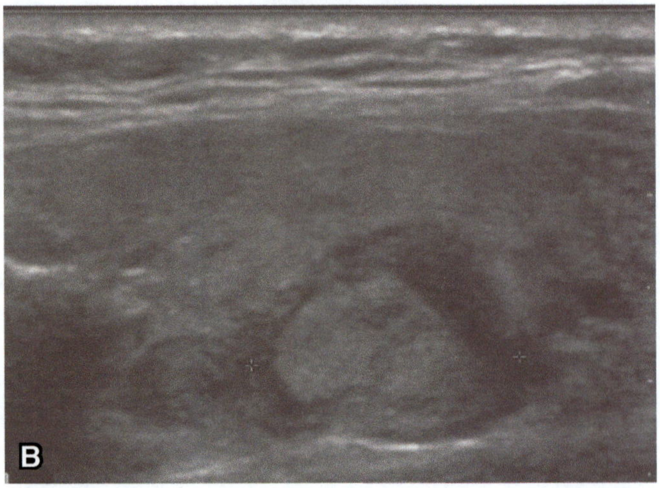

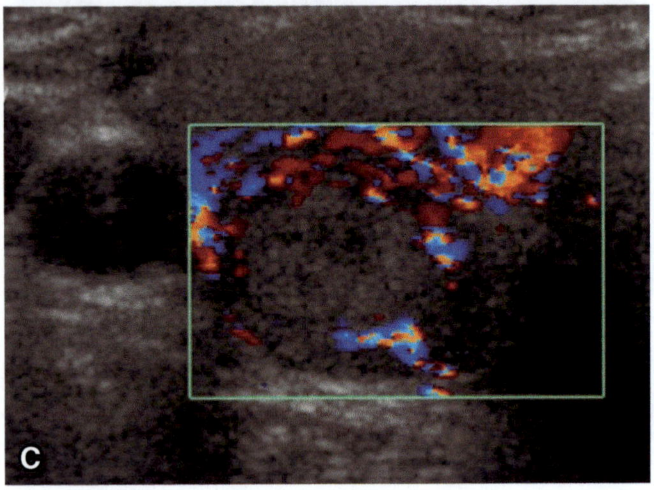

FIGURE 3-56. **A**, Transverse, 10 x 13 mm. **B**, Longitudinal, sagittal diameter: 14 mm. **C**, Color Doppler, transverse.

47-Year-old woman

- **Clinical history:** Nodular goiter and autoimmune thyroiditis for many years.
- **Ultrasound:** Probably papillary thyroid carcinoma left lobe and colloid nodule in right lobe.
- **Cytology:** Hyperplastic nodule.
- **Thyroidectomy:** Papillary carcinoma with follicular differentiation in left lobe. Excessive Hashimoto's thyroiditis. Hyperplastic nodule right lobe.

See also pages 136–137

Features

Hypoechoic like the surrounding thyroid tissue with thyroiditis

Inhomogeneous echo pattern

Well circumscribed

Thick, uneven hypoechoic halo

Less vascular than the surrounding tissue with thyroiditis

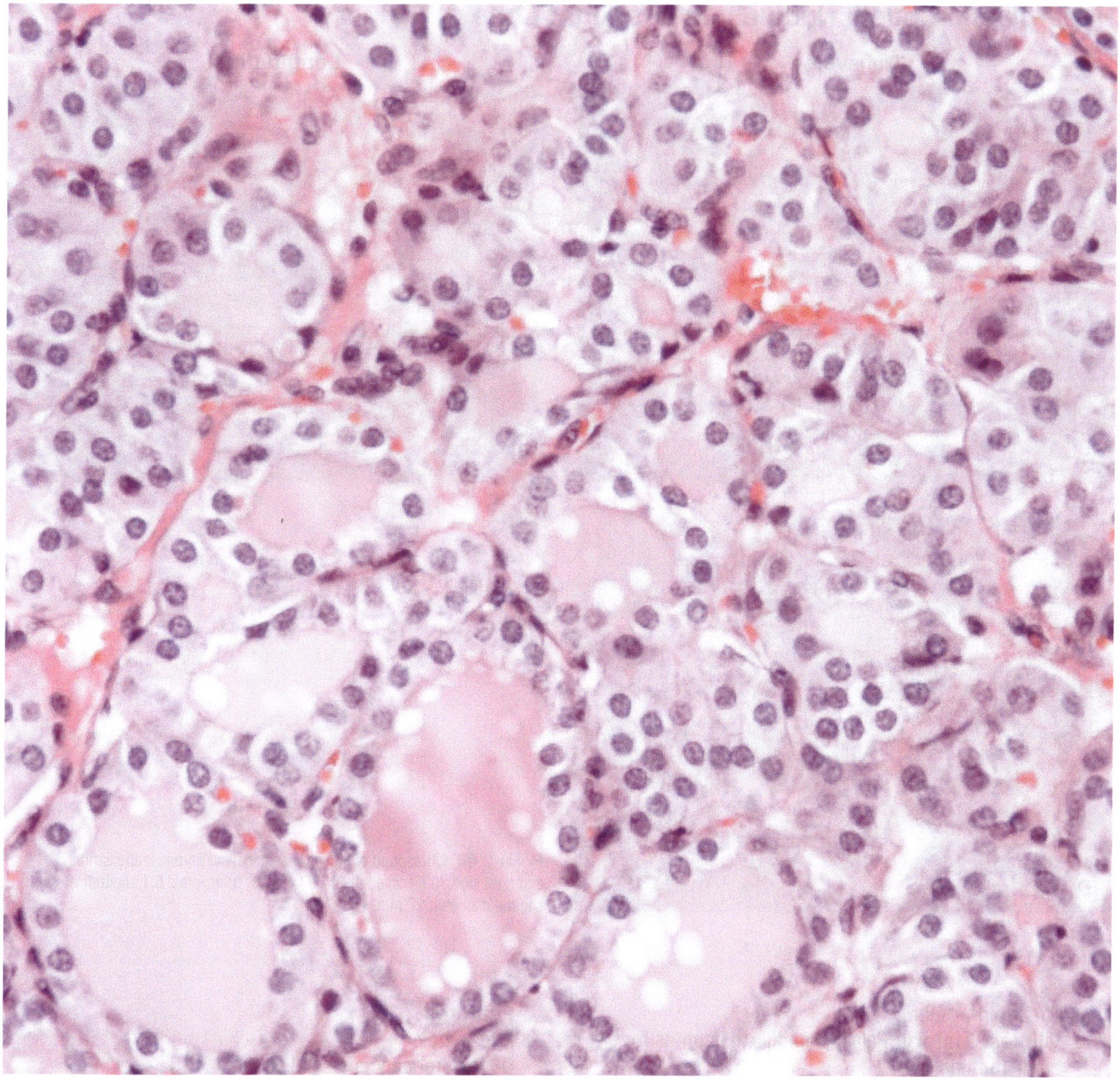

Figure 3-57. Histology: hyperplastic nodule.

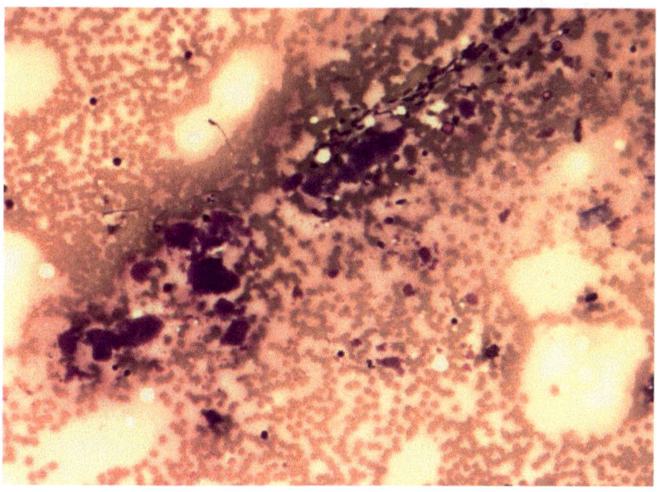

Figure 3-58. Cytology: colloid and some lymphoid cells.

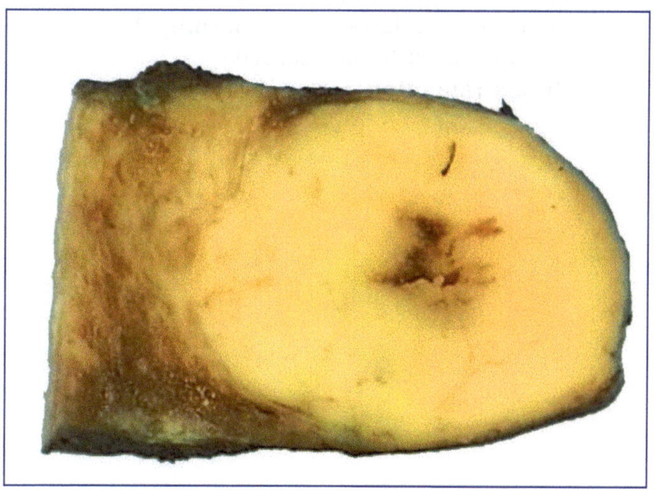

Figure 3-59. Gross section: hyperplastic nodule.

Hyperplastic Colloid Nodule Isthmus/Right Lobe

Transverse | **Longitudinal**

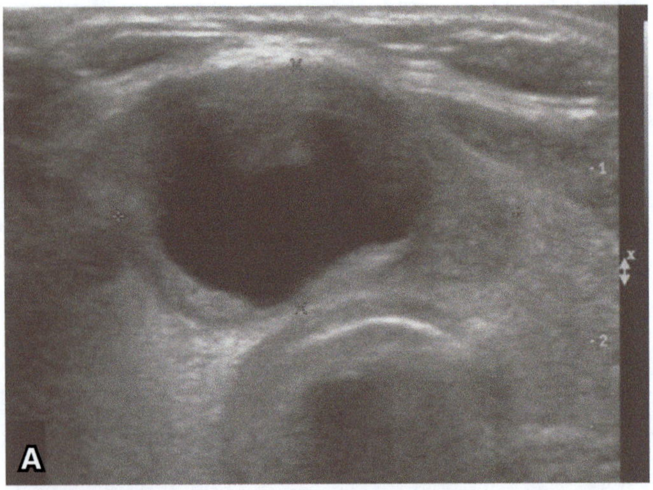

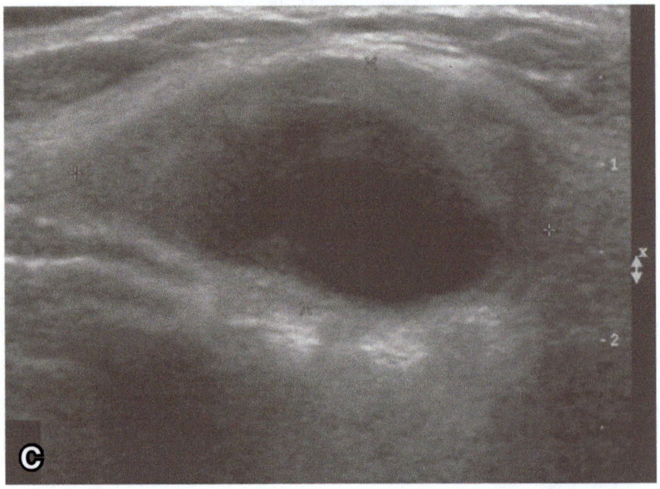

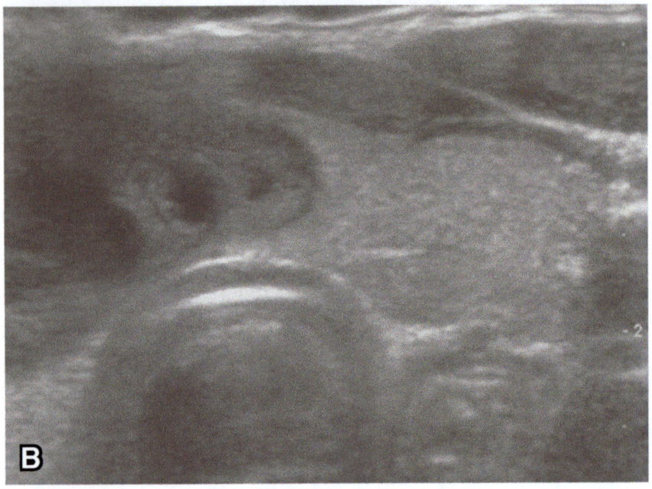

Figure 3-60. Ultrasound of a hyperplastic colloid nodule in the isthmus and right lobe. **A**, Transverse, 14 x 23 mm. **B**, Transverse. **C**, Longitudinal, sagittal diameter: 27 mm.

45-Year-old woman
- **Clinical history:** Palpable nodule in isthmus for some months.
- **Ultrasound:** Probably cystic colloid nodule.
- **Cytology:** Follicular epithelium. Neoplasia?
- **18-Gauge histologic needle biopsy:** Follicular lesion with oncocytic differentiation.
- **Isthmus resection:** Hyperplastic colloid nodule.

Features
Hypoechoic
Quite homogeneous solid tissue
Well circumscribed
Large cyst

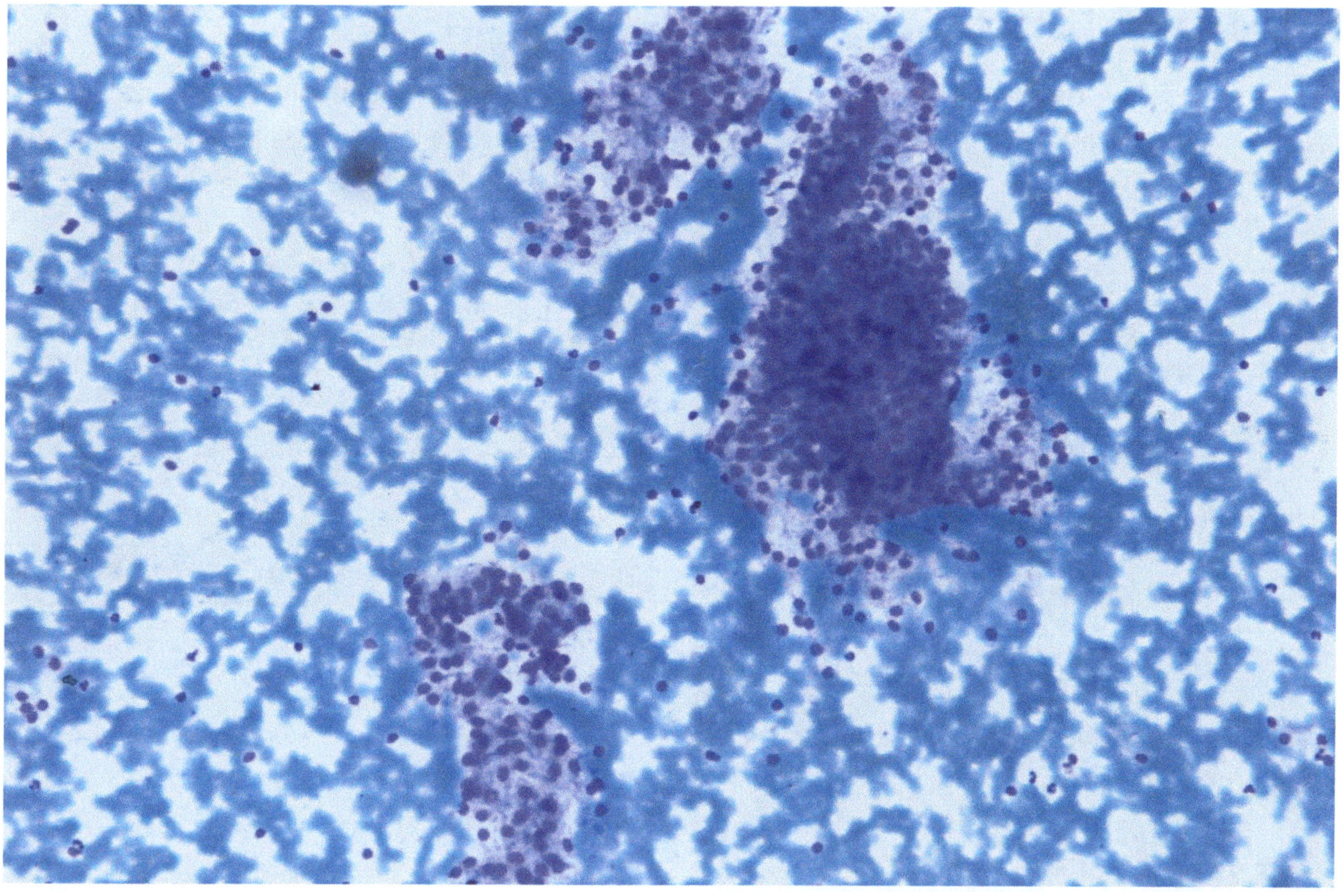

FIGURE 3-61. Cytology: hyperplastic follicular cells.

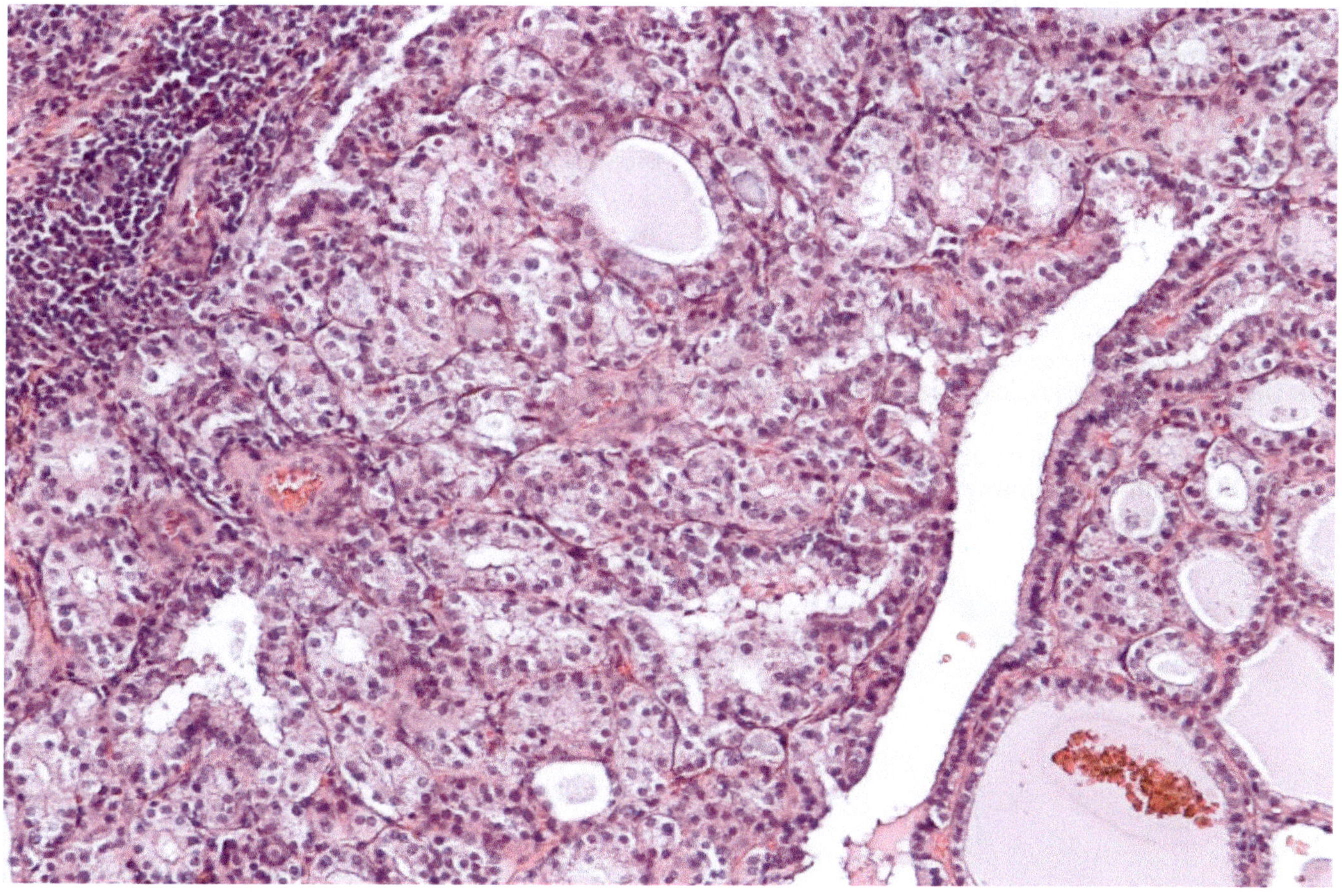

FIGURE 3-62. Histology: adenomatoid colloid nodule.

Colloid Nodule Left Lobe

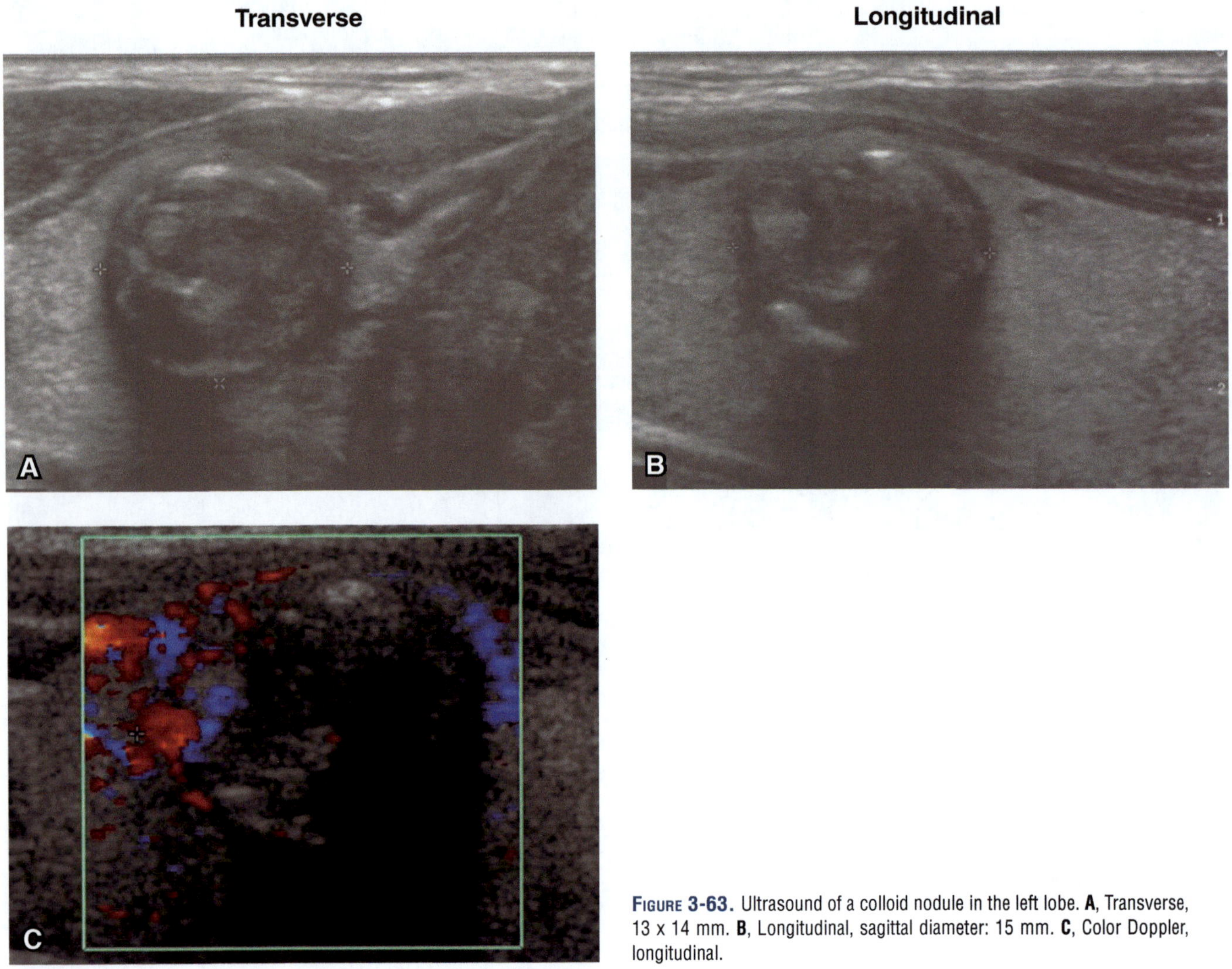

Figure 3-63. Ultrasound of a colloid nodule in the left lobe. **A**, Transverse, 13 x 14 mm. **B**, Longitudinal, sagittal diameter: 15 mm. **C**, Color Doppler, longitudinal.

43-Year-old man

- **Clinical history:** Palpable hard nodule in right lobe for some months.
- **Ultrasound:** Colloid nodule? Papillary thyroid carcinoma?
- **Cytology:** No diagnostic material.
- **Right hemithyroidectomy:** Calcified colloid nodule.

Features

Strongly hypoechoic
Well circumscribed
Inhomogeneous echo pattern
Coarse calcifications with shadowing
Almost avascular

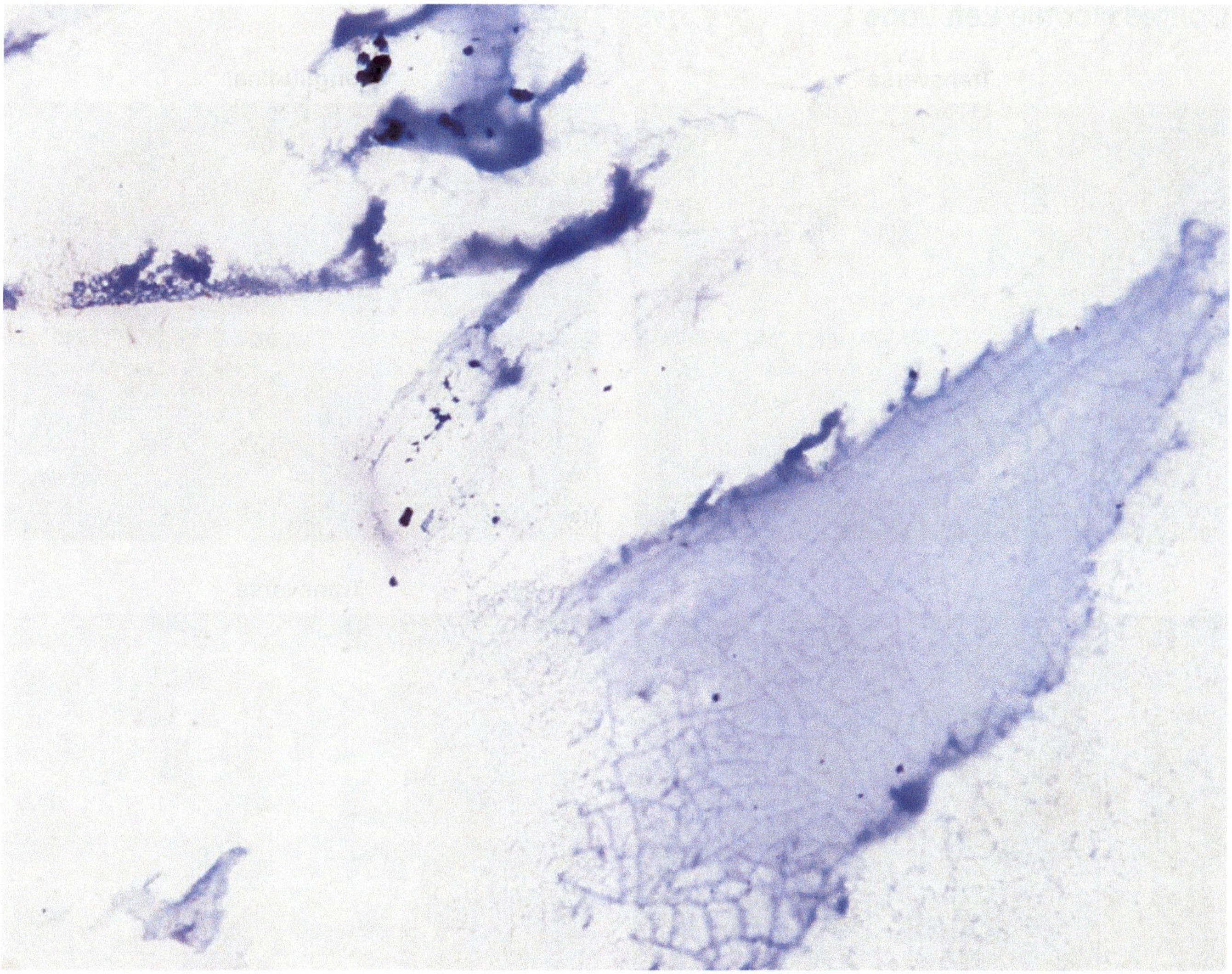

Figure 3-64. Cytology: colloid nodule.

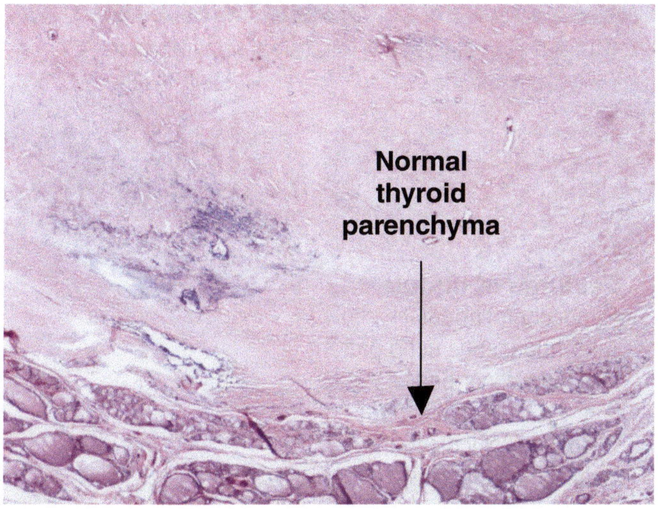

Figure 3-65. Histology: thick capsule, fibrosis, and calcifications.

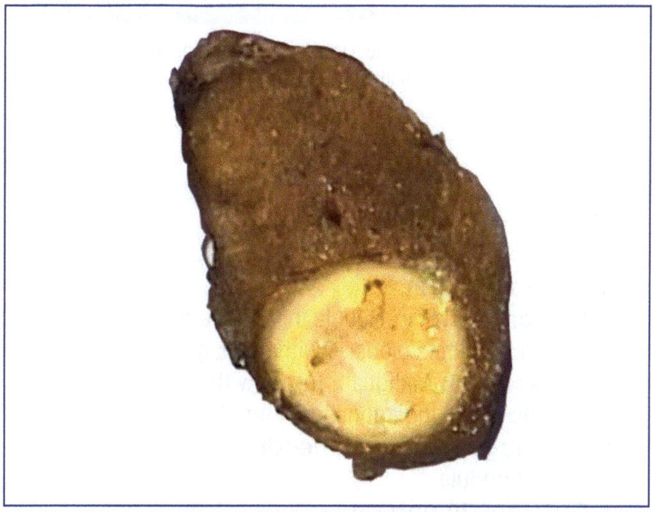

Figure 3-66. Gross section: well-circumscribed lesion.

Colloid Nodule Left Lobe

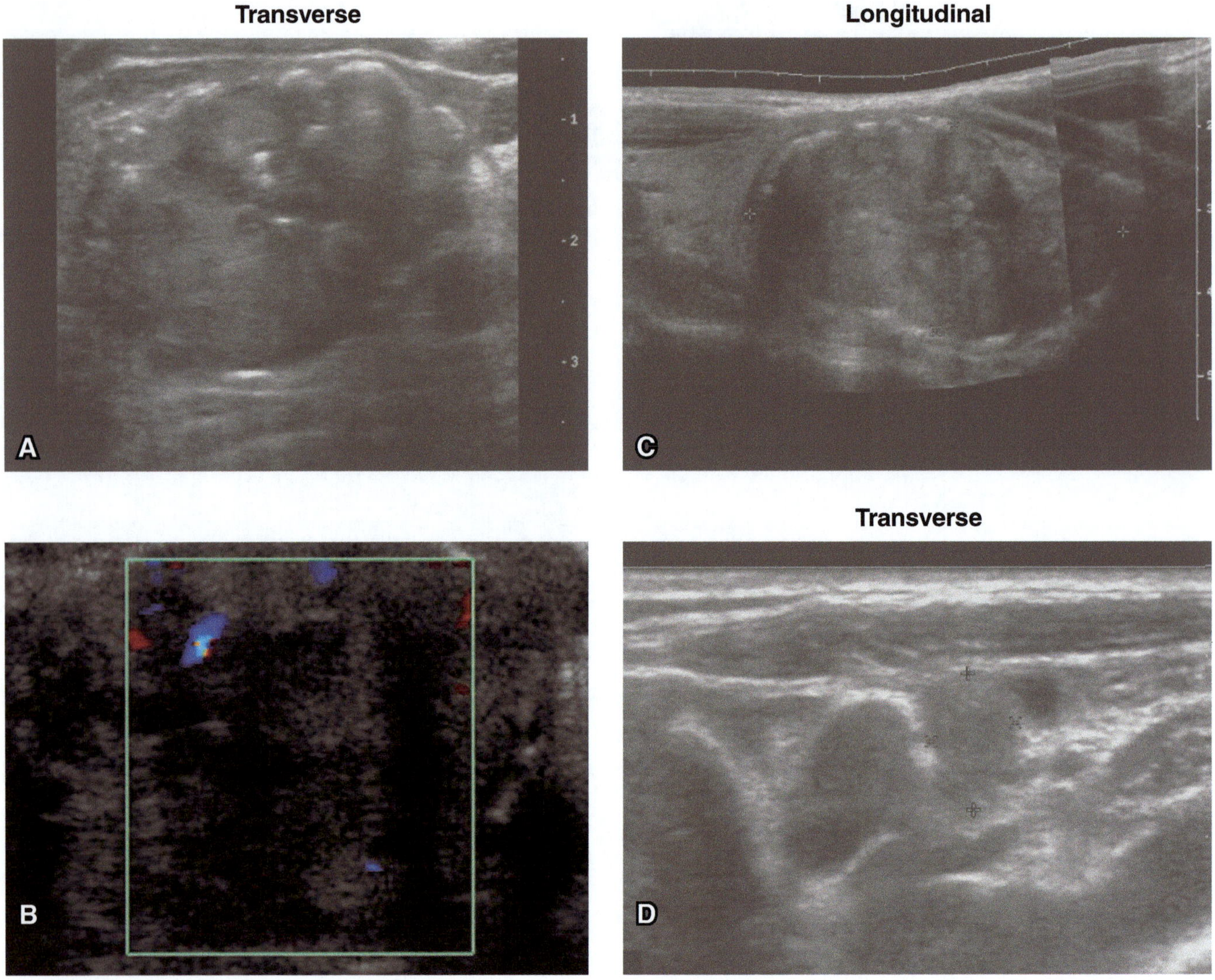

Figure 3-67. Ultrasound of a colloid nodule in the left lobe. **A**, Transverse, 24 x 36 mm. **B**, Color Doppler, transverse. **C**, Longitudinal, sagittal diameter: 44 mm. **D**, Transverse, lymph node 5 x 8 mm, left segment 4.

43-Year-old woman

- **Clinical history:** Nodule in left lobe past 10 years. Several cytologic biopsies without diagnostic material.
- **Ultrasound:** Malignant tumor with metastasis?
- **Cytology:** Nondiagnostic material.
- **16-Gauge histologic needle biopsy:** Colloid nodule.
- **Cytology lymph node:** Normal lymphocytes.
- **Left hemithyroidectomy:** Calcified colloid nodule.

Features of nodule

Hypoechoic, nodular
Inhomogeneous echo pattern
Well circumscribed
A few microcalcifications
"Eggshell" calcifications
Scantly vascularized

Features of lymph node

Taller than wide with blurred margin, "salt and pepper" echo pattern and no fatty hilum

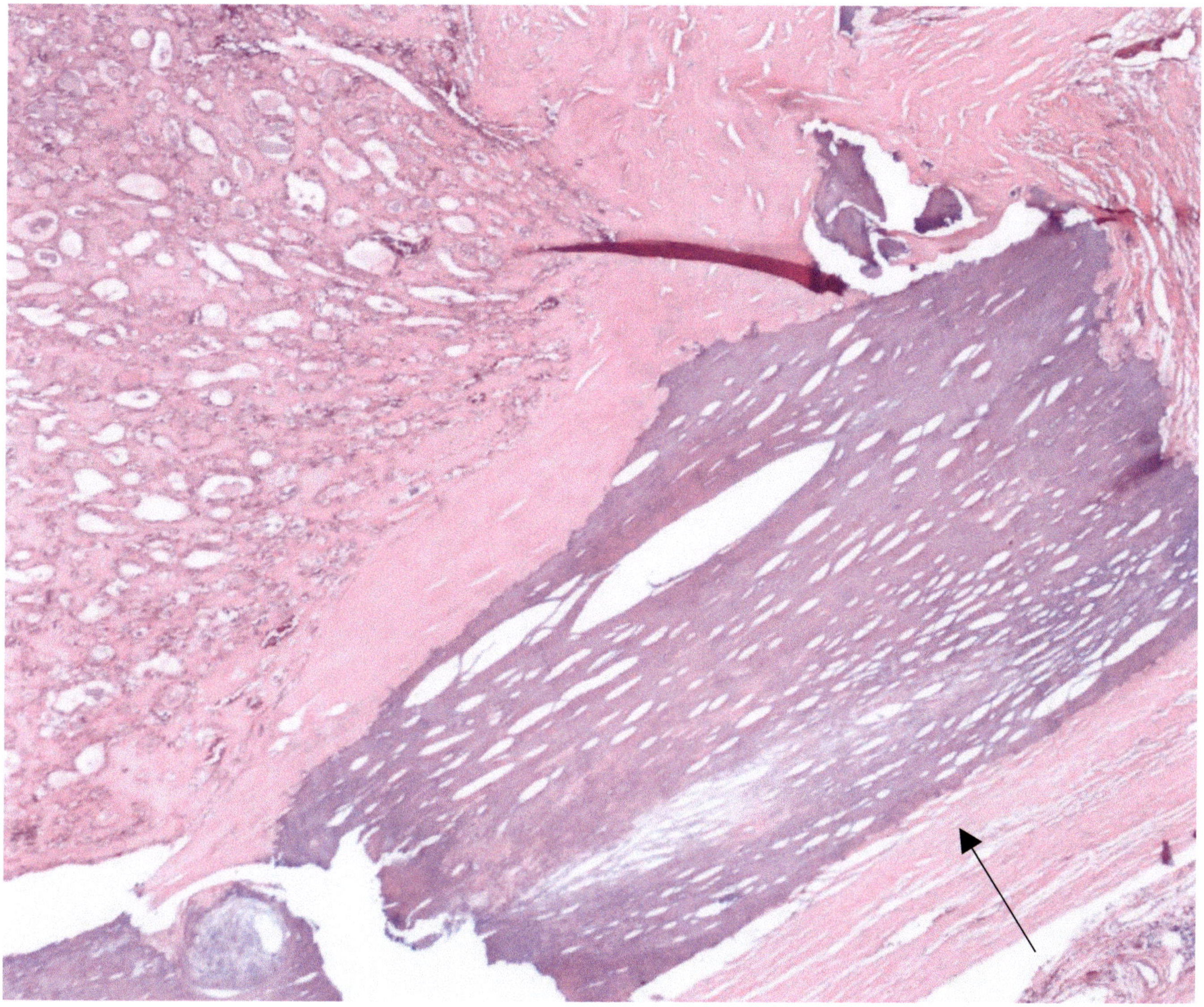

Figure 3-68. Histology: colloid nodule with thick capsule and calcification (*arrow*).

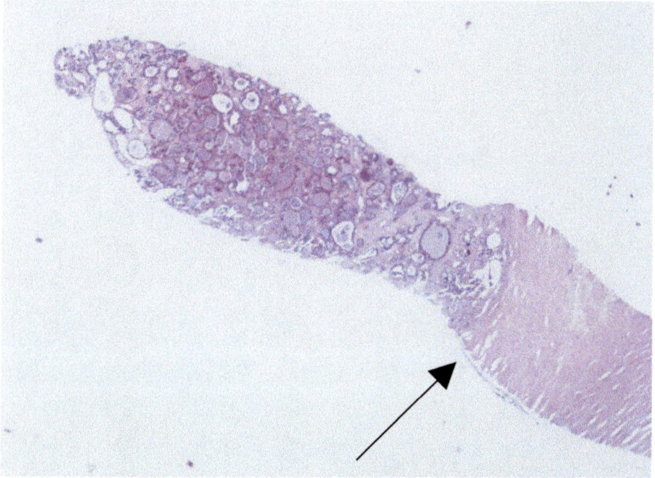

Figure 3-69. Histologic needle biopsy: colloid nodule with thick capsule (*arrow*).

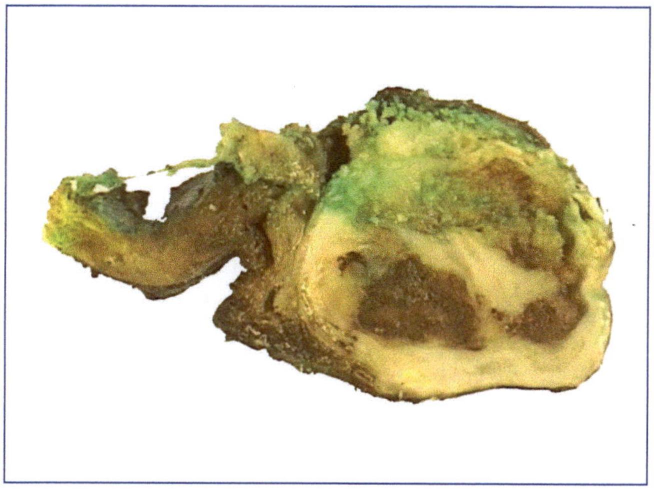

Figure 3-70. Gross section: extensive calcification in the capsule.

4 Follicular Adenoma and Follicular Thyroid Carcinoma

A follicular tumor is often solitary. It often has an egg shape, is well marginated, and has a hypoechoic halo all around the tumor [5,6,10]. Most follicular tumors are solid and have homogeneous echogenicity. They can be hyper-, iso-, hypoechoic, or mixed with well-defined areas of different echogenicity within the tumor. Focal cystic components may be present. They usually have a "spoke-and-wheel-like" vascularity with marked circulation in the peripheral halo with vessels converging toward the tumor center. In our experience carcinomas have a tendency to have more rich and less regular flow in the periphery and inside the tumor compared with the flow in the adenomas. A thick and uneven halo is suspicious for malignancy, and if extrathyroidal infiltration is visualized, the carcinoma diagnosis is obvious.

Common Features of Follicular Adenomas

Solitary
Egg shape
Thin, hypoechoic capsule
Homogeneous echogenicity
Hyper-, iso-, hypoechoic, or mixed
May have cystic degeneration
"Spoke-and-wheel-like" vascularity

Common Features of Follicular Thyroid Carcinomas

Solitary
Egg shape
Thick, uneven hypoechoic capsule
Homogeneous echogenicity
Hyper-, iso-, hypoechoic, or mixed
May have cystic degeneration
Hypervascular
"Spoke-and-wheel-like" vascularity less prominent

Cytologic Morphology

The cytologic picture shows a wide range of variation. Often the material is cellular containing follicular epithelium in a mix of dispersed cells and cells forming follicular formations, sometimes with a "plug" of colloid in the center. As mentioned for oncocytic lesions, the specimen is sometimes rich in blood with only a small amount of epithelium. The differentiation between a highly cellular colloid nodule with adenomatous hyperplasia and a follicular neoplasm may be difficult and sometimes impossible on morphology alone.

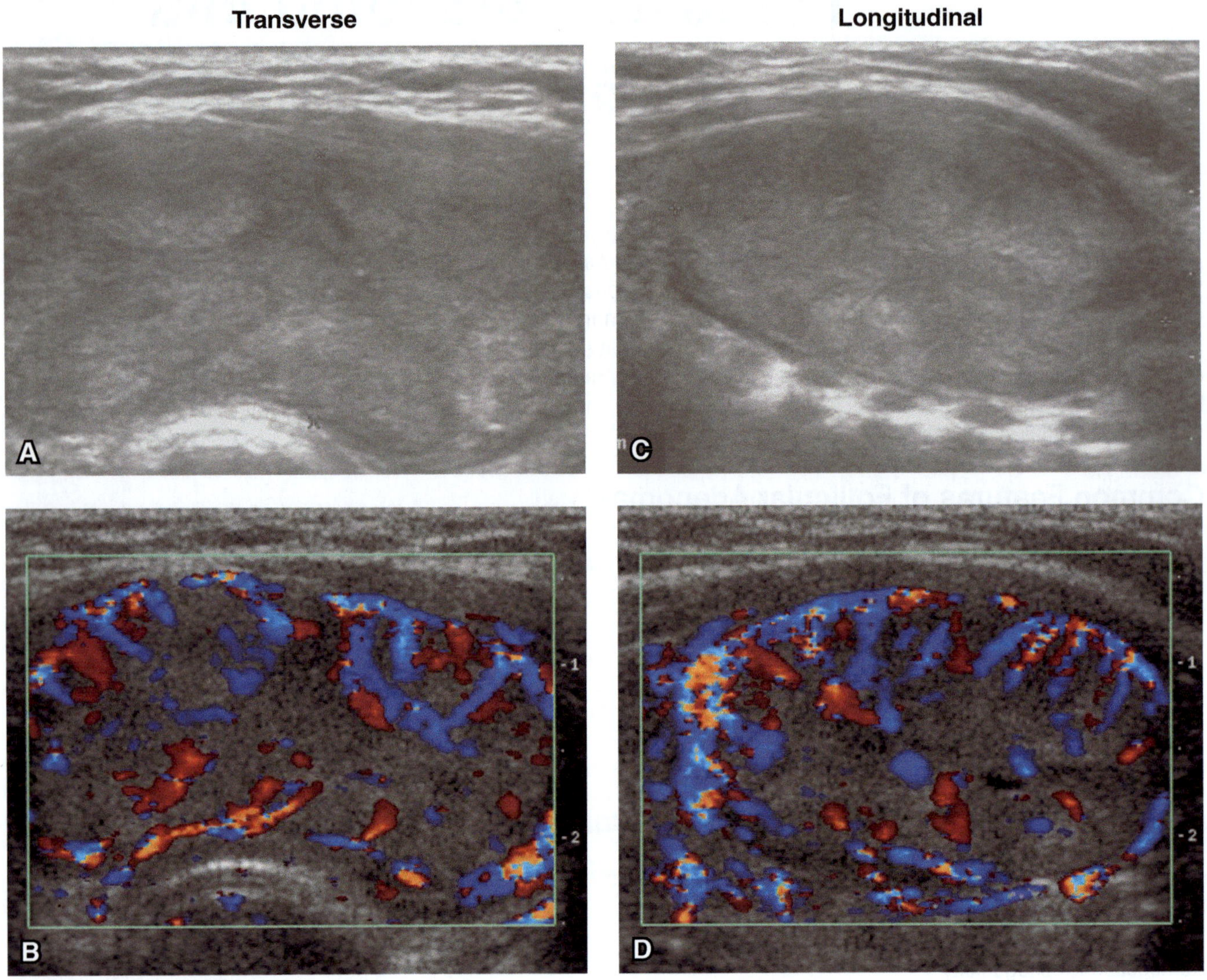

Figure 4-1. Ultrasound of follicular adenoma in the isthmus. **A**, Transverse, 15 x 36 mm. **B**, Color Doppler, transverse. **C**, Longitudinal, sagittal diameter: 30 mm. **D**, Color Doppler, longitudinal.

35-Year-old woman

- **Clinical history:** Autoimmune thyroiditis. Swelling of isthmus for a while.
- **Ultrasound:** Follicular adenoma + thyroiditis.
- **Cytology:** Follicular epithelium with some colloid.
- **16-Gauge histologic needle biopsy:** Follicular lesion.
- **Isthmus and left hemithyroidectomy:** Follicular adenoma. Widespread Hashimoto's thyroiditis.

Features of isthmus tumor

Lobulated with mixed echogenicity
Inhomogeneous echo pattern
Well circumscribed
Partial thin hypoechoic halo
"Spoke-and-wheel-like" vascularity

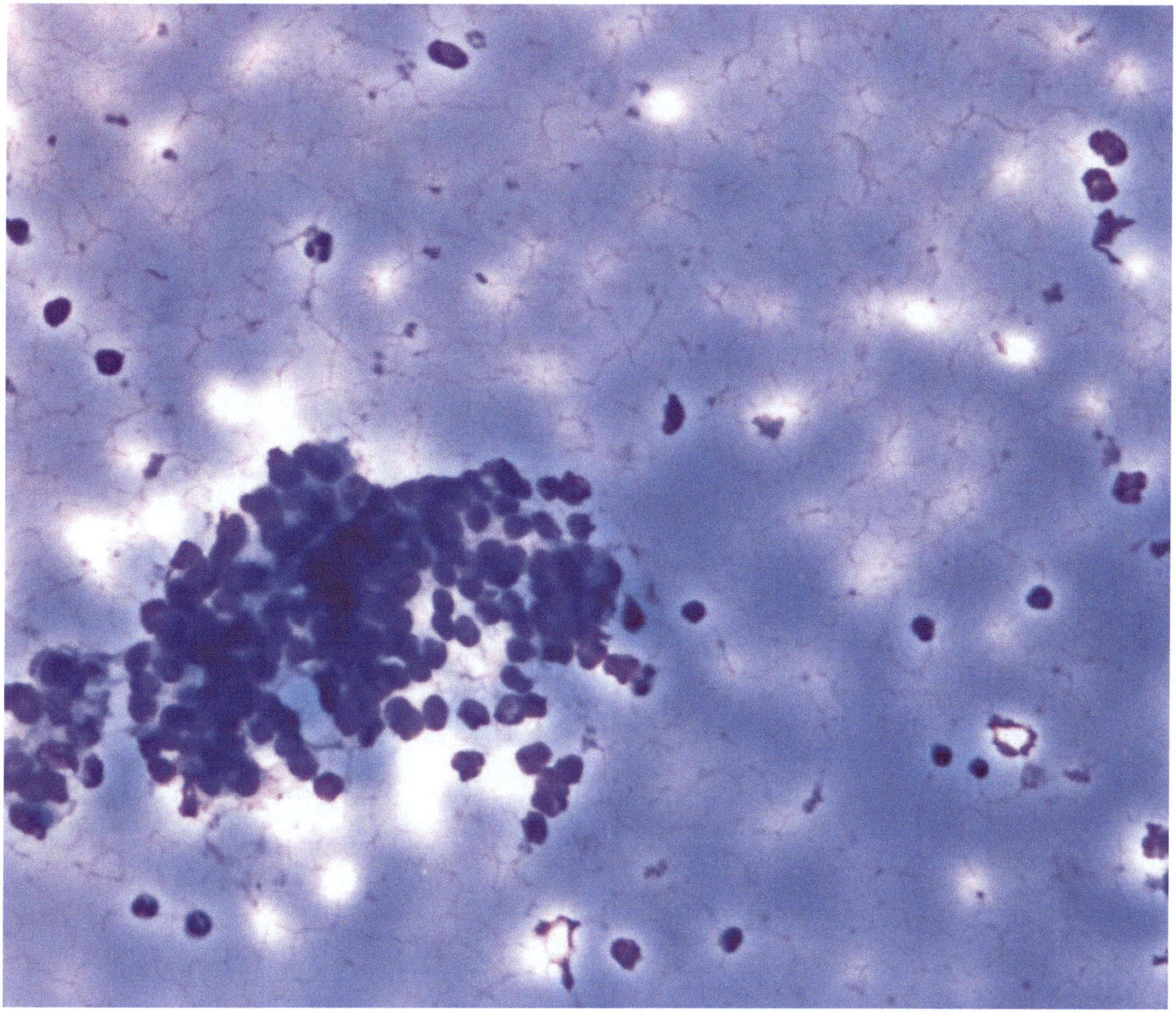

Figure 4-2. Cytology: rich in follicular epithelium.

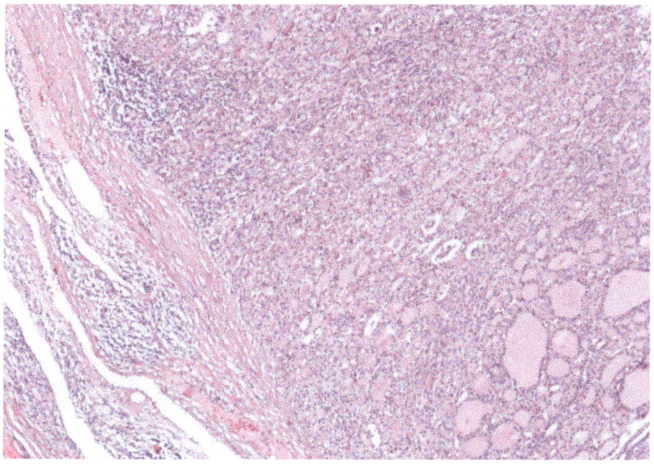

Figure 4-3. Histology: follicular adenoma.

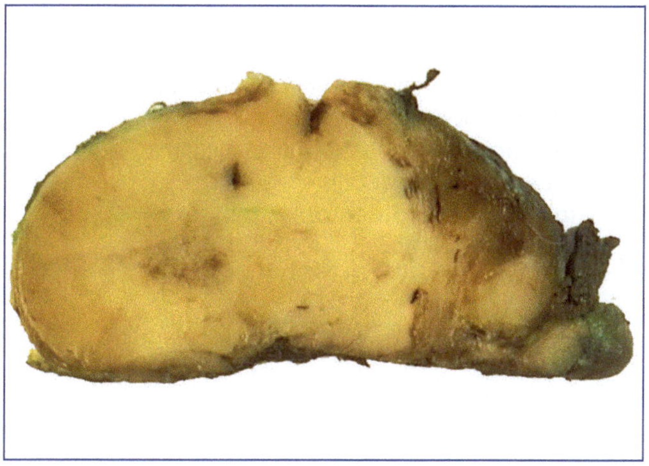

Figure 4-4. Gross section.

Follicular Adenoma Right Lobe/Isthmus

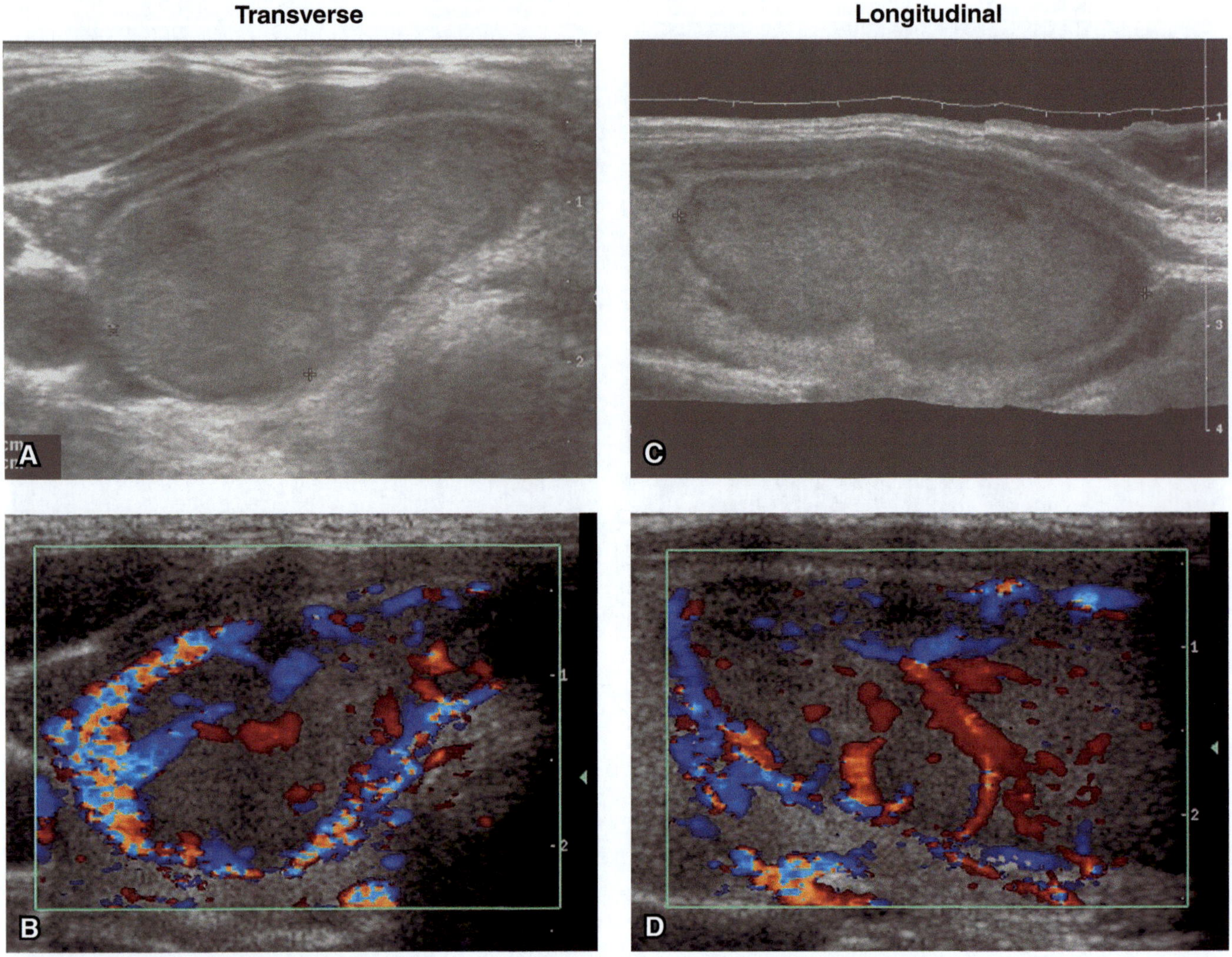

FIGURE 4-5. Ultrasound of follicular adenoma in the right lobe and isthmus. **A**, Transverse, 14 x 29 mm. **B**, Color Doppler, transverse, 15 x 36 mm. **C**, Longitudinal. **D**, Color Doppler, longitudinal.

39-Year-old woman

- **Clinical history:** Tumor in right lobe incidentally revealed on MR.
- **Ultrasound:** Probably follicular adenoma
- **Cytology:** Follicular cells.
- **Right hemithyroidectomy:** Follicular adenoma.

Features

Moderately hypoechoic
Quite homogeneous echo pattern
Well circumscribed
Partial thin uneven hypoechoic halo
"Spoke-and-wheel-like" vascularity

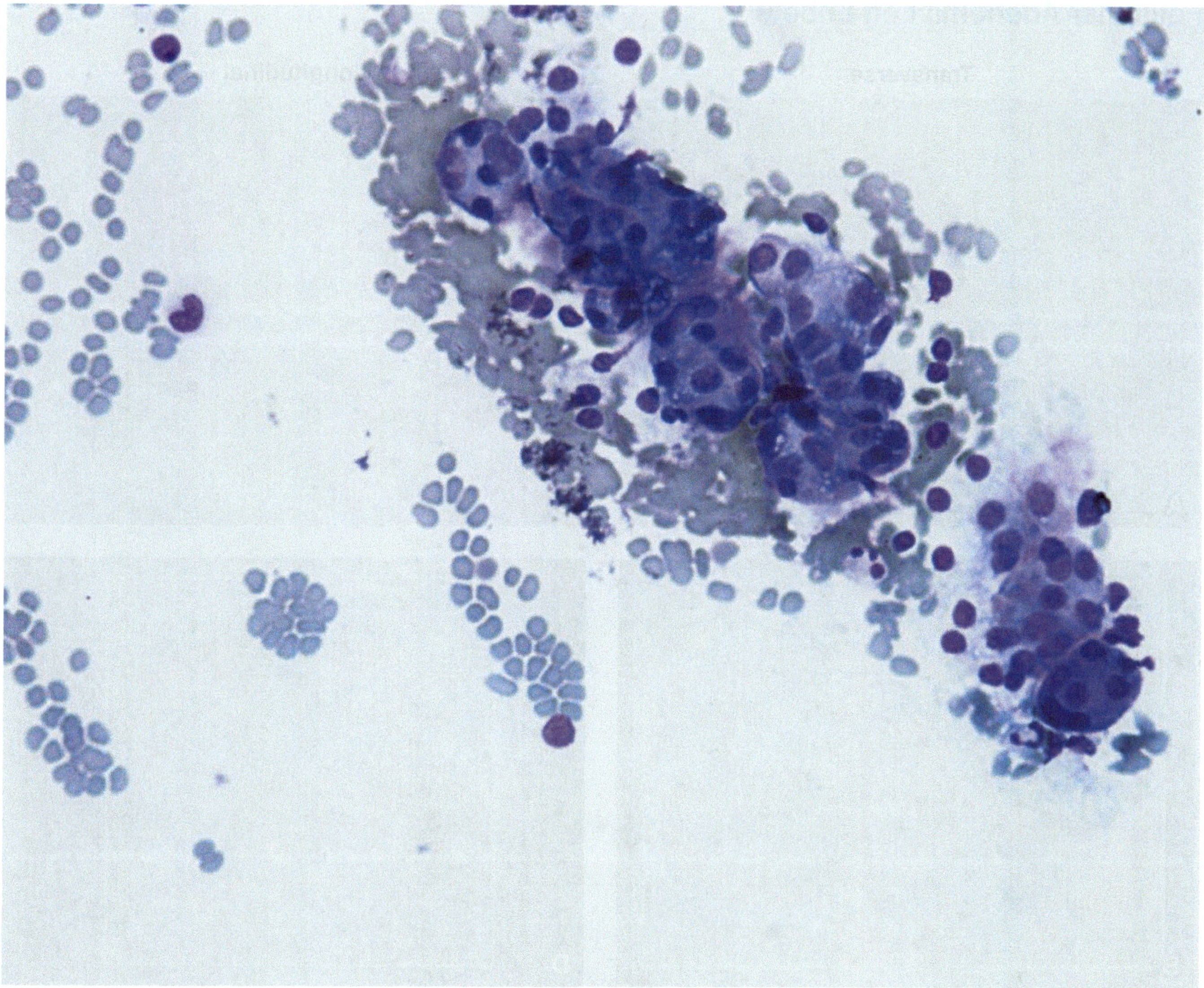

Figure 4-6. Cytology: Predominance of microfollicles. Follicular adenoma cannot be distinguished from follicular carcinoma in cytology.

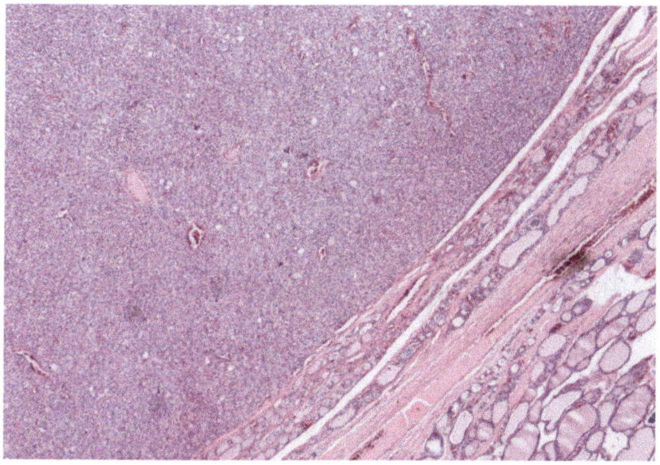

Figure 4-7. Histology: follicular adenoma.

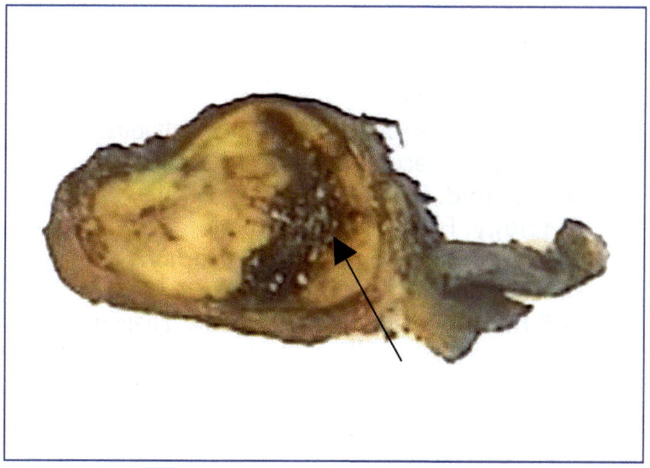

Figure 4-8. Gross section: follicular adenoma with hemorrhage (*arrow*) after histologic needle biopsy.

Follicular Adenoma Left Lobe

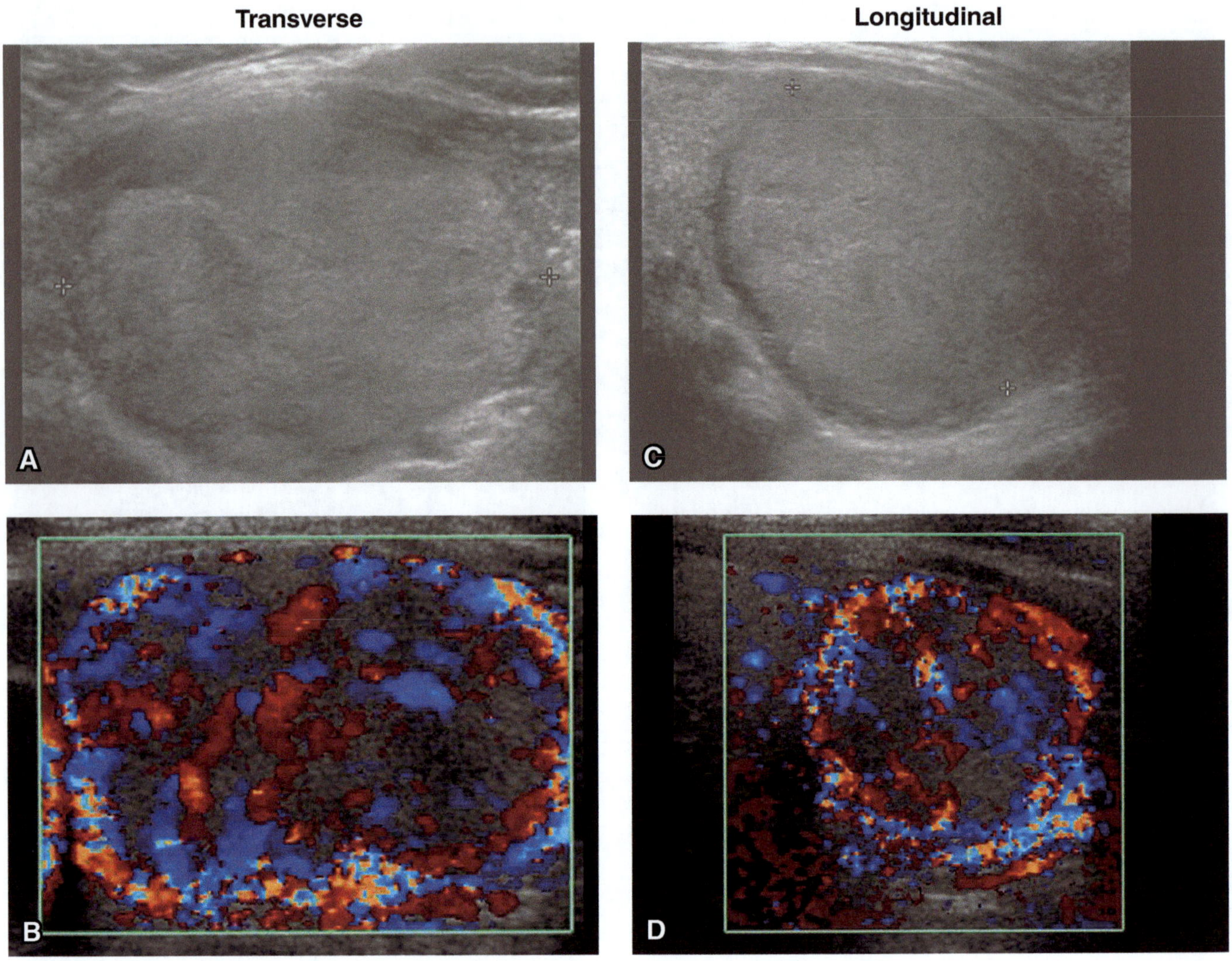

FIGURE 4-9. Ultrasound of follicular adenoma in the left lobe. **A**, Transverse diameter: 33 mm. **B**, Color Doppler, transverse. **C**, Longitudinal, sagittal diameter: 30 mm. **D**, Color Doppler, longitudinal.

62-Year-old woman

- **Clinical history:** Palpable tumor in left lobe. Paresis of left recurrent laryngeal nerve.
- **Ultrasound:** Probably follicular adenoma.
- **Cytology:** Follicular lesion.
- **18-Gauge histologic needle biopsy:** Follicular tumor.
- **Left hemithyroidectomy:** Follicular adenoma.

Features

Slightly hypoechoic
Small hypoechoic areas of variable size in a more smooth, uniform tissue
Well circumscribed
Partial thin hypoechoic halo
Hypervascularized with "spoke-and-wheel-like" appearance

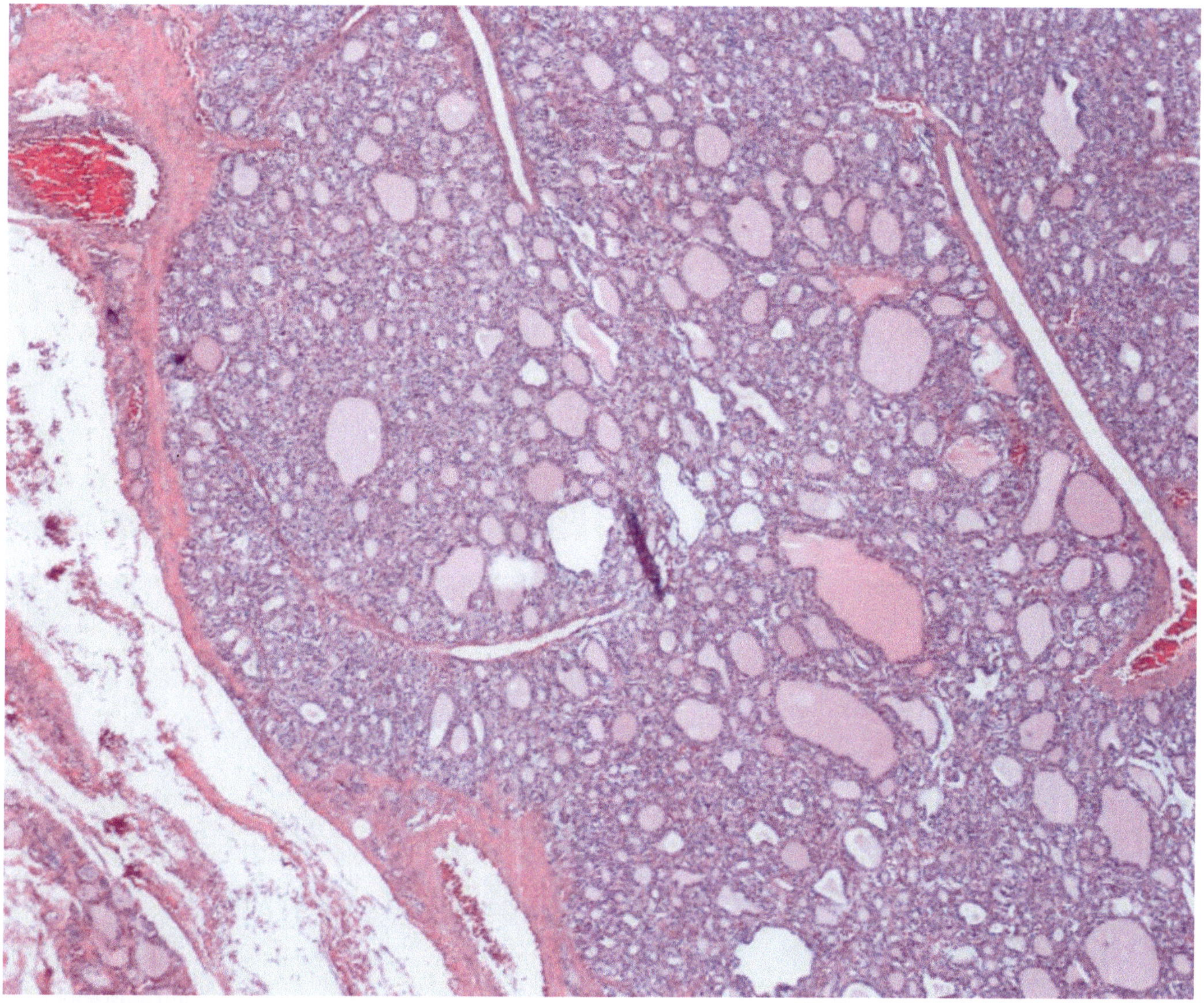

Figure 4-10. Histology: follicular adenoma.

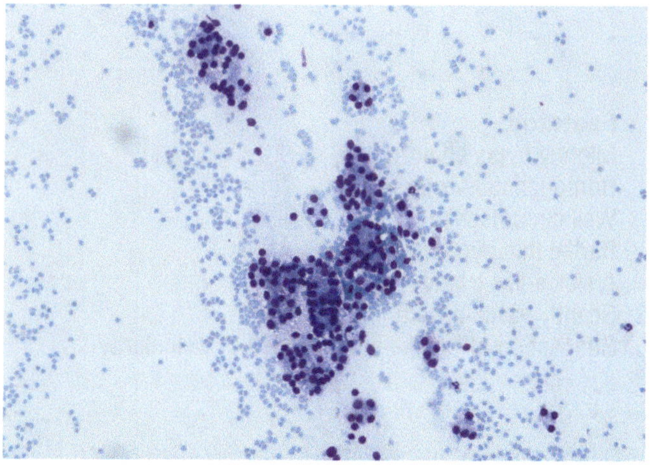

Figure 4-11. Cytology: rich in follicular cells.

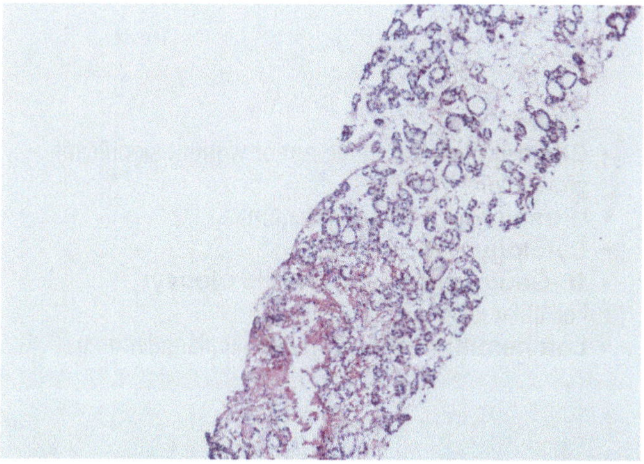

Figure 4-12. Histologic needle biopsy.

Follicular Adenoma Left Lobe

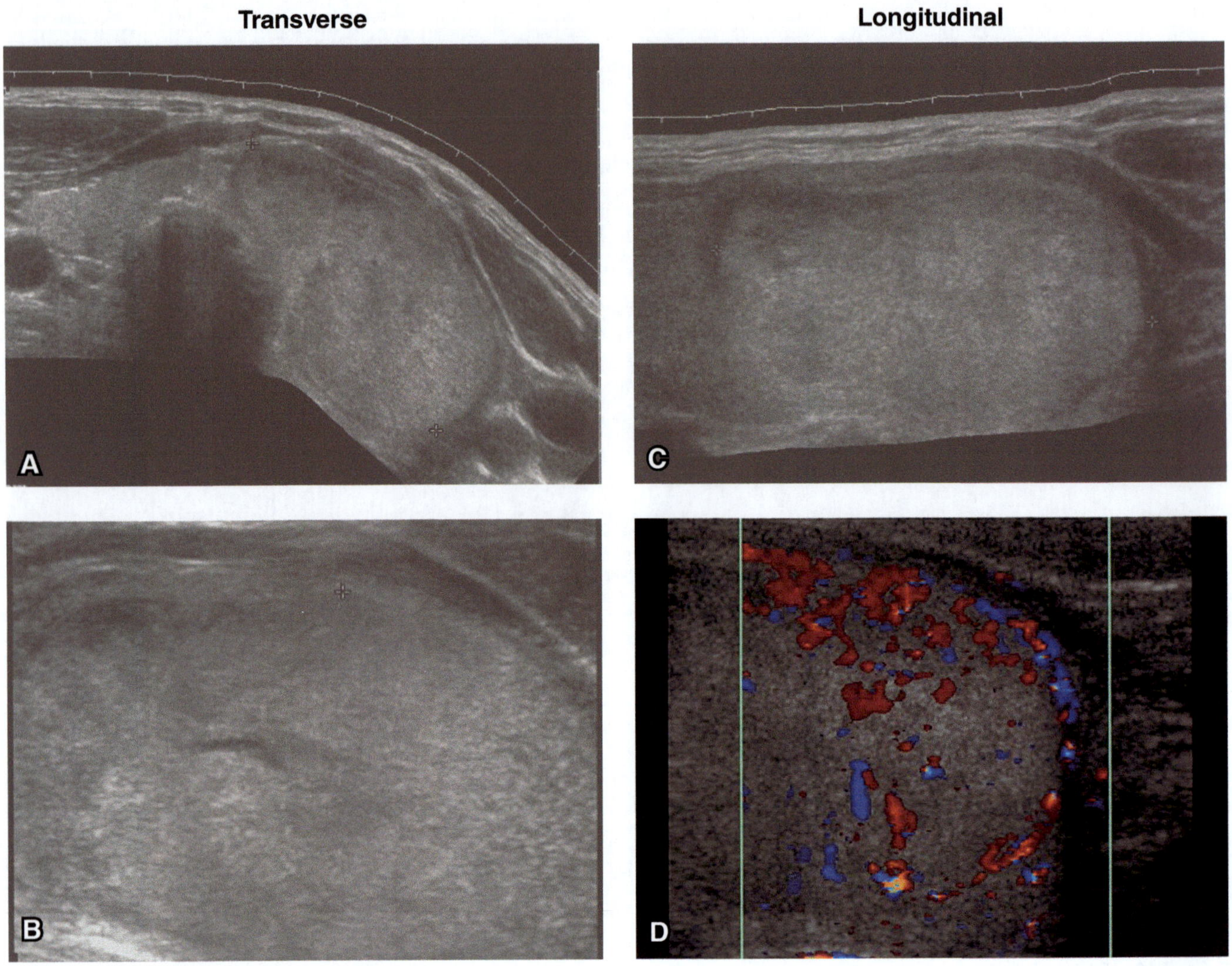

Figure 4-13. Ultrasound of follicular adenoma in the left lobe. **A**, Transverse diameter: 45 mm. **B**, Transverse. **C**, Longitudinal, sagittal diameter: 50 mm. **D**, Color Doppler, longitudinal.

58-Year-old man

- **Clinical history:** Large tumor without significant growth for 1 year.
- **Ultrasound:** Follicular adenoma.
- **Cytology:** Follicular lesion.
- **16-Gauge histologic needle biopsy:** Follicular lesion.
- **Left hemithyroidectomy:** Follicular adenoma.

Features

Slightly hypoechoic
Homogeneous echo pattern
Well circumscribed
Partial thin hypoechoic halo
A sickle-like cystic area
Scantly vascularized
Suggestion of "spoke-and-wheel-like" vascularity

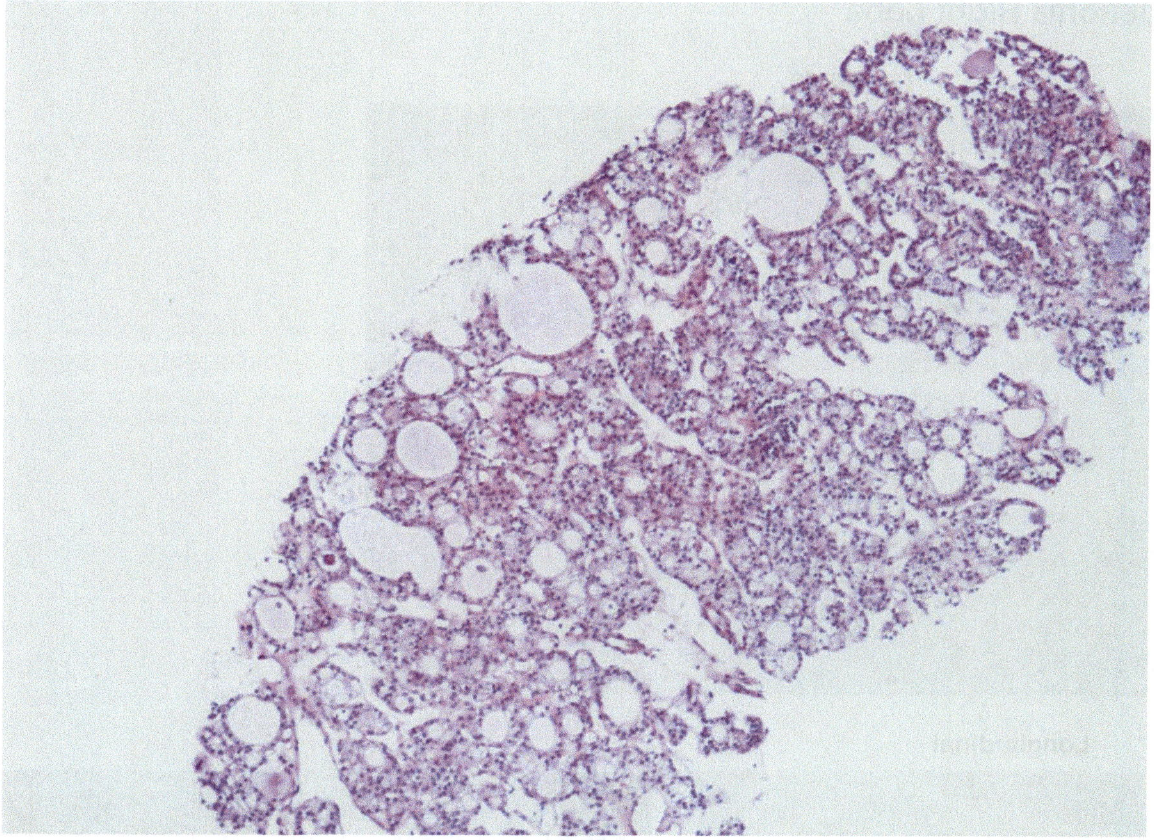

Figure 4-14. Histologic needle biopsy: follicular lesion.

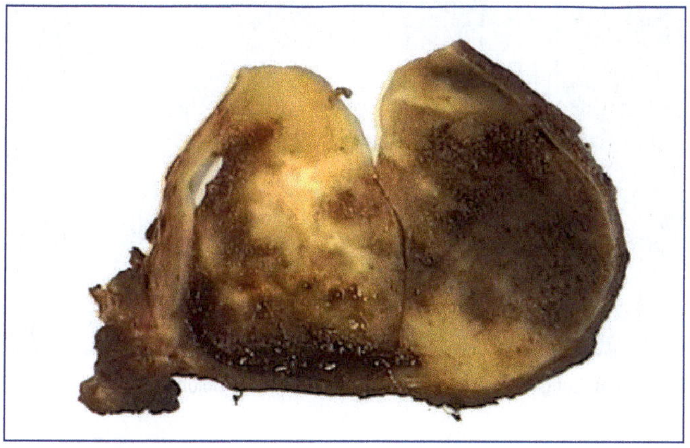

Figure 4-15. Gross section: follicular neoplasia with fibrosis and hemorrhage after histologic needle biopsy.

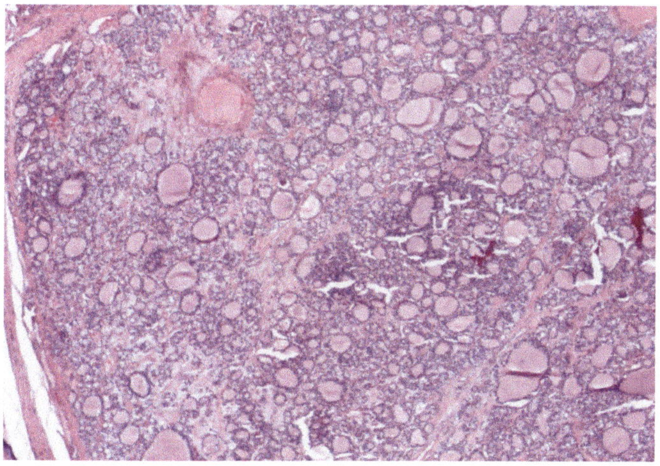

Figure 4-16. Histology: follicular adenoma.

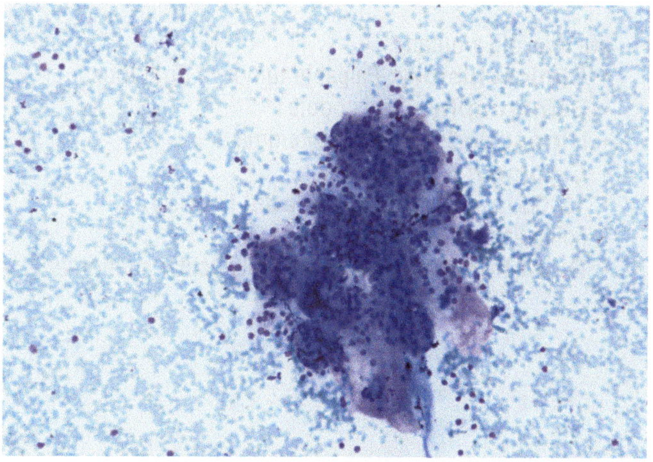

Figure 4-17. Cytology: follicular structure.

Follicular Adenoma Right Lobe

Transverse

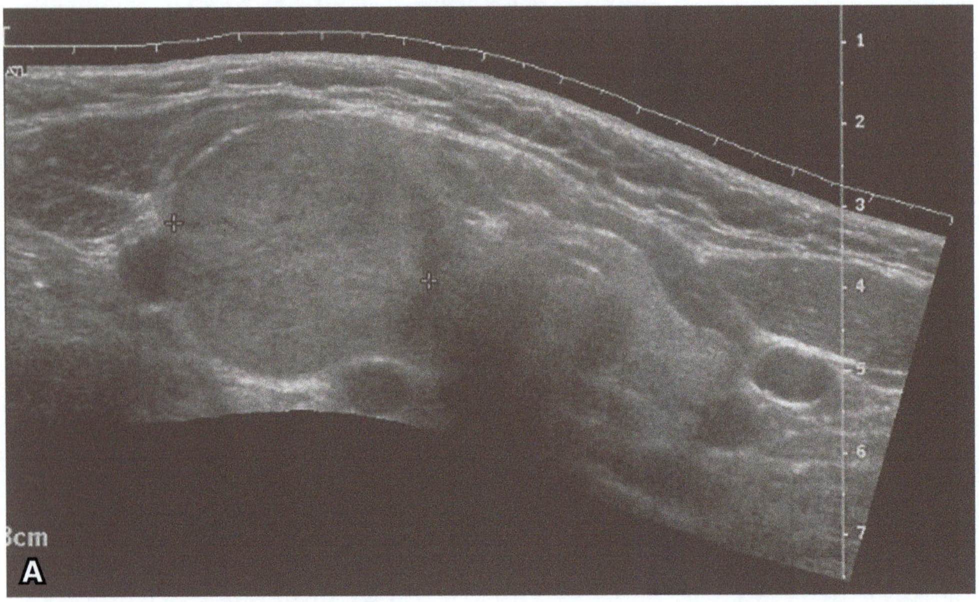

Longitudinal

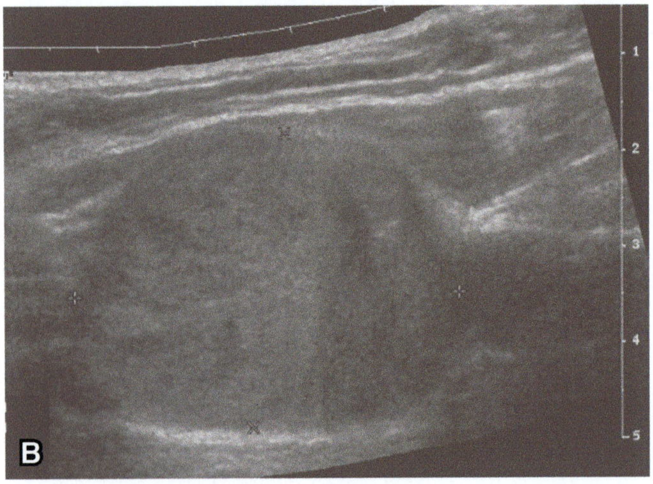

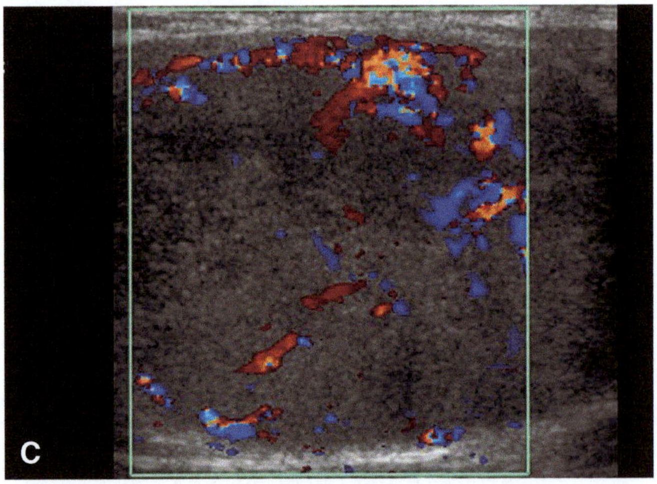

Figure 4-18. Ultrasound of follicular adenoma in the right lobe. **A**, Transverse, 31 x 32 mm. **B**, Longitudinal, sagittal diameter: 40 mm. **C**, Color Doppler.

26-Year-old woman

- **Clinical history:** Palpable tumor in right lobe.
- **Scintigraphy:** Cold nodule.
- **Ultrasound:** Follicular adenoma.
- **Cytology:** Follicular lesion.
- **18-Gauge histologic needle biopsy:** Follicular lesion.
- **Right hemithyroidectomy:** Follicular adenoma.

Features

Slightly hypoechoic

Hypoechoic “spokes” converging toward tumor center between areas with almost isoechoic homogeneous echo pattern

Well circumscribed

Scantly vascularized

Suggestion of “spoke-and-wheel-like” vascularity

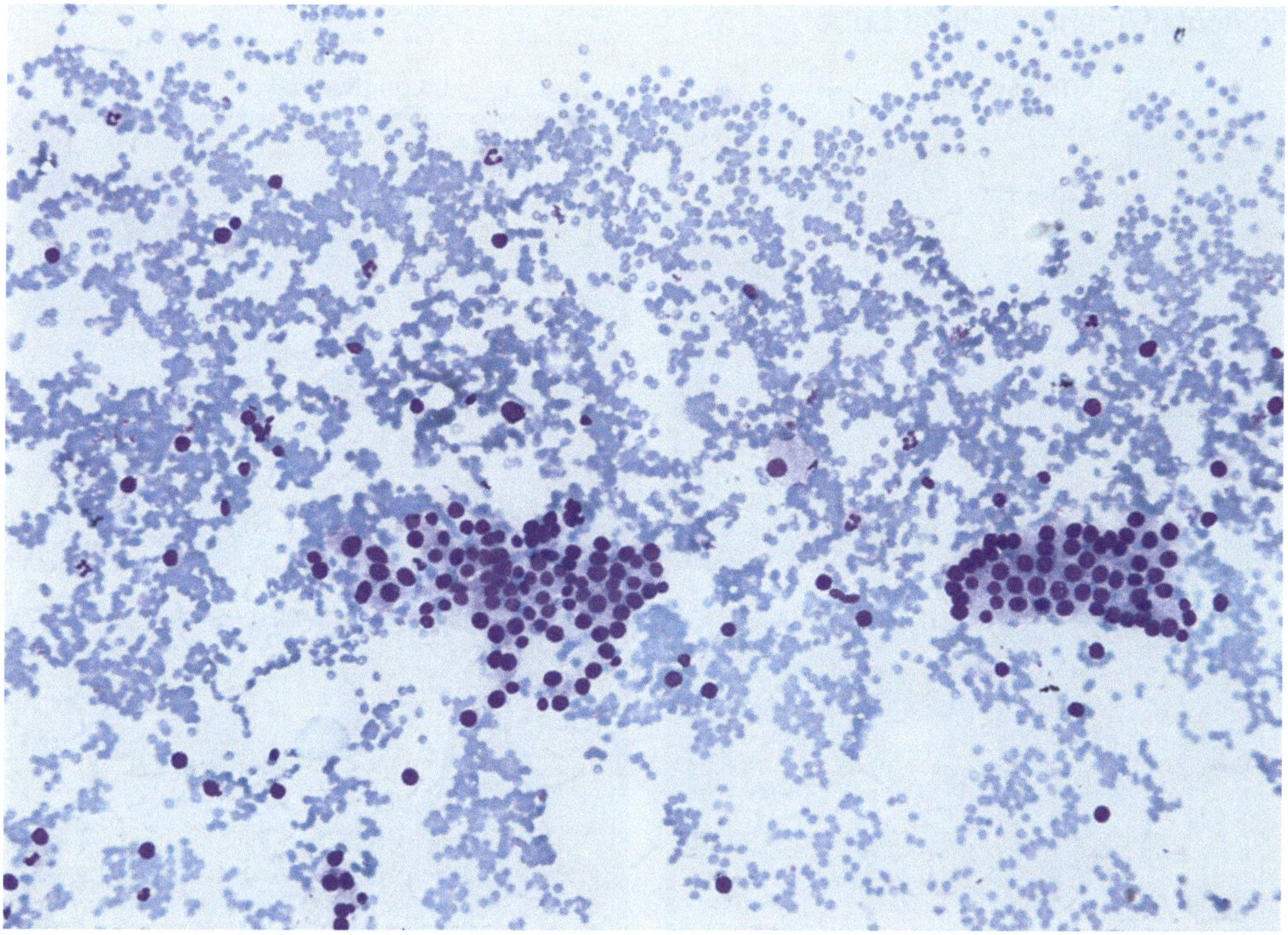

FIGURE 4-19. Cytology: rich in follicular cells.

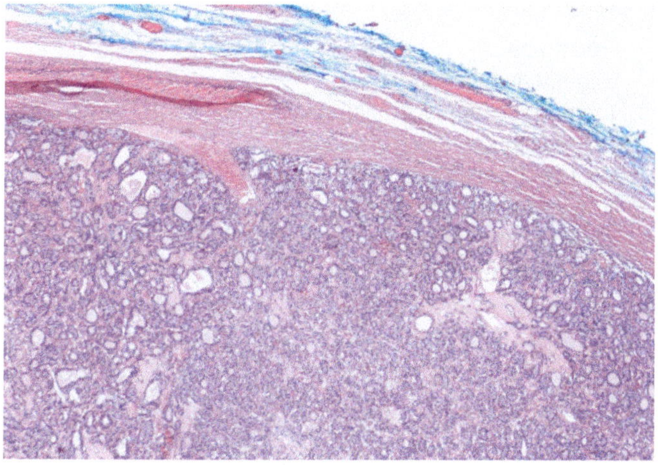

FIGURE 4-20. Histology: follicular adenoma.

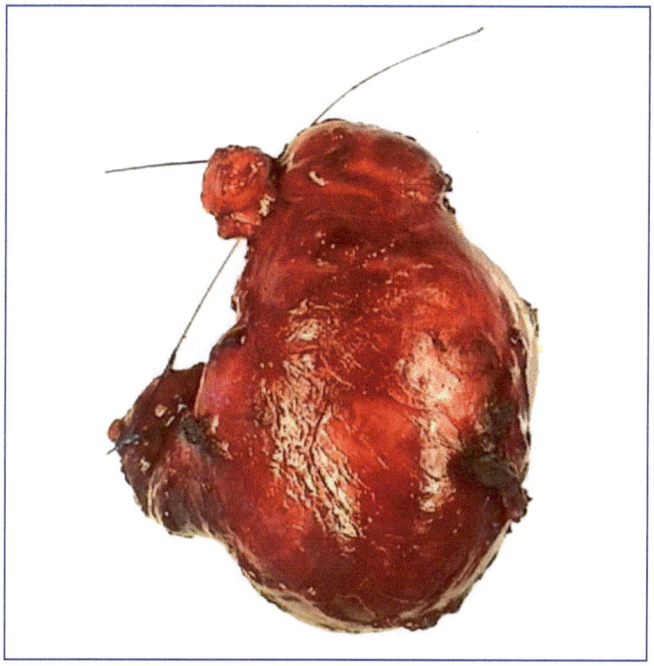

FIGURE 4-21. Gross section: fresh surgical specimen.

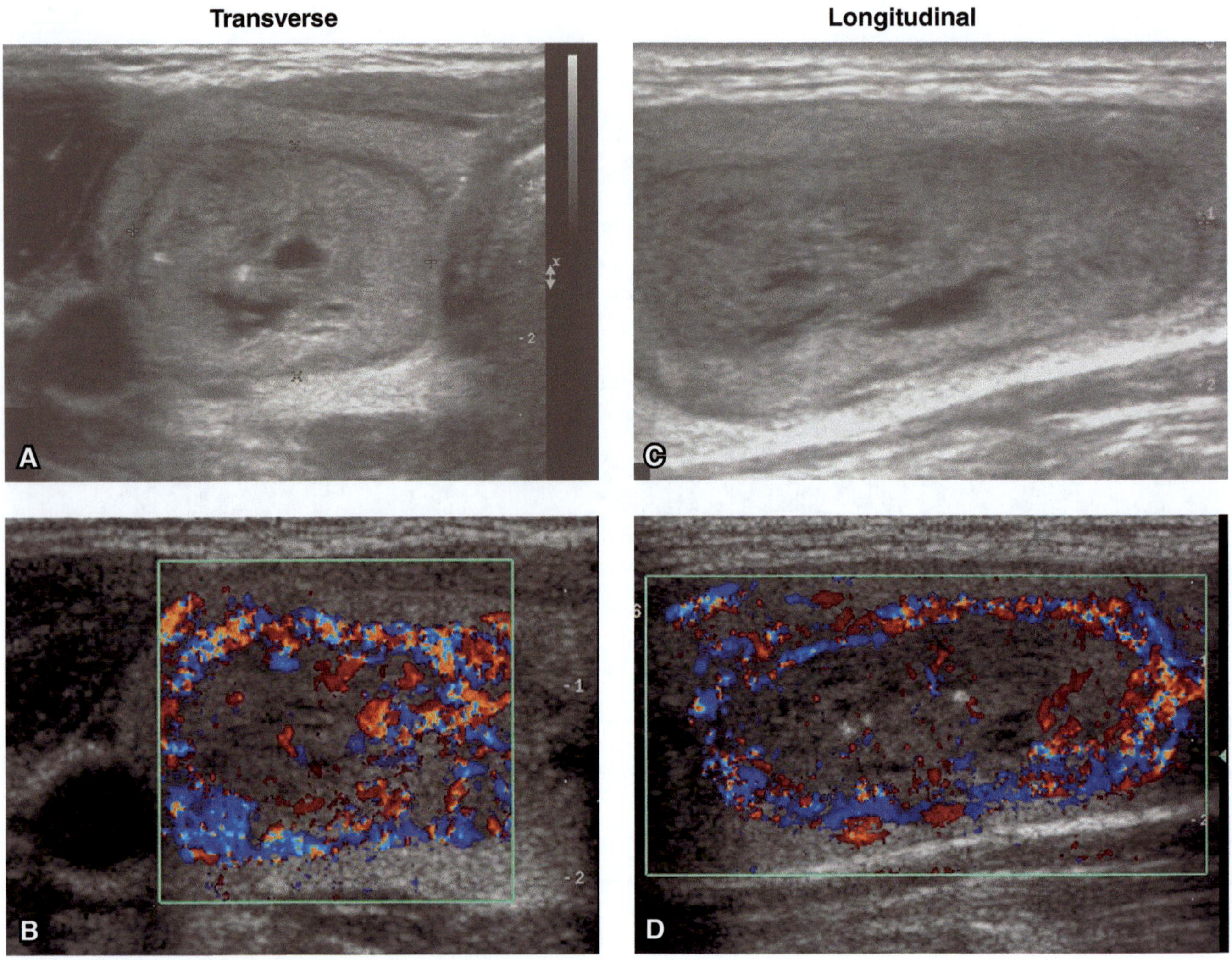

Figure 4-22. Ultrasound of follicular adenoma in the right lobe. **A**, Transverse, 15 x 20 mm. **B**, Color Doppler, transverse. **C**, Longitudinal, sagittal diameter: 36 mm. **D**, Color Doppler, longitudinal.

37-Year-old woman

- **Clinical history:** Incidentally found tumor in right lobe.
- **Ultrasound:** Probably follicular adenoma.
- **Cytology:** Suspicious for follicular neoplasia.
- **18-Gauge histology:** Probably follicular adenoma.
- **Right hemithyroidectomy:** Follicular adenoma.

Features

Slightly hypoechoic
Inhomogeneous echo pattern
Somewhat spongy apperance
Well circumscribed
A few microcalcifications
Thin hypoechoic halo
"Spoke-and-wheel-like" vascularity

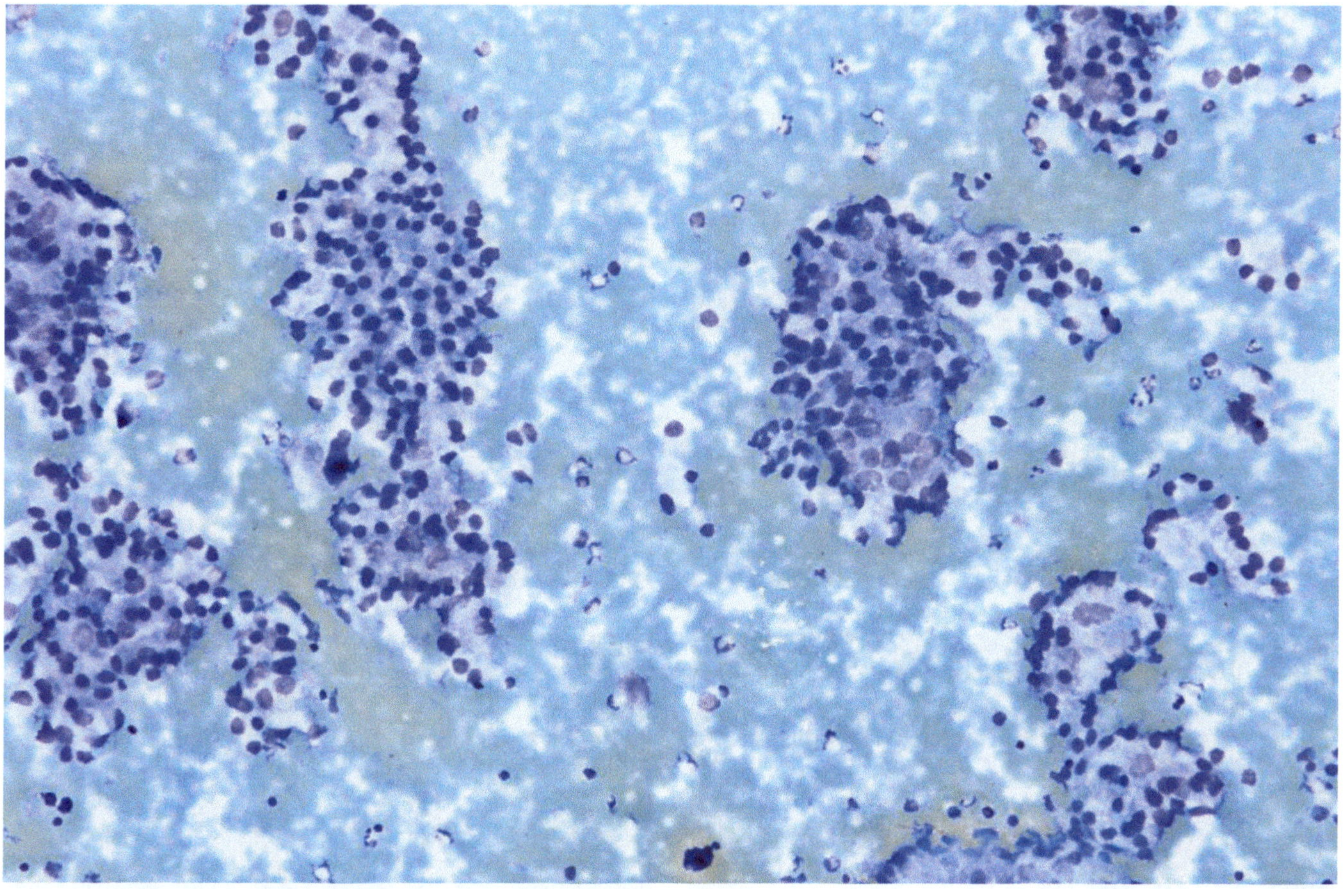

Figure 4-23. Cytology: rich in follicular epithelium. No colloid.

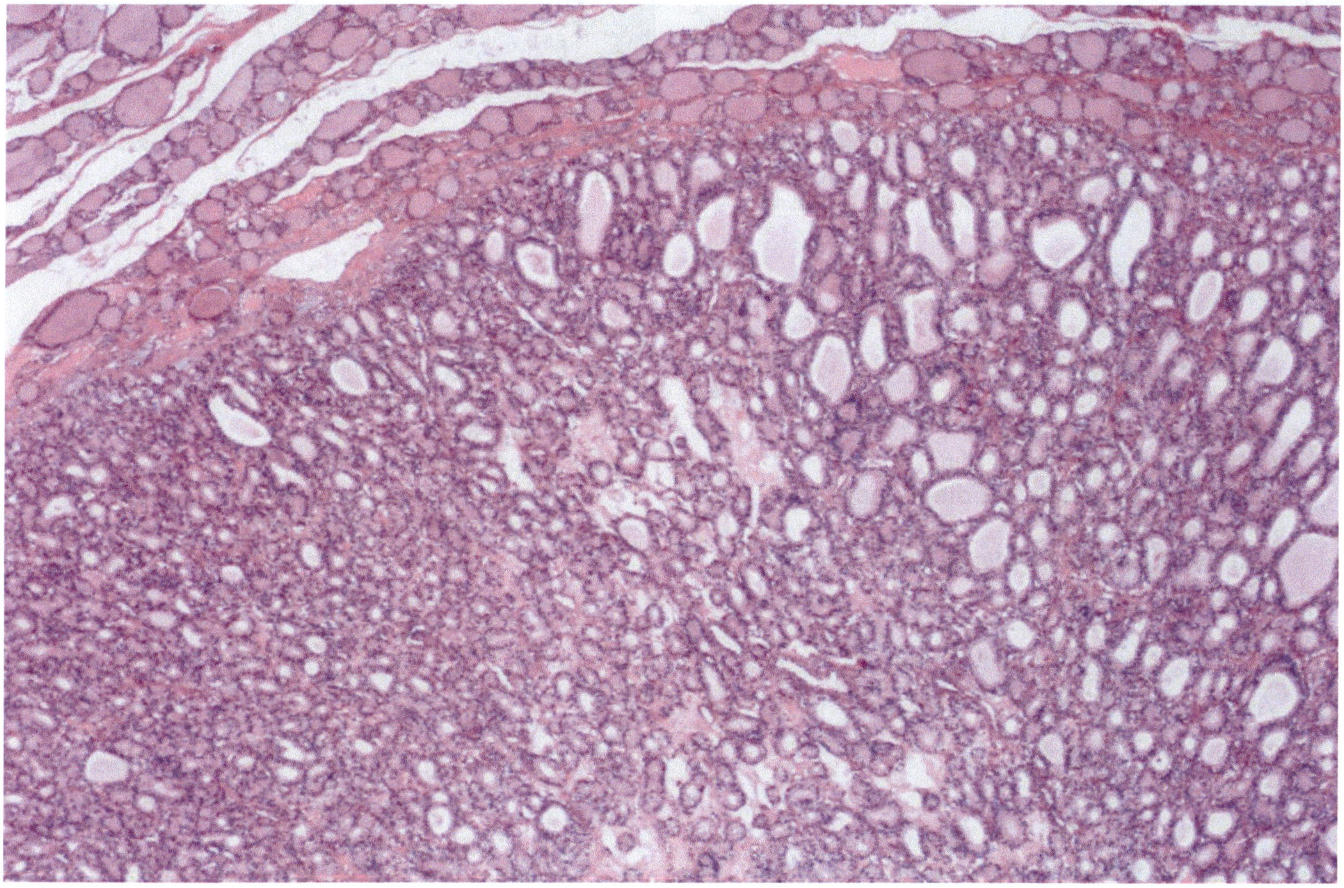

Figure 4-24. Histology: follicular adenoma.

Follicular Adenoma Left Lobe

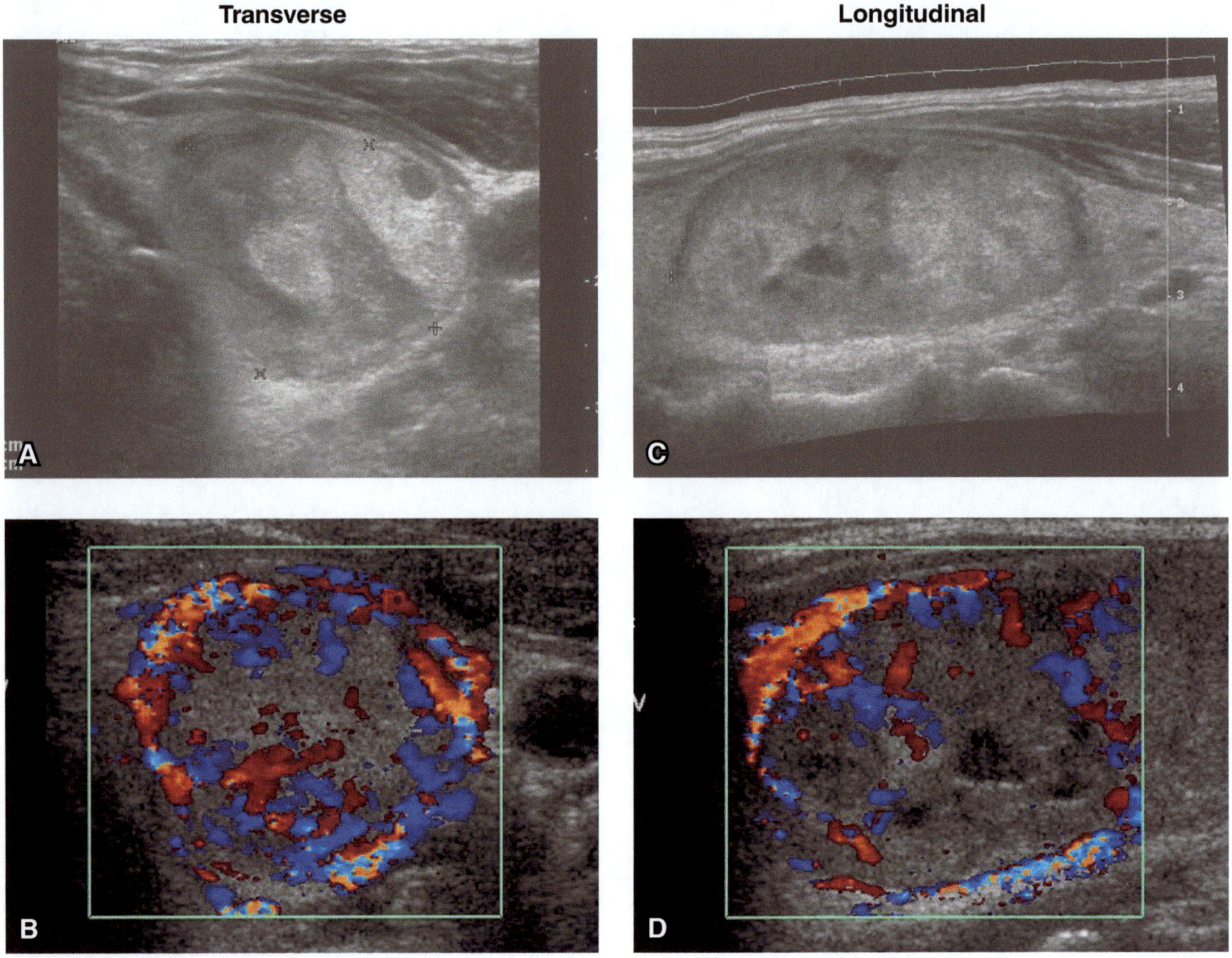

Figure 4-25. Ultrasound of follicular adenoma in the left lobe. **A**, Transverse, 12 x 13 mm. **B**, Color Doppler, transverse. **C**, Longitudinal, sagittal diameter: 44 mm. **D**, Color Doppler, longitudinal.

52-Year-old man

- **Clinical history:** Palpable tumor in left lobe for some weeks.
- **Ultrasound:** Follicular tumor.
- **Cytology:** Follicular epithelium.
- **18-Gauge histologic needle biopsy:** Follicular lesion.
- **Left hemithyroidectomy:** Follicular adenoma.

Features

Iso- and slightly hypoechoic
Geographic inhomogeneous echo pattern
Small cystic areas
Well circumscribed
Partial thin hypoechoic halo
"Spoke-and-wheel-like" vascularity

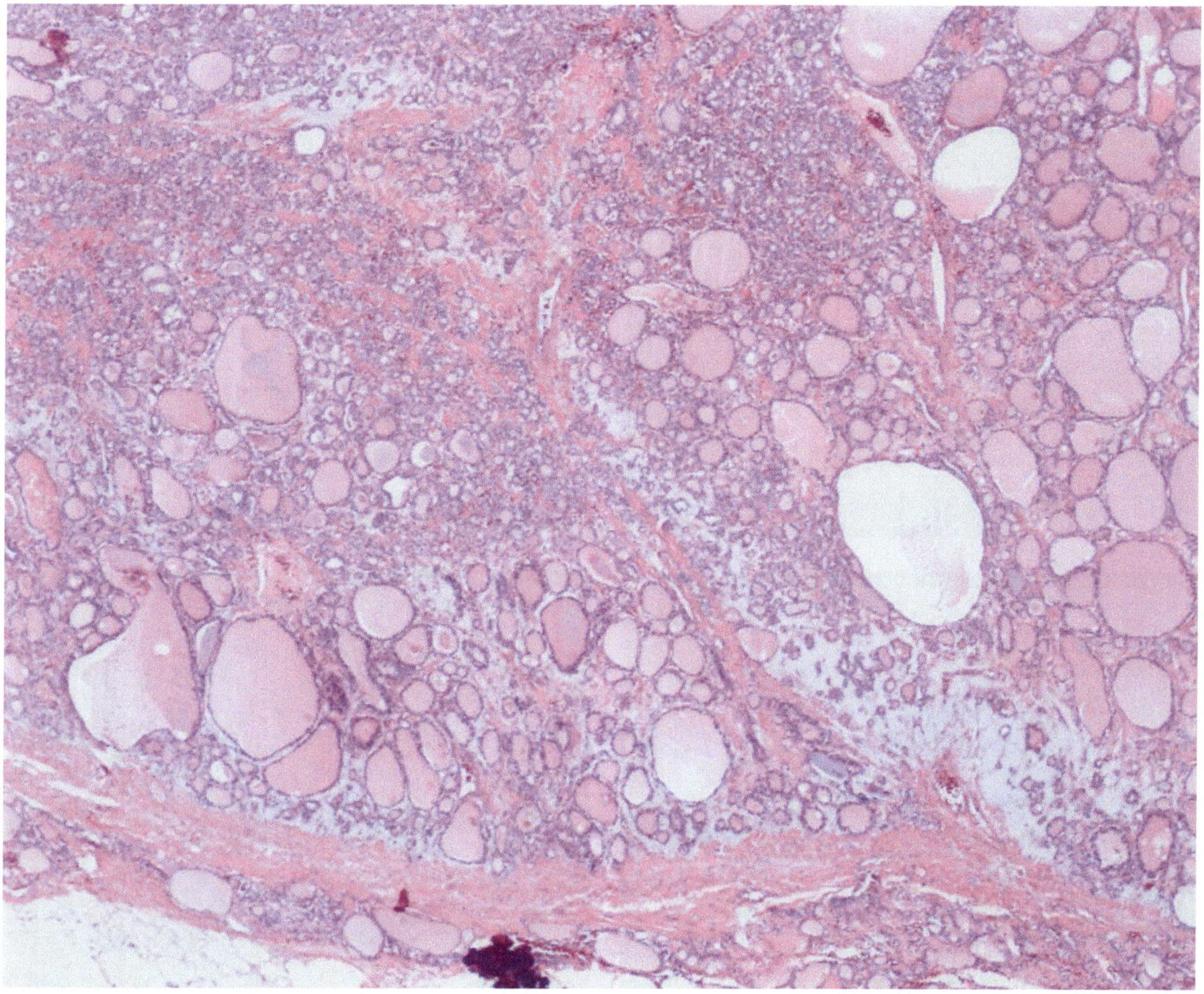

FIGURE 4-26. Histology: follicular adenoma.

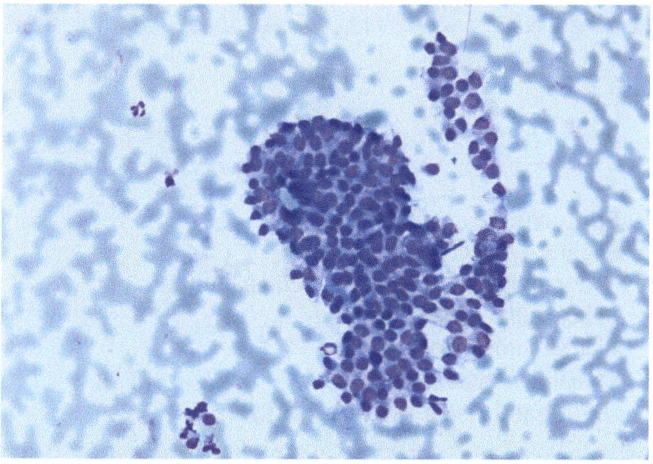

FIGURE 4-27. Cytology: rich in follicular epithelium. No colloid.

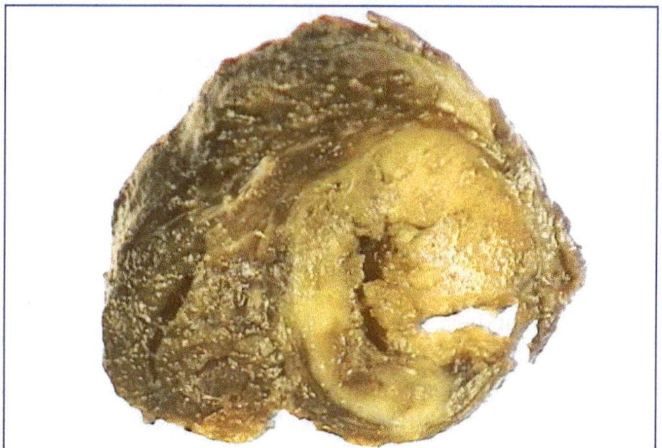

FIGURE 4-28. Gross section.

Follicular Adenoma Left Lobe

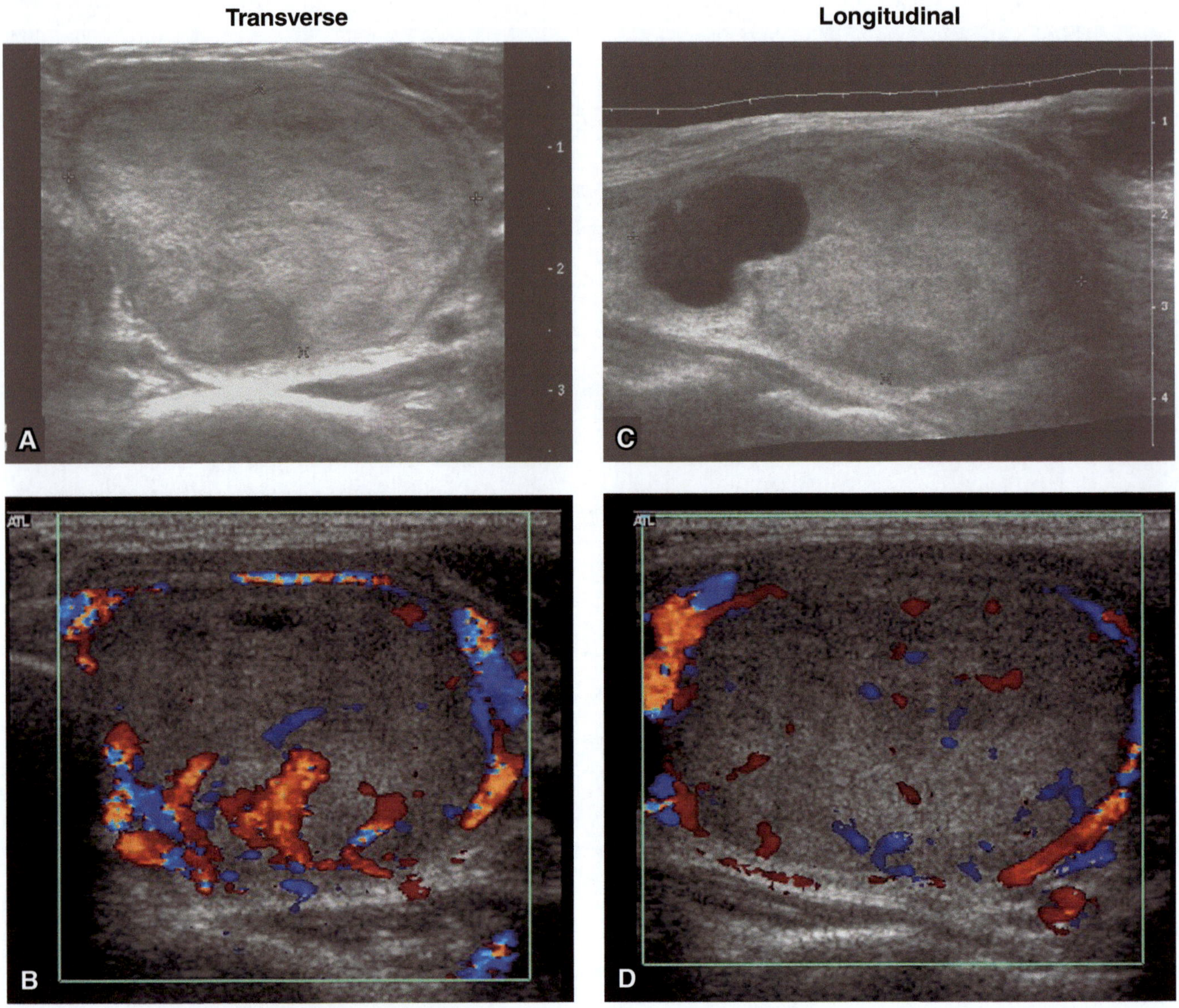

Figure 4-29. Ultrasound of follicular adenoma in the left lobe. **A**, Transverse, 22 x 34 mm. **B**, Color Doppler, transverse. **C**, Longitudinal, sagittal diameter: 49 mm. **D**, Color Doppler, longitudinal.

53-Year-old woman

- **Clinical history:** Node in left lobe past 11 years. Presently growing slowly. Cold nodule at scintigraphy.
- **Ultrasound:** Probably cystic follicular adenoma.
- **Cytology:** Follicular lesion with cyst.
- **Left hemithyroidectomy:** Follicular adenoma.

Features

Slightly hypoechoic
Geographic inhomogeneous echo pattern
Subcapsular cyst
Well circumscribed
Partial thin hypoechoic halo
"Spoke-and-wheel-like" vascularity

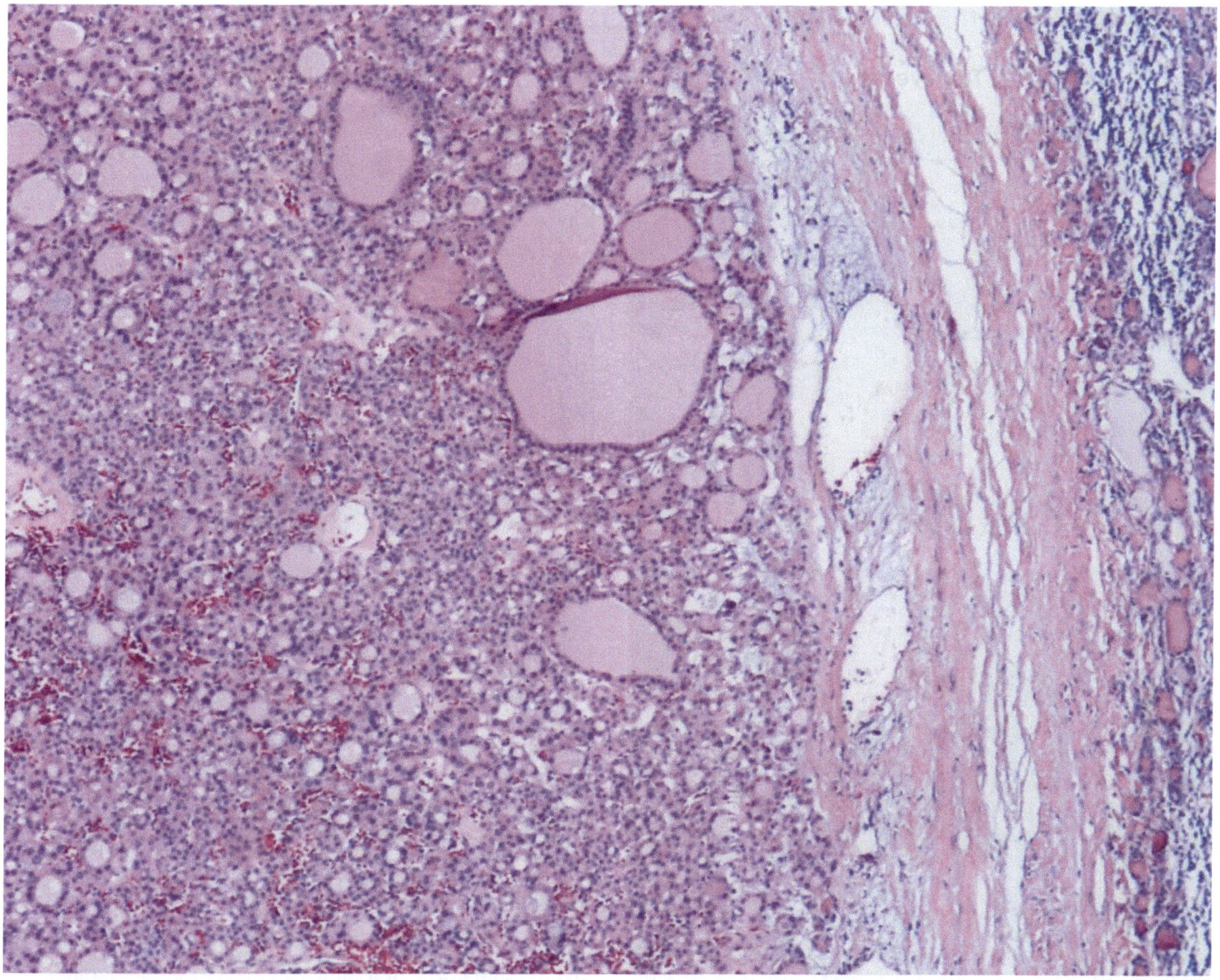

Figure 4-30. Histology: follicular adenoma. Thick fibrous capsule.

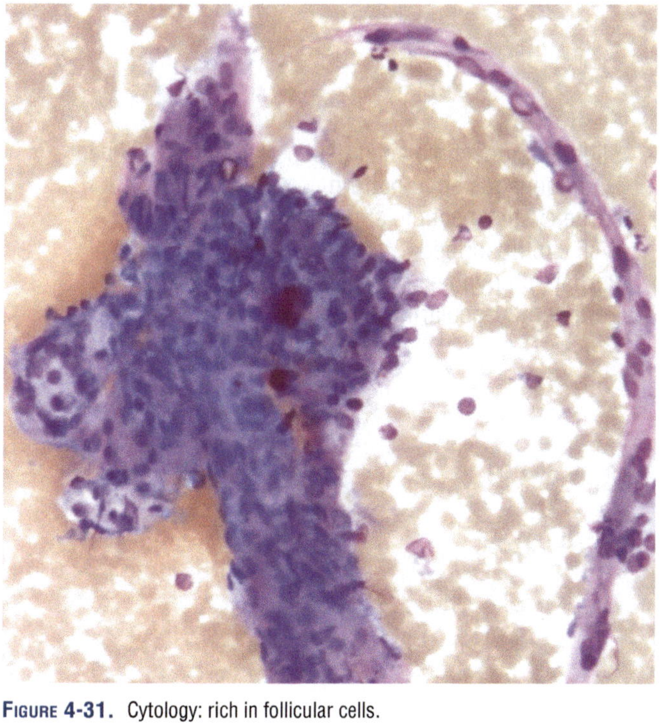

Figure 4-31. Cytology: rich in follicular cells.

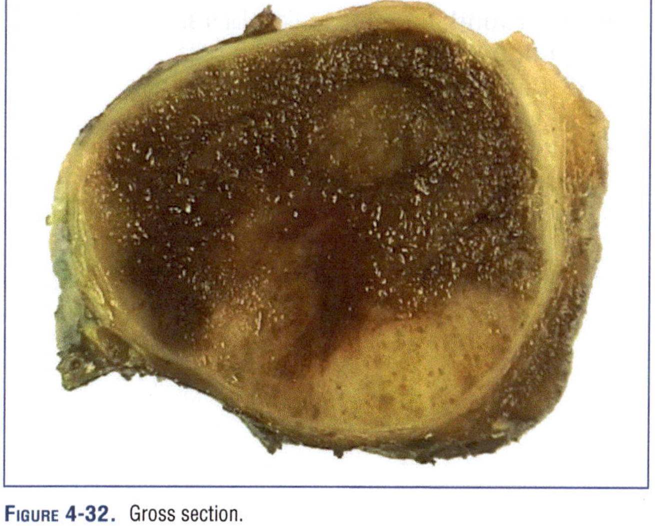

Figure 4-32. Gross section.

Follicular Adenoma Left Lobe

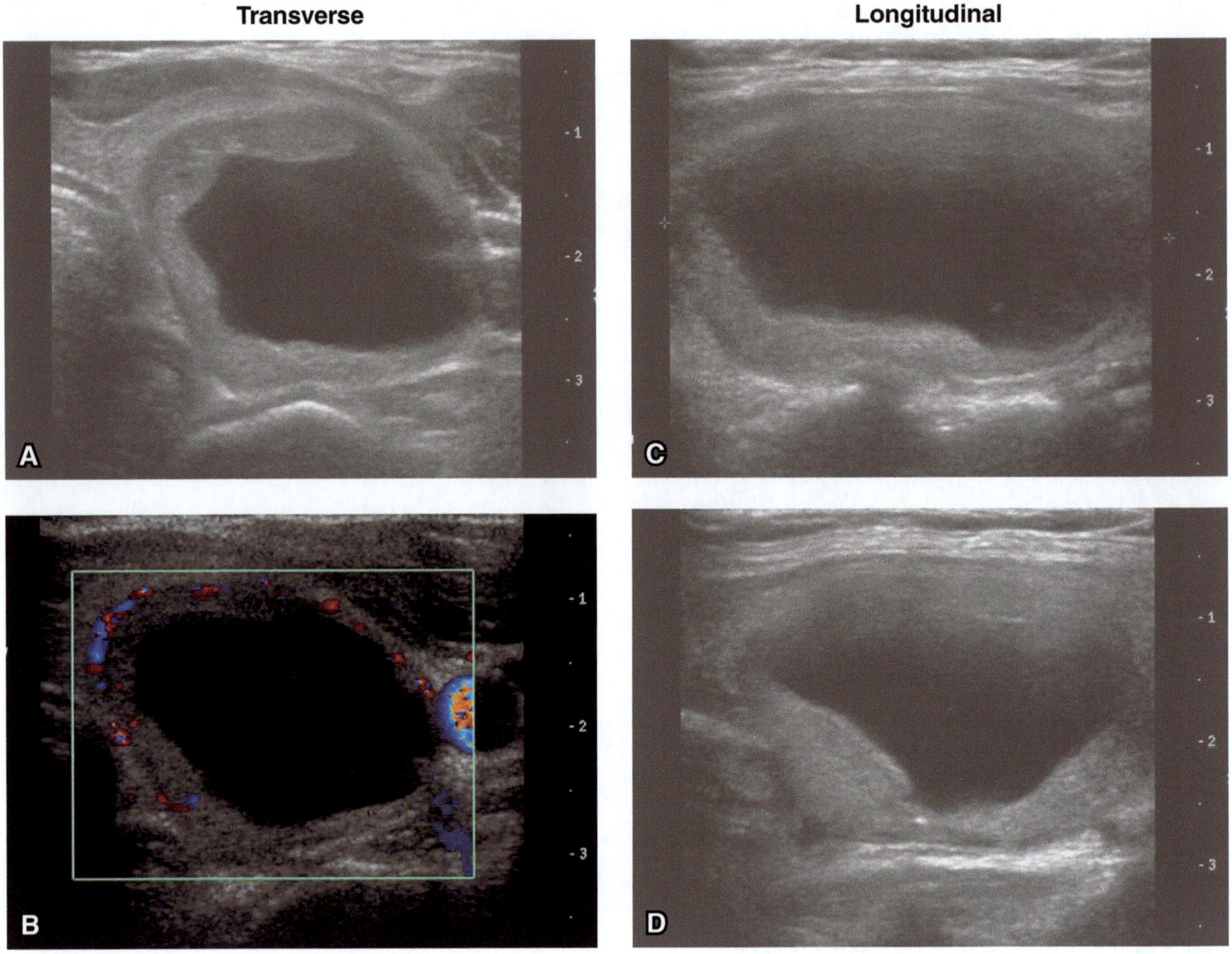

Figure 4-33. Ultrasound of follicular adenoma in the left lobe. **A**, Transverse. **B**, Color Doppler, transverse. **C**, Longitudinal, sagittal diameter: 40 mm. **D**, Longitudinal.

36-Year-old woman

- **Clinical history:** Palpable node in left lobe for a short time.
- **Ultrasound:** Probably cystic follicular adenoma
- **Cytology:** Cyst fluid and reactive cells.
- **18-Gauge histologic needle biopsy:** Thyroid tissue.
- **Left hemithyroidectomy:** Follicular adenoma with cystic degeneration.

Features

Slightly hypoechoic solid tissue of variable thickness
Homogeneous echo pattern
Large cystic anechoic area centrally
Well circumscribed
Partial thin hypoechoic halo
Peripheral vascularity

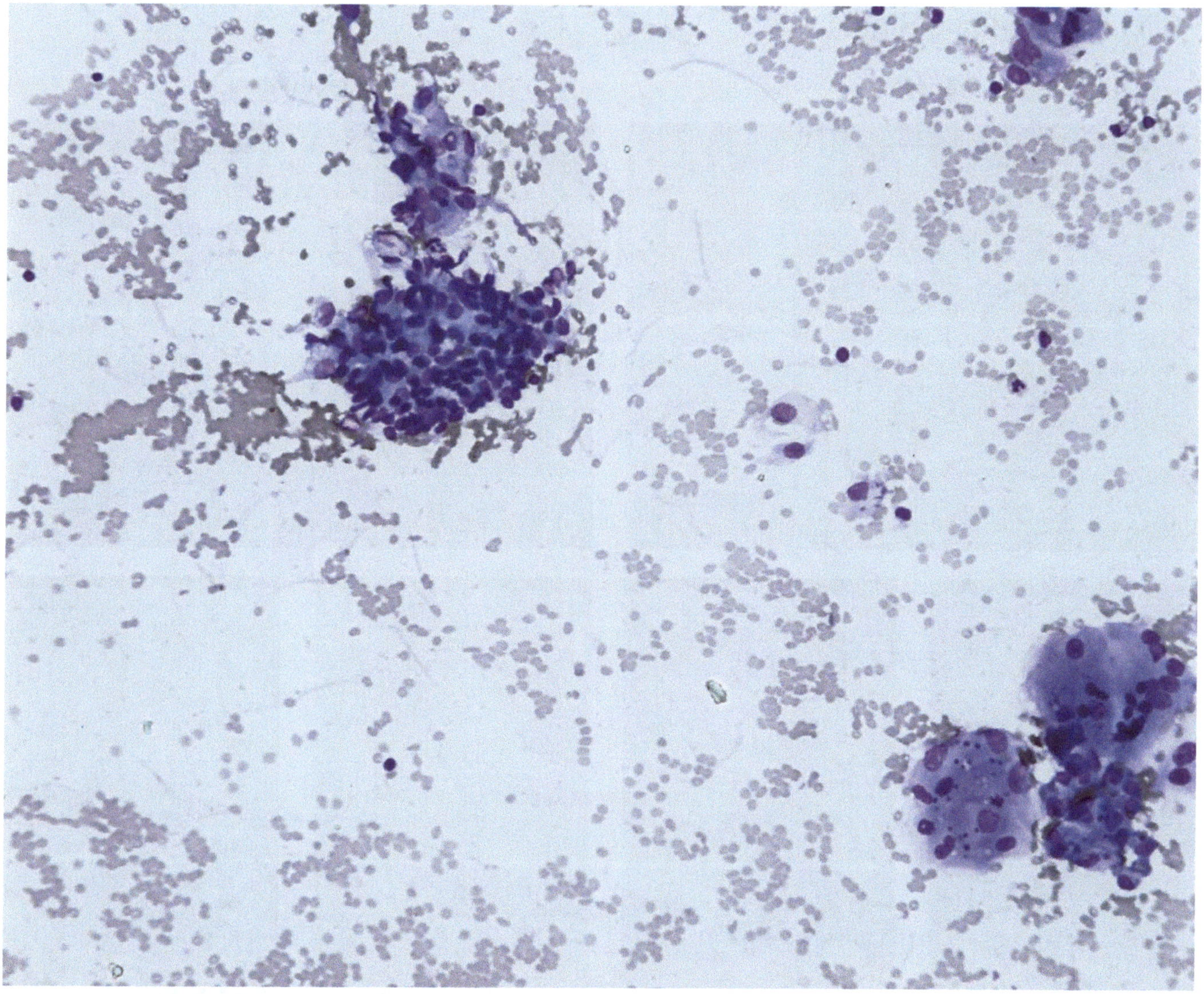

Figure 4-34. Cytology: cystic fluid with follicular cells.

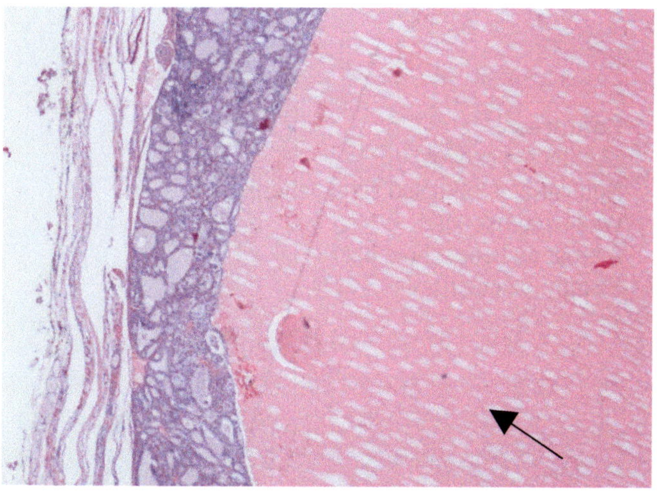

Figure 4-35. Histology: follicular adenoma with cyctic degeneration in the center (*arrow*).

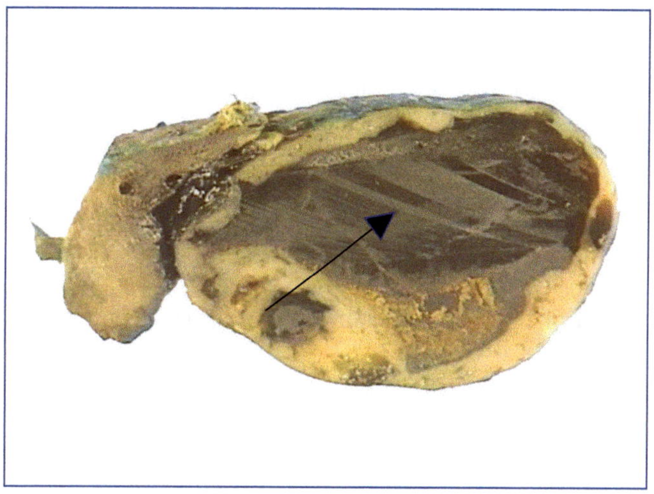

Figure 4-36. Gross section. Cystic degeneration (*arrow*).

Follicular Adenoma Right Lobe

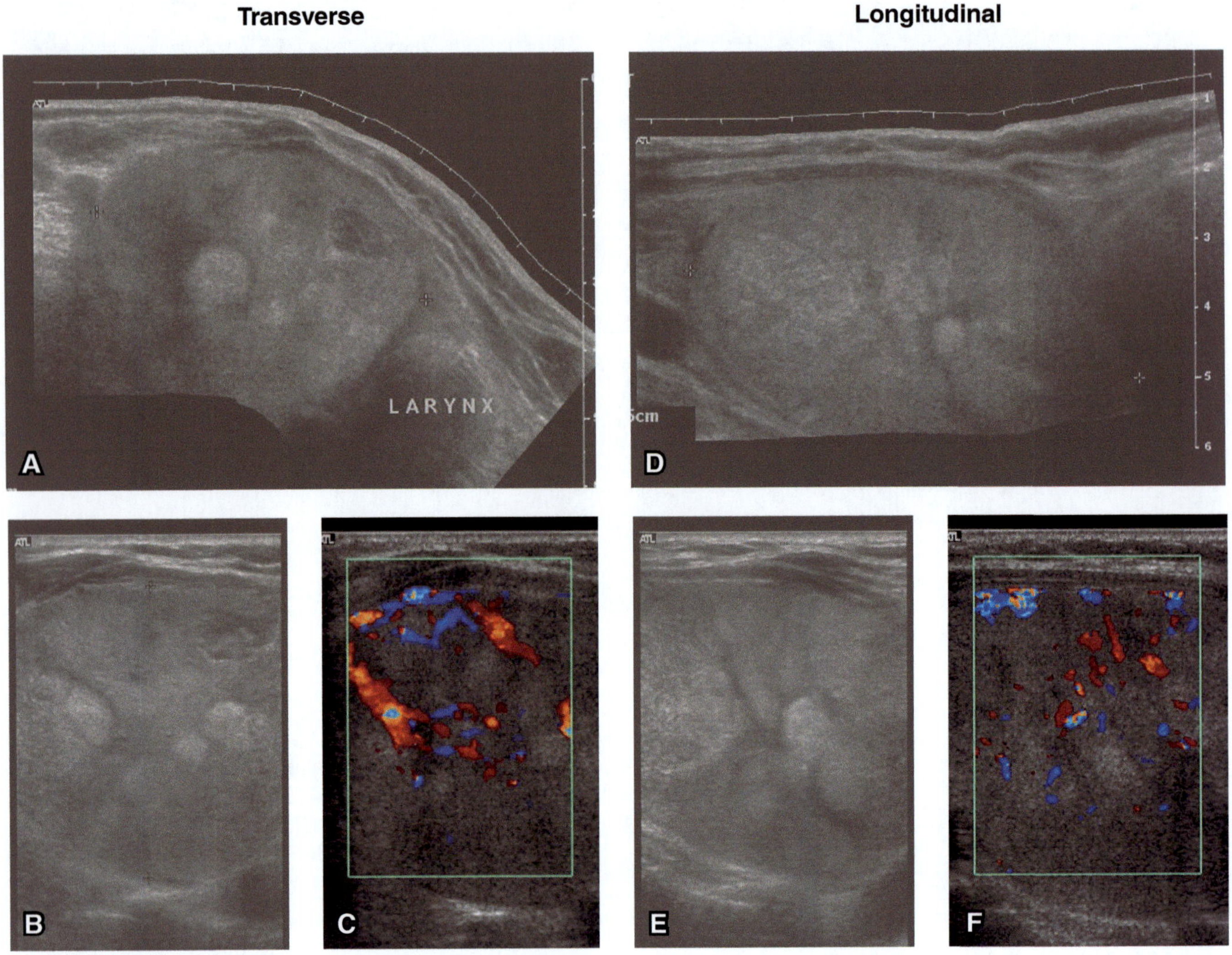

Figure 4-37. Ultrasound of follicular adenoma in the right lobe. **A**, Transverse, 40 x 50 mm. **B**, Transverse. **C**, Color Doppler, transverse. **D**, Longitudinal, sagittal diameter: 66 mm. **E**, Longitudinal. **F**, Color Doppler, longitudinal.

76-Year-old woman

- **Clinical history:** Nodular goiter for some years.
- **Ultrasound:** Probably follicular adenoma.
- **Cytology:** Follicular neoplasia?
- **16-Gauge histologic needle biopsy:** Follicular tumor.
- **Right hemithyroidectomy:** Follicular adenoma.

Features

Slightly hypoechoic
Nodular and lobulated echo pattern
Well circumscribed
Almost no hypoechoic halo
Scantly vascularized

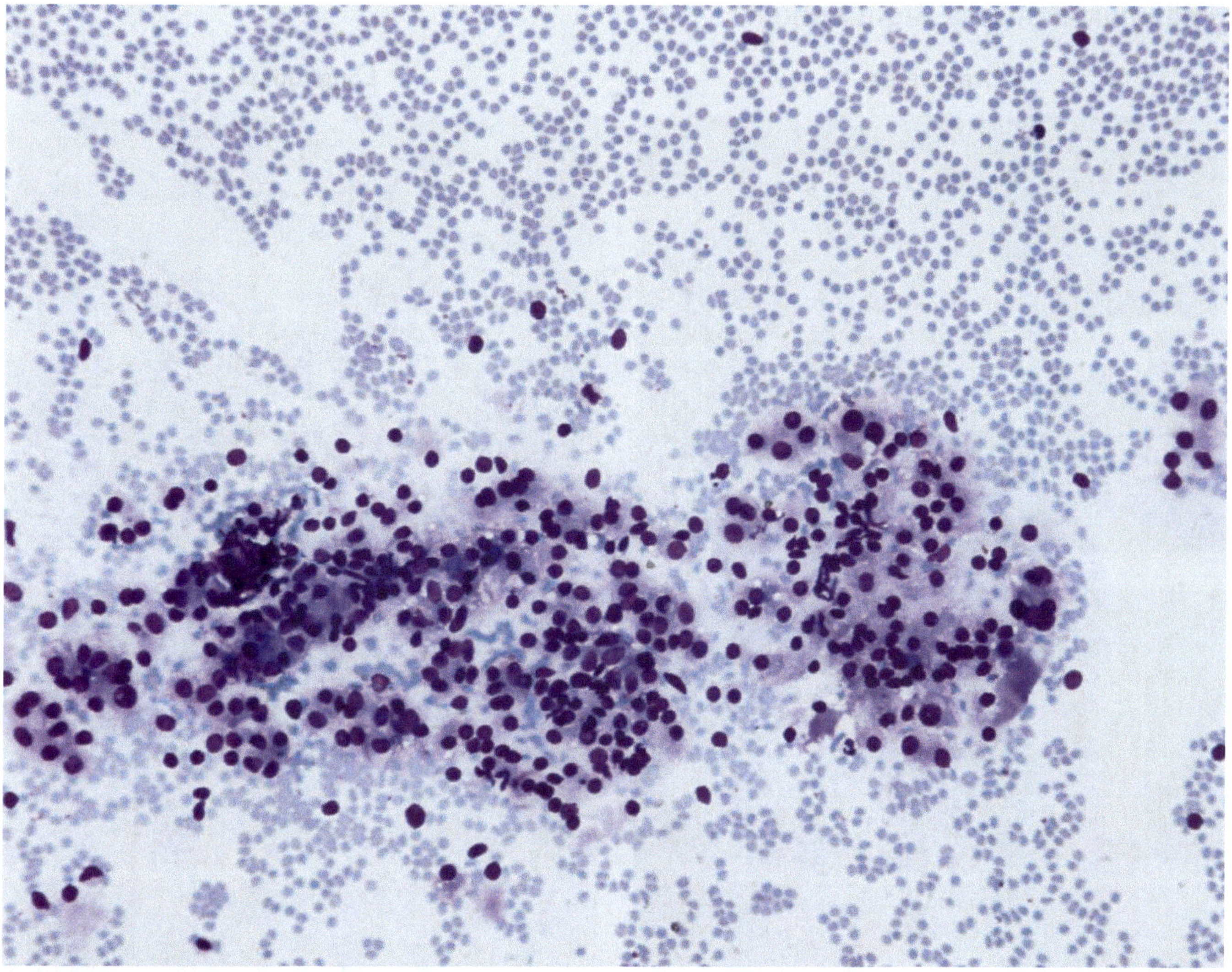

Figure 4-38. Cytology: suspicious for follicular neoplasia.

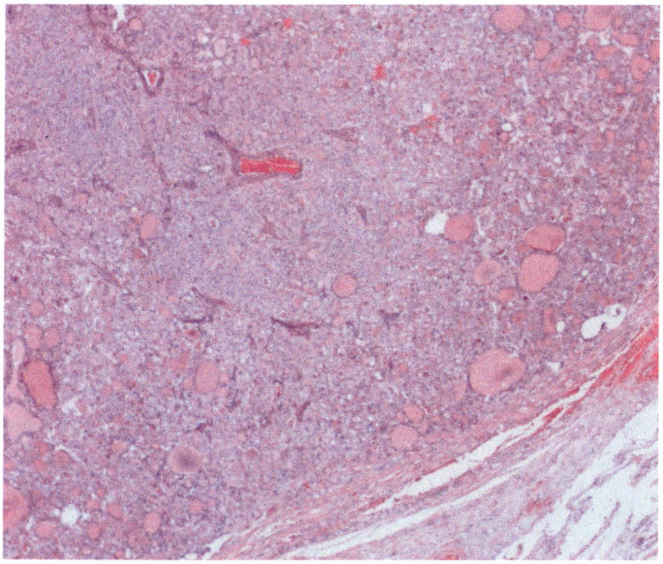

Figure 4-39. Histology: follicular adenoma.

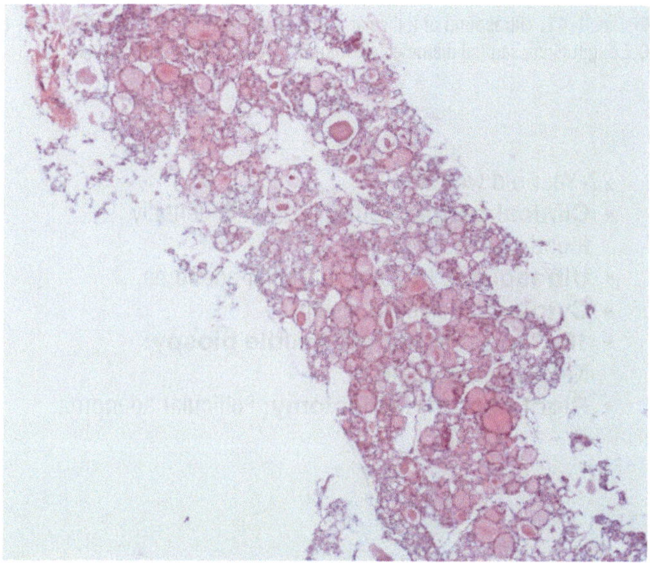

Figure 4-40. Histologic needle biopsy: follicular lesion.

Follicular Adenoma Right Lobe

Transverse **Longitudinal**

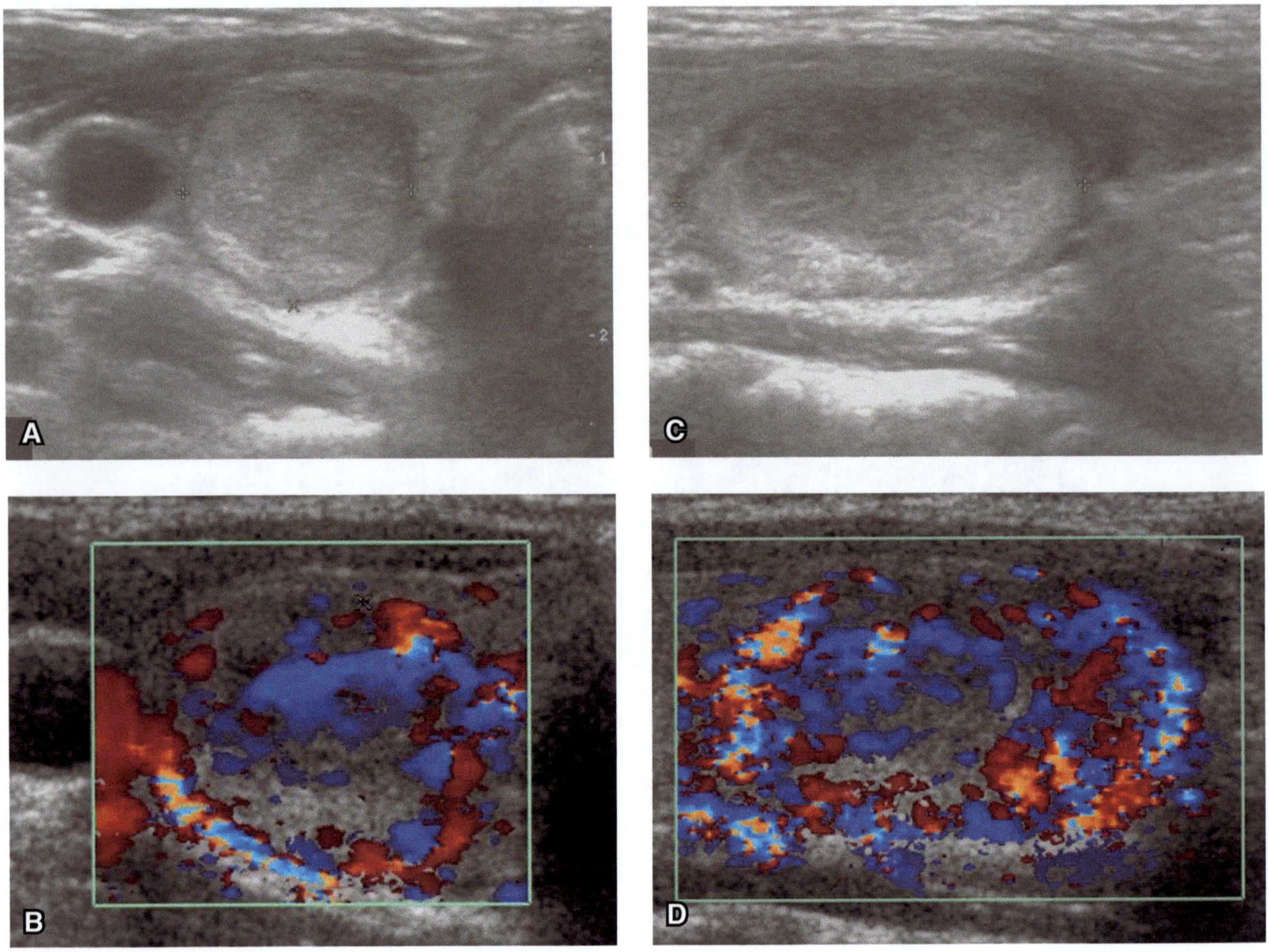

FIGURE 4-41. Ultrasound of follicular adenoma in the right lobe. **A**, Transverse, 12 x 13 mm. **B**, Color Doppler, transverse. **C**, Longitudinal, sagittal diameter: 22 mm. **D**, Color Doppler, longitudinal.

27-Year-old woman

- **Clinical history:** Small tumor incidentally found on MR.
- **Ultrasound:** Probably follicular adenoma.
- **Cytology:** Follicular lesion.
- **18-Gauge histologic needle biospy:** Not diagnostic material.
- **Right hemithyroidectomy:** Follicular adenoma.

Features

Slightly hypoechoic
Geographic inhomogeneous echo pattern
Well circumscribed
Thin hypoechoic halo
Microcalcifications?
Hypervascularized
Suggestion of "spoke-and-wheel-like" vascularity

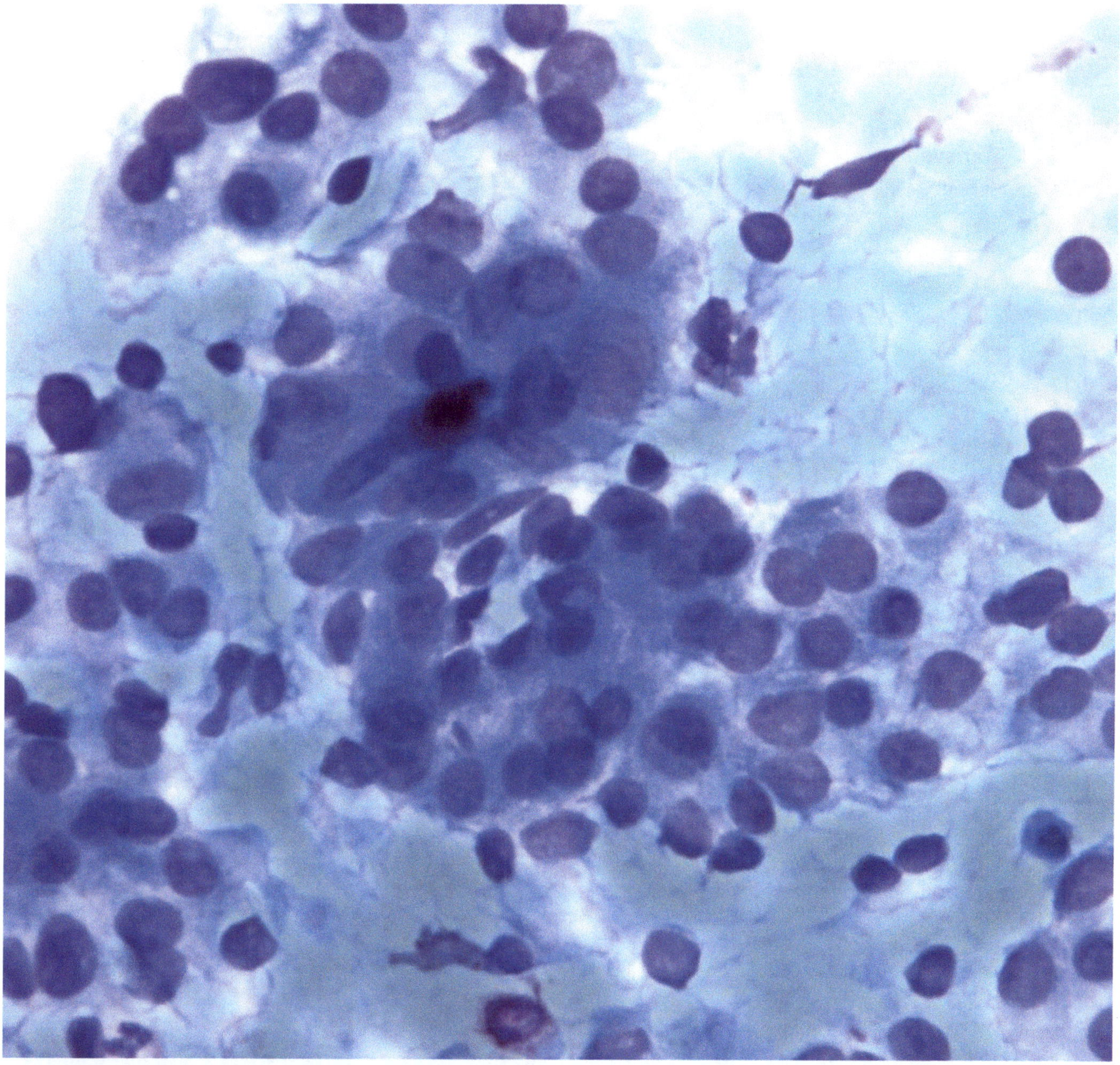

FIGURE 4-42. Cytology: follicular structures with central colloid.

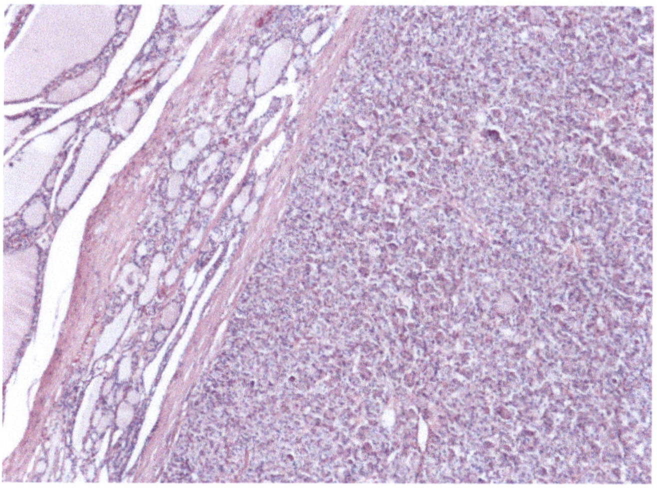

FIGURE 4-43. Histology: follicular neoplasia adjacent to normal thyroid tissue.

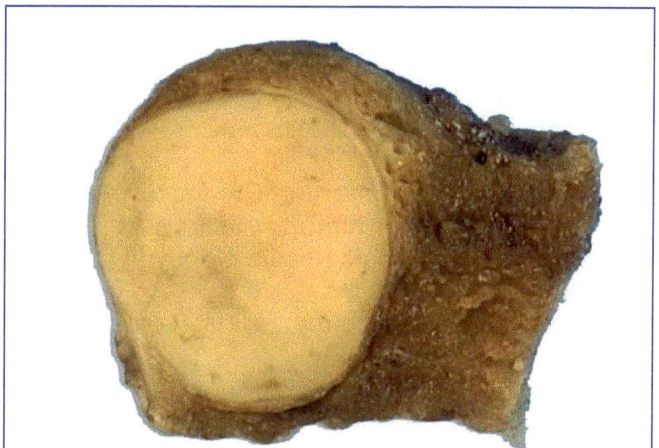

FIGURE 4-44. Gross section: well-circumscribed lesion.

Follicular Adenomas Left Lobe

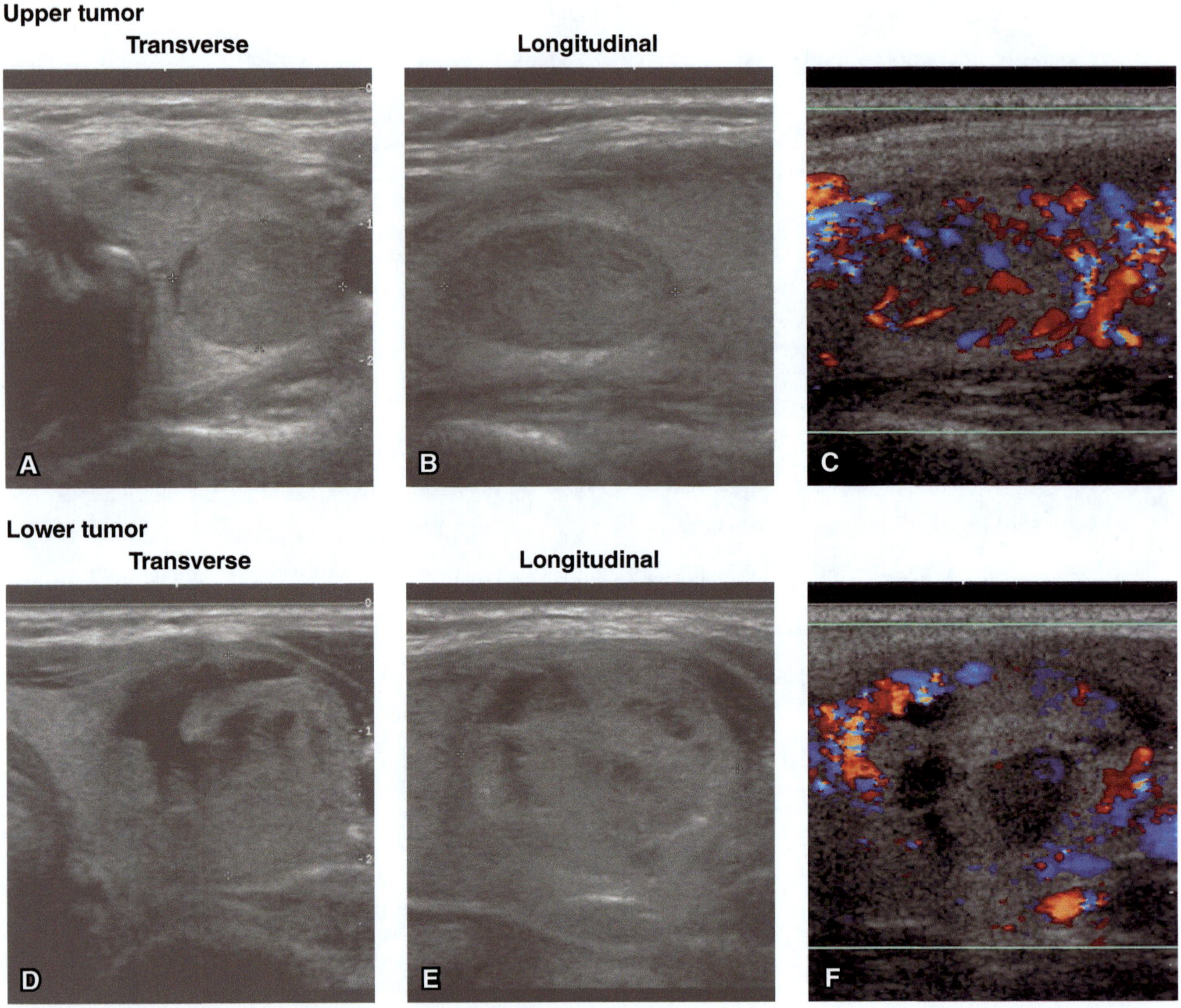

FIGURE 4-45. Ultrasound of follicular adenomas in the left lobe. **A**, Upper tumor, transverse: 9 x 12 mm. **B**, Upper tumor, longitudinal, sagittal diameter: 17 mm. **C**, Upper tumor, color Doppler. **D**, Lower tumor, transverse: 17 x 20 mm. **E**, Lower tumor, longitudinal, sagittal diameter: 21 mm. **F**, Lower tumor, color Doppler.

50-Year-old woman

- **Clinical history:** Palpable nodule in right lobe for some months.
- **Ultrasound:** Colloid nodules? Follicular adenomas?
- **Cytology of lower tumor:** Follicular lesion.
- **18-Gauge histologic needle biopsy:** Macro- and microfollicles.
- **Left hemithyroidectomy:** Follicular adenomas.

Features of upper tumor
Moderately hypoechoic
Inhomogeneous echo pattern
Well circumscribed
Suggestion of "spoke-and-wheel-like" vascularity

Features of lower tumor
Slightly hypoechoic
Inhomogeneous echo pattern
Cystic areas
Quite well circumscribed
A few microcalcifications
Peripheral vascularity

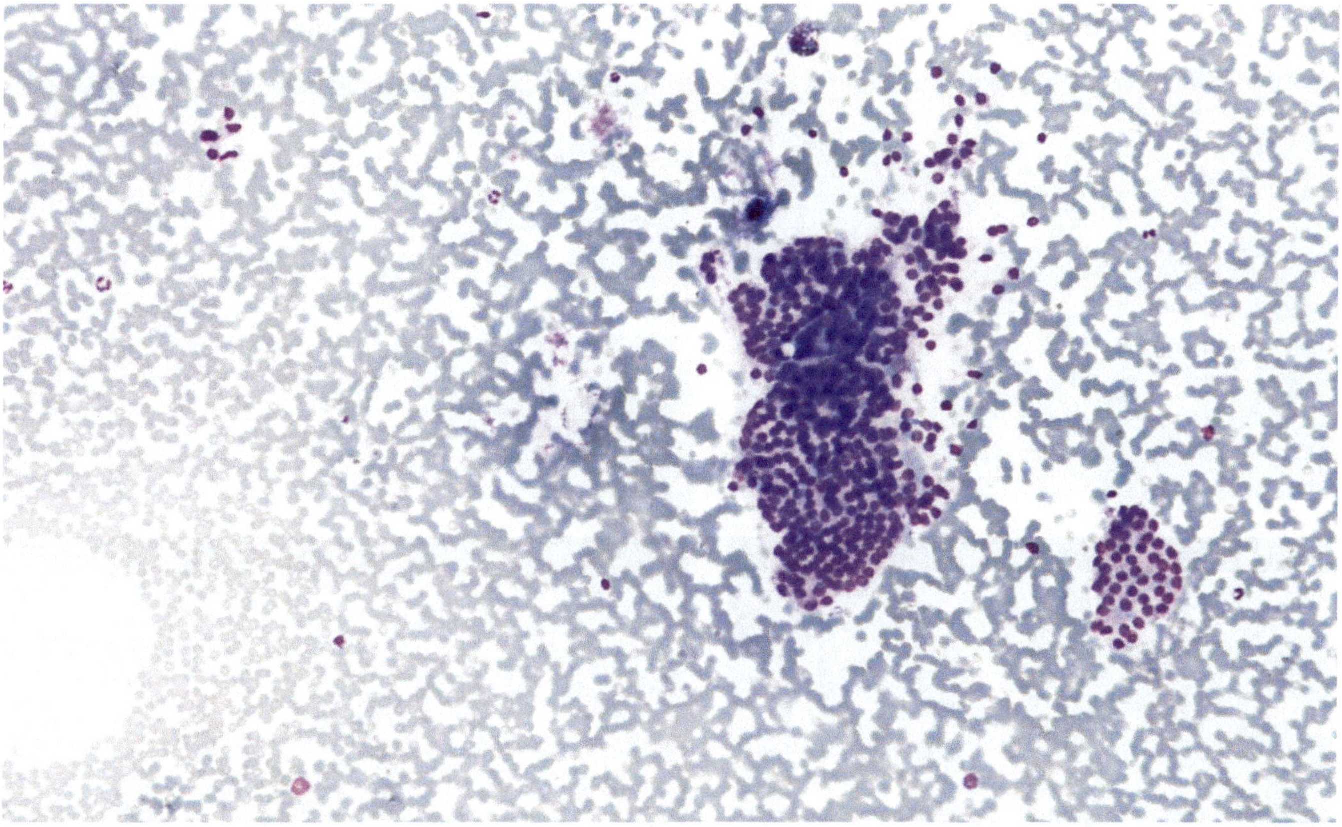

Figure 4-46. Cytology: rich in follicular cells.

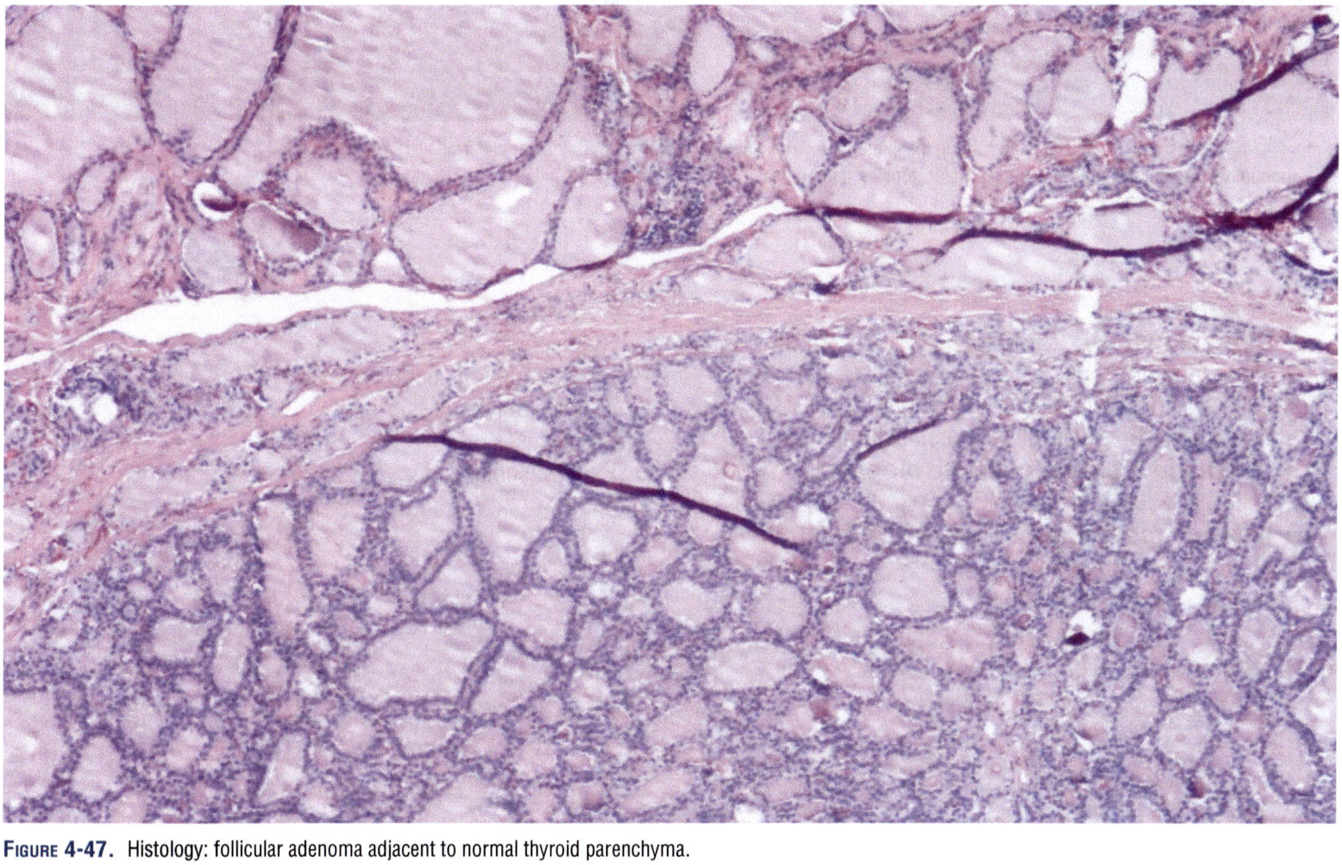

Figure 4-47. Histology: follicular adenoma adjacent to normal thyroid parenchyma.

Follicular Adenoma Isthmus

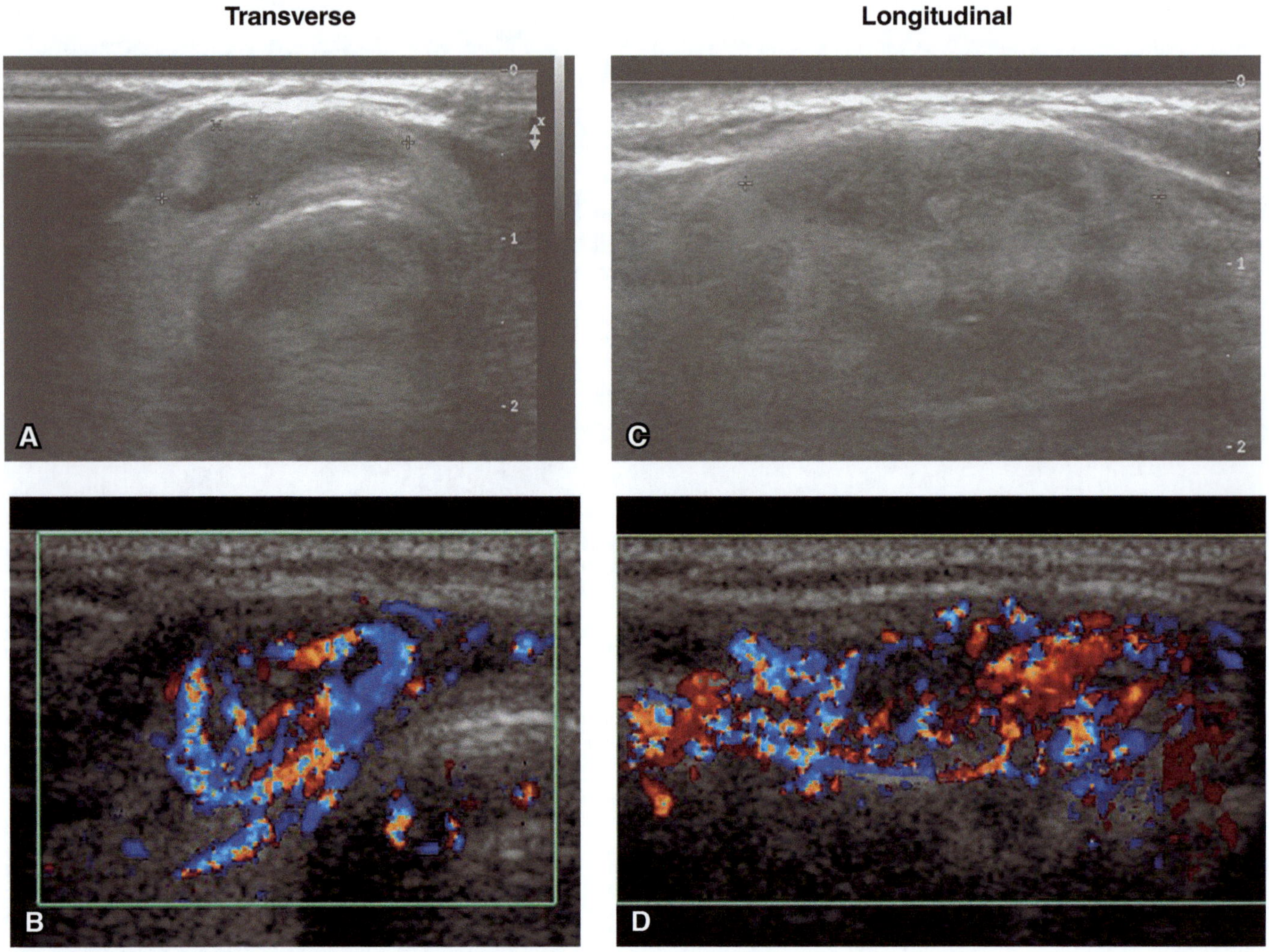

Figure 4-48. Ultrasound of follicular adenoma in the isthmus. **A**, Transverse, 5 x 15 mm. **B**, Color Doppler, transverse. **C**, Longitudinal, sagittal diameter: 22 mm. **D**, Color Doppler, longitudinal.

56-Year-old woman

- **Clinical history:** Palpable nodule for some months.
- **Ultrasound:** Tumor of uncertain nature.
- **Cytology:** Irregular follicular epithelium.
- **16-Gauge histologic needle biopsy:** Follicular neoplasia.
- **Isthmus resection:** Follicular adenoma.

Features

Hypoechoic
Inhomogeneous echo pattern
Mostly well circumscribed
Small cyst
Hypervascularized

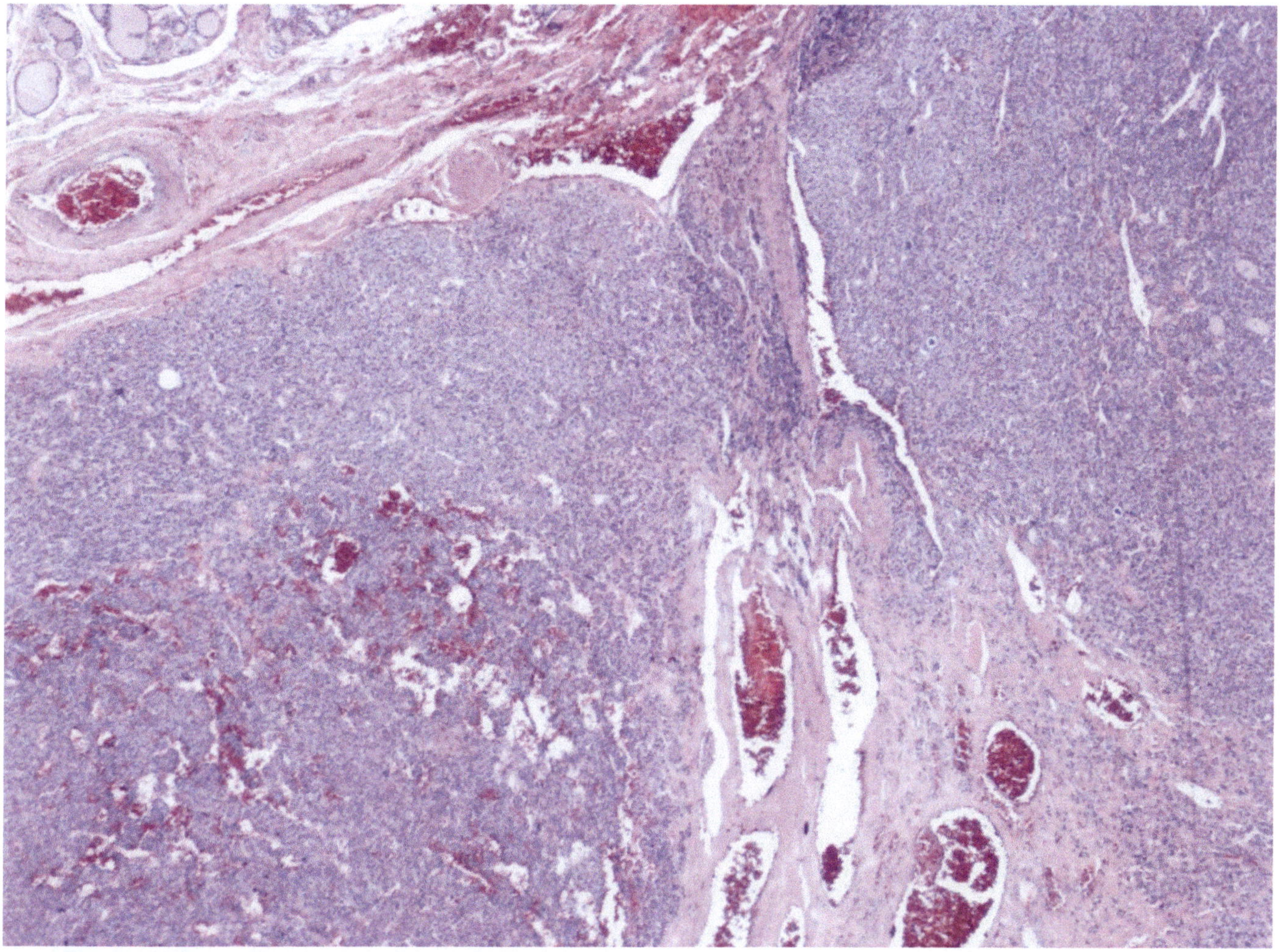

FIGURE 4-49. Histology: follicular adenoma.

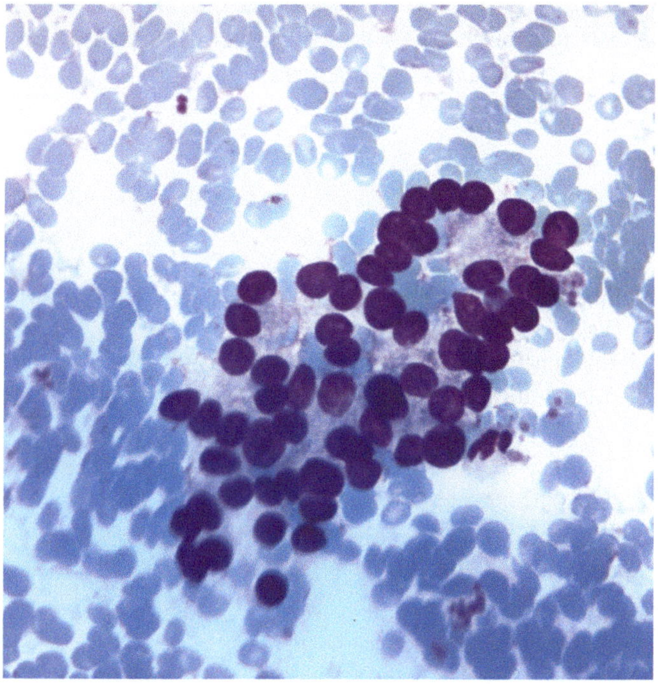

FIGURE 4-50. Cytology: follicular structures.

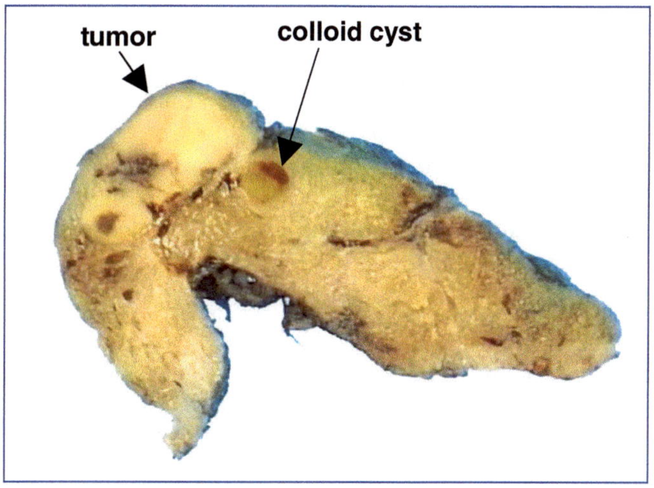

FIGURE 4-51. Gross section: tumor in isthmus.

Follicular Adenoma Right Lobe/Isthmus

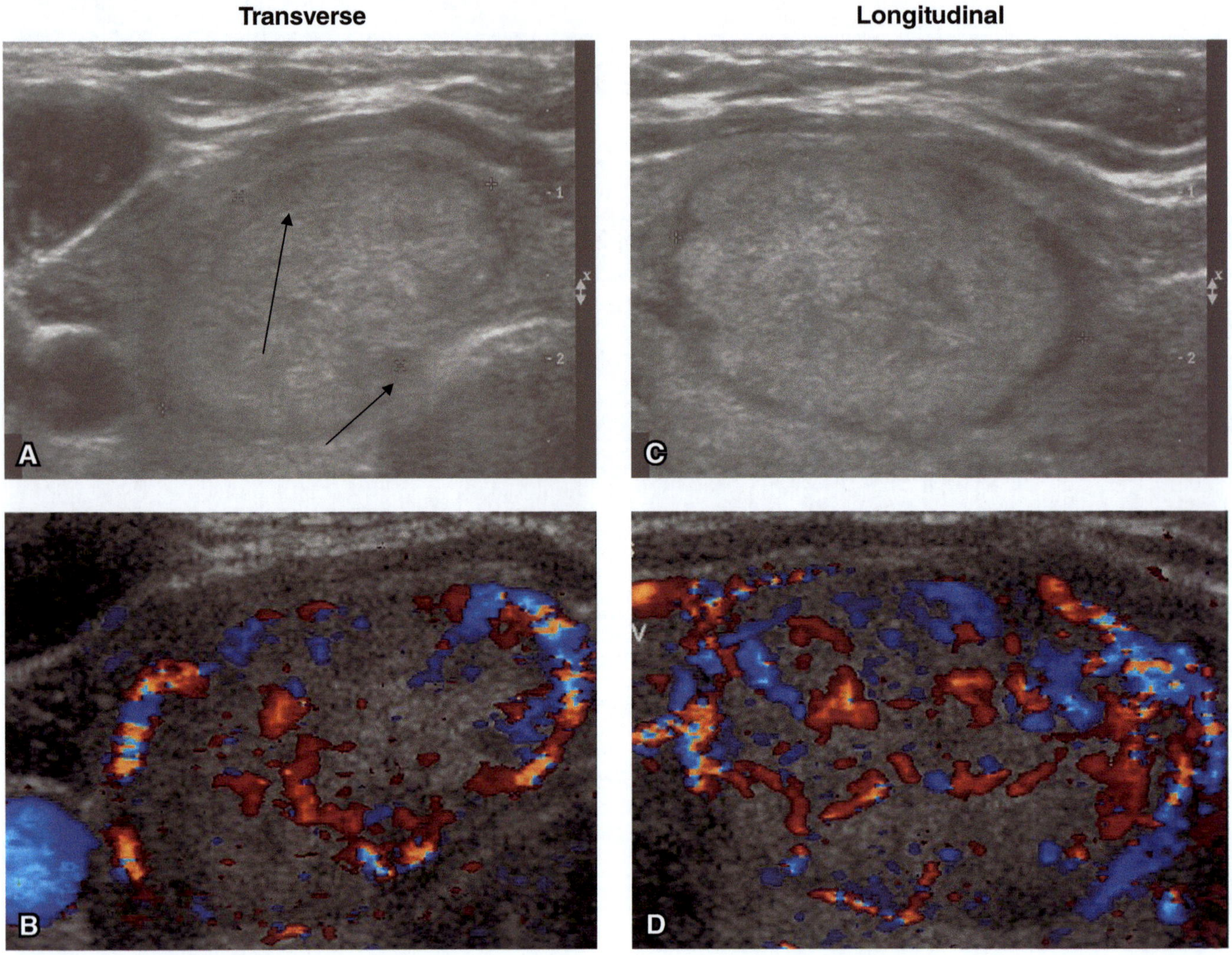

FIGURE 4-52. Ultrasound of follicular adenoma in the right lobe and isthmus. **A**, Transverse, 14 x 24 mm. *Arrows* show hemorrhages. **B**, Color Doppler, transverse. **C**, Longitudinal, sagittal diameter: 25 mm. **D**, Color Doppler, longitudinal.

39 Year-old woman

- **Clinical history:** Palpable tumor for some months.
- **Ultrasound:** Follicular tumor. Malignant?
- **Cytology:** Follicular lesion.
- **16-Gauge histologic needle biopsy:** Follicular lesion.
- **Right hemithyroidectomy:** Follicular adenoma.

Features

Almost isoechoic
Inhomogeneous echo pattern
Well circumscribed
Thin, uneven hypoechoic halo
"Spoke-and-wheel-like" vascularity

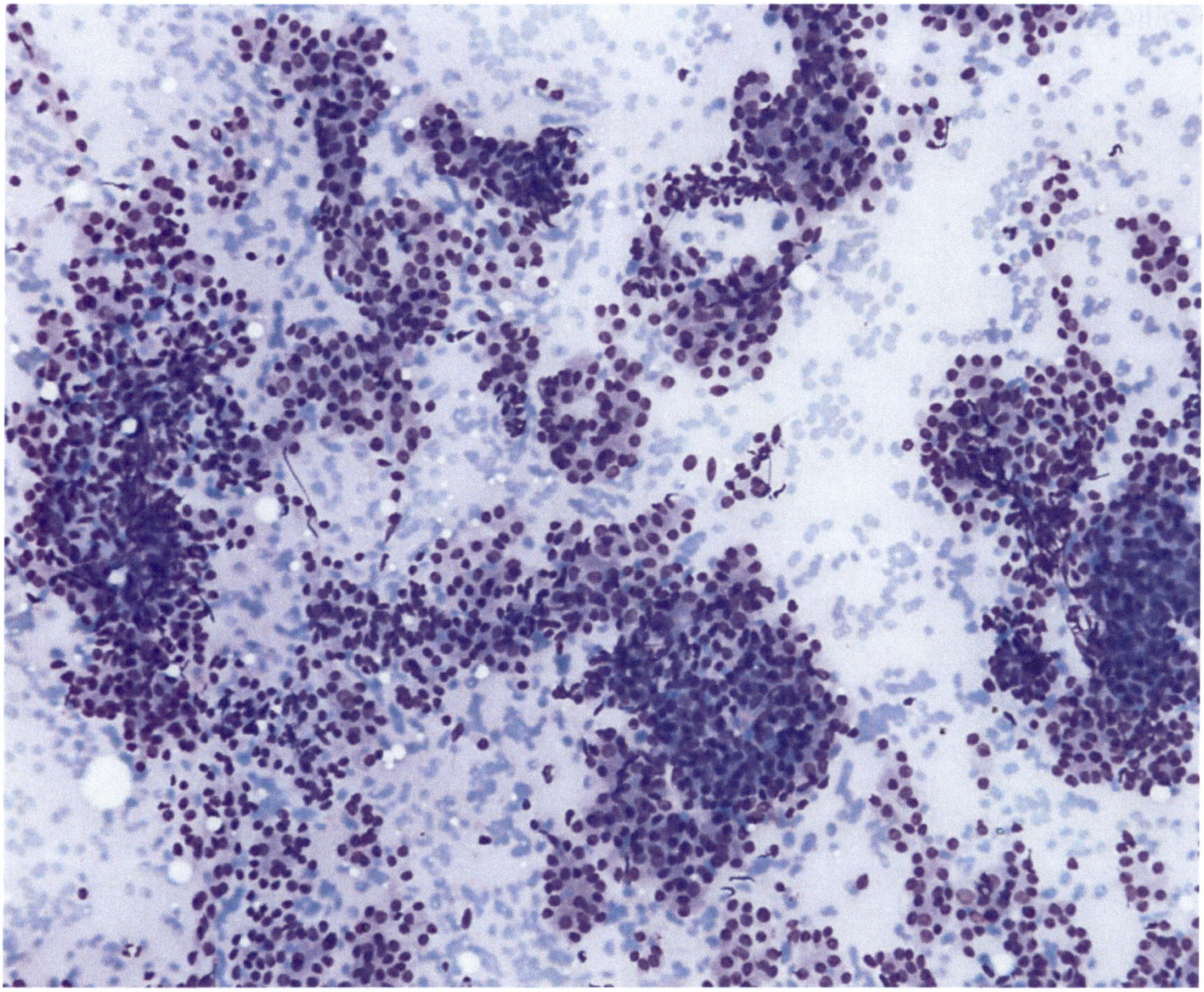

Figure 4-53. Cytology: rich in follicular epithelium, favors follicular neoplasia.

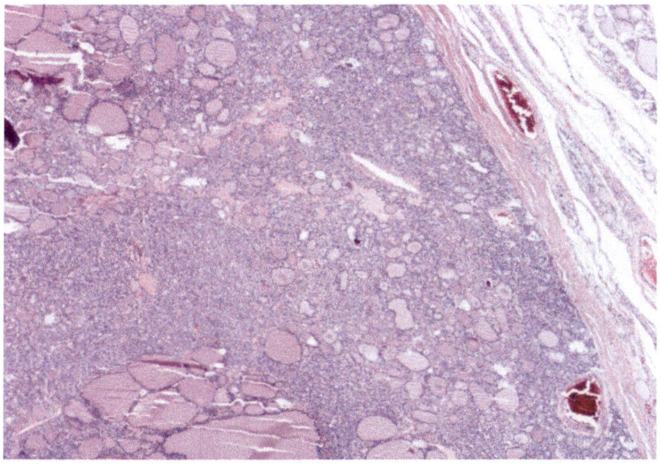

Figure 4-54. Histology: follicular adenoma.

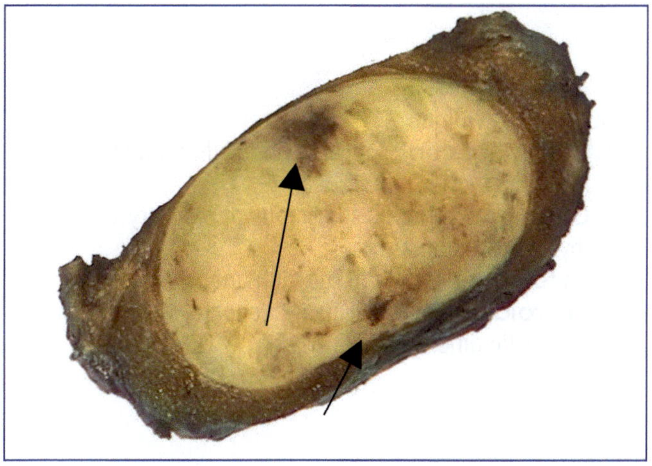

Figure 4-55. Gross section: well-circumscribed nodule with hemorrhages (*arrows*) in the right lobe. Good correlation with US image.

Follicular Adenoma Right Lobe

Transverse | Longitudinal

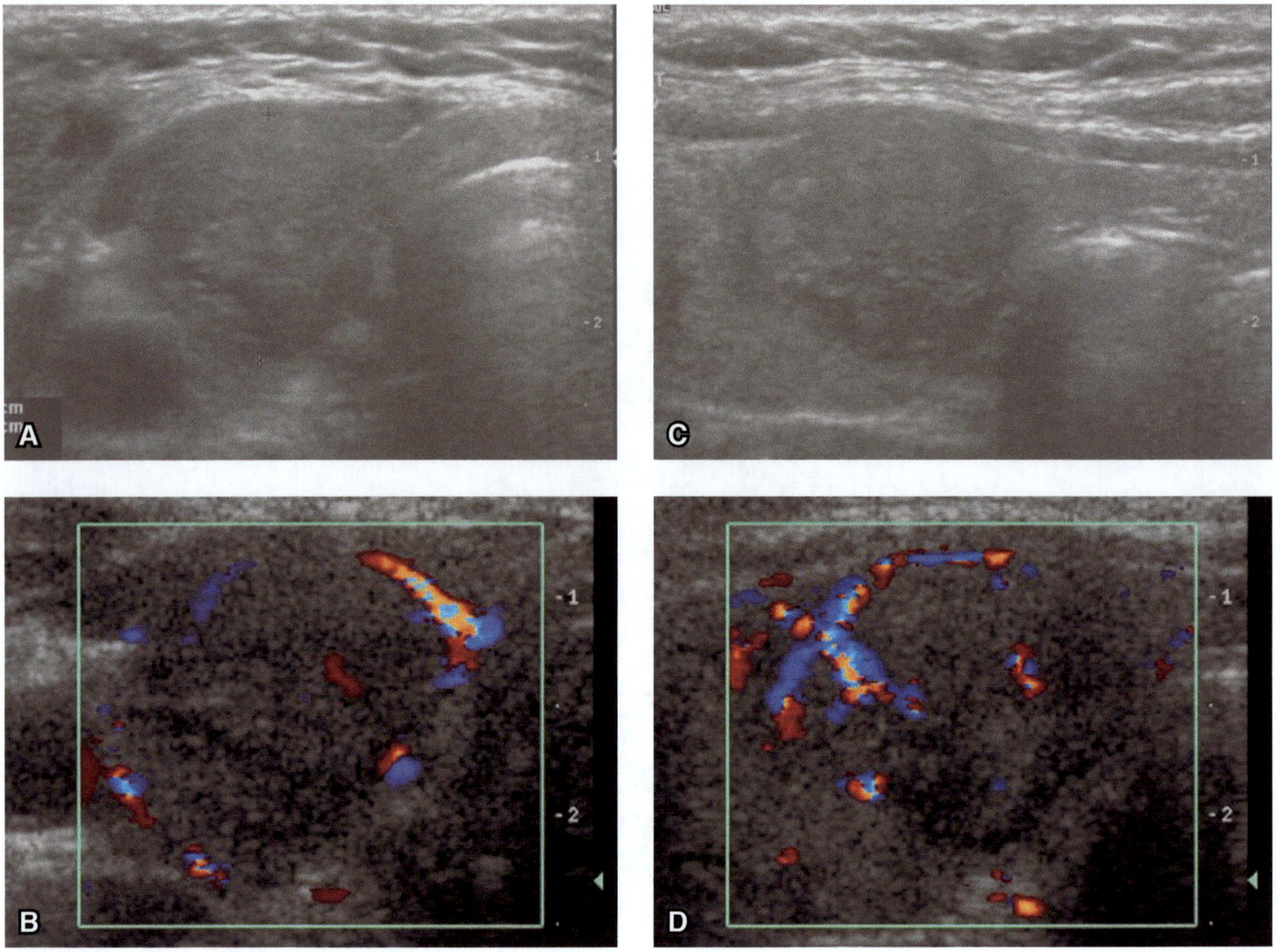

Figure 4-56. Ultrasound of follicular adenoma in the right lobe. **A**, Transverse, 15 x 15 mm. **B**, Color Doppler, transverse. **C**, Longitudinal, sagittal diameter: 17 mm. **D**, Color Doppler, longitudinal.

66-Year-old woman

- **Clinical history:** Palpable nodule in right lobe for some months.
- **Ultrasound:** Highly suspicious of papillary thyroid carcinoma.
- **Cytology:** Necrotic tissue with oncocytic cells.
- **Thyroidectomy:** Follicular adenoma with oncocytic differentiation.

Features

Strongly hypoechoic
Inhomogeneous echo pattern
Blurred margins
Microcalcifications
Scantly vascularized

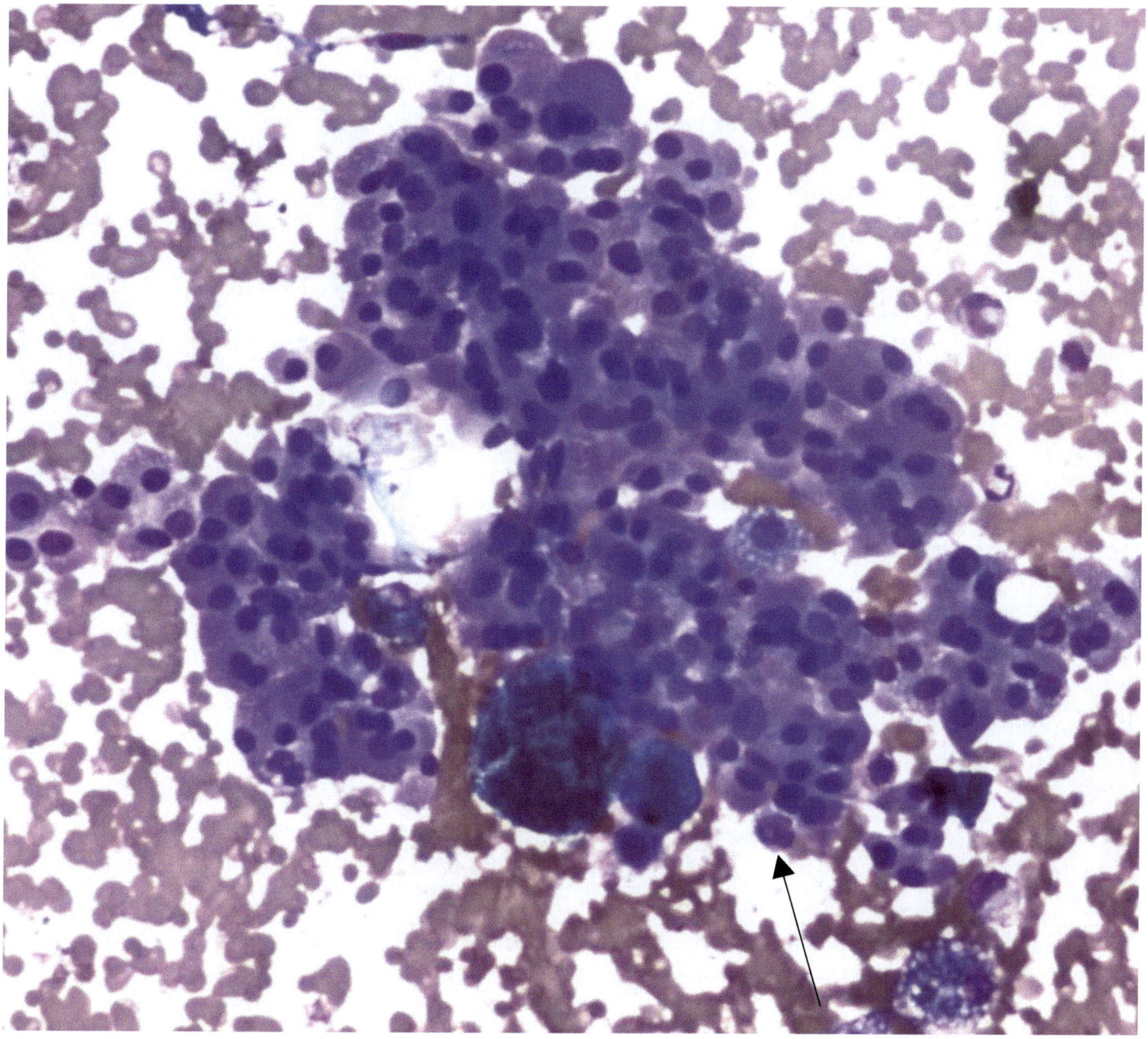

Figure 4-57. Cytology: oncocytic epithelium (*arrow*).

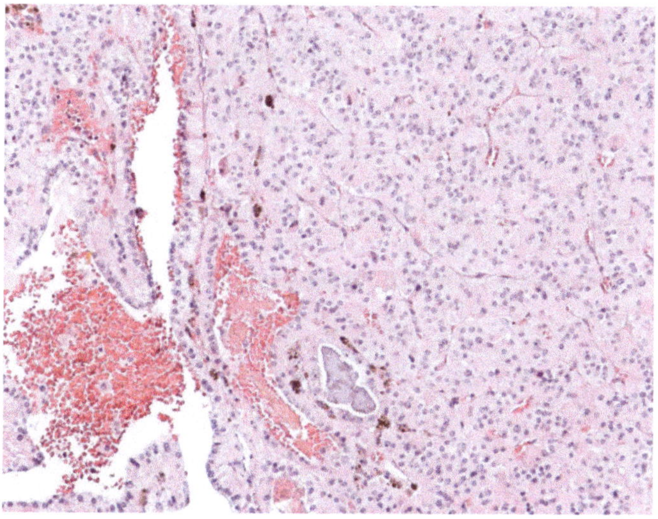

Figure 4-58. Histology: area with oncocytic cells within tumor.

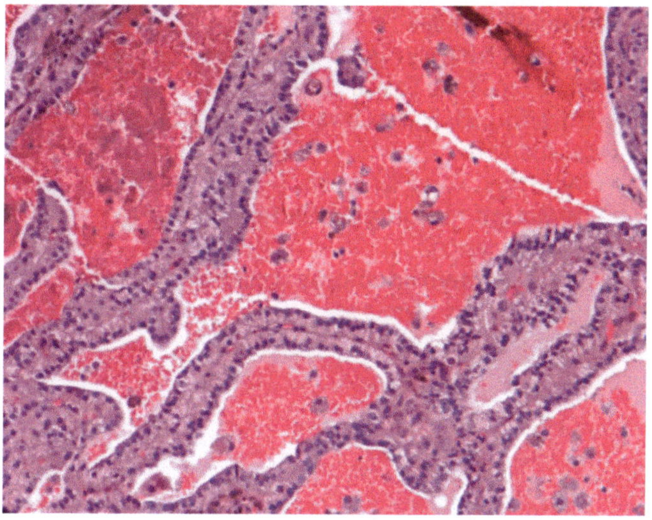

Figure 4-59. Histology: area with papillary growth pattern and bleeding. Note: often areas of bleeding in oncocytic variants of follicular neoplasia.

Follicular Adenoma Left Lobe

Transverse **Longitudinal**

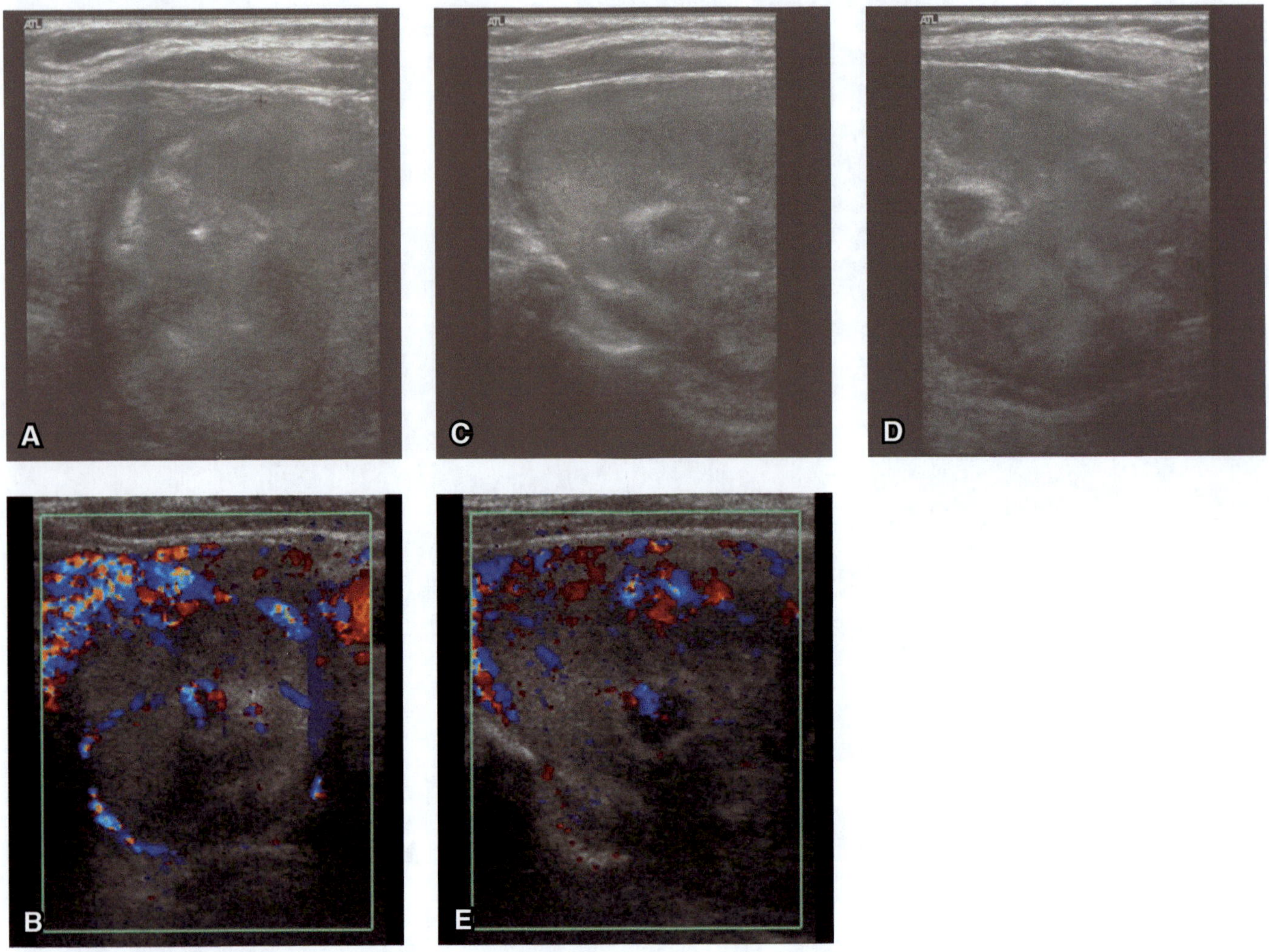

FIGURE 4-60. Ultrasound of follicular adenoma in the left lobe. **A**, Transverse, 27 x 39 mm. **B**, Color Doppler, transverse. **C**, Upper part, longitudinal. **D**, Lower part, longitudinal. **E**, Color Doppler, longitudinal.

76-Year-old woman

- **Clinical history:** Tumor in right lobe incidentally found on CT. No palpable mass.
- **Ultrasound:** Follicular variant of papillary thyroid carcinoma?
- **Cytology:** Follicular lesion.
- **18-Gauge histologic needle biopsy:** Follicular lesion.
- **Left hemithyroidectomy:** Follicular adenoma + Hashimoto's thyroiditis.

Features

Slightly hyperechoic compared with hypoechoic thyroid tissue due to Hashimoto's thyroiditis
Inhomogeneous echo pattern, but also areas with quite uniform echo texture
Well circumscribed
Both coarse calcifications and microcalcifications
Thin hypoechoic halo
"Spoke-and-wheel-like" hypervascularity

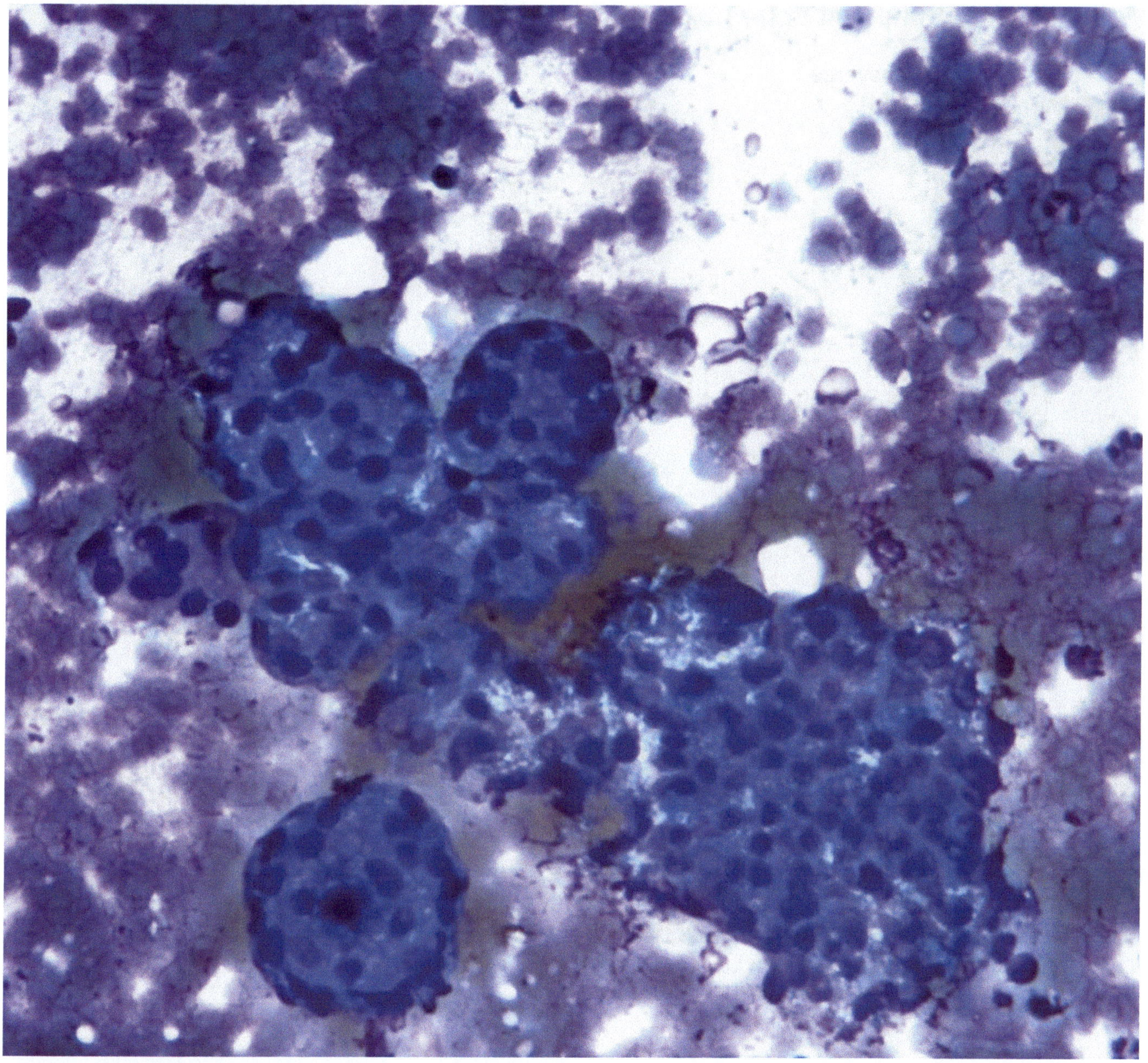

Figure 4-61. Cytology: follicular structures.

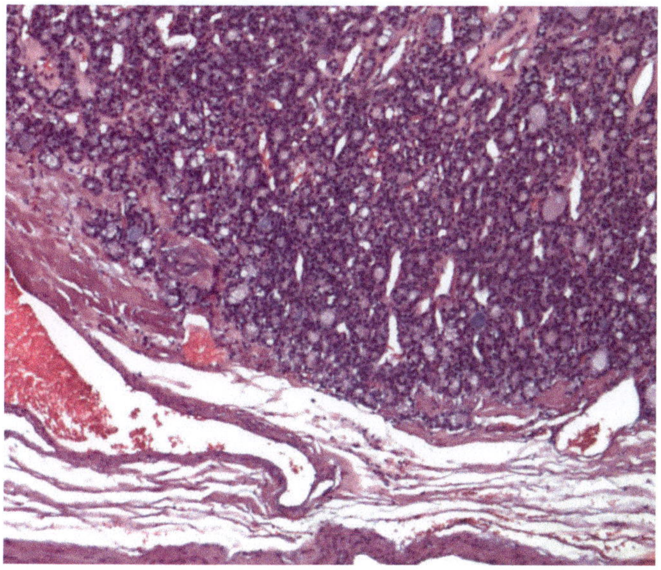

Figure 4-62. Histology: follicular adenoma.

Follicular Adenoma Left Lobe

Transverse | **Longitudinal**

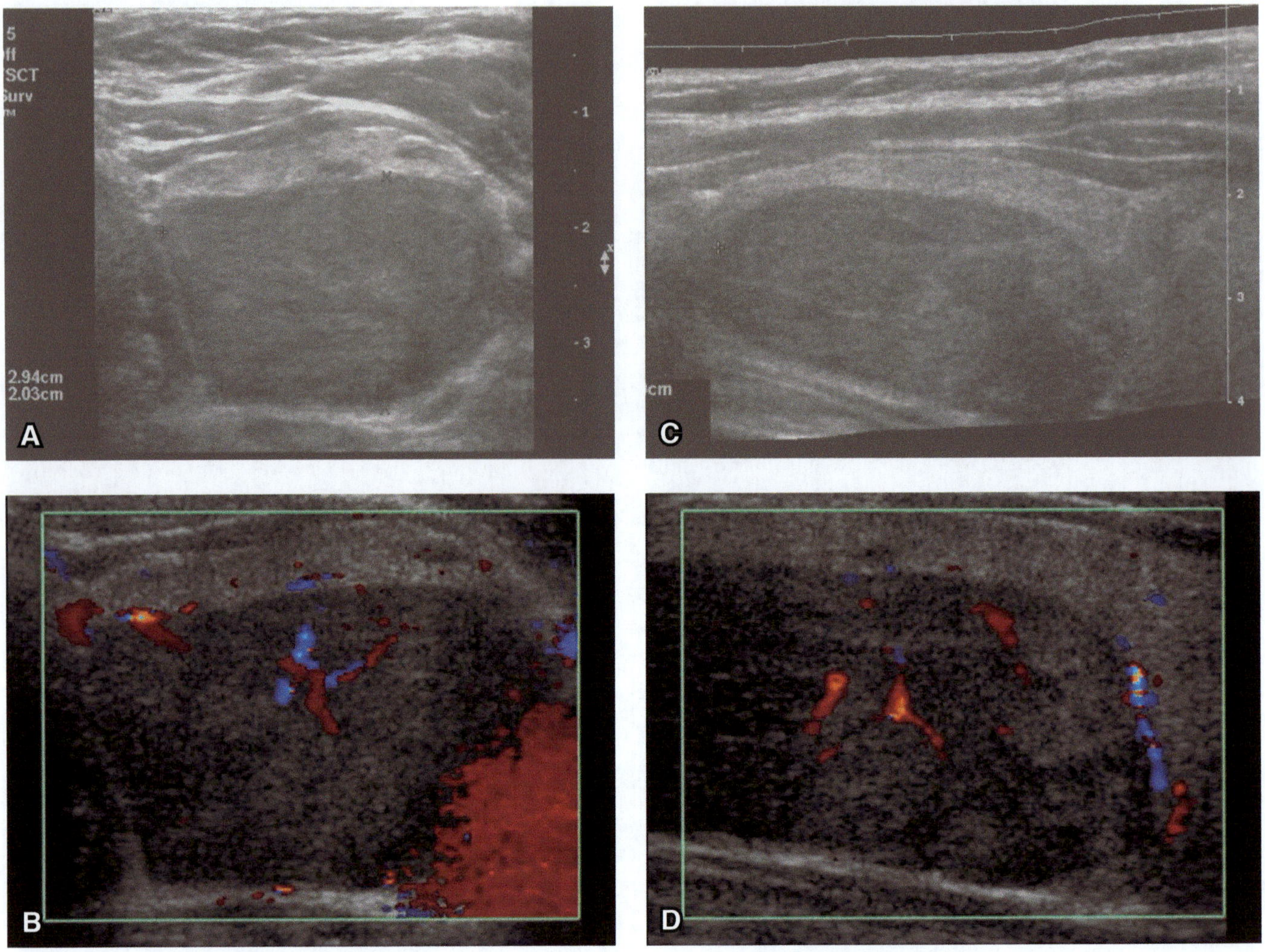

Figure 4-63. Ultrasound of follicular adenoma in the left lobe. **A**, Transverse, 20 x 29 mm. **B**, Color Doppler, transverse. **C**, Longitudinal, sagittal diameter: 40 mm. **D**, Color Doppler, longitudinal.

49-Year-old woman

- **Clinical history:** Right hemithyroidectomy 10 years ago. Nodular goiter past 3 years.
- **Ultrasound:** Unspecified. Lymphoma?
- **Cytology:** Suspicious for follicular neoplasia with oncocytic differentiation.
- **Left hemthyroidectomy:** Follicular adenoma with oncocytic differentiation.

Features

Strongly hypoechoic
Quite homogeneous echo pattern
Sharply circumscribed
Scantly vascularized

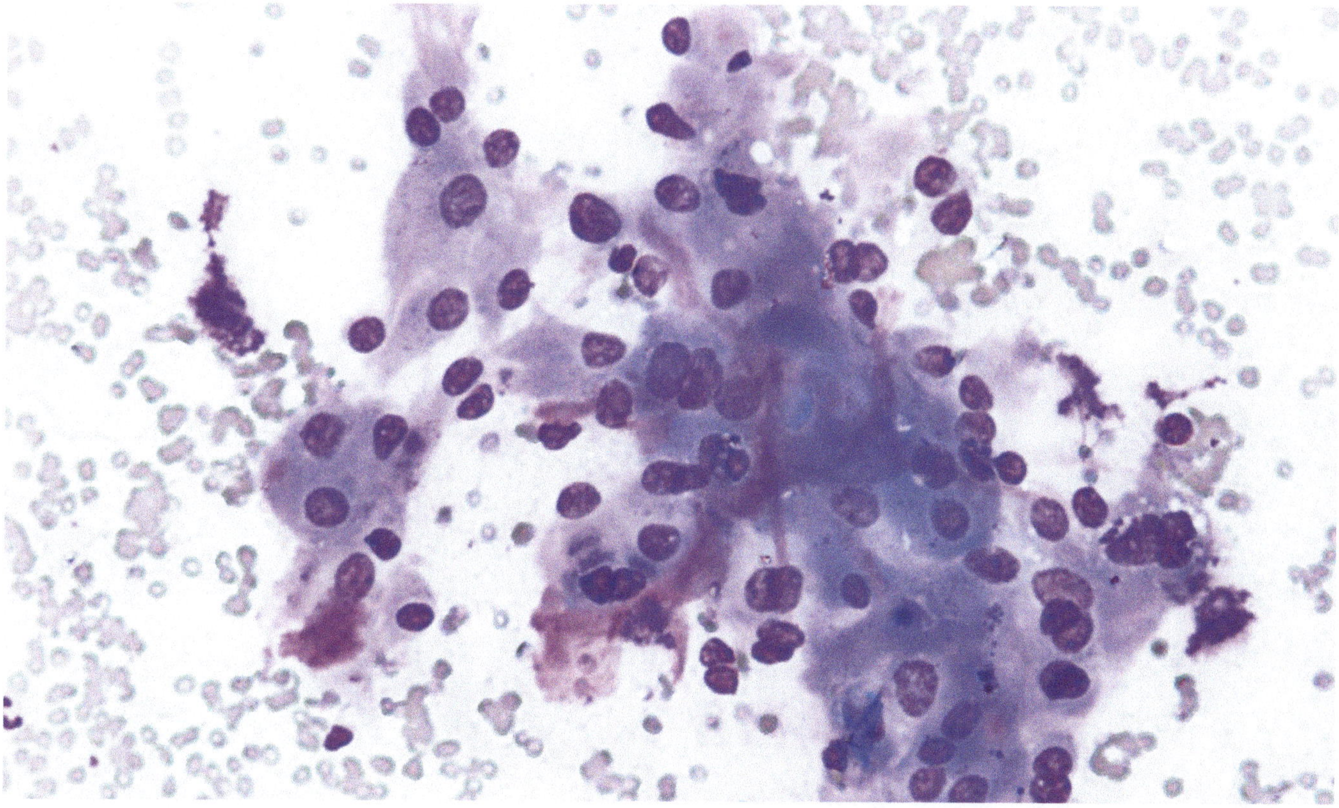

Figure 4-64. Cytology: oncocytic cells.

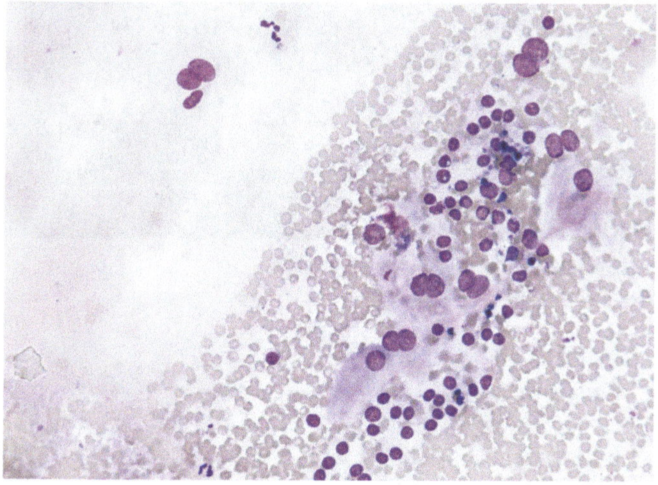

Figure 4-65. Cytology: some oncocytic cells and some follicular cells of normal size.

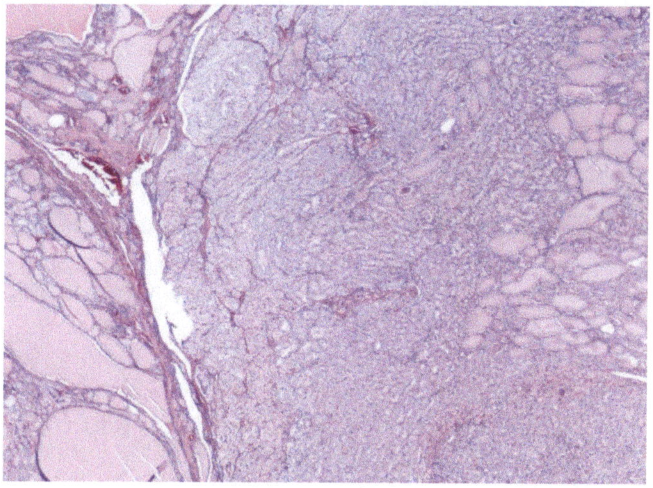

Figure 4-66. Histology: follicular adenoma.

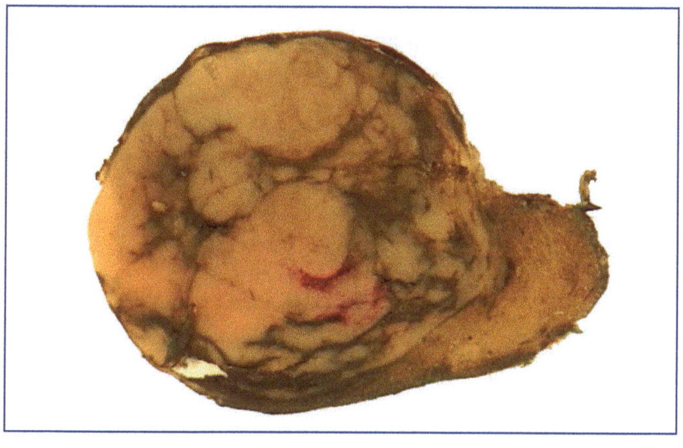

Figure 4-67. Gross section: solid tumor with lobulation.

Follicular Thyroid Carcinoma Isthmus

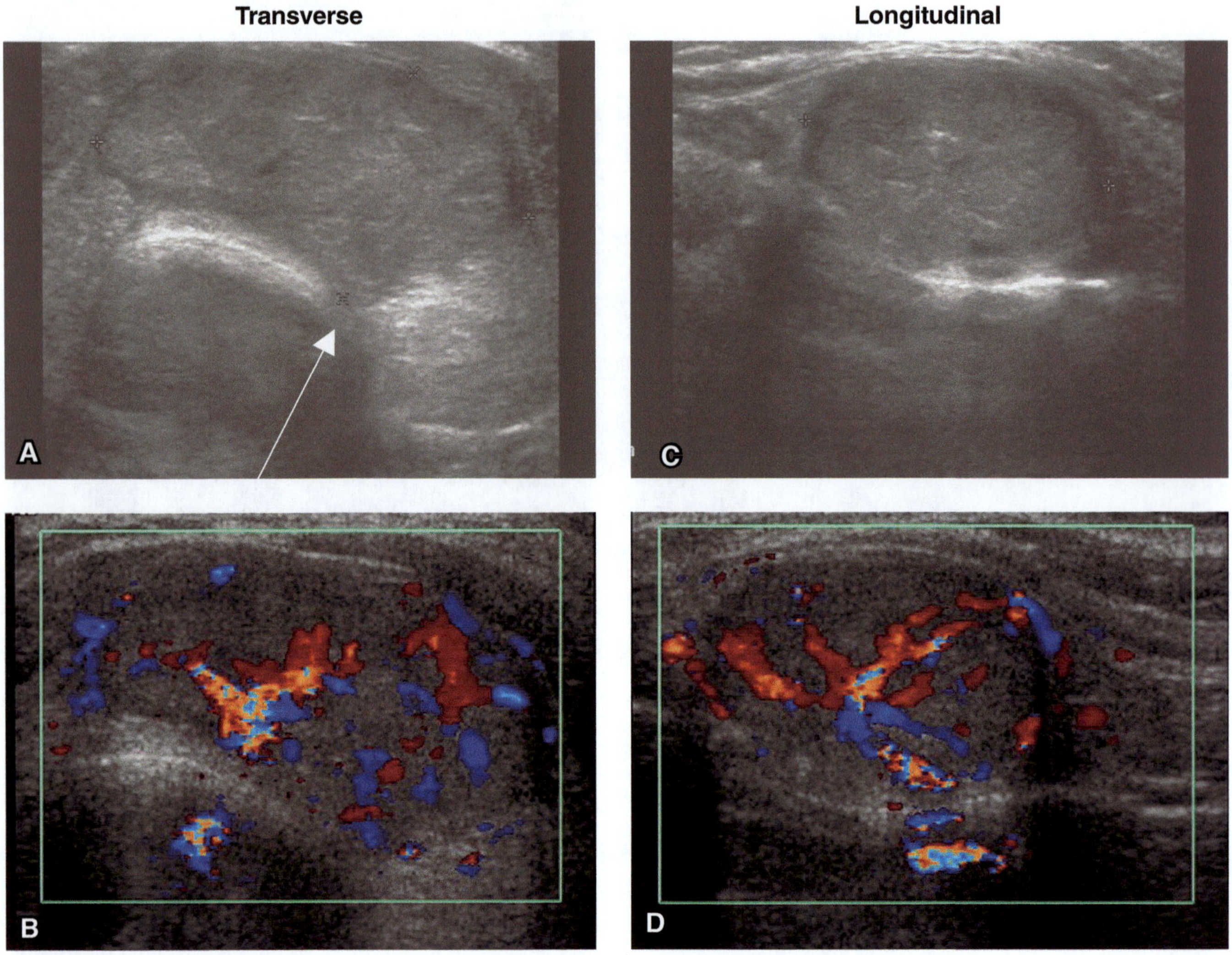

FIGURE 4-68. Ultrasound of follicular thyroid carcinoma in the isthmus. **A**, Transverse, 18 x 32 mm. Infiltration (*arrow*) through the capsule. **B**, Color Doppler, transverse. **C**, Longitudinal, sagittal diameter: 23 mm. **D**, Color Doppler, longitudinal.

53-Year-old man

- **Clinical history:** Right hemithyroidectomy 10 years ago. Nodular goiter past 3 years.
- **Ultrasound:** Probably malignant tumor suspicious for infiltration in trachea.
- **Cytology:** Oncocytic tumor. Follicular neoplasia?
- **18-Gauge histologic needle biopsy:** Oncocytic tumor.
- **Left hemithyroidectomy:** Follicular thyroid carcinoma with oncocytic differentiation. Widely invasive. Not free resectional border posteriorly. Infiltration in fatty tissue.

Features

Hypoechoic
Inhomogeneous echo pattern
Sharply circumscribed
Probably perithyroidal infiltration
Partial uneven hypoechoic halo
Scant vascularity
Suggestion of "spoke-and-wheel-like" vascularity

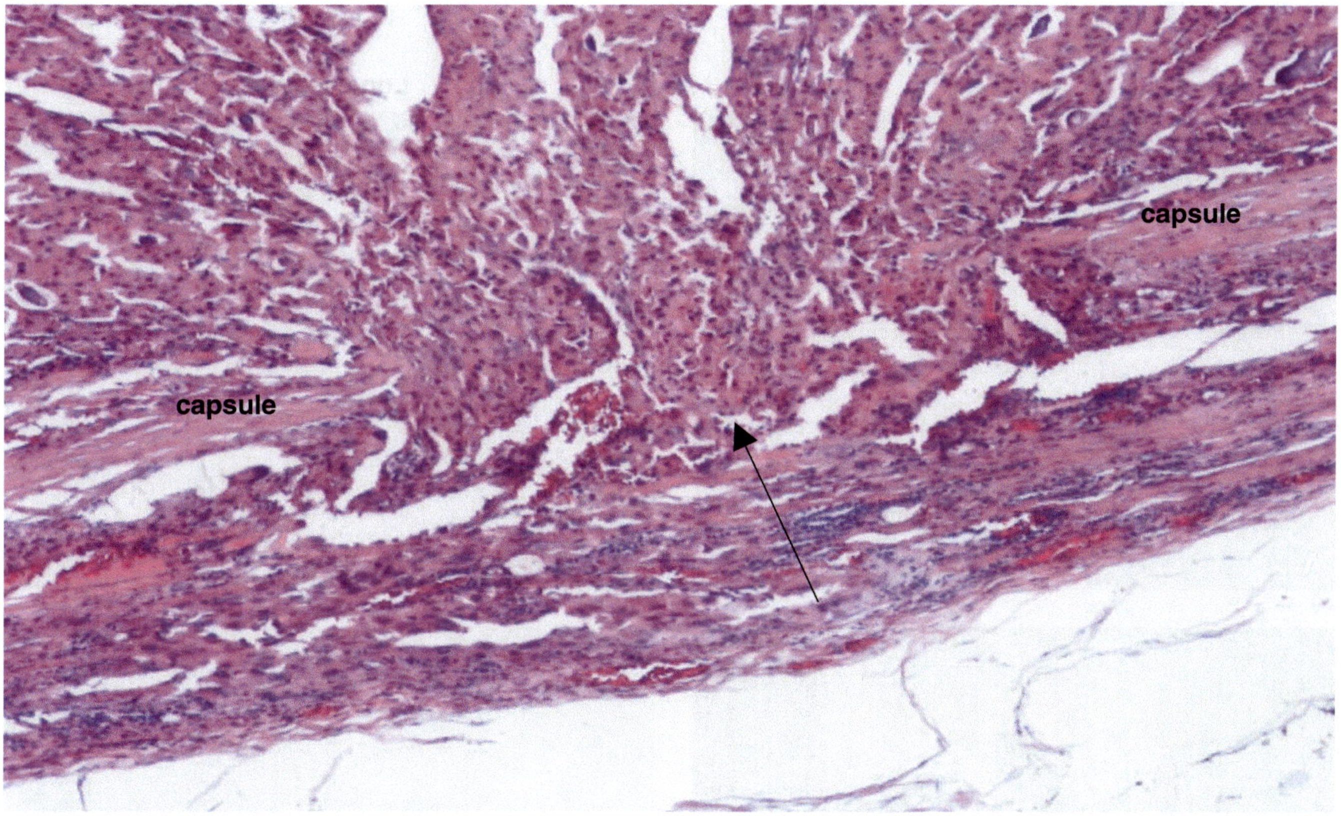

Figure 4-69. Histology: Infiltration through the capsule.

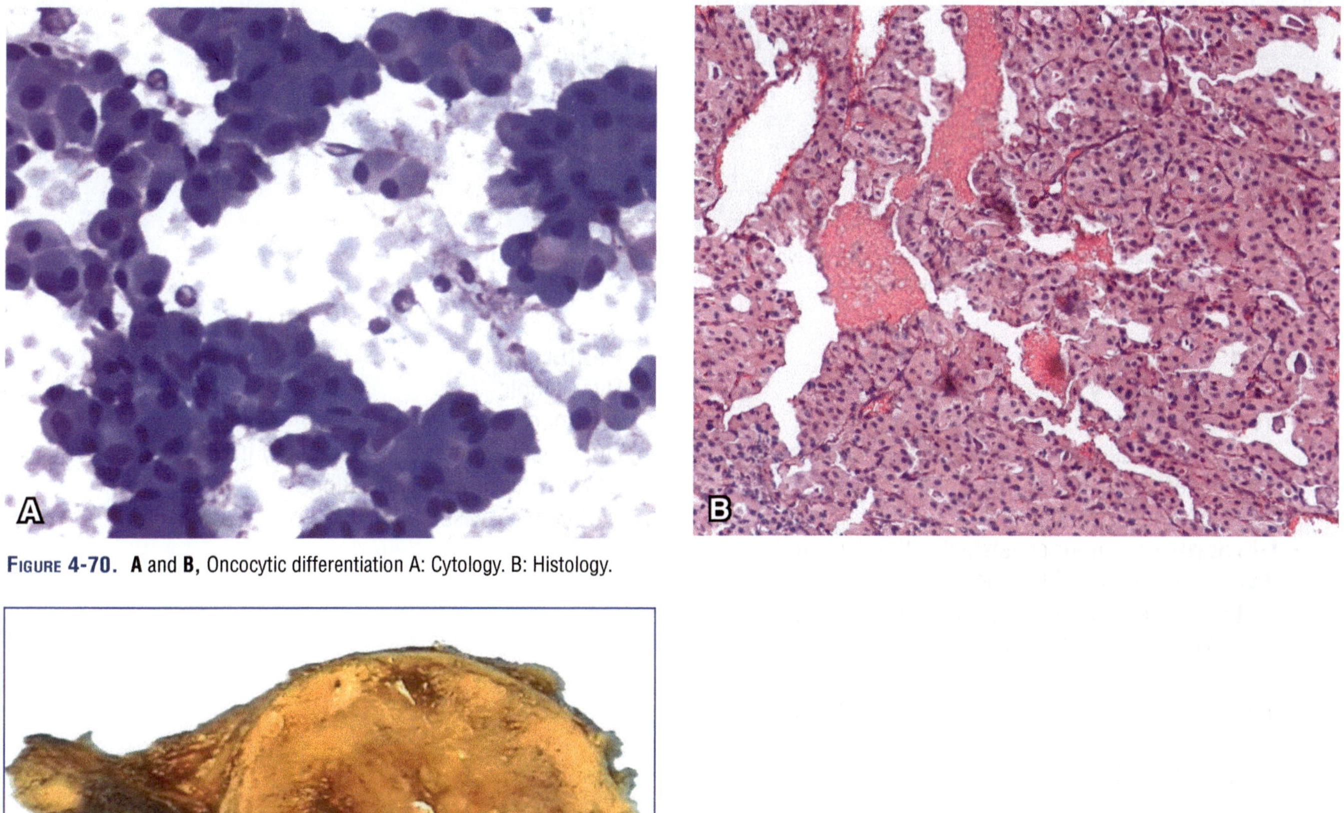

Figure 4-70. **A** and **B,** Oncocytic differentiation A: Cytology. B: Histology.

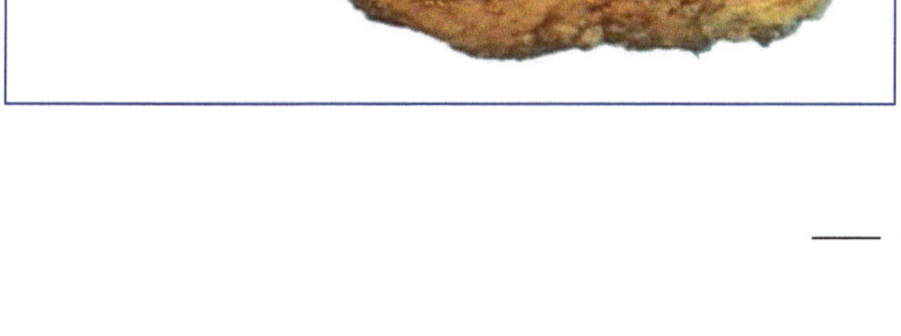

Figure 4-71. Gross section: no radical resection.

Follicular Thyroid Carcinoma Left Lobe

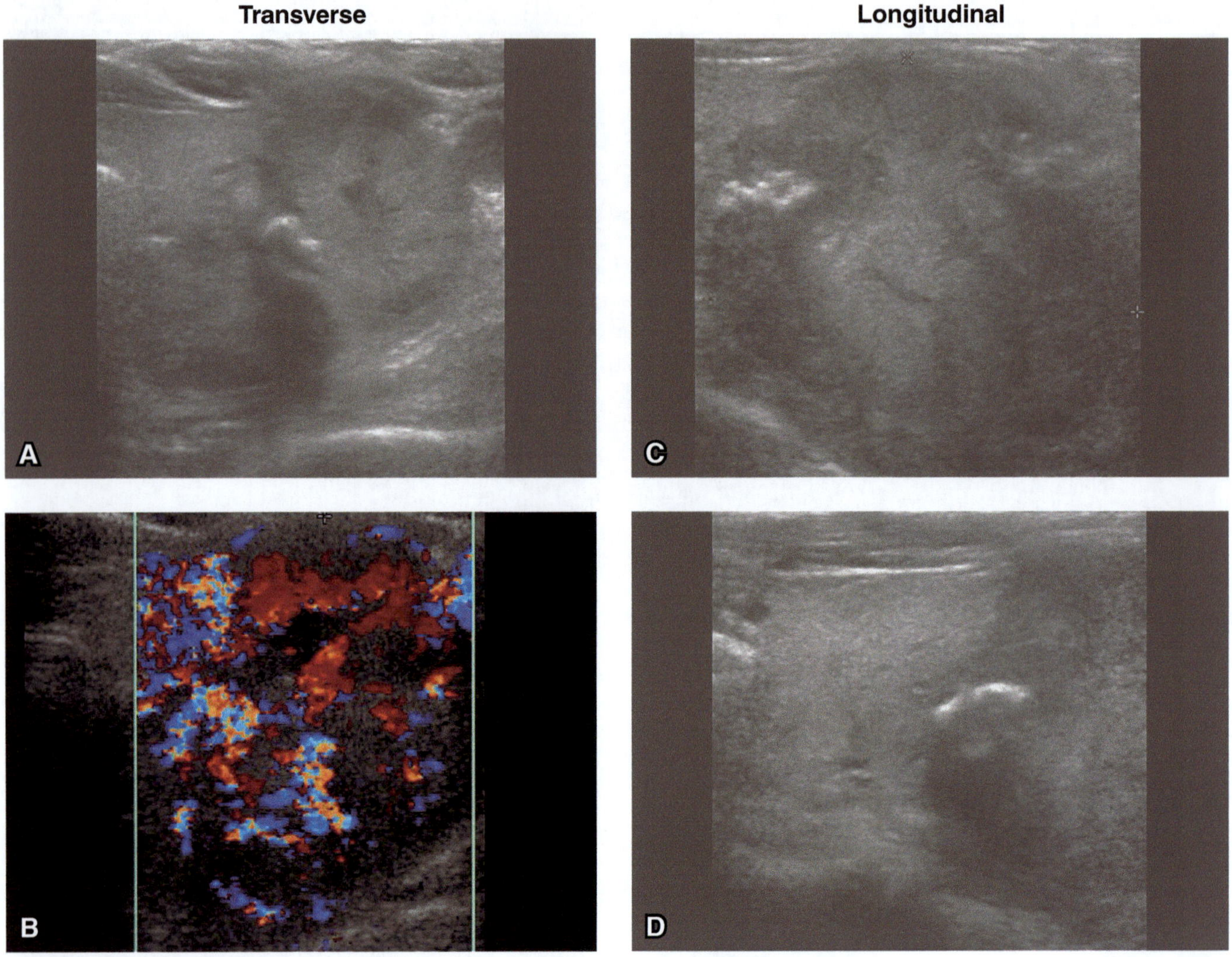

Figure 4-72. Ultrasound of follicular thyroid carcinoma in the left lobe. **A**, Transverse. **B**, Color Doppler, transverse. **C**, Longitudinal, sagittal diameter: 39 mm. **D**, Longitudinal.

65-Year-old woman

- **Clinical history:** About 10 years ago iodine treatment because of hyperparathyroidism. Presently nodular goiter. Metastasis from follicular thyroid carcinoma in left iliac bone revealed 2 weeks before examination.
- **Ultrasound:** Tumor consistent with follicular thyroid carcinoma (FTC) in left lobe.
- **Cytology left lobe:** Follicular tumor consistent with FTC according to information about bone metastasis.
- **Thyroidectomy:** Widely invasive FTC left lobe.

See also pages 28–29

Features

Hypoechoic
Inhomogeneous echo pattern
Quite well circumscribed, but very irregular border
Coarse and microcalcifications
Partial hypervascularity

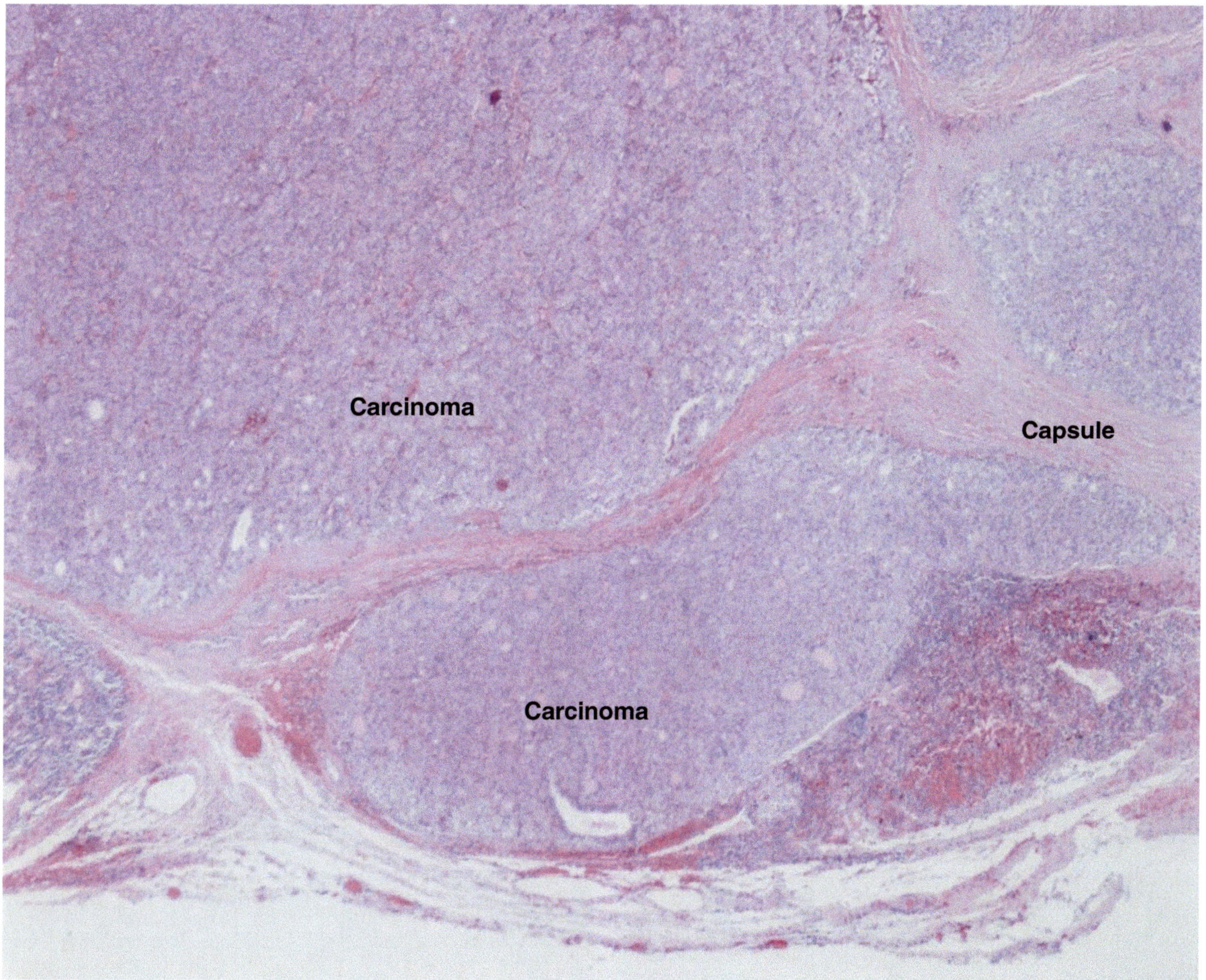

Figure 4-73. Histology: follicular thyroid carcinoma with infiltration through the capsule.

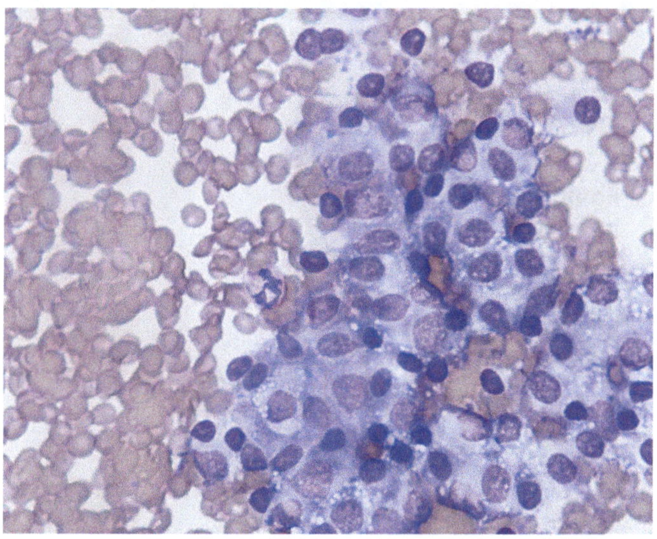

Figure 4-74. Cytology: follicular cells, follicular neoplasia.

Follicular Thyroid Carcinoma Left Lobe

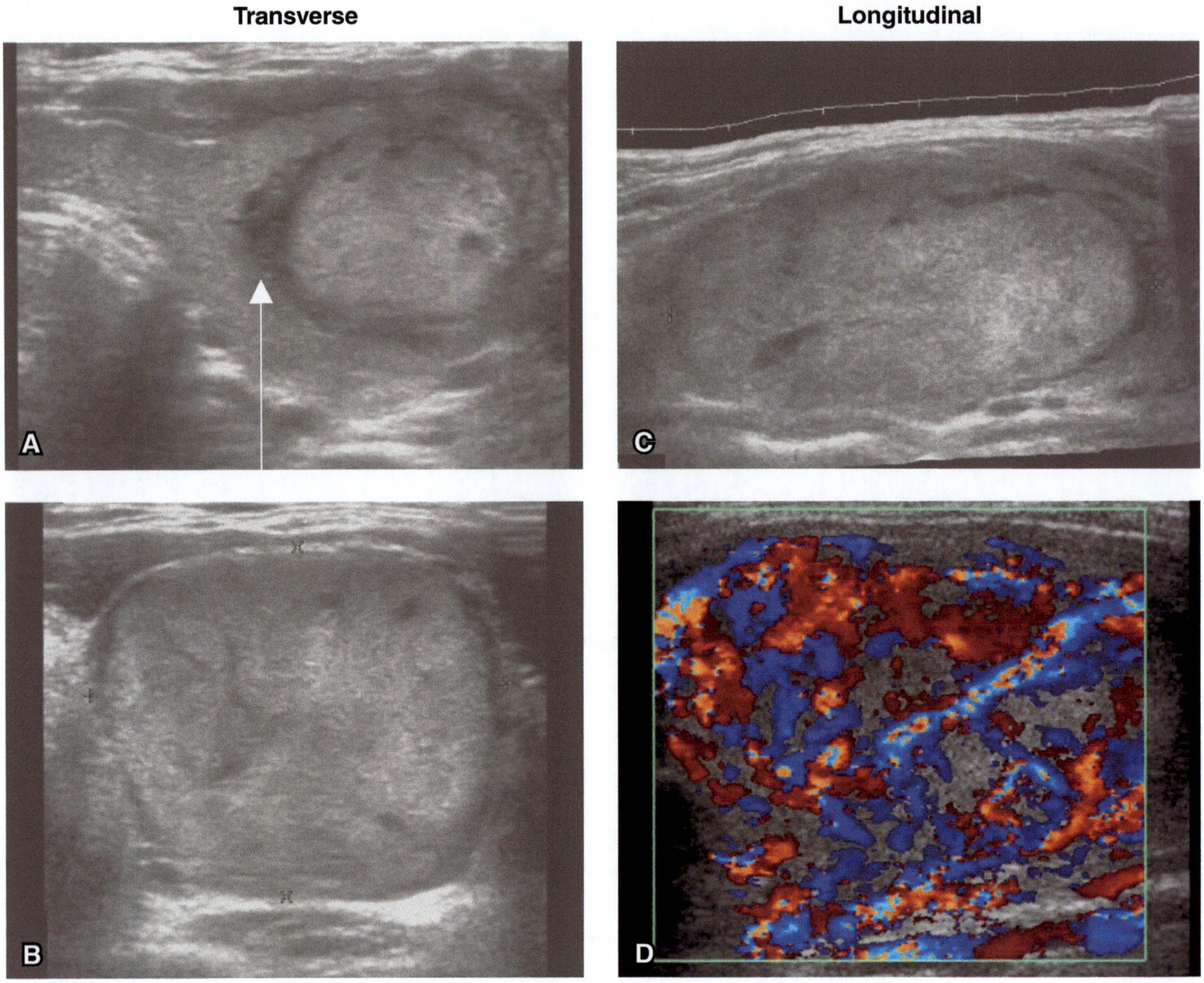

Figure 4-75. Ultrasound of follicular thyroid carcinoma in the left lobe. **A**, Transverse, 18 x 32 mm. The arrow indicates the most suspicious area. **B**, Transverse. **C**, Longitudinal, sagittal diameter: 23 mm. **D**, Color Doppler, longitudinal.

44-Year-old woman

- **Clinical history:** Increased thyroid stimulating hormone, anti thyroid peroxidase. Endocrinologist found tumor.
- **Ultrasound:** Follicular tumor. Malignant?
- **Cytology:** Follicular neoplasia.
- **18-Gauge histologic needle biopsy:** Follicular tumor.
- **Left hemithyroidectomy:** Follicular thyroid carcinoma.

Features

Isoechoic
Inhomogeneous echo pattern
Well circumscribed
Uneven, partially thick hypoechoic halo
Hypervascular
Suggestion of "spoke-and-wheel-like" vascularity

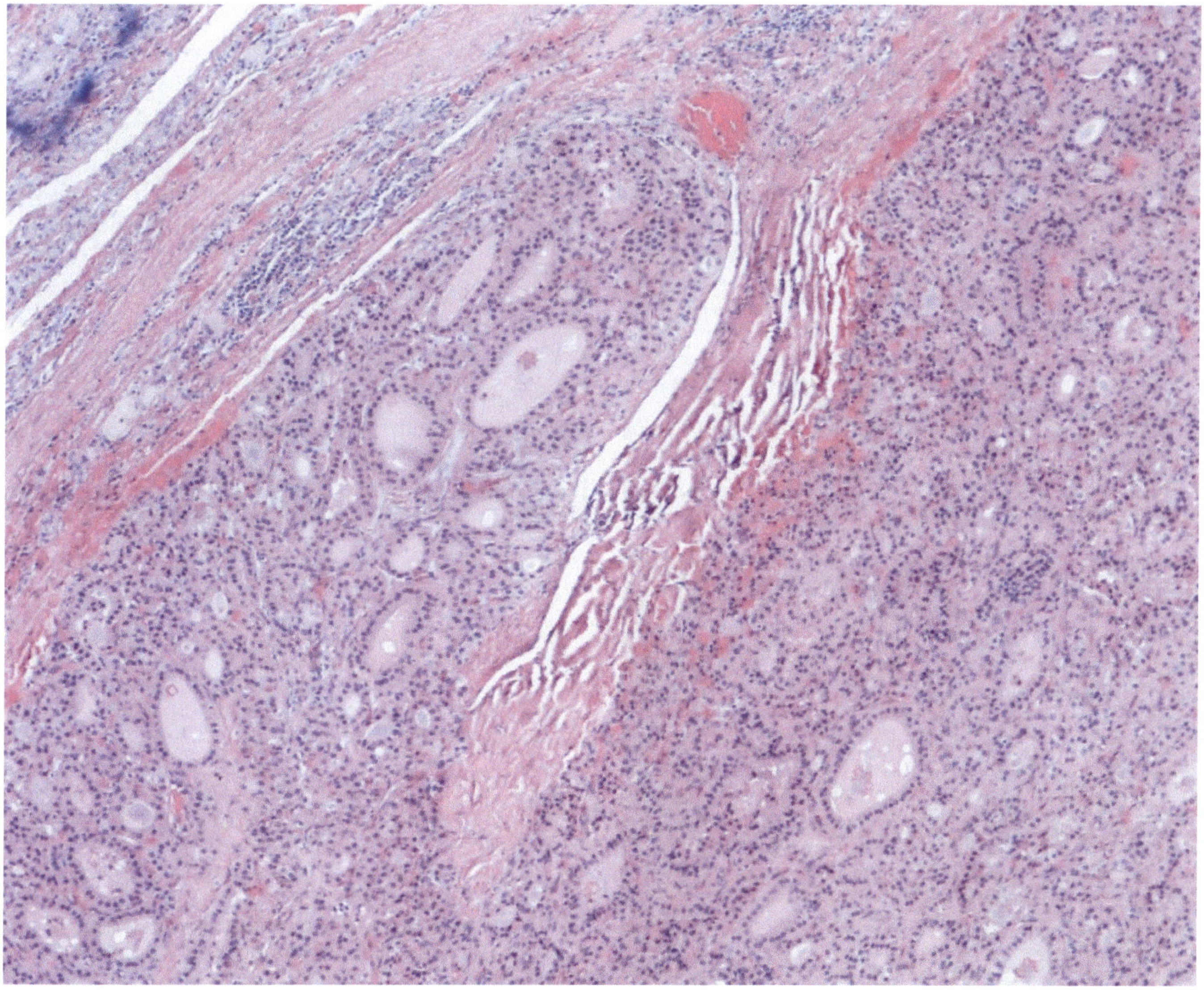

Figure 4-76. Histology: follicular thyroid carcinoma, minimally invasive type. Tumor demonstrates complete penetration of the capsule and has a mushroom-like configuration.

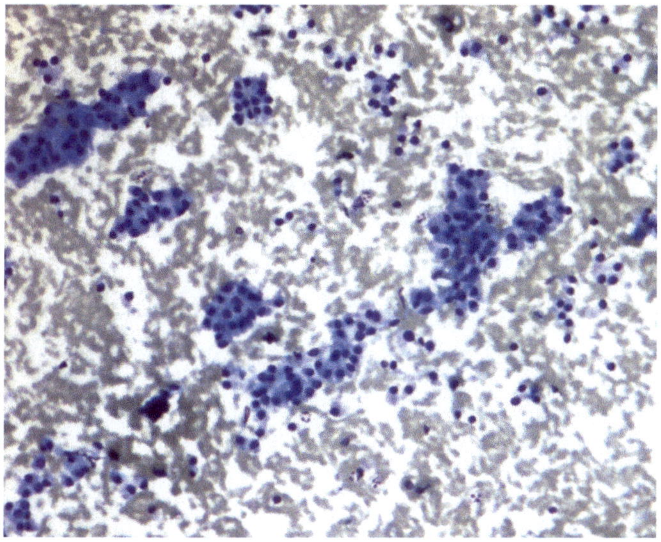

Figure 4-77. Cytology: follicular structure, follicular neoplasia.

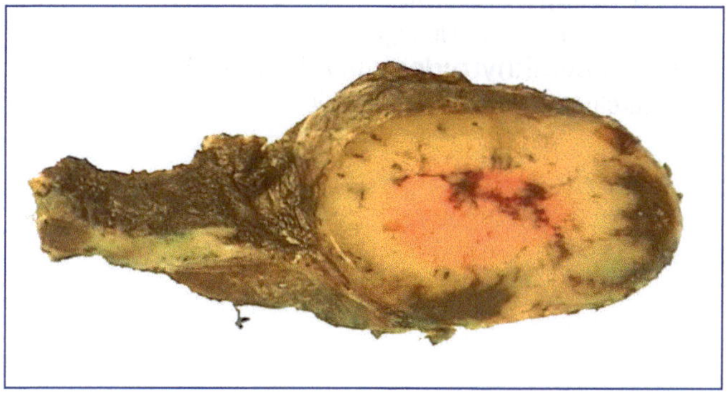

Figure 4-78. Gross section: minimally invasive tumors are often indistinguishable grossly from follicular adenoma.

Follicular Thyroid Carcinoma Left Lobe

Transverse

Longitudinal

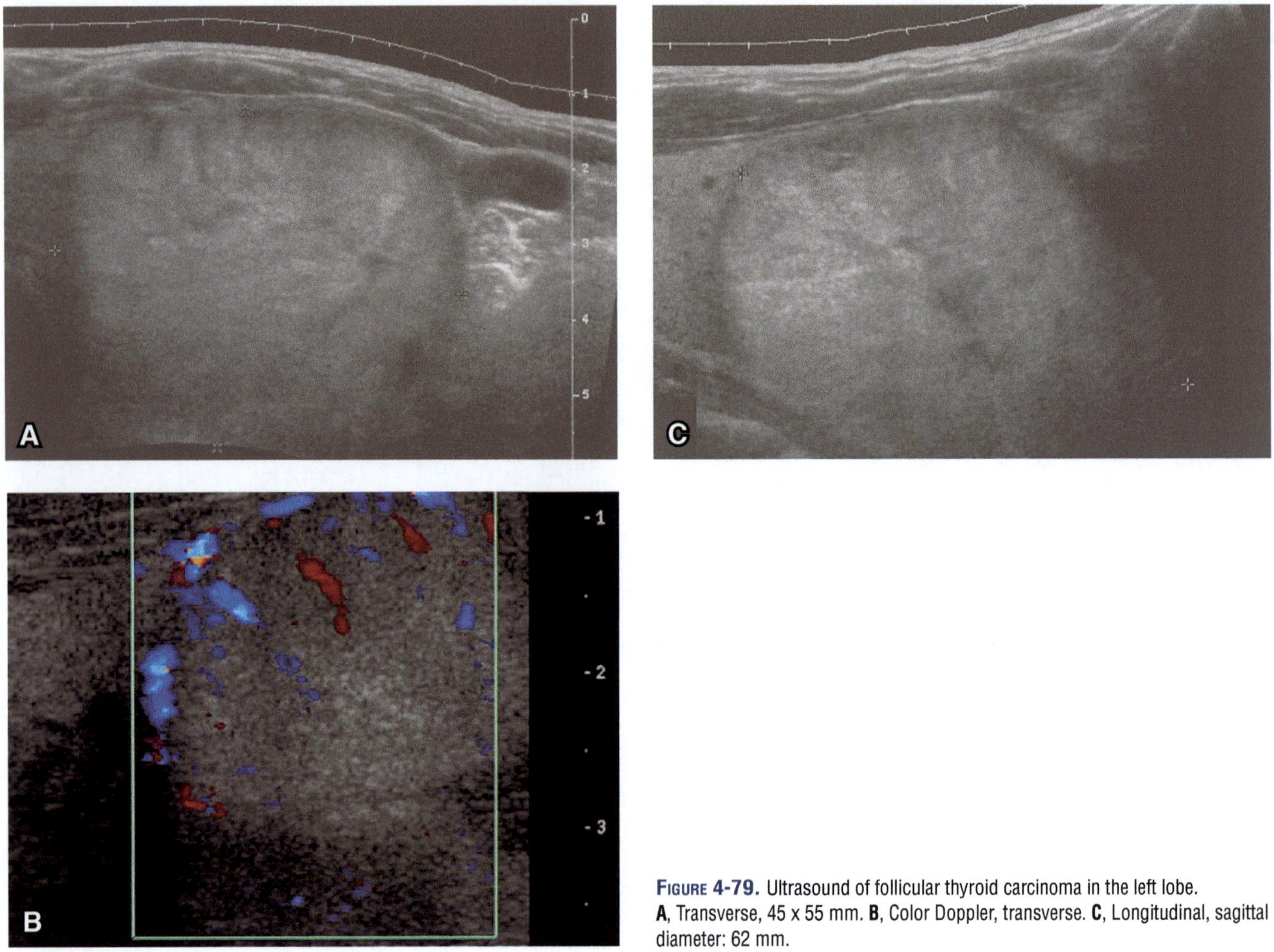

Figure 4-79. Ultrasound of follicular thyroid carcinoma in the left lobe. **A**, Transverse, 45 x 55 mm. **B**, Color Doppler, transverse. **C**, Longitudinal, sagittal diameter: 62 mm.

41-Year-old man

- **Clinical history:** Neck pain for a while. Incidentaloma on MR.
- **Ultrasound:** Follicular adenoma.
- **Cytology:** Follicular epithelium.
- **18-Gauge histologic needle biopsy:** Follicular lesion. No sign of malignancy.
- **Left hemithyroidectomy:** Follicular thyroid carcinoma, minimally invasive.

Features

Slightly hypoechoic
Inhomogeneous echo pattern
Well circumscribed
Thin uneven hypoechoic halo
Suggestion of "spoke-and-wheel-like" scant vascularity

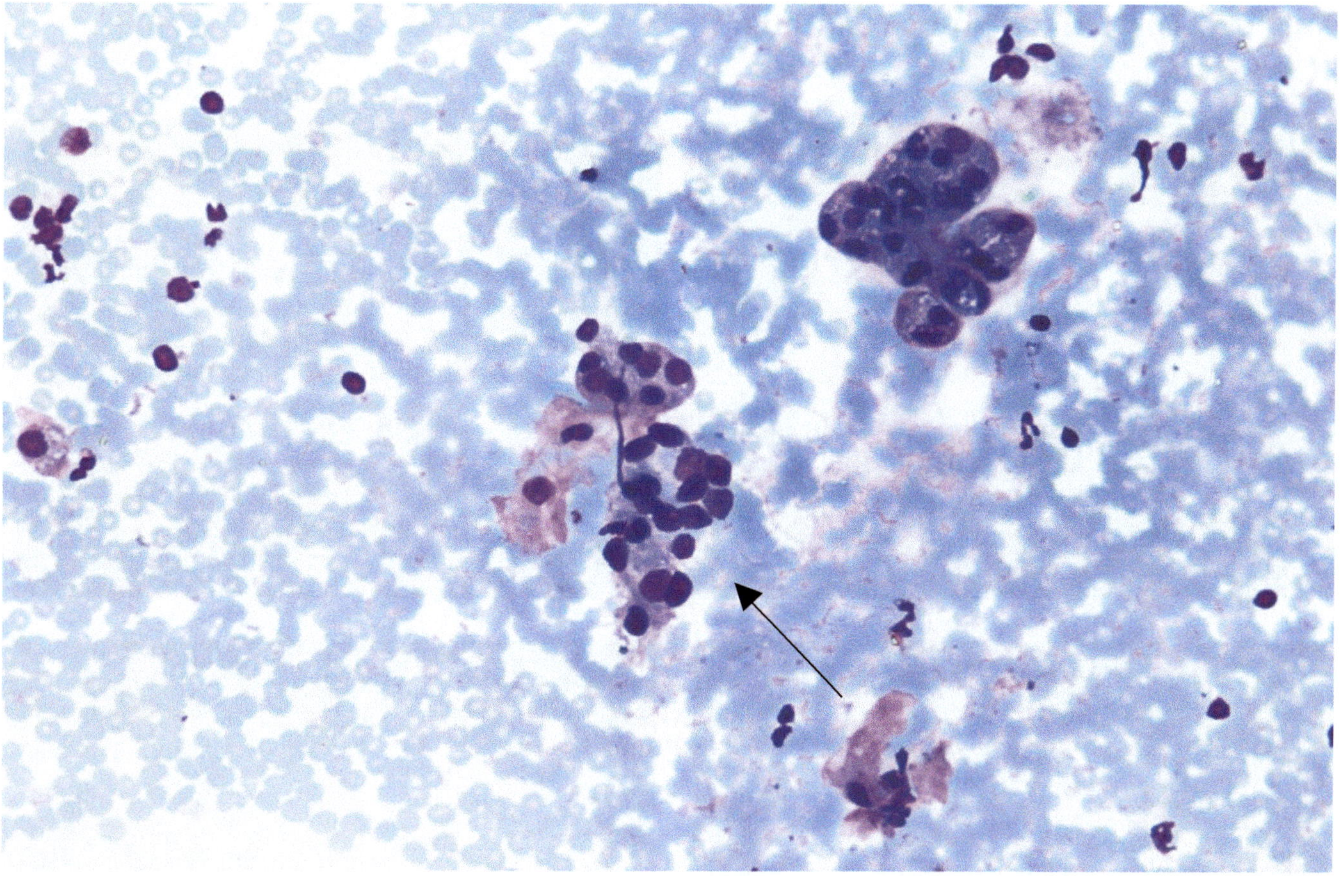

FIGURE 4-80. Cytology: follicular structure (arrow).

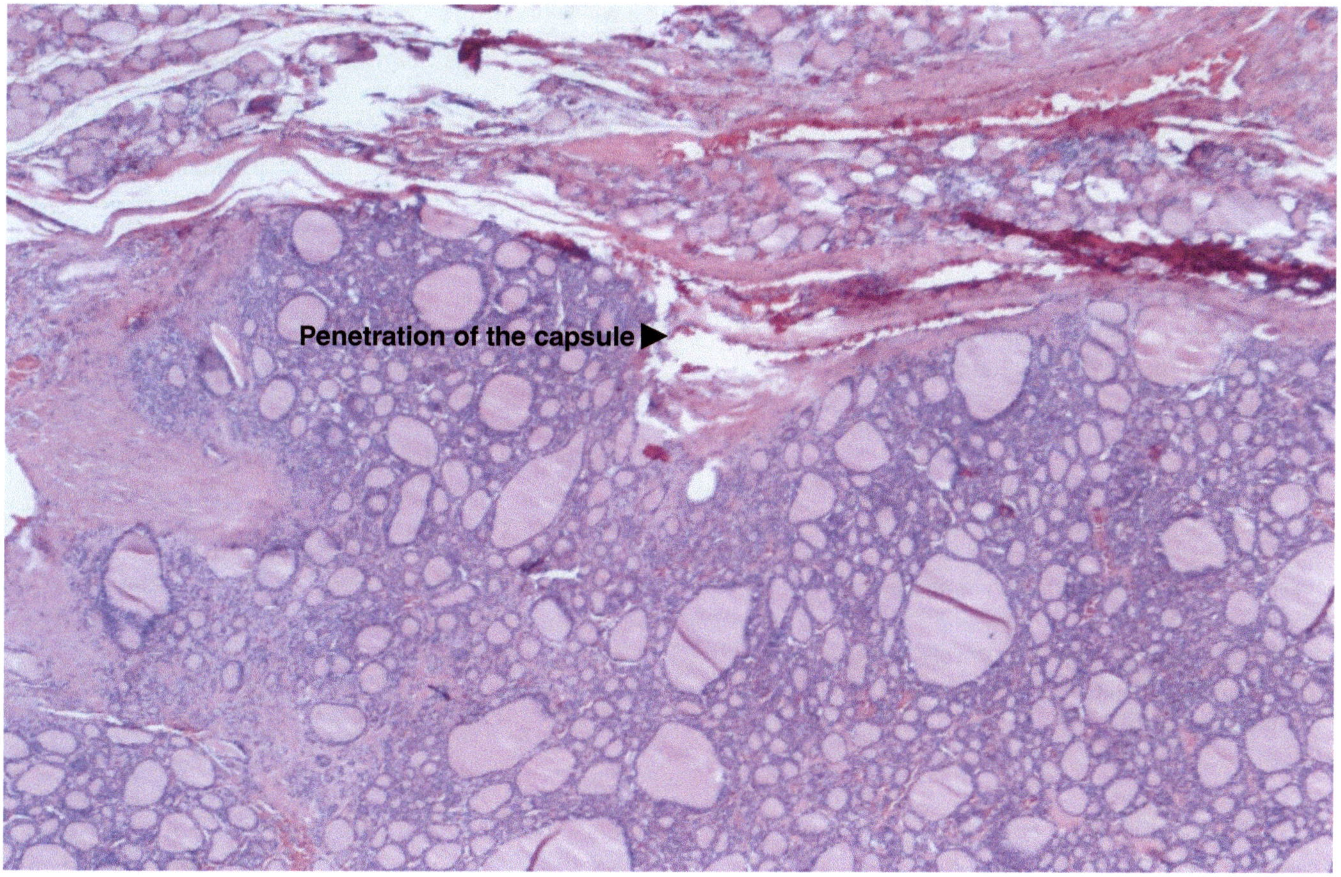

FIGURE 4-81. Histology: follicular thyroid carcinoma, minimally invasive.

Follicular Thyroid Carcinoma Isthmus

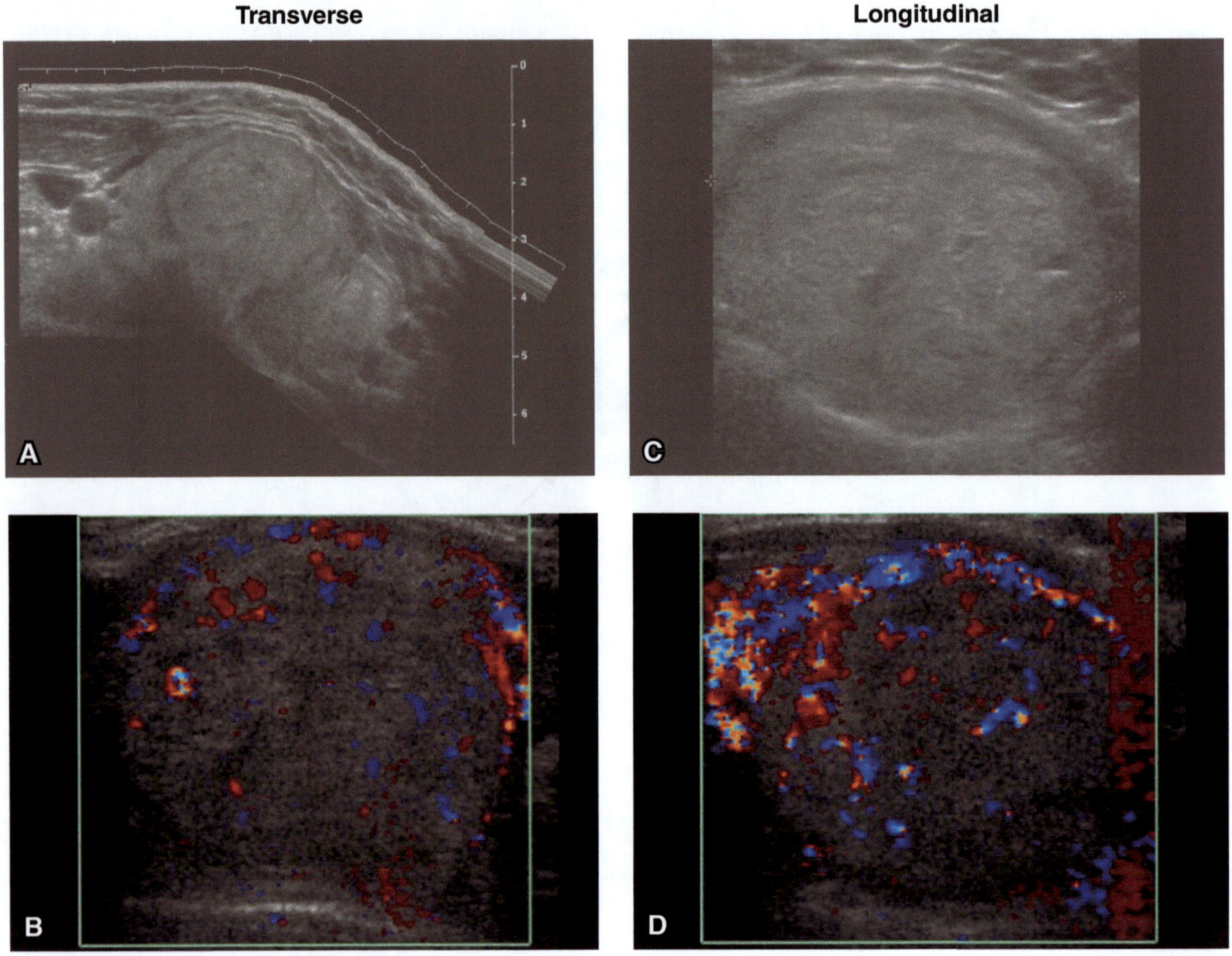

Figure 4-82. Ultrasound of follicular thyroid carcinoma in the isthmus. **A**, Transverse. **B**, Color Doppler, transverse. **C**, Longitudinal, sagittal diameter: 38 mm. **D**, Color Doppler, longitudinal.

47-Year-old woman

- **Clinical history:** Large tumor in isthmus with compression of trachea.
- **Ultrasound:** Follicular adenomas in isthmus and left lobe.
- **16-Gauge histologic needle biopsy:** Encapsulated follicular lesion with tumor infiltration in the capsule.
- **Cytology:** Follicular lesion of undetermined significance.
- **Left hemithyroidectomy:** Follicular thyroid carcinoma, minimally invasive in isthmus plus colloid nodule.

Features

Moderately hypoechoic
Quite homogeneous echo pattern
Well circumscribed
Suggestion of "spoke-and-wheel-like" scant vascularity

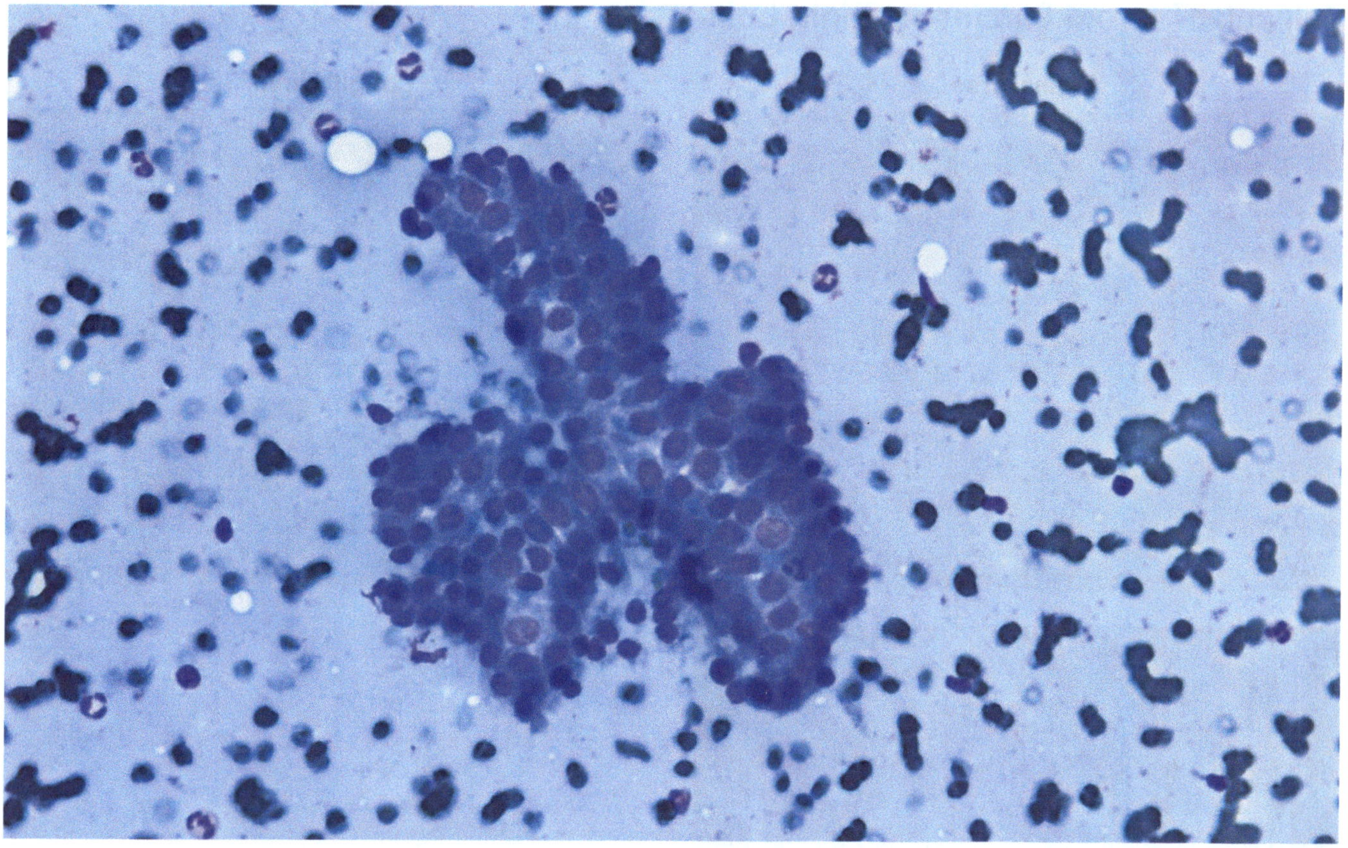

FIGURE 4-83. Cytology: follicular structure, follicular neoplasia/lesion.

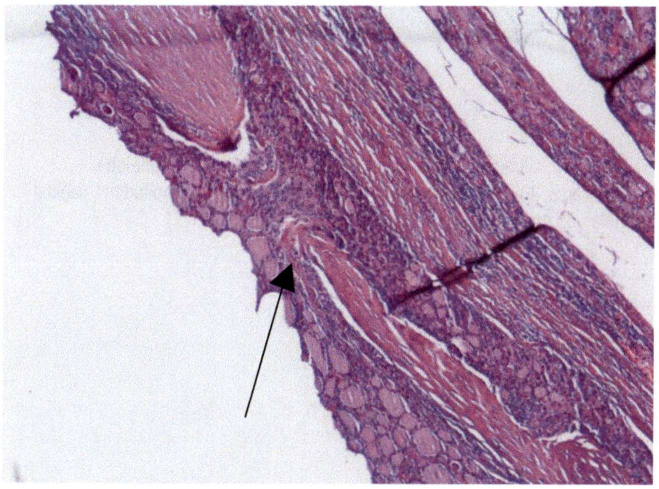

FIGURE 4-84. Histology: infiltration through the capsule (*arrow*).

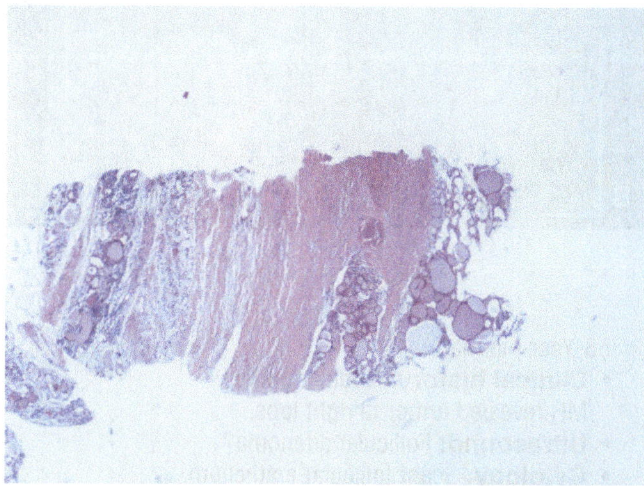

FIGURE 4-85. Histologic needle biopsy: focus of infiltration in the capsule.

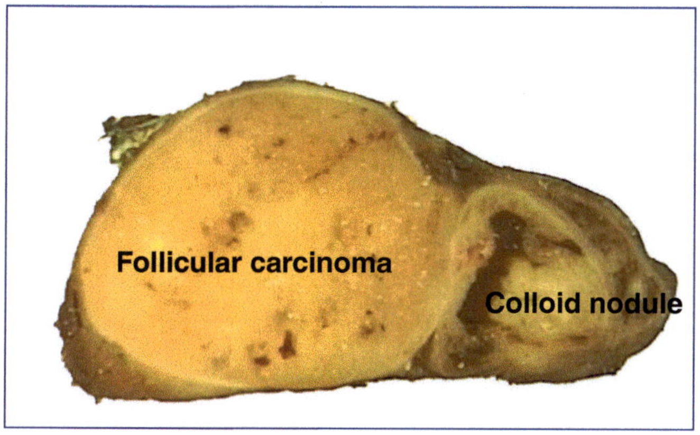

FIGURE 4-86. Gross examination.

Follicular Thyroid Carcinoma Right Lobe

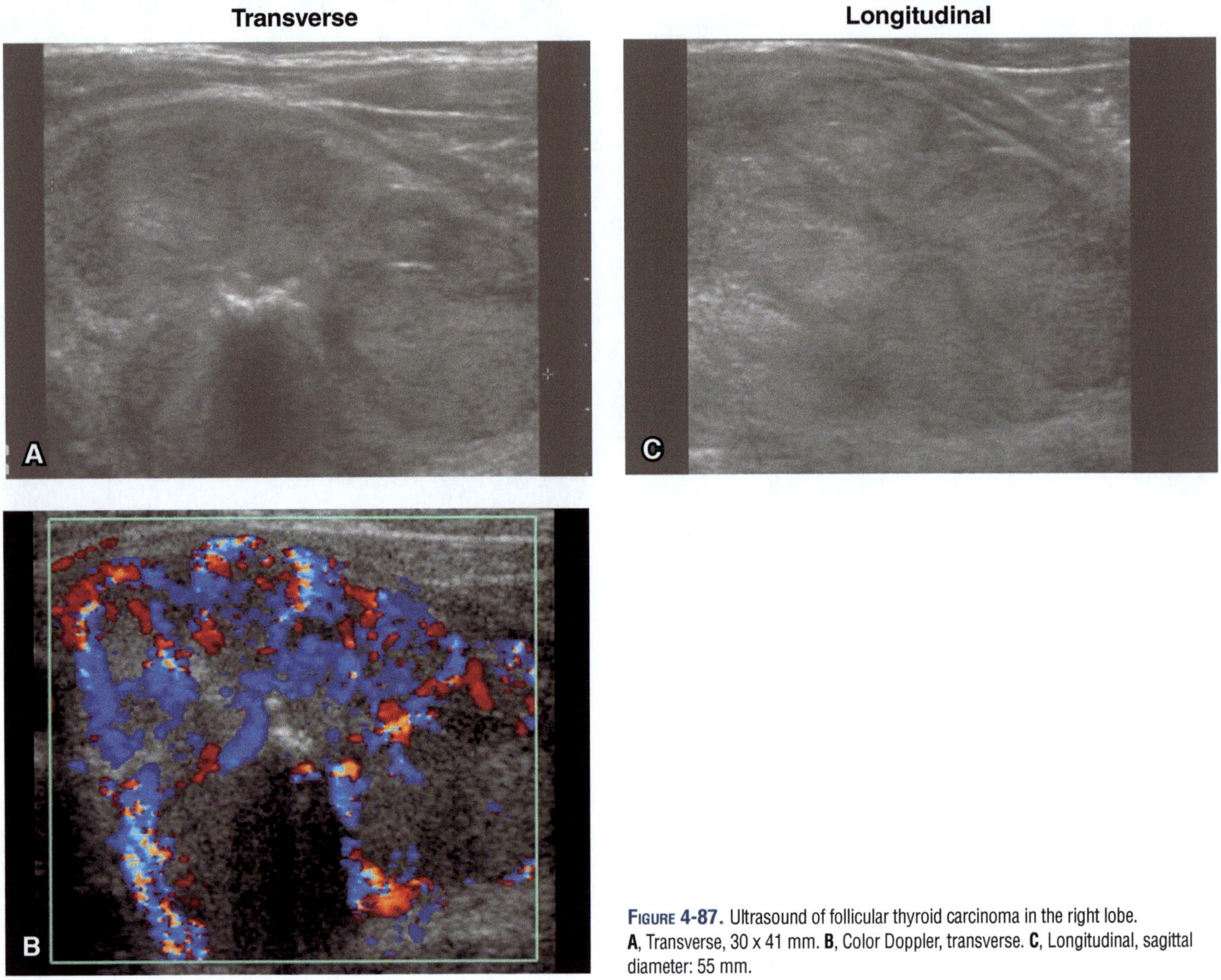

Figure 4-87. Ultrasound of follicular thyroid carcinoma in the right lobe. **A**, Transverse, 30 x 41 mm. **B**, Color Doppler, transverse. **C**, Longitudinal, sagittal diameter: 55 mm.

56-Year-old man

- **Clinical history:** Nodular goiter. MR revealed tumor in right lobe.
- **Ultrasound:** Follicular adenoma?
- **Cytology:** Scant follicular epithelium.
- **16-Gauge histologic needle biopsy:** Follicular lesion with fibrosis.
- **Right hemithyroidectomy:** Follicular thyroid carcinoma, minimally invasive.

Features

Hypoechoic, lobulated
Inhomogeneous echo pattern
Well circumscribed
Coarse calcifications
Lobulated vascularity
Hypervascular

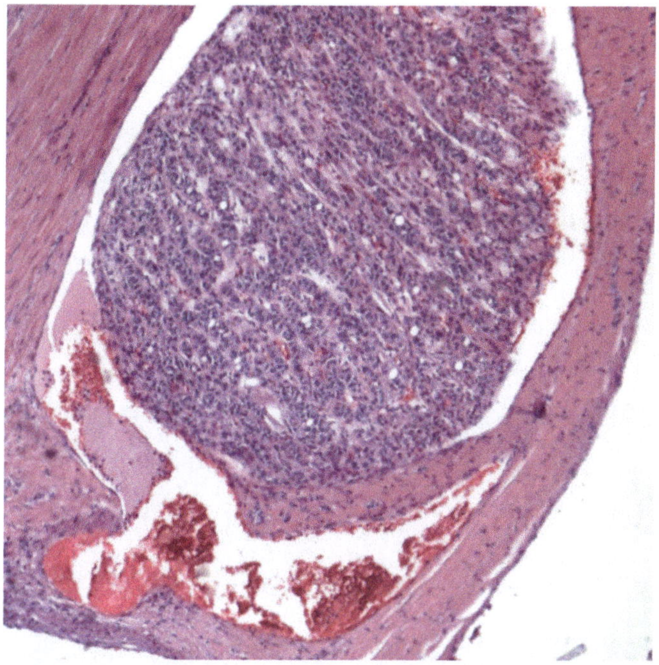

Figure 4-88. Histology: tumor invasion in a vessel.

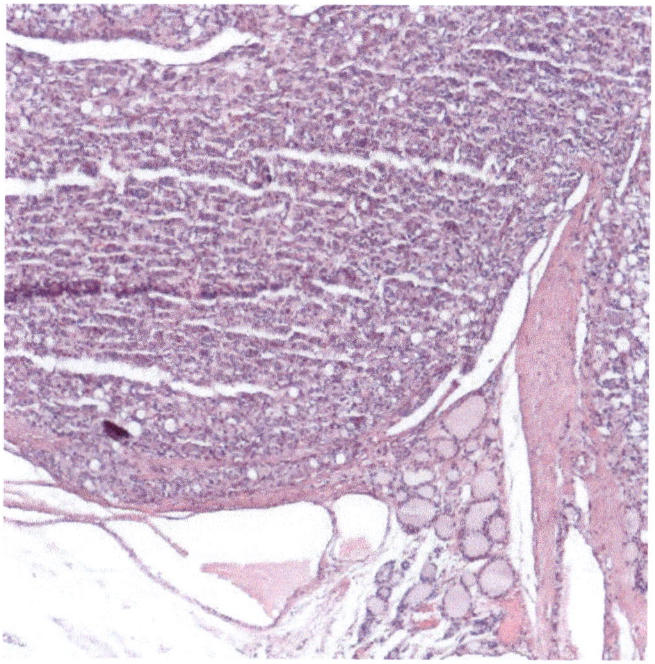

Figure 4-89. Histology: follicular thyroid carcinoma.

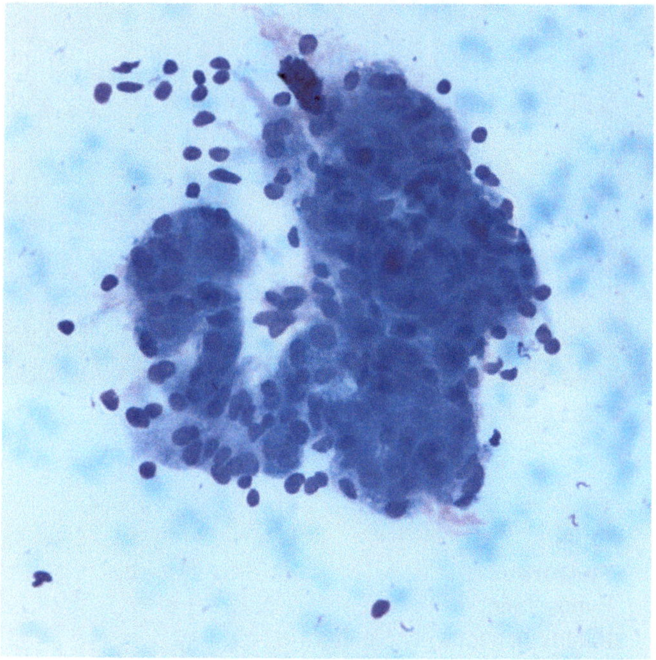

Figure 4-90. Cytology: follicular neoplasia.

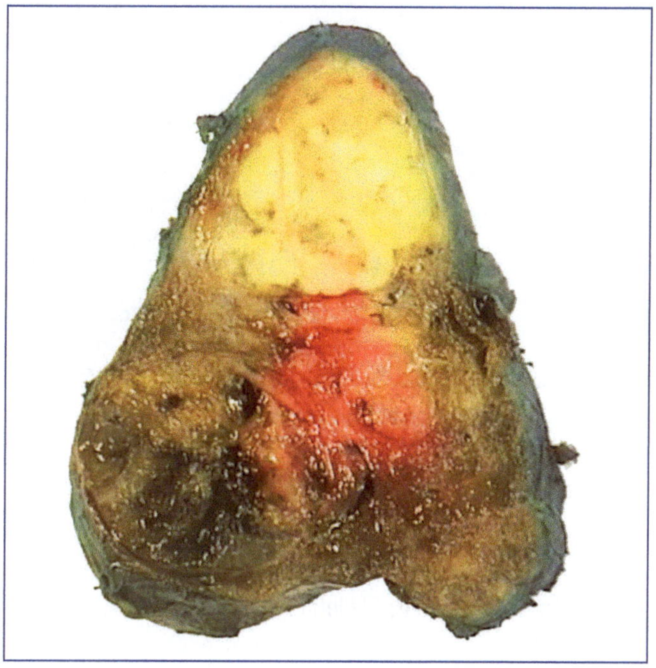

Figure 4-91. Gross section: not encapsulated tumor.

Follicular Thyroid Carcinoma Right Lobe

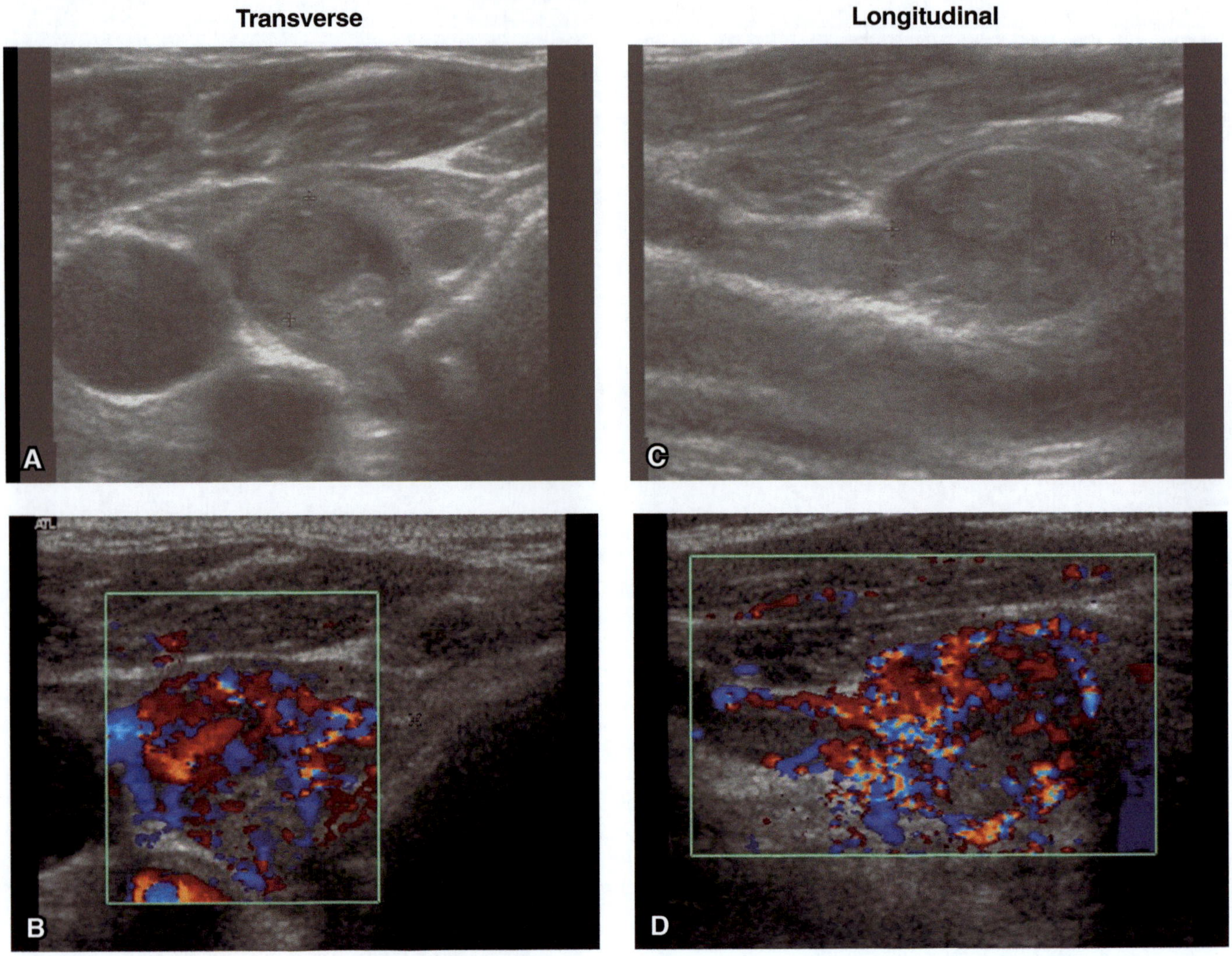

Figure 4-92. Ultrasound of follicular carcinoma in the right lobe. **A**, Transverse, 10 x 14 mm. **B**, Color Doppler, transverse. **C**, Longitudinal, sagittal diameter: 16 mm. **D**, Color Doppler, longitudinal.

75-Year-old man

- **Clinical history:** Skeletal metastasis revealed on MR.
- **Bone biopsy:** Probably follicular thyroid carcinoma.
- **Ultrasound:** Probably papillary thyroid carcinoma.
- **Cytology:** Follicular neoplasia.
- **Thyroidectomy:** Follicular thyroid carcinoma, widely invasive.

Features

Hypoechoic
Inhomogeneous echo pattern
Quite well circumscribed
Microcalcifications
Hypervascular
Suggestion of "spoke-and-wheel-like" vascularity

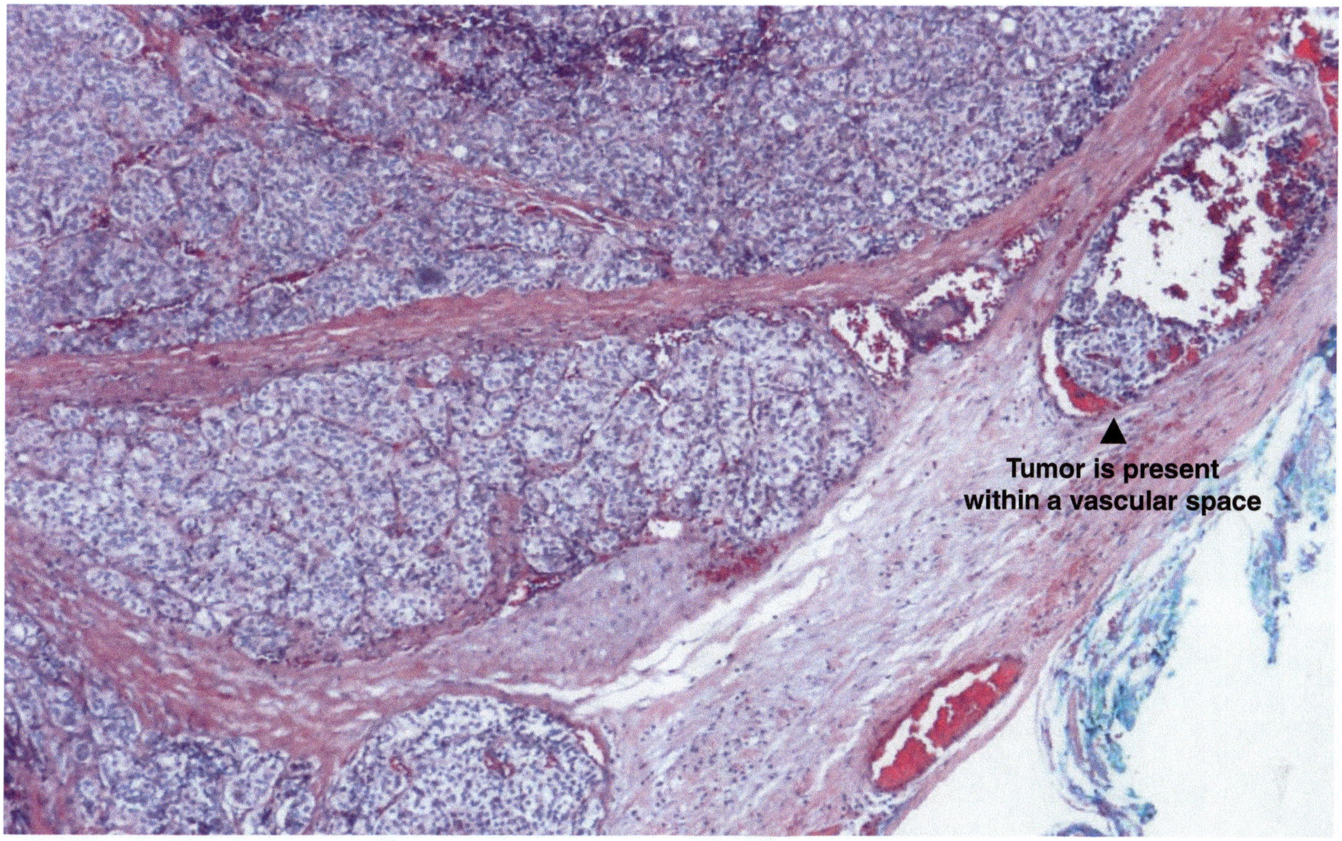

Figure 4-93. Histlogy: follicular thyroid carcinoma, widely invasive type. Tumor demonstrates both capsular and vascular invasion.

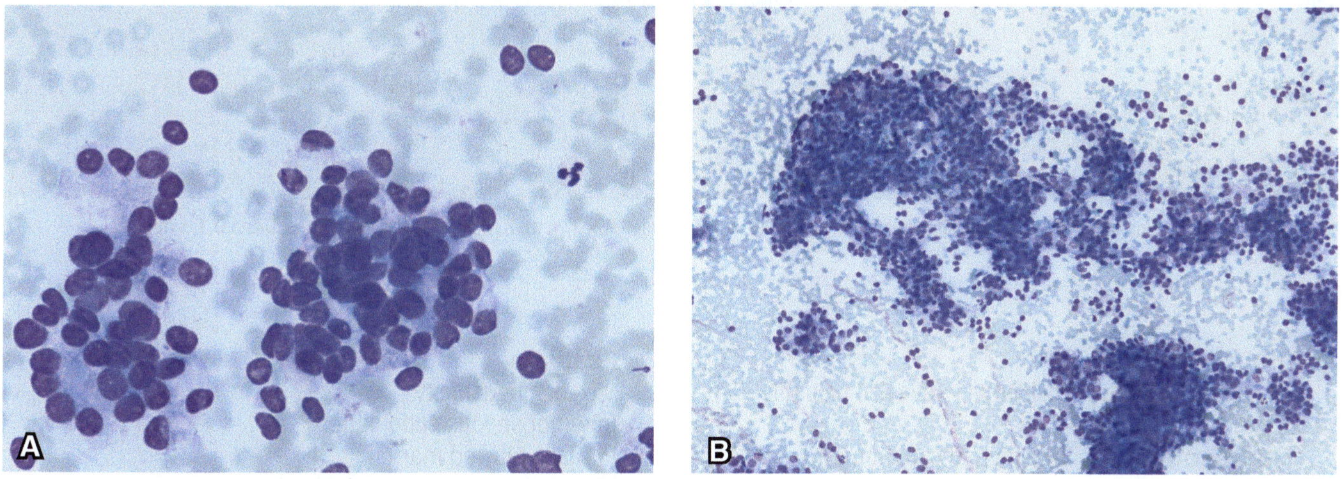

Figure 4-94. **A** and **B**, Cytology: material rich in follicular epithelium.

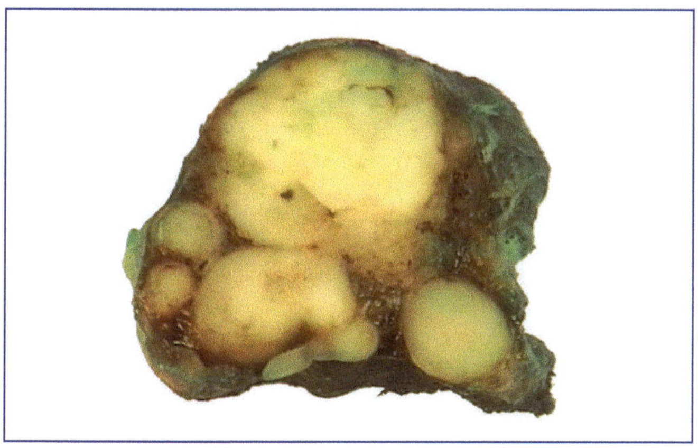

Figure 4-95. Gross section: several nodules and no distinct tumor capsule. The entire lobe is replaced with tumor.

Follicular Thyroid Carcinoma Right Lobe

Transverse | **Longitudinal**

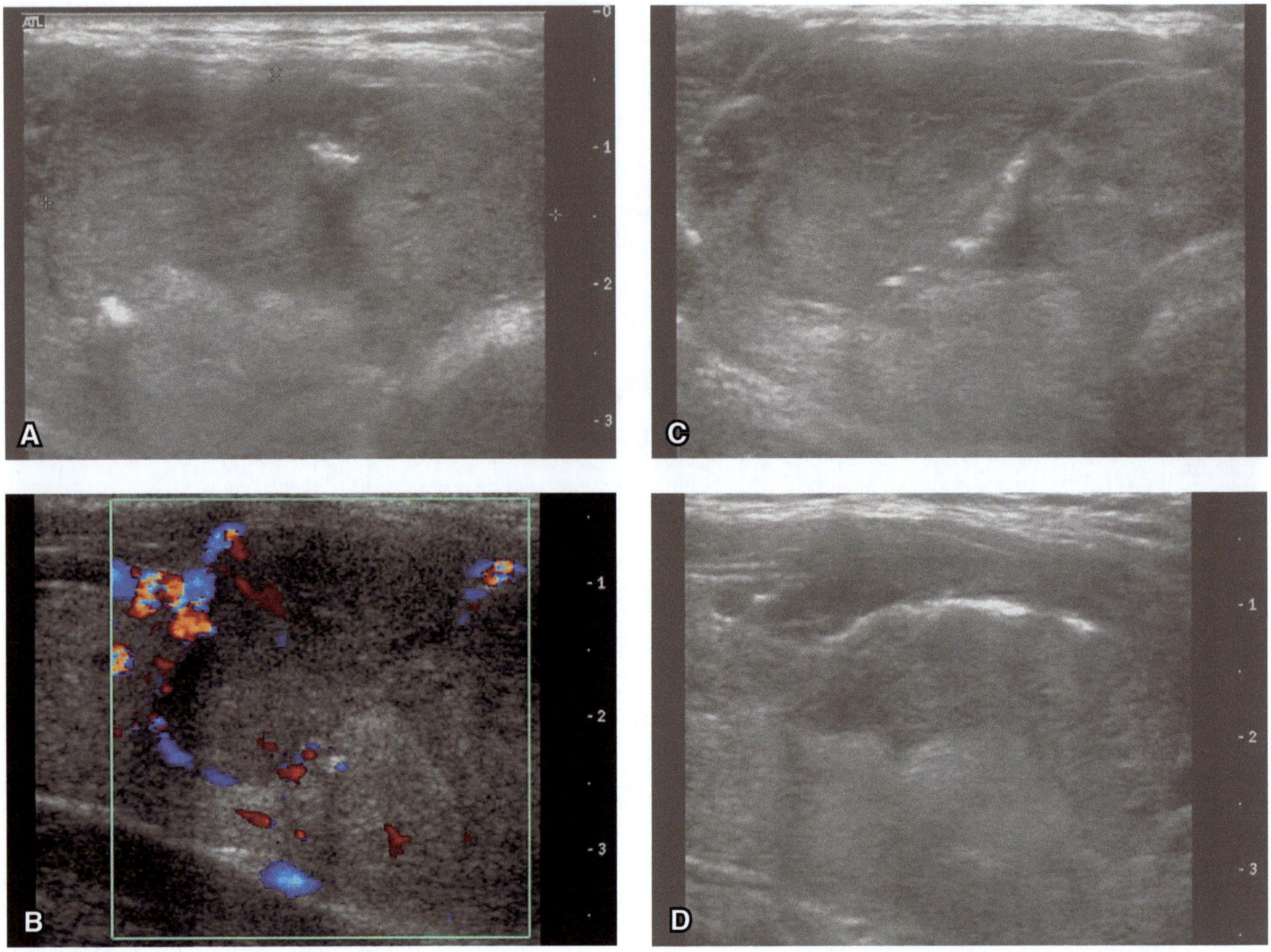

Figure 4-96. Ultrasound of follicular thyroid carcinoma in the right lobe. **A**, Transverse, 31 x 37 mm. **B**, Color Doppler, transverse. **C** and **D**, Longitudinal.

46-Year-old man

- **Clinical history:** Incidentally revealed palpable tumor.
- **Ultrasound:** Papillary thyroid carcinoma? Colloid nodule?
- **Cytology:** Rich in follicular cells. Hyperplasia? Neoplasia?
- **16-Gauge histologic needle biopsy:** Suspicious for follicular neoplasia.
- **Right hemithyroidectomy:** Follicular thyroid carcinoma, widely invasive.

Features

Mixed echogenicity
Inhomogeneous echo pattern
Partially blurred margin
"Eggshell" and coarse calcifications
Scant vascularity

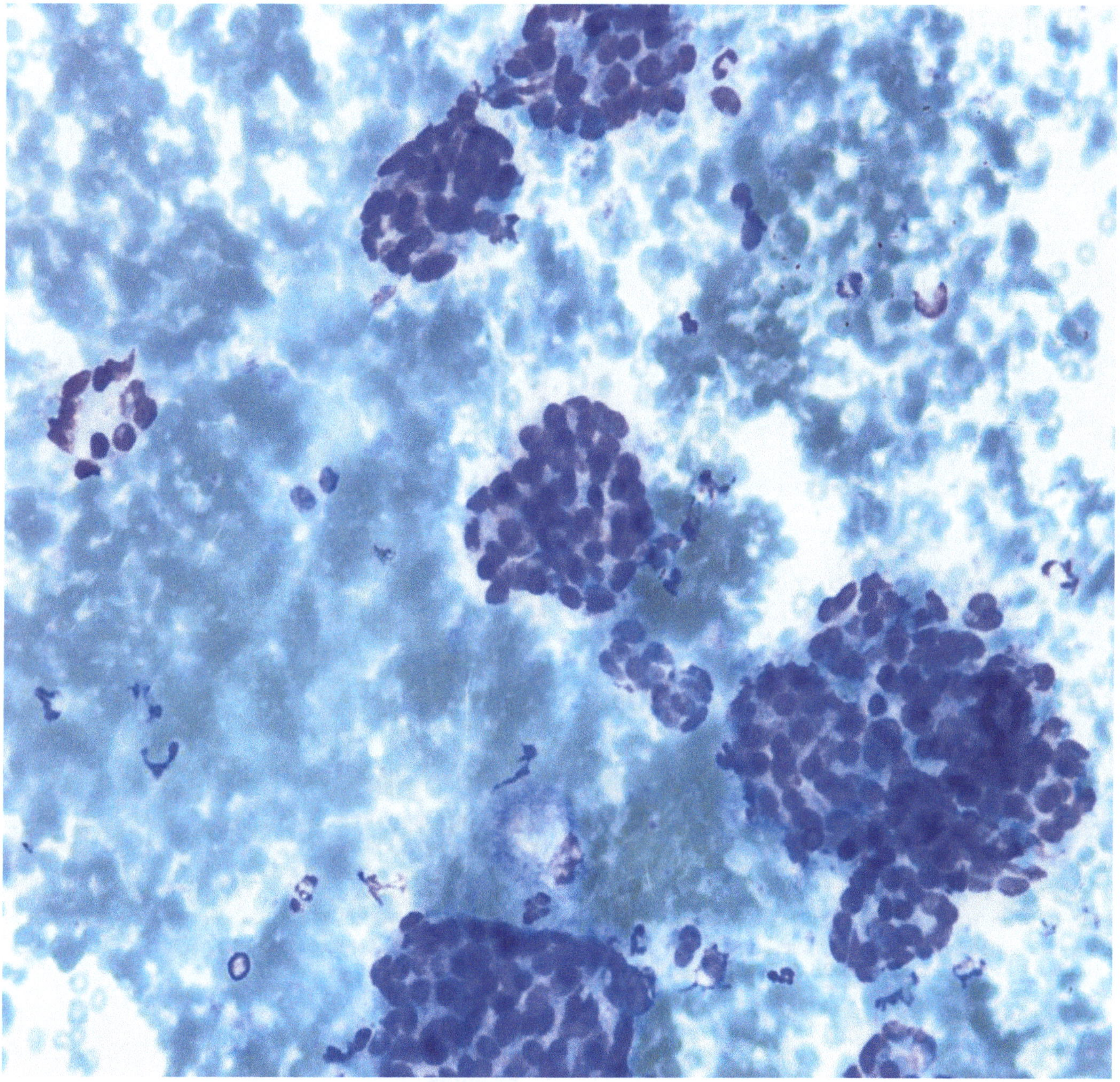

Figure 4-97. Cytology: rich in follicular epithelium.

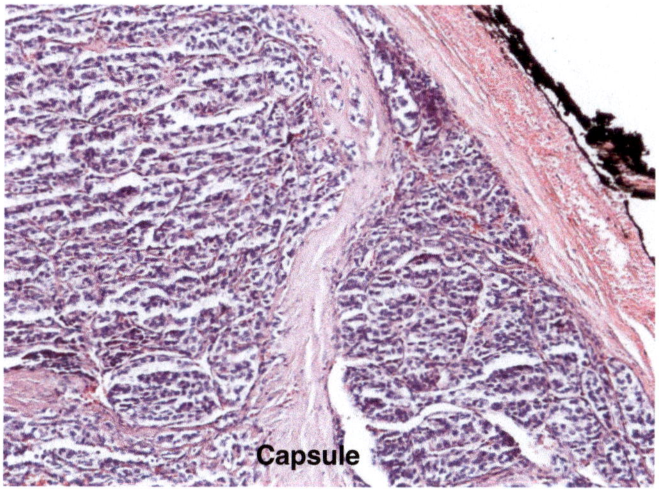

Figure 4-98. Histology: penetration through the capsule.

Follicular Thyroid Carcinoma Right Lobe

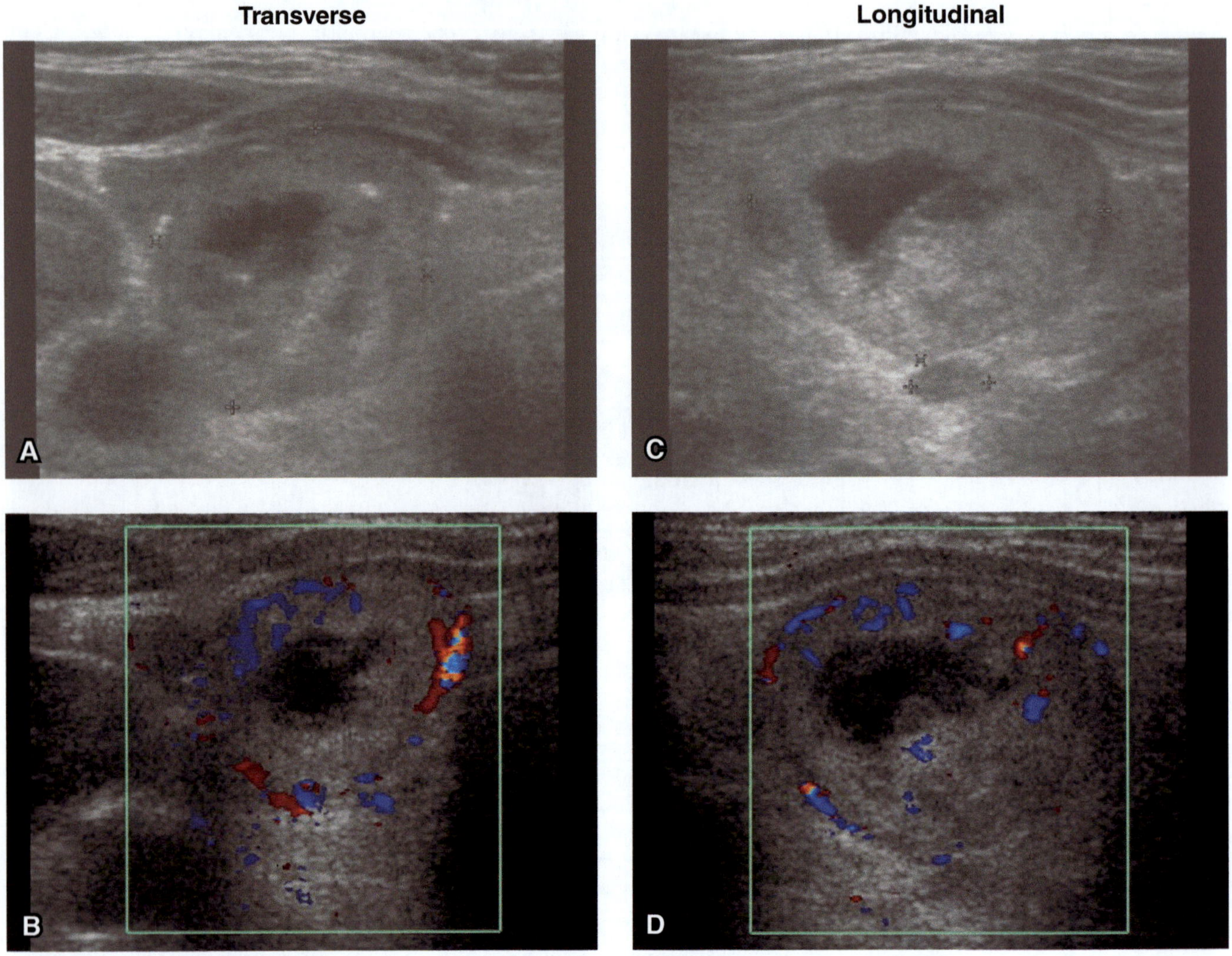

Figure 4-99. Ultrasound of follicular thyroid carcinoma in the right lobe. **A**, Transverse, 20 x 21 mm. **B**, Color Doppler, transverse. **C**, Longitudinal, sagittal diameter: 26 mm. **D**, Color Doppler, longitudinal.

77-Year-old man

- **Clinical history:** Skeletal metastasis in left iliac bone from follicular thyroid carcinoma (FTC).
- **Ultrasound:** Papillary thyroid carcinoma?
- **Cytology:** Follicular neoplasia.
- **Thyroidectomy:** FTC.

Features

Slightly hypoechoic
Inhomogeneous echo pattern
Partial hypoechoic halo
Cystic areas
Well circumscribed
Some microcalcifications
Scant peripheral vascularity

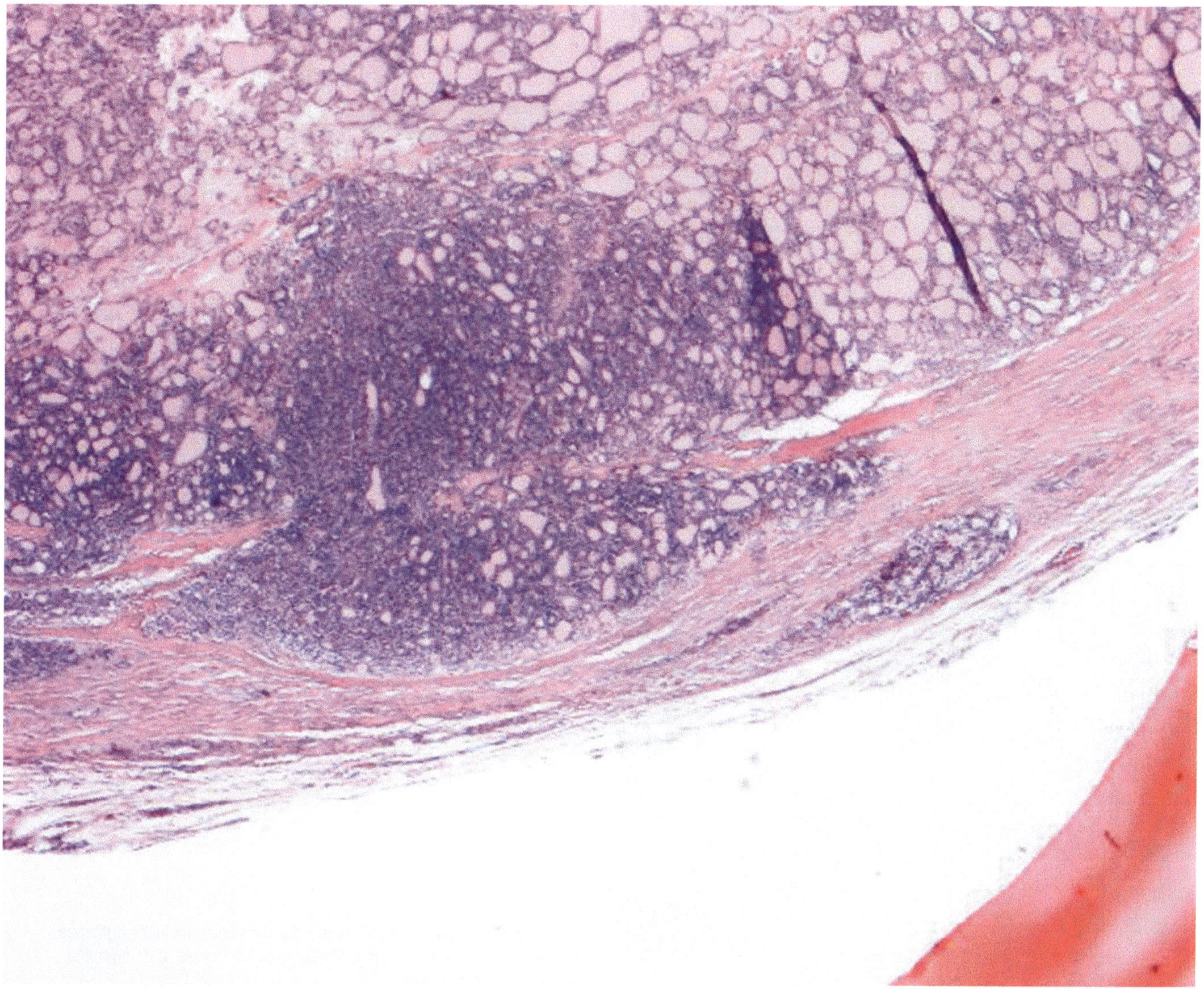

Figure 4-100. Histology: infiltration through the capsule.

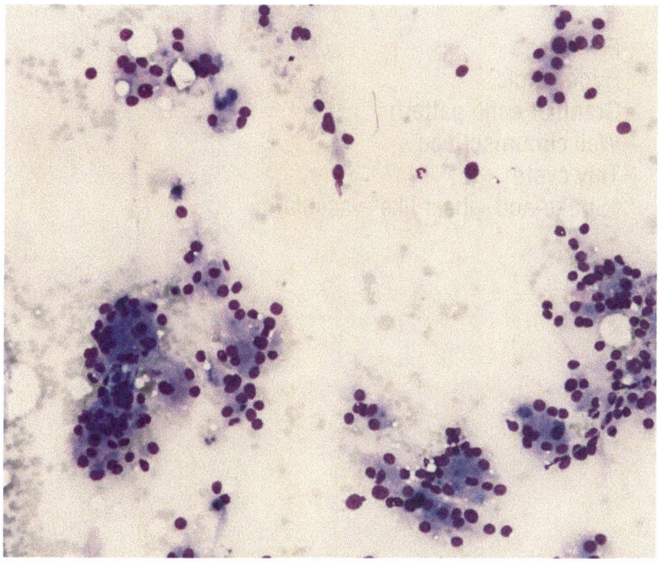

Figure 4-101. Cytology: several follicular structures.

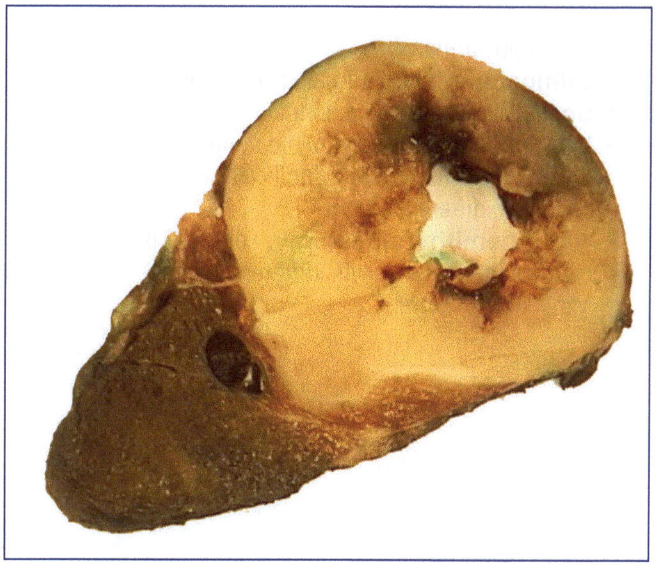

Figure 4-102. Gross section: penetration through the capsule.

Follicular Thyroid Carcinoma Right Lobe

Transverse | **Longitudinal**

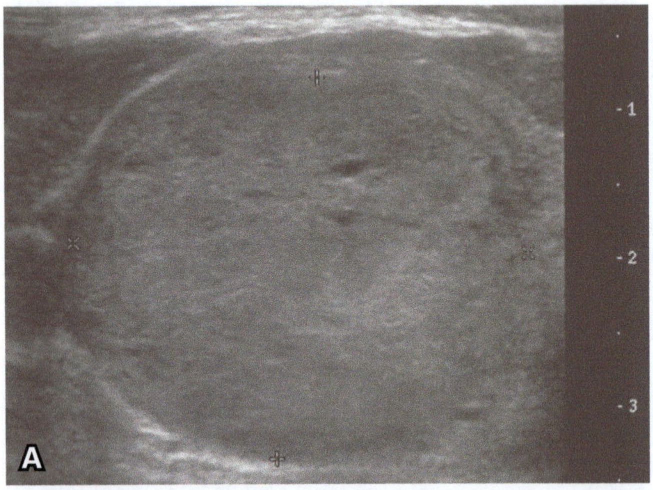

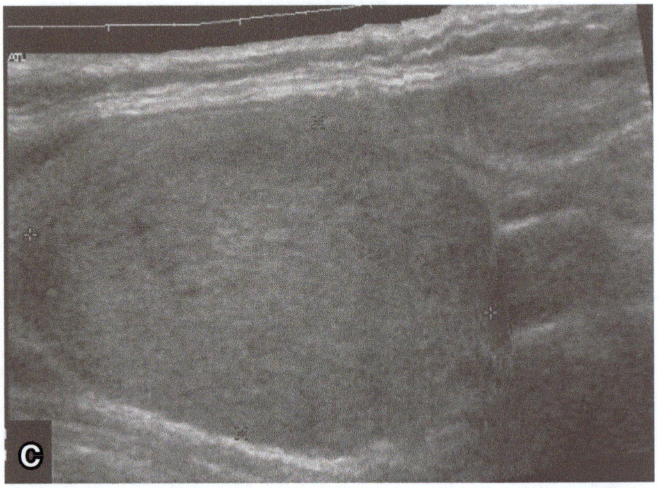

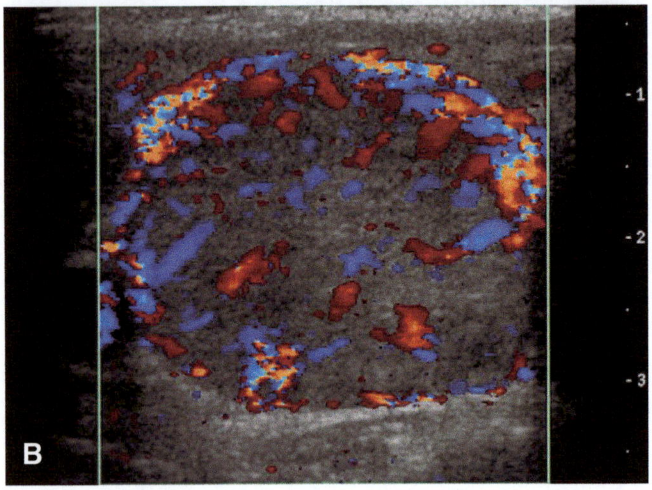

Figure 4-103. Ultrasound of follicular thyroid carcinoma in the right lobe. **A**, Transverse, 26 x 31 mm. **B**, Color Doppler, transverse. **C**, Longitudinal, sagittal diameter: 35 mm.

61-Year-old woman

- **Clinical history:** Soft palpable tumor in left lobe.
- **Scintigraphy:** Colloid nodule.
- **Ultrasound:** Probably colloid nodule.
- **Cytology:** Suspicious for follicular tumor with oncocytic differentiation.
- **Right hemithyroidectomy:** Follicular thyroid carcinoma with oncocytic differentiation. Minimally invasive.

Features
Hypoechoic
Granular echo pattern
Well circumscribed
Tiny cysts
"Spoke-and-wheel-like" vascularity

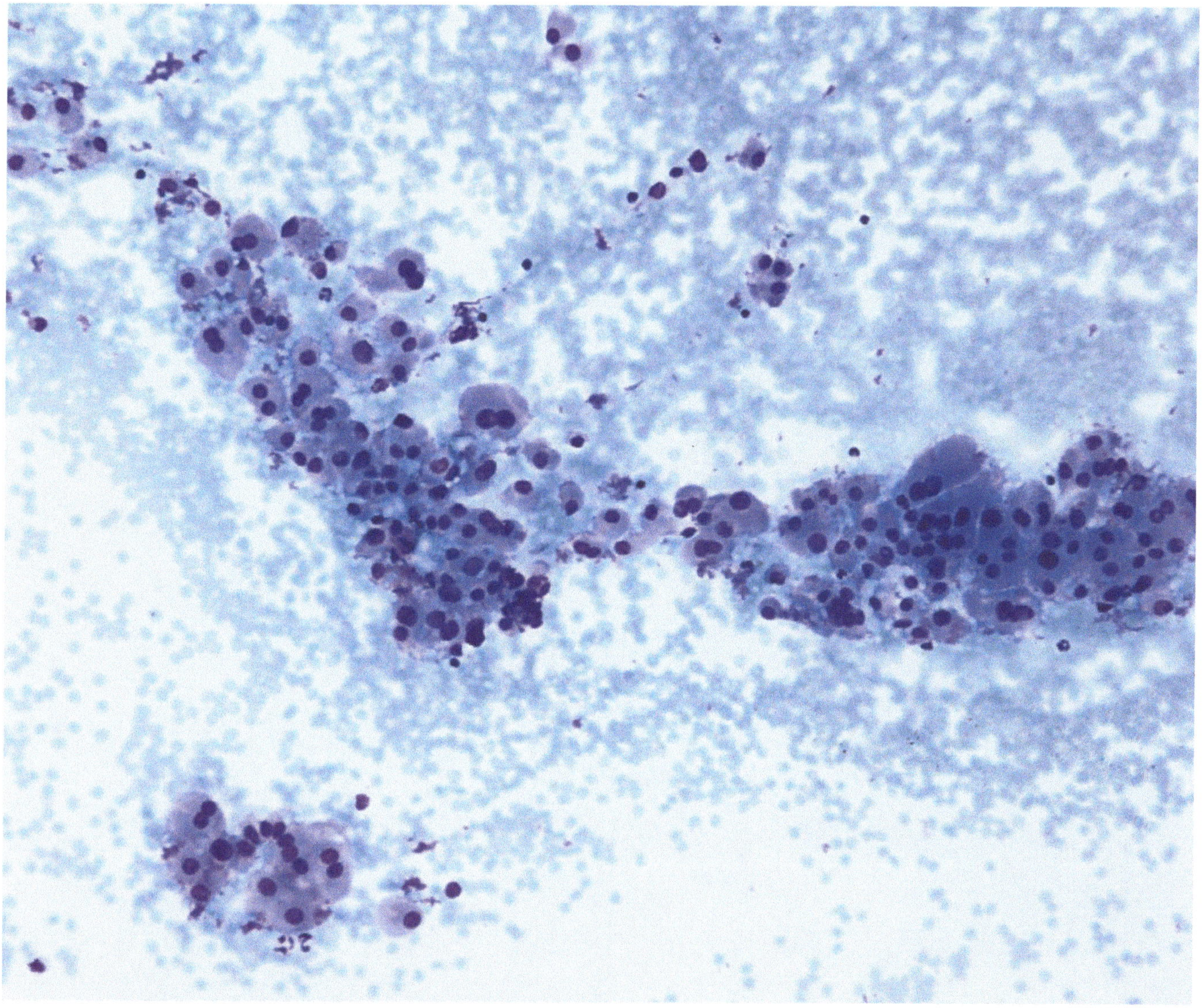

Figure 4-104. Cytology: oncocytic follicular epithelium.

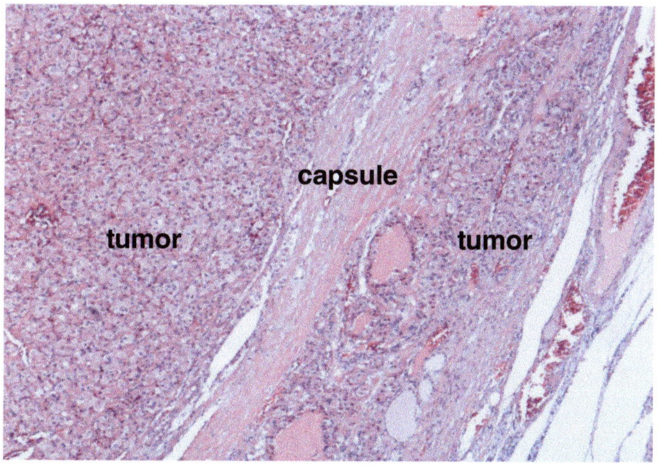

Figure 4-105. Histology: Follicular thyroid carcinoma with oncocytic differentiation. Infiltration through the capsule.

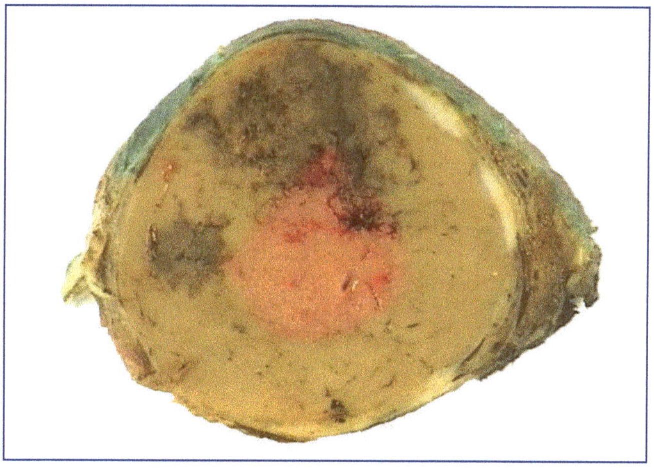

Figure 4-106. Gross section: mahogany brown appearance of the tumor.

5 Oncocytic Nodule/ Hürtle Cell Tumors

Formerly oncocytic lesions were regarded as a definite entity, but this classification is no longer used. Cytopathologists define oncocytic cells as follows: "Oncocytic follicular cells in the thyroid, known as Hürtle cells, are characterized by large size, polygonal to square shape, distinct cell borders, voluminous granular and eosinophilic cytoplasm, and a large, often hyperchromatic nucleus with prominent cherry pink macronucleoli". The proliferation of oncocytes gives rise to hyperplastic and neoplastic nodules. Oncocytic cells may behave as follicular thyroid carcinomas including capsular and vascular invasion, or they may behave as papillary thyroid carcinomas showing papillary architecture.

Features

It is unlikely that oncocytic nodules will have any specific characteristics on ultrasound.

Cytologic Morphology

The material is often cellular containing oncocytic cells with characteristic abundant eosinophilic cytoplasm and round nuclei with fine dispersed chromatin. The material is either devoid of colloid or contains just a sparse amount. As for follicular neoplasm with ordinary follicular epithelium, the finding of some colloid in material rich with oncocytic epithelium does not exclude a diagnosis of neoplasm. From many follicular lesions the yield of material may be bloody and the amount of epithelium scant. Puncture with a 27-gauge needle without aspiration may reduce the amount of blood and achieve a more cellular specimen.

Examples of oncocytic cells can be found on the following pages: Colloid nodules, page 59; in follicular adenomas, pages 95, 99; in follicular thyroid carcinomas, pages 101, 109, 119; in follicular variant of papillary thyroid carcinoma, page 139; and in thyroiditis, pages 237, 241.

6 Follicular Variant of Papillary Thyroid Carcinoma

Morphologically, follicular variant of papillary thyroid carcinoma (FVPTC) may appear partially or completely encapsulated and can be misdiagnosed as follicular adenoma or follicular carcinoma pathologically and on ultrasound examination. They can be hyper-, iso-, hypoechoic, or mixed with an uneven hypoechoic capsule that is hypervascular with a "spoke-and-wheel-like" appearance. Some have sharply marginated areas of different echogenicity within the tumor, a feature we introduce as geographic echo pattern (*see page* 9). If microcalcifications are found inside the tumor, FVPTC is more likely the diagnosis. These encapsulated FVPTC are often solitary. If they are not encapsulated, they often look like an ordinary PTC both pathologically and on US examination [17].

Pathologic Morphology

Among the different subtypes of PTC, FVPTC is the most frequent after the classical variant. FVPTC demonstrates a follicular growth pattern and the follicles are lined by cells with the characteristic features of PTC. In some cases, the classic nuclear features are only present in small areas of tumor, and quite often these features are missing in cytologic smears. When the radiologic investigation shows a tumor suspicious for FVPTC, one should look at the smears thoroughly and try to find nuclear grooves and/or inclusions. There has been some debate concerning how to classify follicular neoplasias with foci of nuclei consistent with PTC. According to recent recommendations, all patients with these types of tumors should be treated as though they had PTC of classic variant.

Pathologically, the most important criteria for diagnosis of FVPTC are cytoplasmic invagination into the nucleus, abundant nuclear grooves, ground glass nuclei, psammoma bodies, enlarged overlapping nuclei, and irregularly shaped nuclei.

Common Features of Encapsulated Follicular Variant of Papillary Thyroid Carcinoma

Solitary
Well circumscribed
Uneven complete or partial hypoechoic halo
Homogeneous or geographic echo pattern
Mixed echogenicity
Hypervascular with suggestion of "spoke-and-wheel-like" vascularity

Common Features of Not Encapsulated Follicular Variant of Papillary Thyroid Carcinoma

Irregular borders, blurred margins
Absence of peripheral halo
Inhomogeneous echo pattern
Mixed echogenicity
Microcalcifications
Often intranodular hypervascularity

Follicular Variant of Papillary Thyroid Carcinoma Right Lobe

Transverse | **Longitudinal**

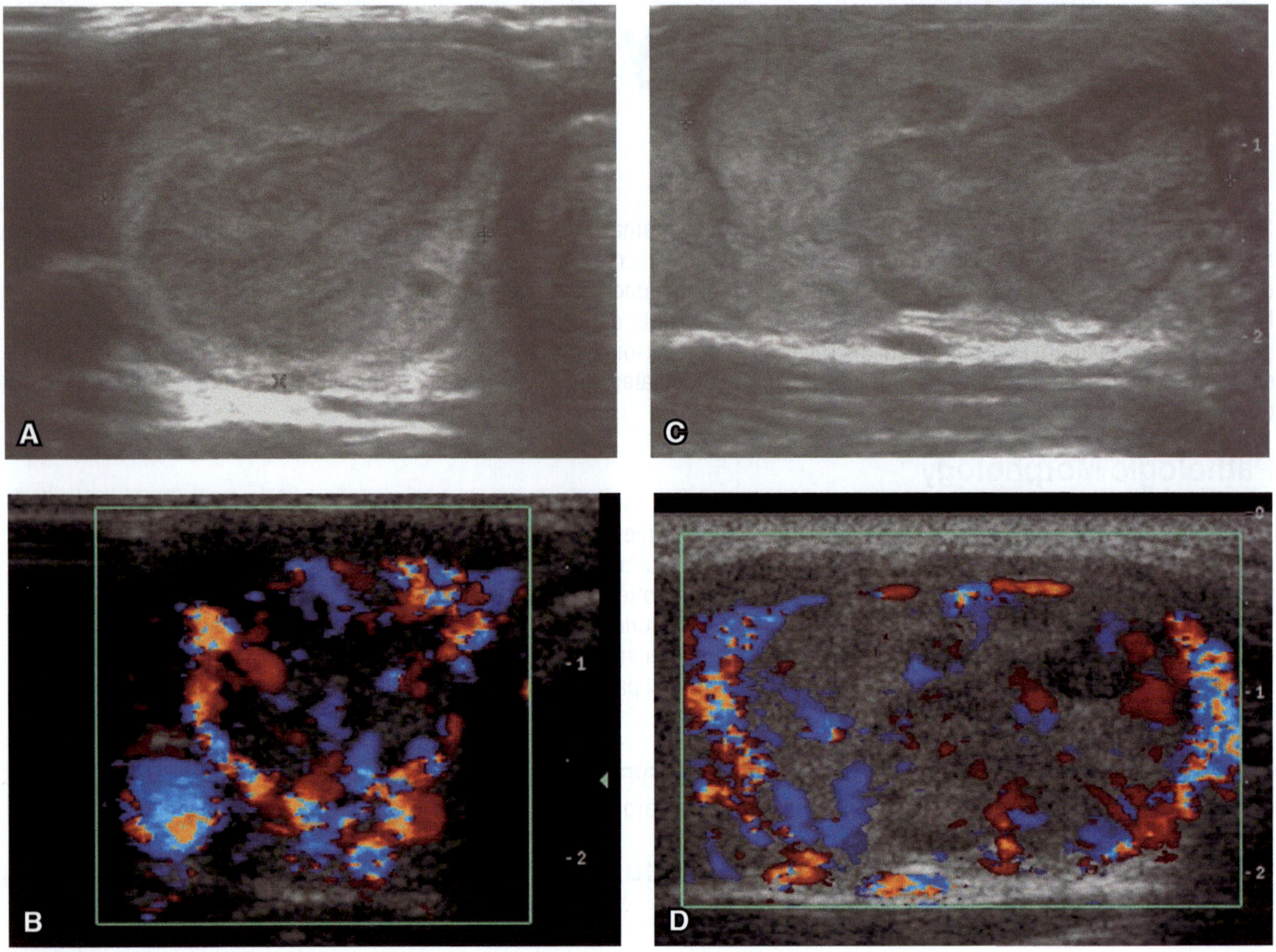

FIGURE 6-1. Ultrasound of follicular variant of papillary thyroid carcinoma in the right lobe. **A**, Transverse, 17 x 19 mm. **B**, Color Doppler, transverse. **C**, Longitudinal, sagittal diameter: 28 mm. **D**, Color Doppler, longitudinal.

39-Year-old woman

- **Clinical history:** Palpable nodule in right thyroid lobe for some months. Euthyroid.
- **Scintigraphy:** Cold nodule.
- **Ultrasound:** Follicular tumor. Malignant?
- **Cytology:** Follicular lesion.
- **Right hemithyroidectomy:** Follicular variant of papillary thyroid carcinoma.

Features

Mixed echogenicity
Geographic, inhomogeneous echo pattern
Well circumscribed
Partial thin hypoechoic halo
Hypervascular with “spoke-and-wheel-like” appearance

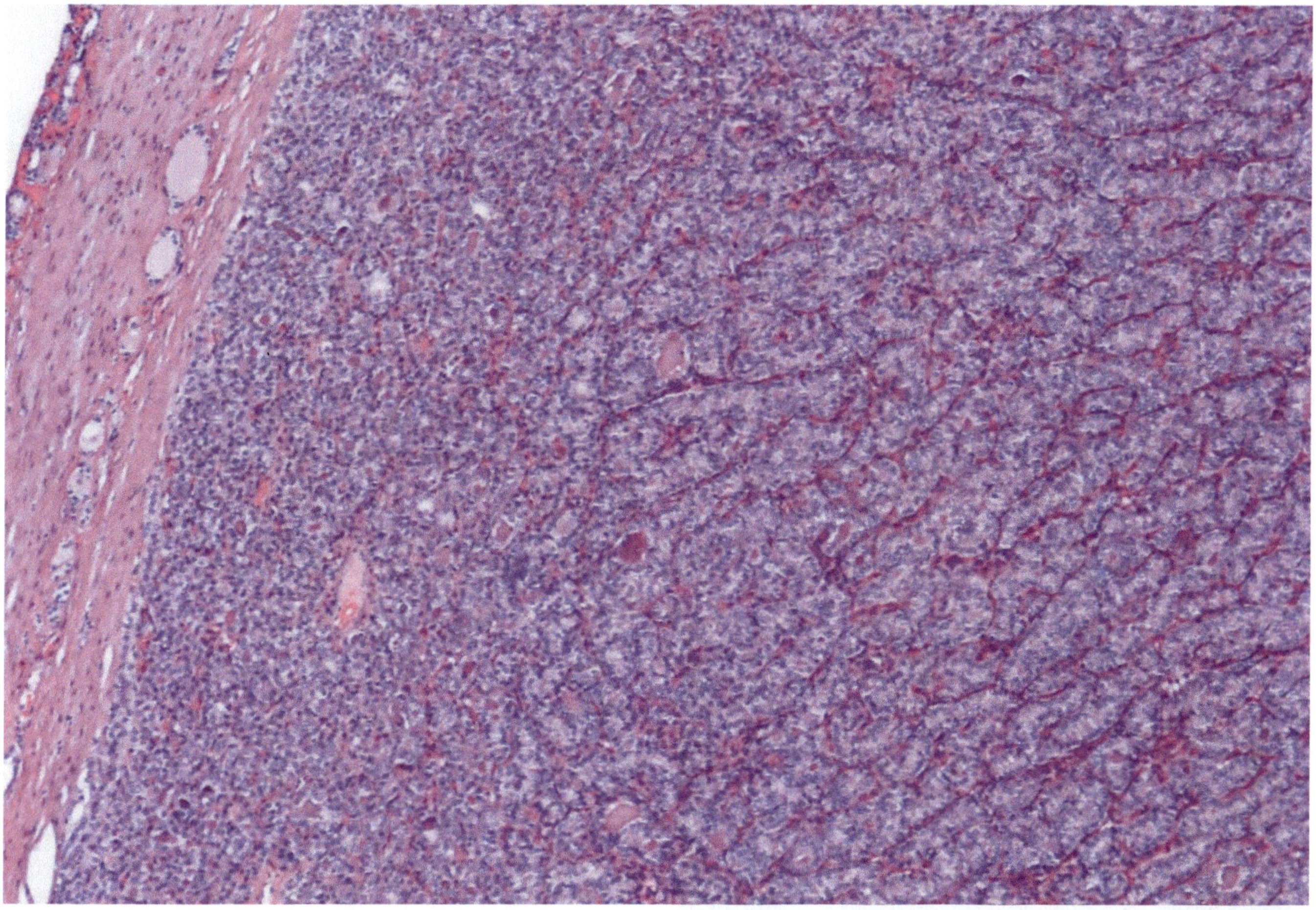

Figure 6-2. Histology: follicular variant of papillary thyroid carcinoma.

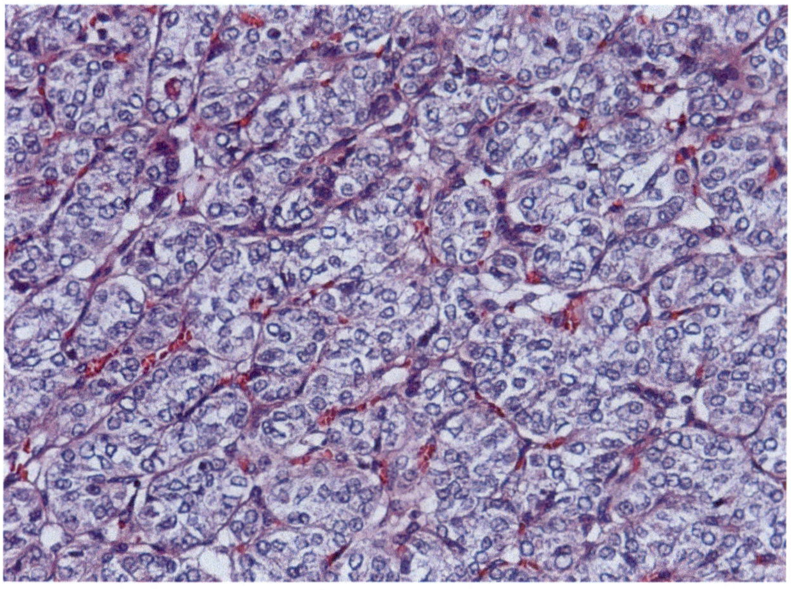

Figure 6-3. Histology: nuclear features of papillary thyroid carcinoma.

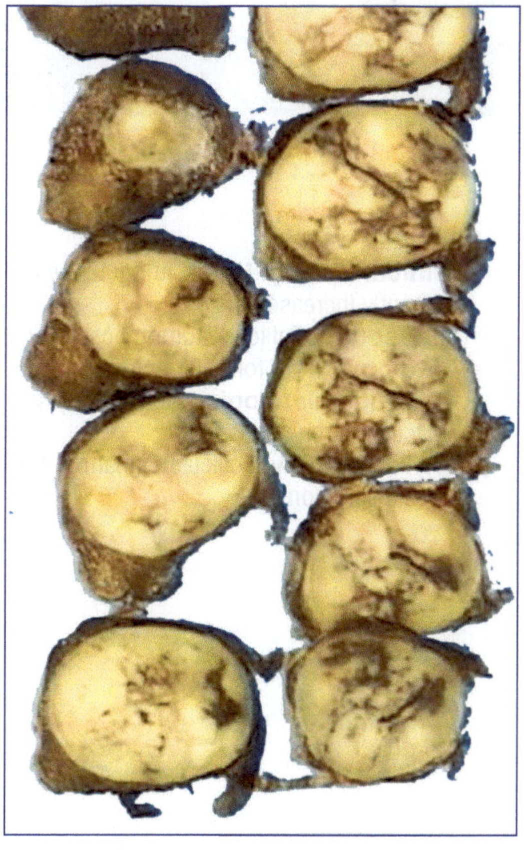

Figure 6-4. Gross section: several slices through the tumor.

Follicular Variant of Papillary Thyroid Carcinoma Right Lobe

Transverse **Longitudinal**

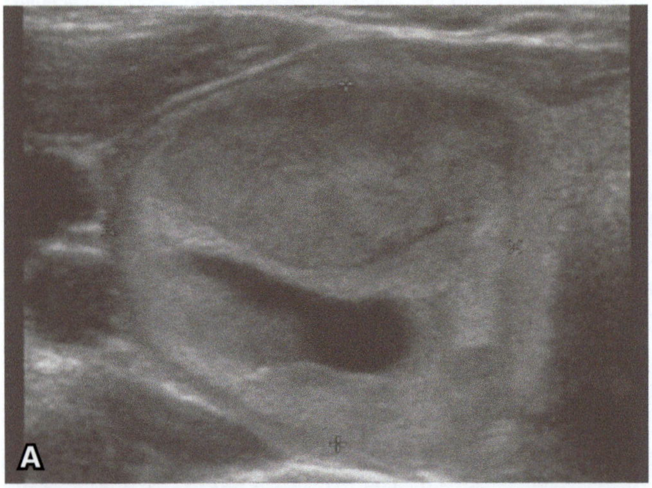

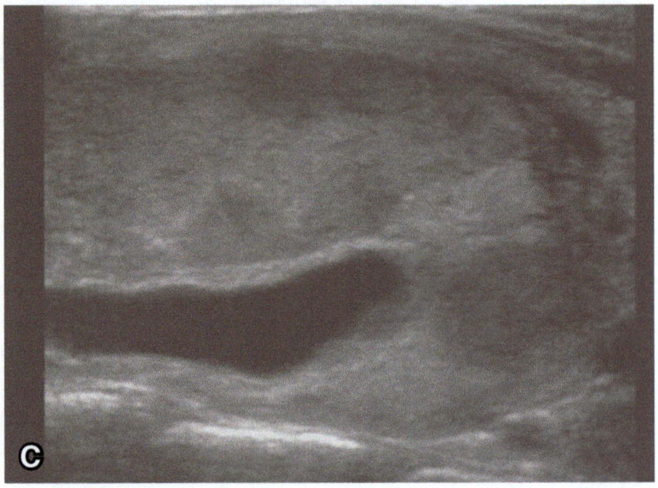

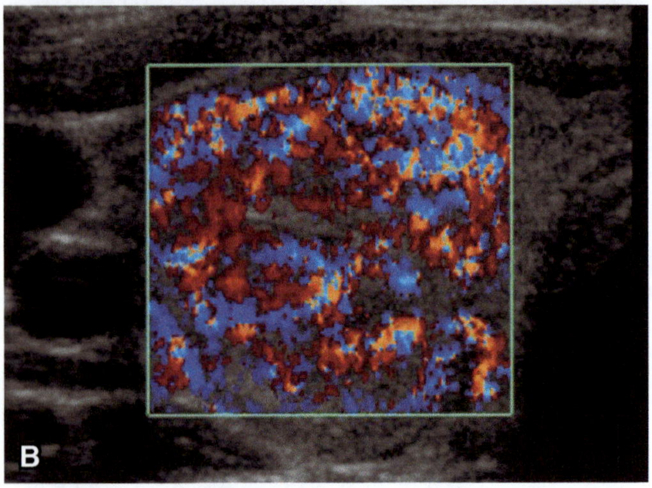

Figure 6-5. Ultrasound of follicular variant of papillary thyroid carcinoma in the right lobe. **A**, Transverse, 23 x 26 mm. **B**, Color Doppler, transverse. **C**, Longitudinal.

29-Year-old woman

- **Clinical history:** Nodule in right lobe for a while. Presently increased size.
- **Ultrasound:** Follicular tumor, possibly malignant.
- **Cytology:** Scant follicular epithelium.
- **18-Gauge histologic needle biopsy:** Follicular parenchyma.
- **Thyroidectomy:** Follicular variant of papillary thyroid carcinoma.

Features

Geographic, inhomogeneous echo pattern with hypoechoic, isoechoic, and cystic well marginated areas

Well circumscribed

Uneven, partially thick hypoechoic halo

Highly hypervascular

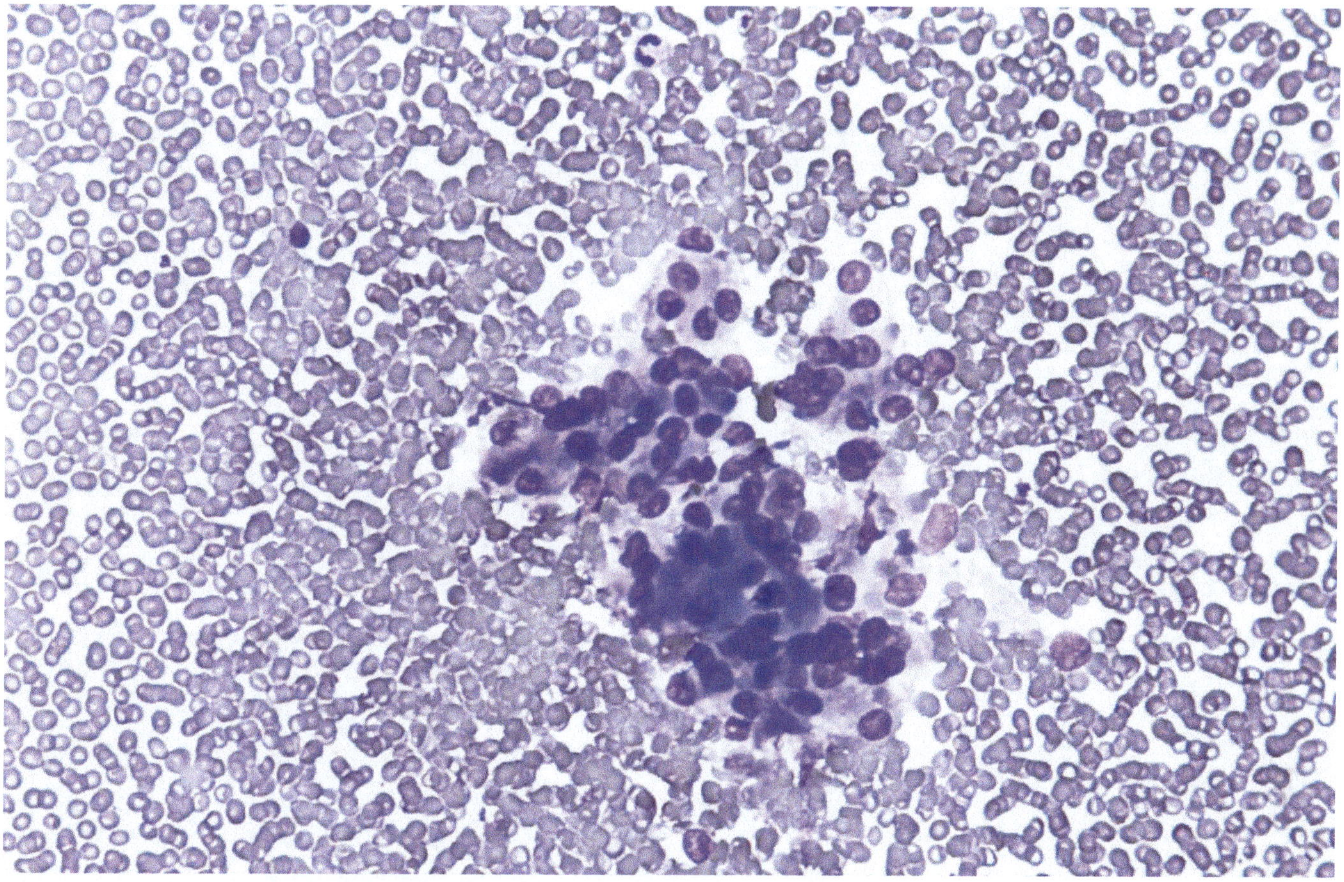

Figure 6-6. Cytology: follicular cells with no obvious features of papillary thyroid carcinoma (PTC).

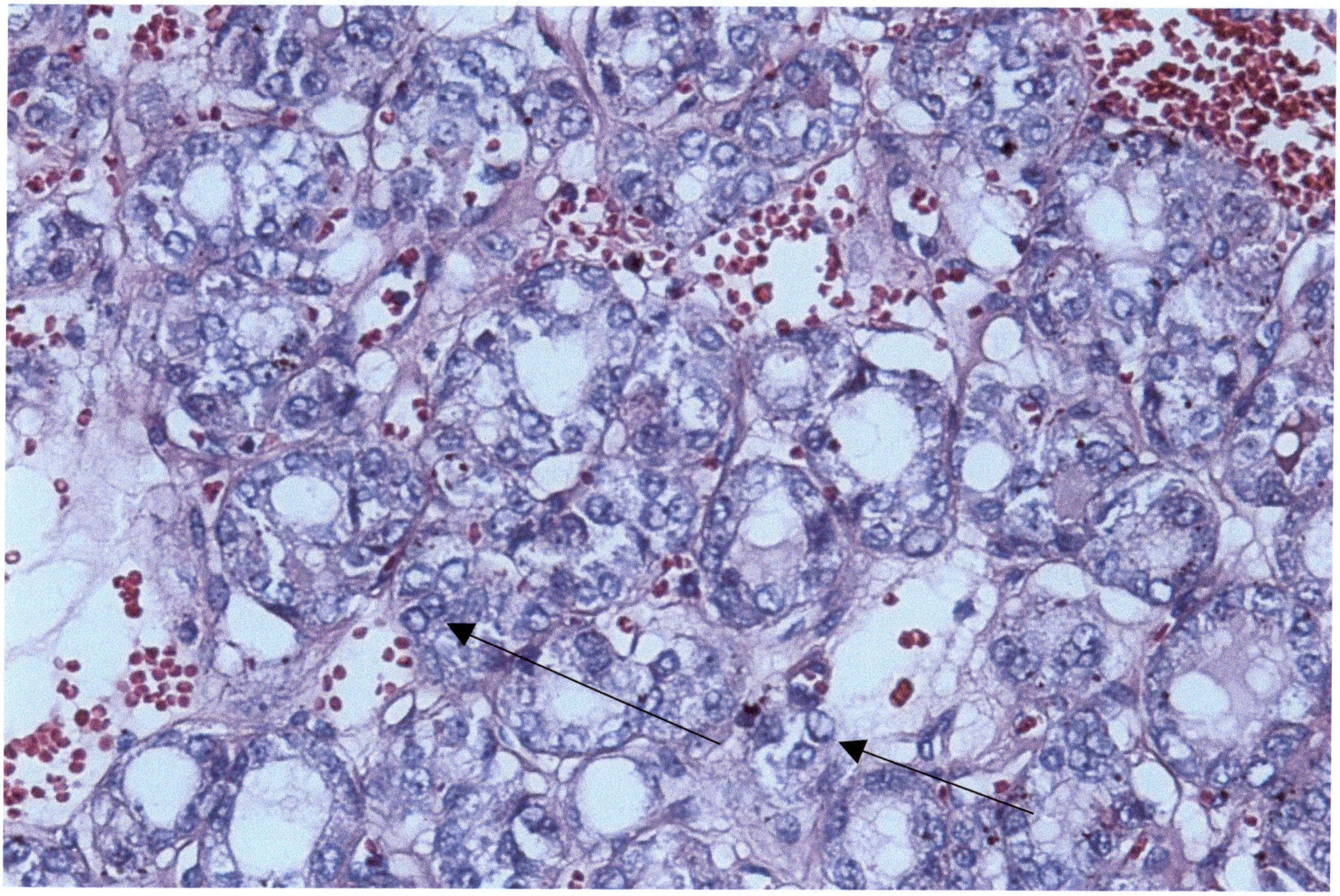

Figure 6-7. Histology: follicular growth pattern, nuclear features of PTC. Nuclear clearings (*left arrow*). Nuclear groove (*right arrow*).

Follicular Variant of Papillary Thyroid Carcinoma Left Lobe

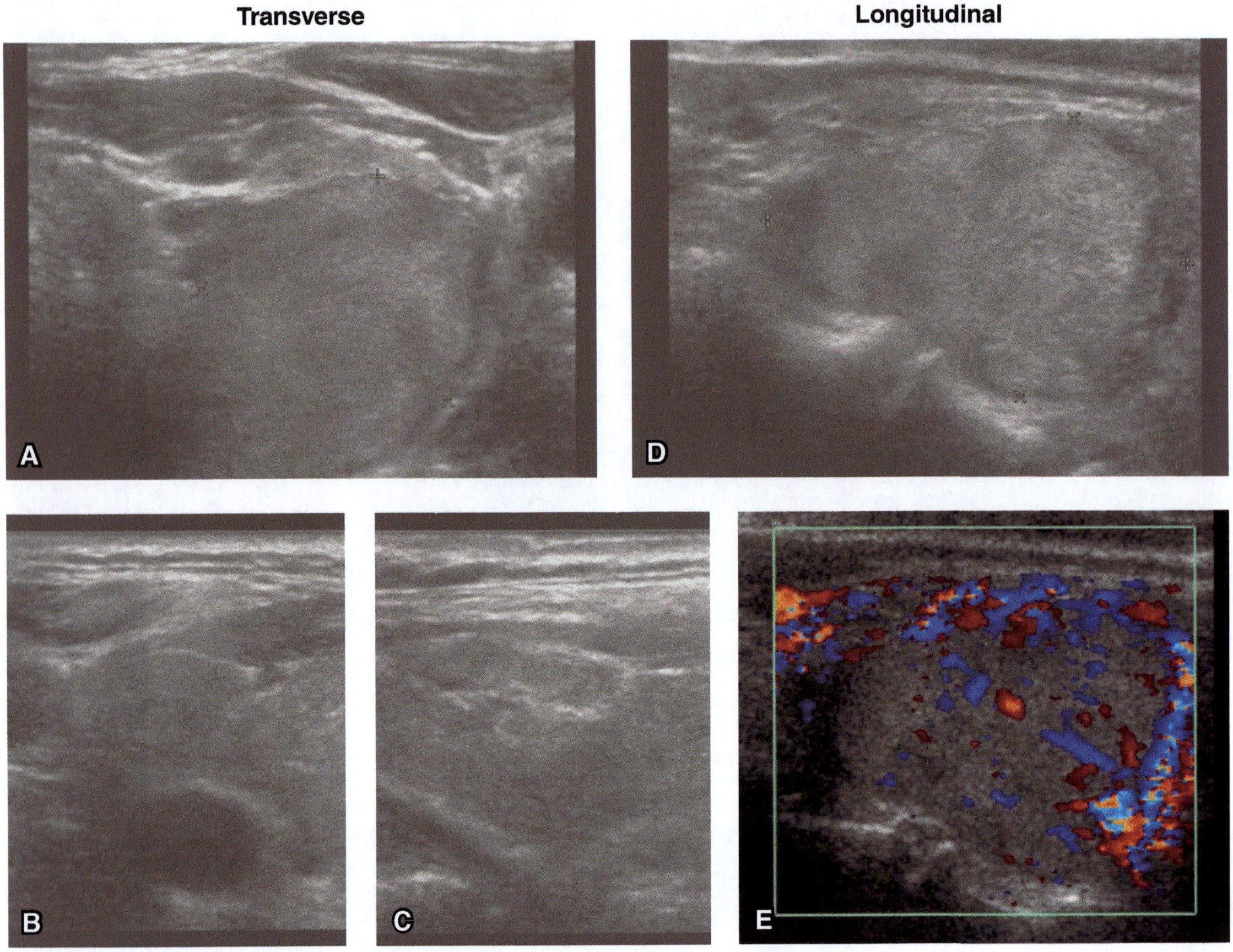

Figure 6-8. Ultrasound of follicular variant of papillary thyroid carcinoma in the left lobe. **A**, Transverse, 19 x 24 mm. **B**, Right lobe transverse. **C**, Transverse. **D**, Longitudinal, sagittal diameter: 39 mm. **E**, Color Doppler, longitudinal.

73-Year-old woman

- **Clinical history:** Goiter, most prominent in left lobe.
- **Ultrasound:** Follicular tumor suspicious for malignancy + thyroiditis.
- **Cytology:** Papillary thyroid carcinoma (PTC).
- **Thyroidectomy:** Follicular variant of PTC. Hashimoto's thyroiditis.

Features

Slightly hypoechoic
Slightly inhomogenous echo pattern
Mostly well circumscribed, but blurred margin medially and upper part
Partial thin hypoechoic halo
Somewhat hypervascularized with suggestion of "spoke-and-wheel-like" appearance

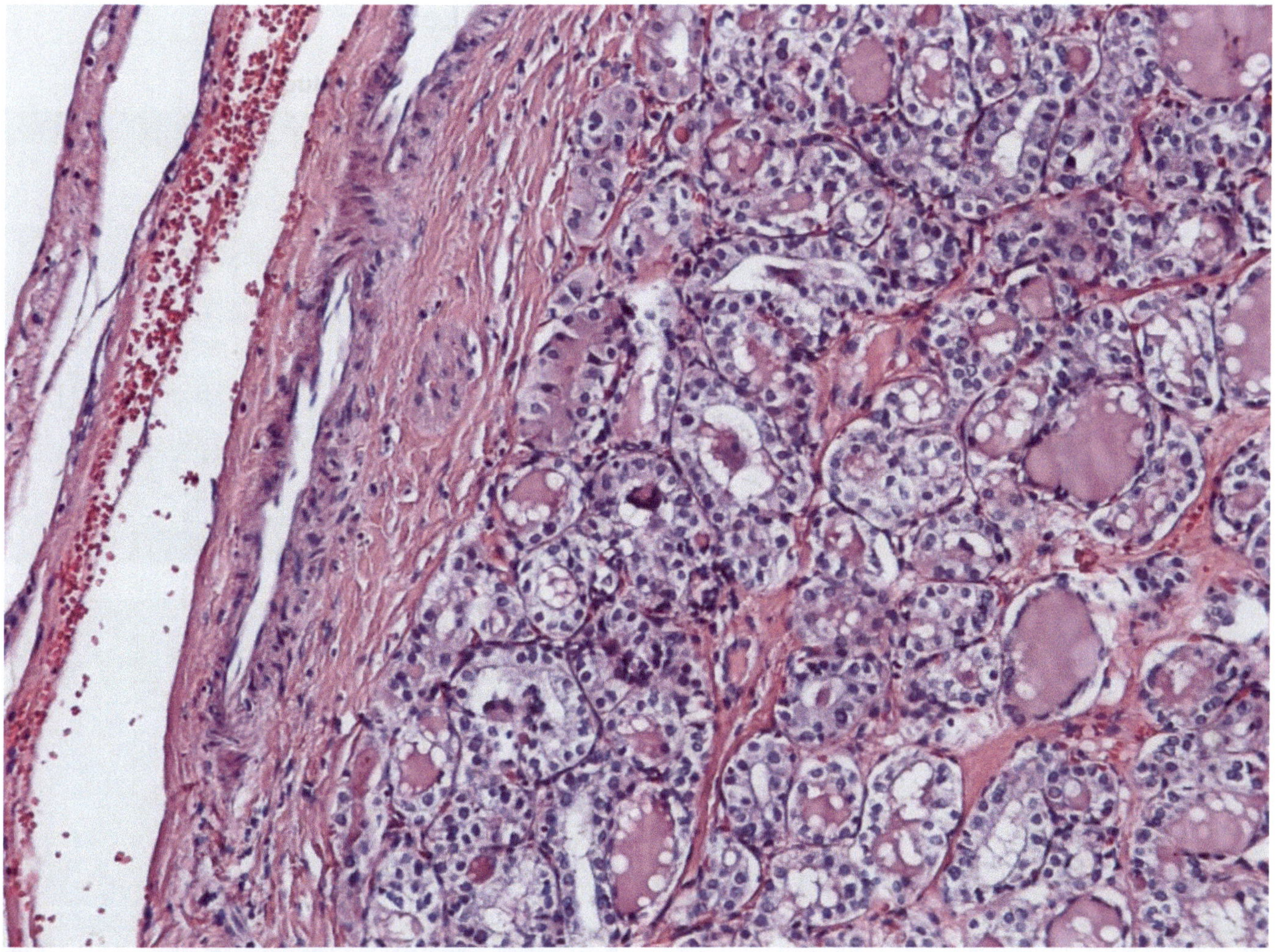

Figure 6-9. Histology: follicular variant of papillary thyroid carcinoma.

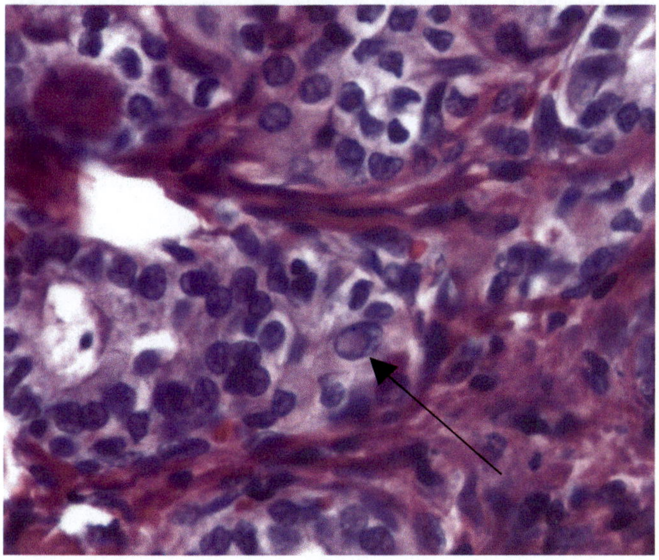

Figure 6-10. Histology: optically clear nucleus (*arrow*).

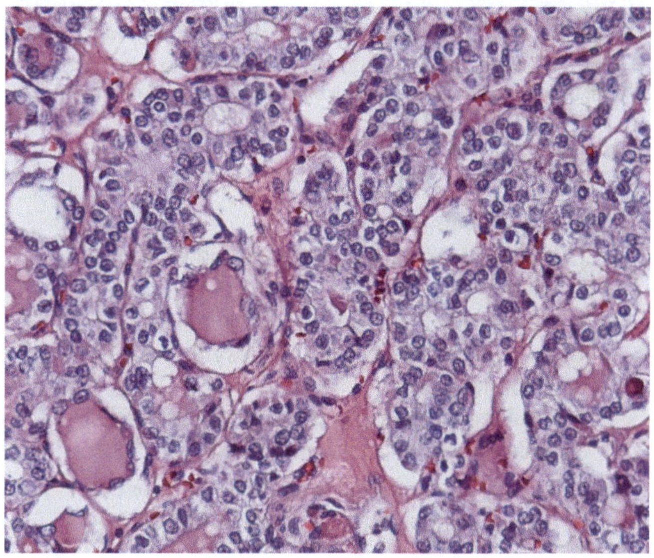

Figure 6-11. Histology: follicular variant of papillary thyroid carcinoma.

Follicular Variant of Papillary Thyroid Carcinoma Left Lobe

Transverse | Longitudinal

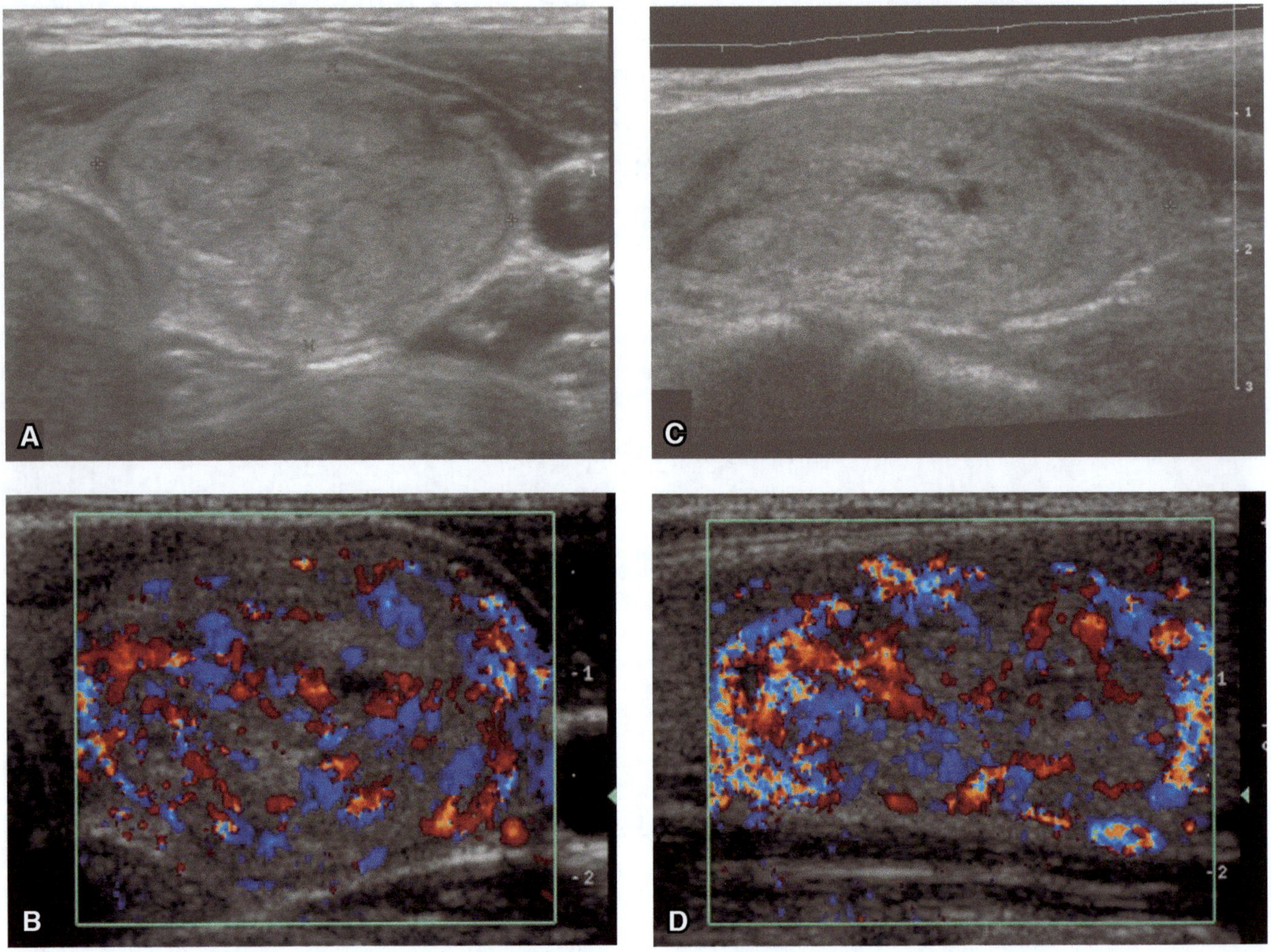

FIGURE 6-12. Ultrasound of follicular variant of papillary thyroid carcinoma in the left lobe. **A**, Transverse, 17 x 25 mm. **B**, Color Doppler, transverse. **C**, Longitudinal, sagittal diameter: 39 mm. **D**, Color Doppler, longitudinal.

29-Year-old woman

- **Clinical history:** Growing tumor in left lobe past 2 months.
- **Ultrasound:** Probably follicular adenoma.
- **Cytology:** Suspicious for papillary thyroid carcinoma (PTC).
- **16-Gauge histologic needle biopsy:** PTC.
- **Thyrectomy:** Follicular variant of PTC.

Features

Almost isoechoic
Inhomogeneous echo pattern
Well circumscribed
Partial thin, uneven hypoechoic halo
Some small cysts
A few microcalcifications?
Suggestion of "spoke-and-wheel-like" hypervascularity

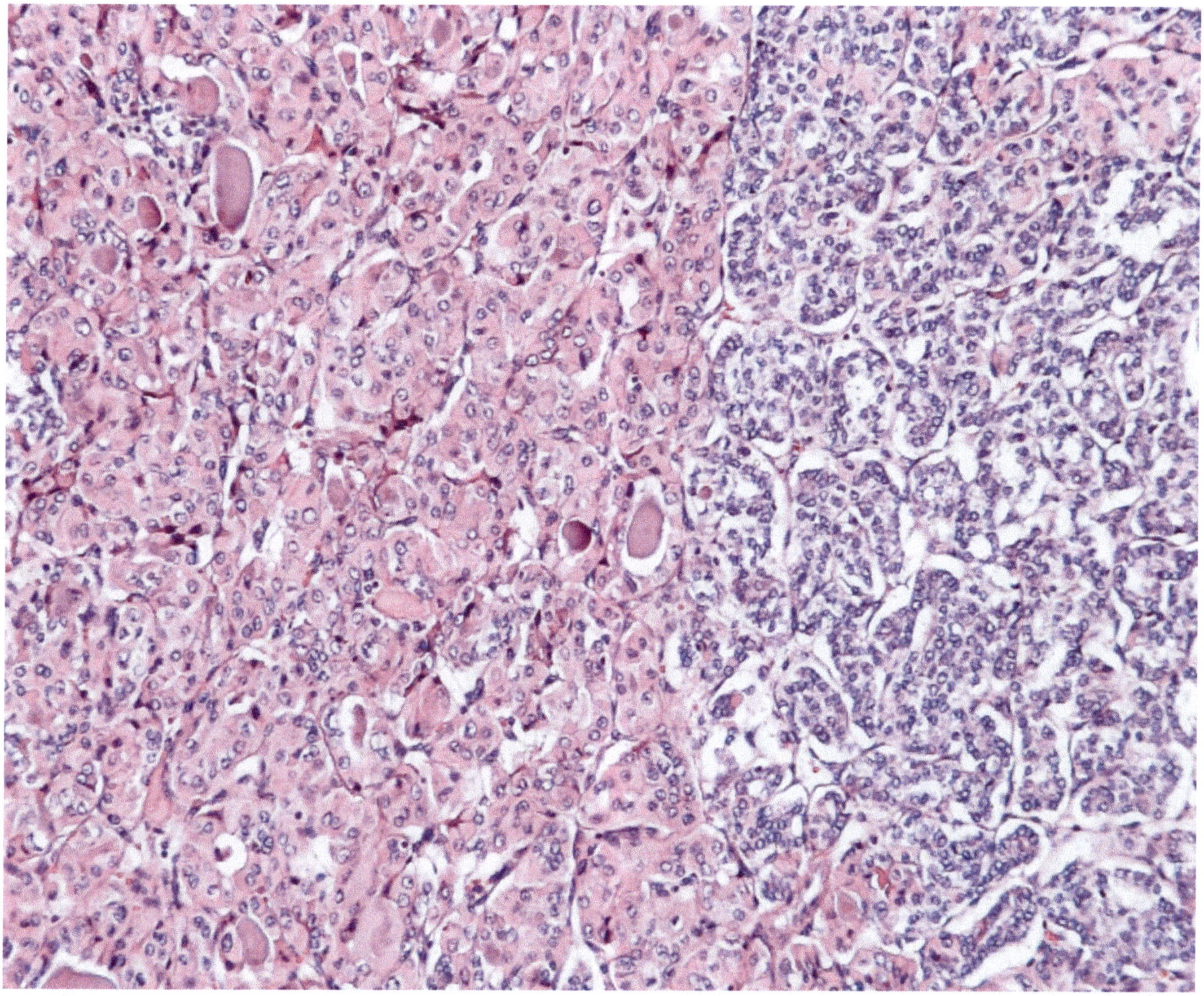

Figure 6-13. Histology: nuclear features of follicular variant of papillary thyroid carcinoma. Area with oncocytic differentiations to the left.

Follicular Variant of Papillary Thyroid Carcinoma Both Lobes

Right lobe transverse **Left lobe transverse**

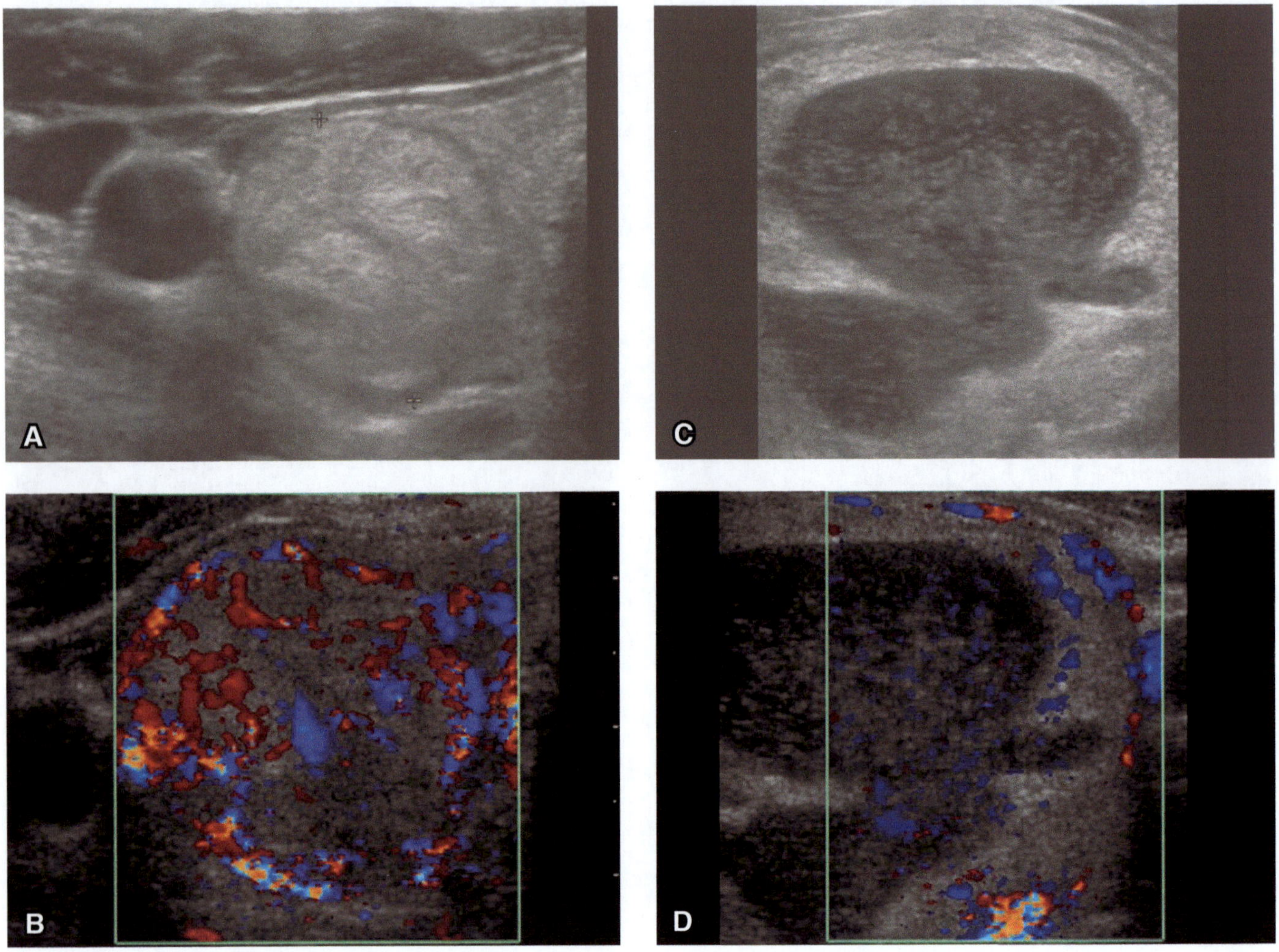

Figure 6-14. Ultrasound of follicular variant of papillary thyroid carcinoma in both lobes. **A**, Right lobe transverse, 23 x 24 mm. **B**, Color Doppler, right lobe transverse. **C**, Left lobe transverse, anteroposterior diameter: 42 mm. **D**, Color Doppler, left lobe transverse.

44-Year-old man

- **Clinical history:** Thyroid carcinoma in his family. Nodule in left lobe.
- **Ultrasound right lobe:** Probably follicular adenoma.
- **Ultrasound left lobe:** Probably cystic colloid nodule.
- **Cytology right lobe:** Suspicious for follicular neoplasia.
- **Cytology left lobe:** Cystic lesion with necrosis. Tumor?
- **16-Gauge histologic needle biopsy right lobe:** Inadequate biopsy.
- **16-Gauge histologic needle biopsy left lobe:** Normal thyroid tissue.
- **Thyroidectomy:** Follicular variant of papillary thyroid carcinoma in both lobes.

Features right lobe

Isoechoic, slightly inhomogeneous echo pattern
Well circumscribed
Thin hypoechoic halo
Some microcalcifications
Somewhat hypervascularized with suggestion of “spoke-and-wheel-like” appearance

Features left lobe

Hyperechoic, homogeneous solid tissue
Cystic degeneration probably with hematoma
Scant peripheral vascularity

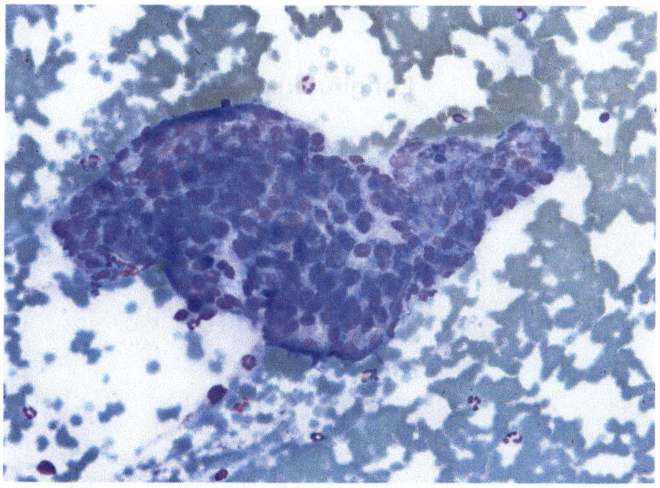

Figure 6-15. Cytology (right lobe): follicular neoplasia.

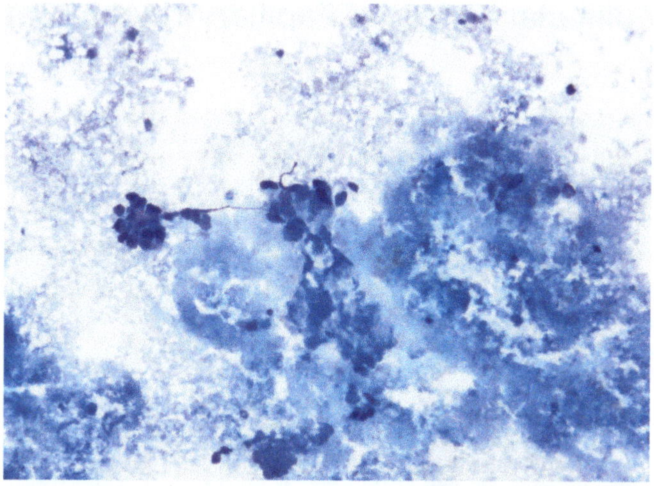

Figure 6-16. Cytology (left lobe): necrosis and some irregular epithelial cells.

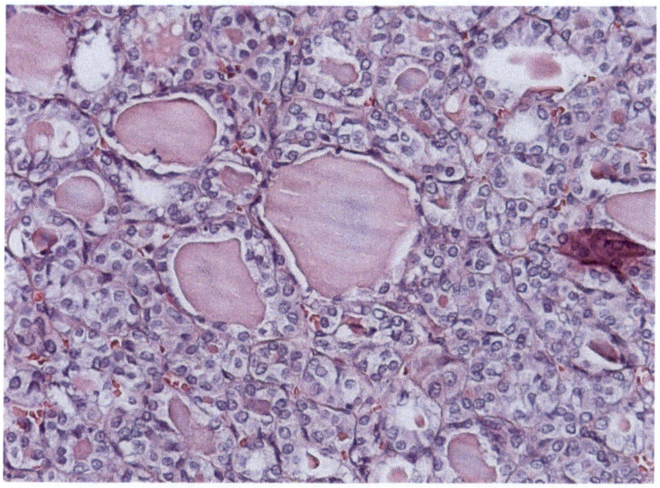

Figure 6-17. Histology (right lobe) : follicular variant of papillary thyroid carcinoma.

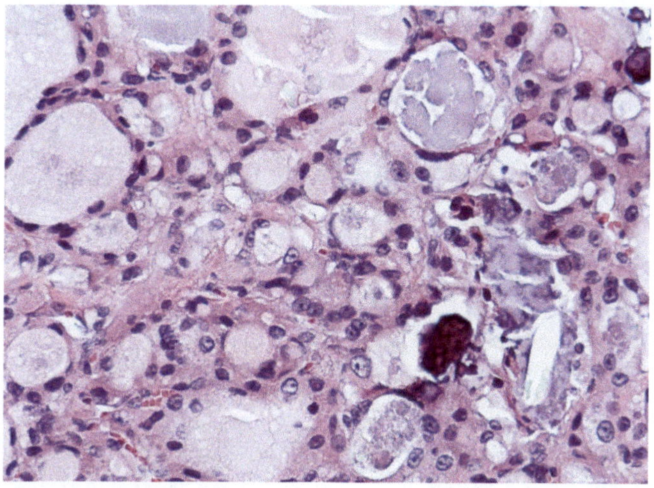

Figure 6-18. Histology (left lobe): psamomma calcification and nuclei with characteristic inclusions.

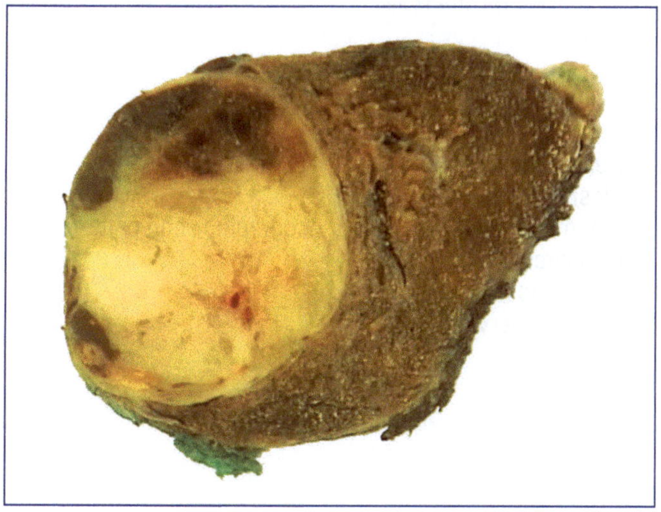

Figure 6-19. Gross section (right lobe): heterogenic, well-demarcated tumor.

Follicular Variant of Papillary Thyroid Carcinoma Right Lobe

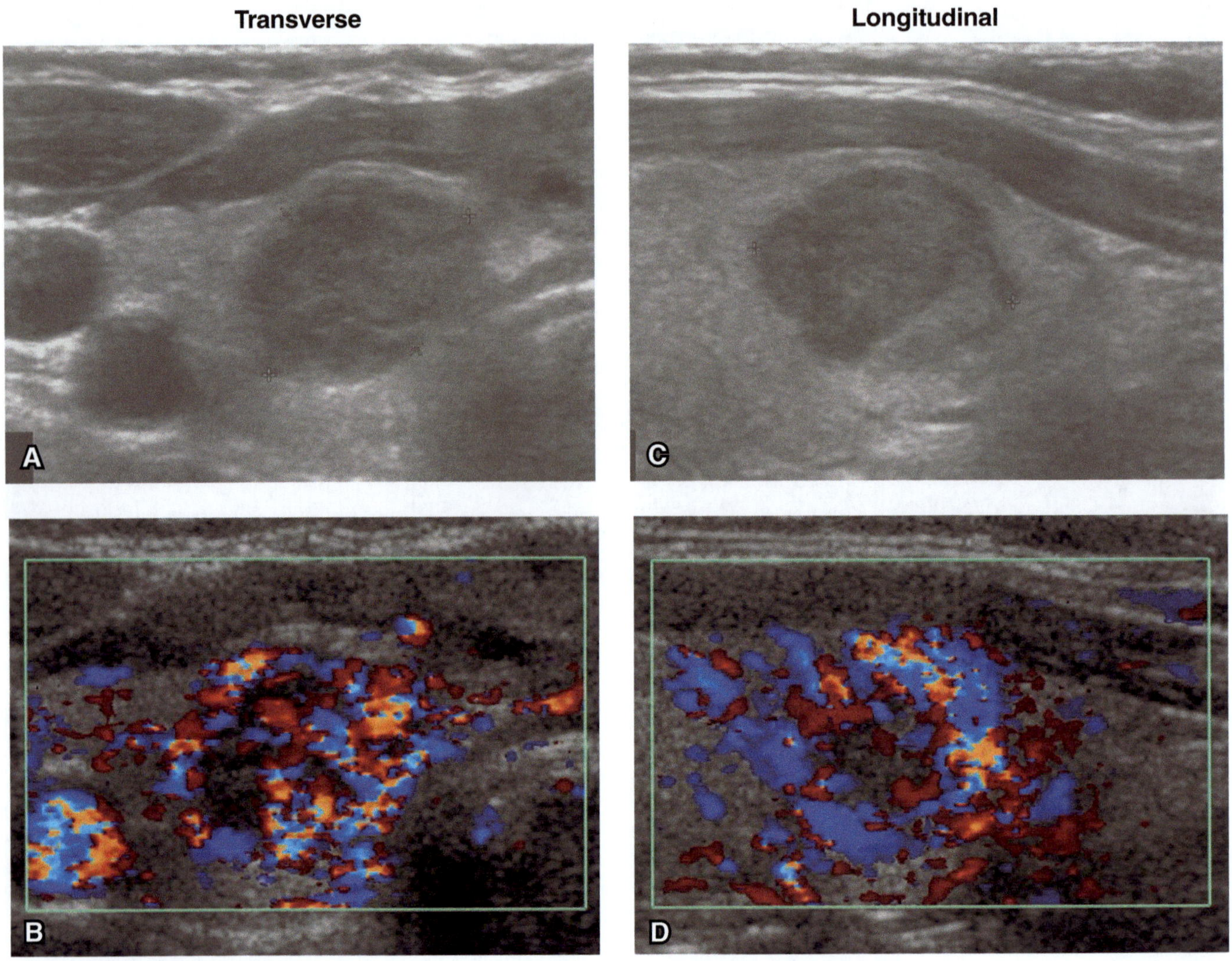

Figure 6-20. Ultrasound of follicular variant of papillary thyroid carcinoma in the right lobe. **A**, Transverse, 10 x 14 mm. **B**, Color Doppler, transverse. **C**, Longitudinal, sagittal diameter: 14 mm. **D**, Color Doppler, longitudinal.

73-Year-old woman

- **Clinical history:** Nodular goiter unraveled 5 months ago. Scintigraphy showed hot nodule in isthmus.
- **Ultrasound:** Probably papillary thyroid carcinoma (PTC).
- **Cytology:** Nondiagnostic material.
- **18-Gauge histologic needle biopsy:** Follicular neoplasia.
- **Thyroidectomy:** Follicular variant of PTC.

Features

Mostly hypoechoic
Inhomogeneous, somewhat geographic echo pattern
Well circumscribed
Not encapsulated
Highly hypervascular

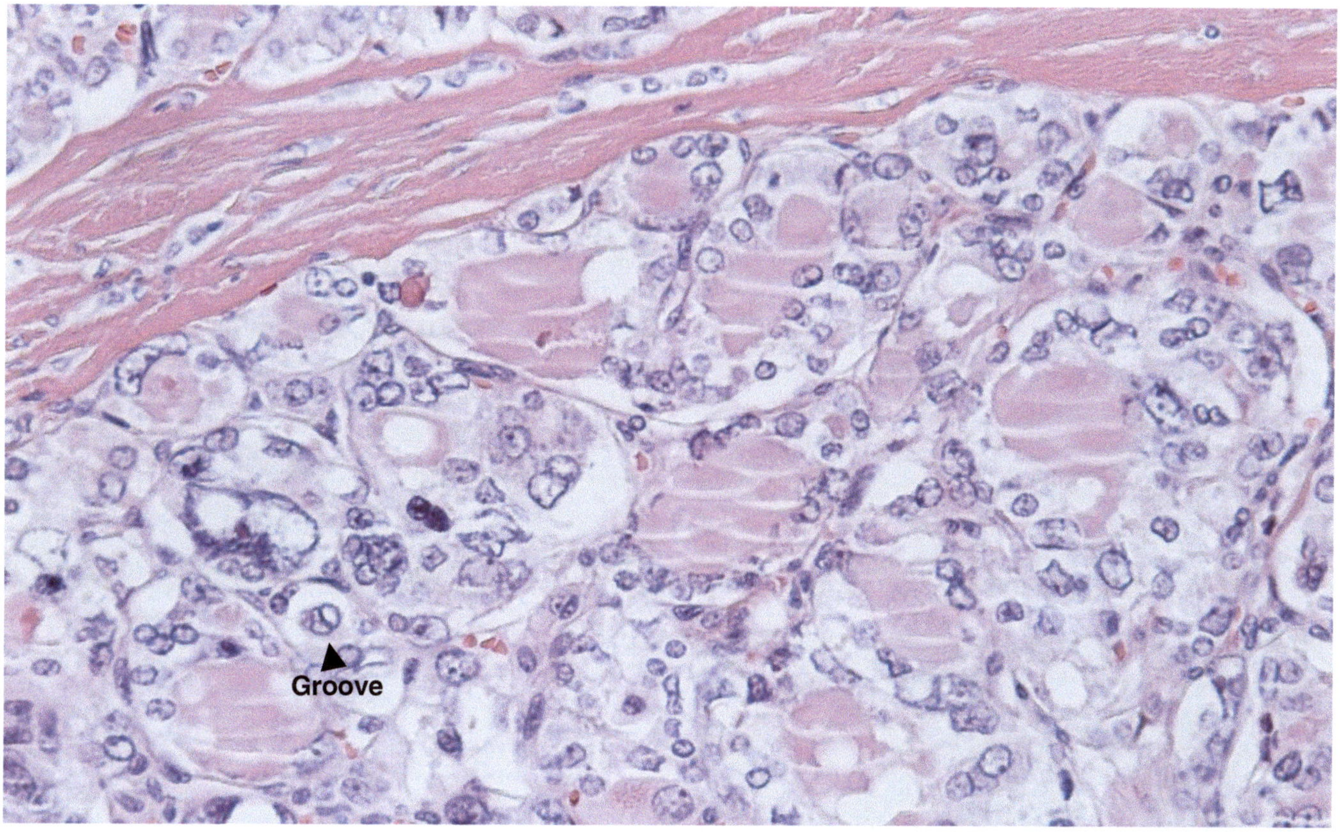

Figure 6-21. Histology: follicular growth pattern. Nuclei consistent with papillary carcinoma.

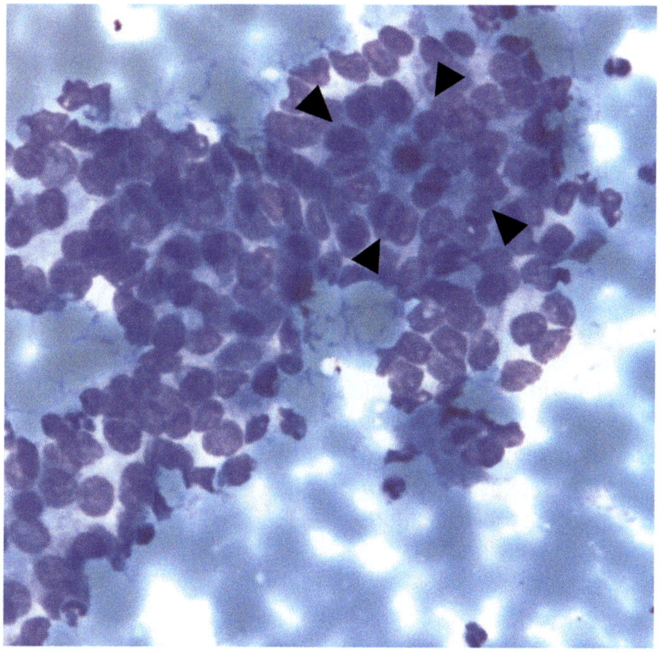

Figure 6-22. Cytology: papillary pattern with one follicular structure (*arrowheads*).

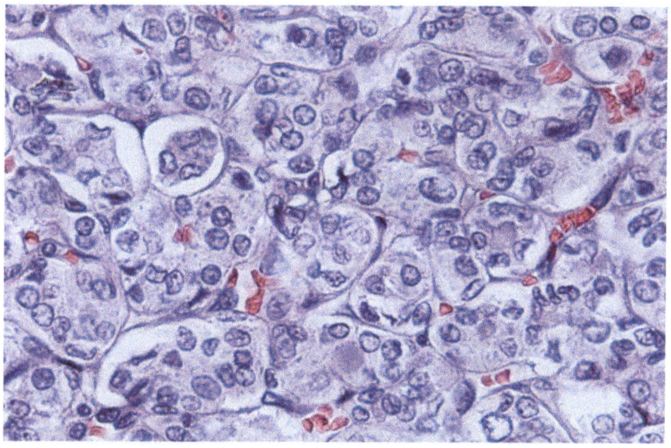

Figure 6-23. Histology: follicular growth pattern. Nuclei consistent with papillary carcinoma.

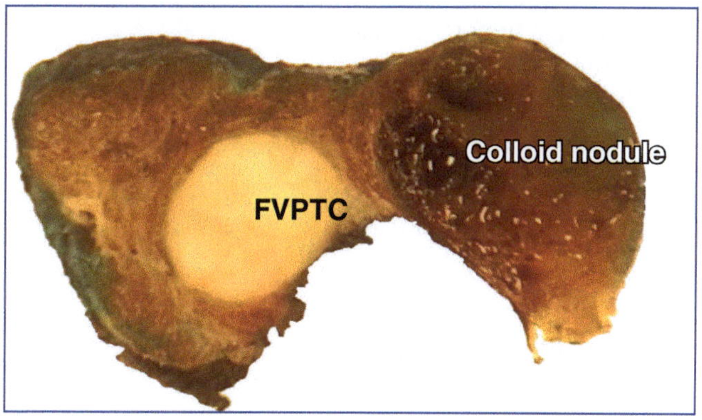

Figure 6-24. Gross section. Follicular variant of papillary thyroid carcinoma (FVPTC).

Follicular Variant of Papillary Thyroid Carcinoma Left Lobe

Transverse

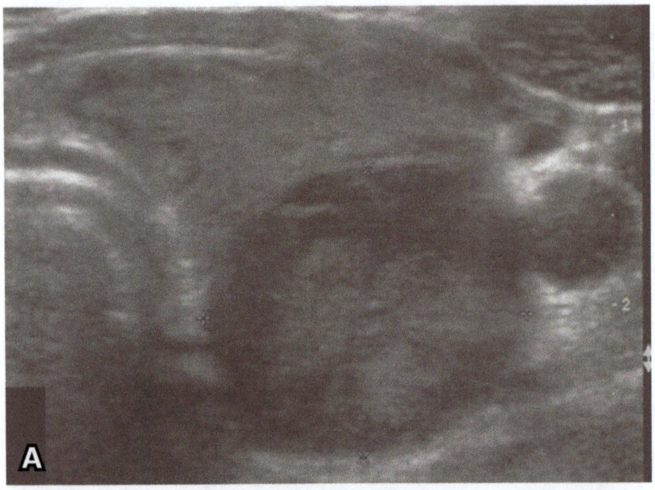

Longitudinal

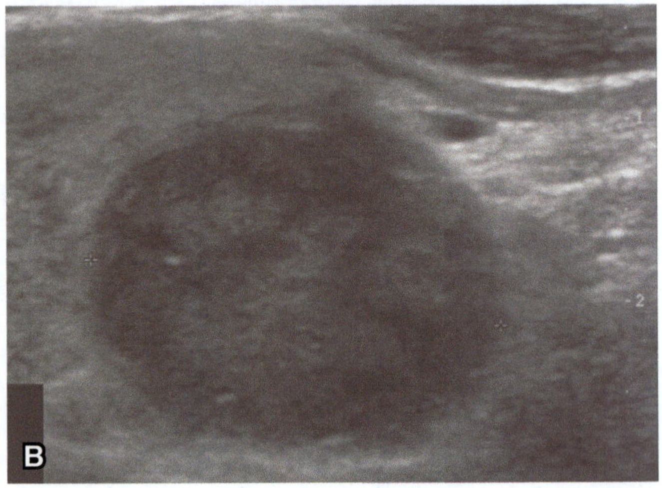

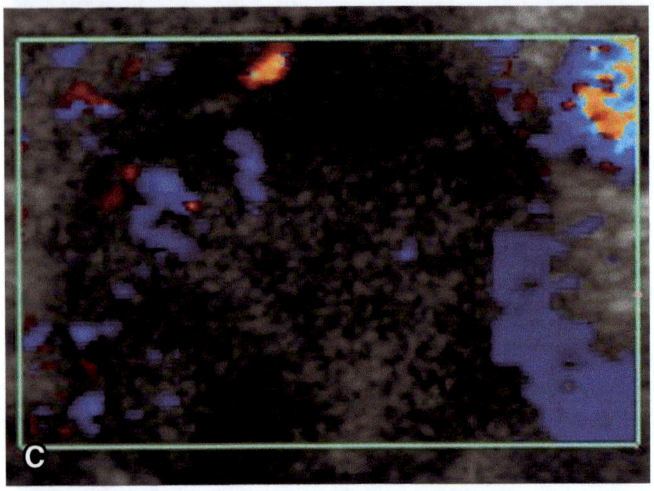

Figure 6-25. Ultrasound of follicular variant of papillary thyroid carcinoma in the left lobe. **A**, Transverse, 16 x 18 mm. **B**, Longitudinal, sagittal diameter: 23 mm. **C**, Color Doppler, longitudinal.

47-Year-old woman

- **Clinical history:** Nodular goiter and autoimmune thyroiditis for many years.
- **Ultrasound:** Probably papillary thyroid carcinoma (PTC).
- **Cytology:** Hashimoto's thyroiditis.
- **18-Gauge histologic needle biopsy:** Malignant tumor. Follicular? Chronic inflammation.
- **Thyroidectomy:** Follicular variant of PTC. Excessive Hashimoto's thyroiditis.

See also pages 56–57

Features

Inhomogeneous echo pattern with concentric hypoechoic bars in less hypoechoic tissue surrounded by a thick, uneven highly hypoechoic halo

Well circumscribed

Not encapsulated

A few microcalcifications

Scant vascularity

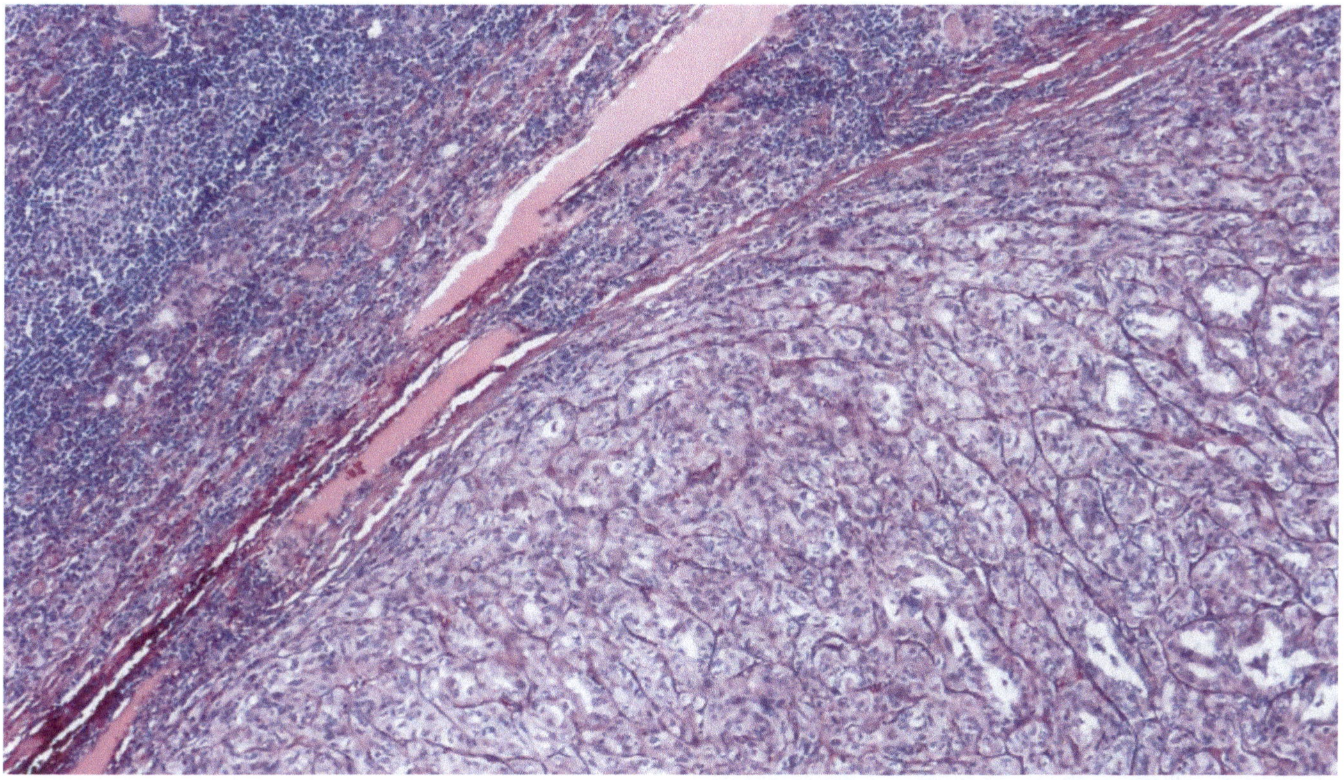

Figure 6-26. Histology: thyroiditis plus follicular variant of papillary thyroid carcinoma.

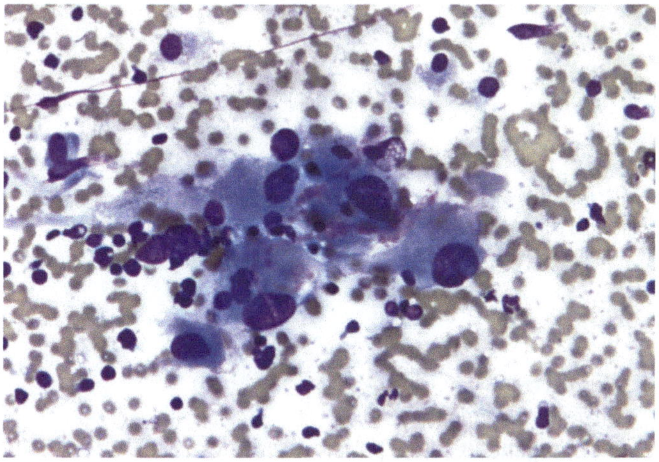

Figure 6-27. Cytology: no distinct characteristics indicating papillary carcinoma.

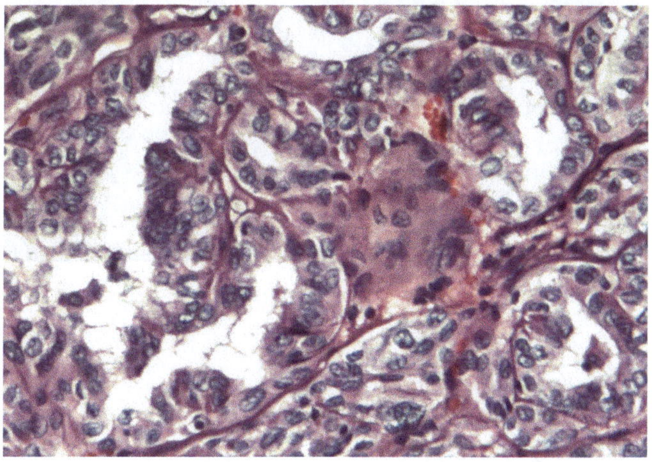

Figure 6-28. Histology: features of follicular variant of papillary thyroid carcinoma.

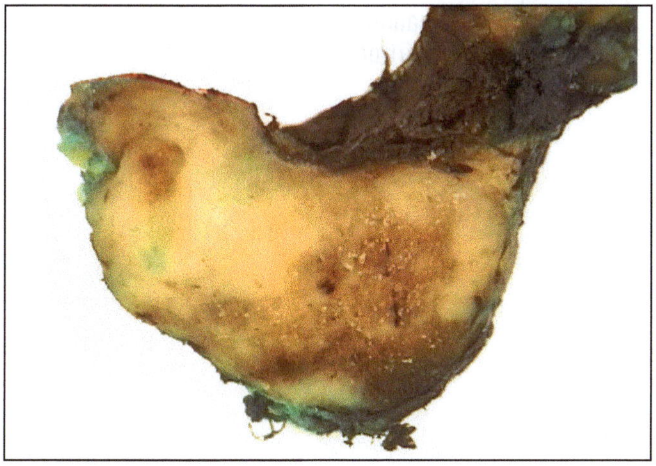

Figure 6-29. Gross section: infiltrating tumor and Hashimoto's thyroiditis.

Follicular Variant of Papillary Thyroid Carcinoma Right Lobe

Transverse

Longitudinal

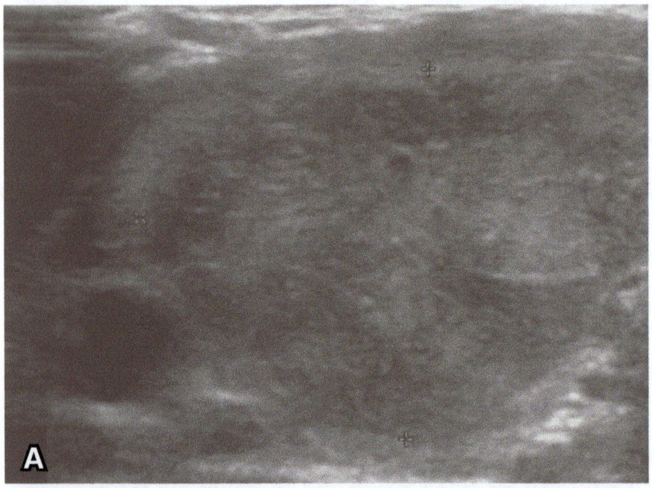

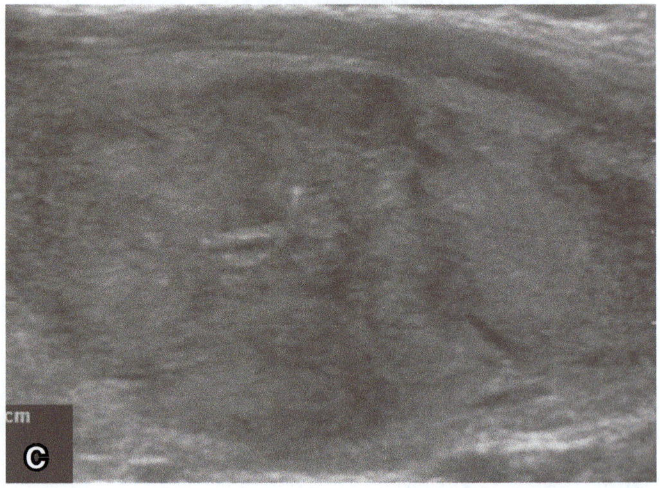

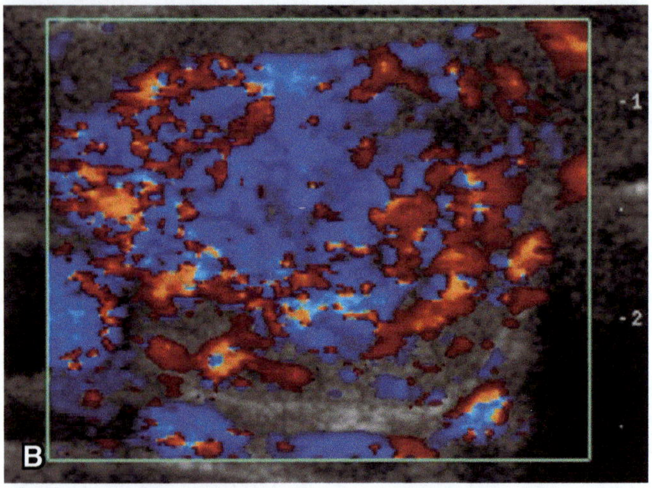

Figure 6-30. Ultrasound of follicular variant of papillary thyroid carcinoma in the right lobe. **A**, Transverse, 19 x 22 mm. **B**, Color Doppler, transverse. **C**, Longitudinal, sagittal diameter: 38 mm.

22-Year-old woman

- **Clinical history:** Nodule in right lobe for many years.
- **Ultrasound:** Papillary thyroid carcinoma (PTC).
- **Cytology:** Highly suspicious for PTC.
- **Thyroidectomy:** Follicular variant of PTC.

Features

Mixed echogenicity
Inhomogeneous echo pattern
Partly blurred margins
Not encapsulated
A few microcalcifications
Highly hypervascularized

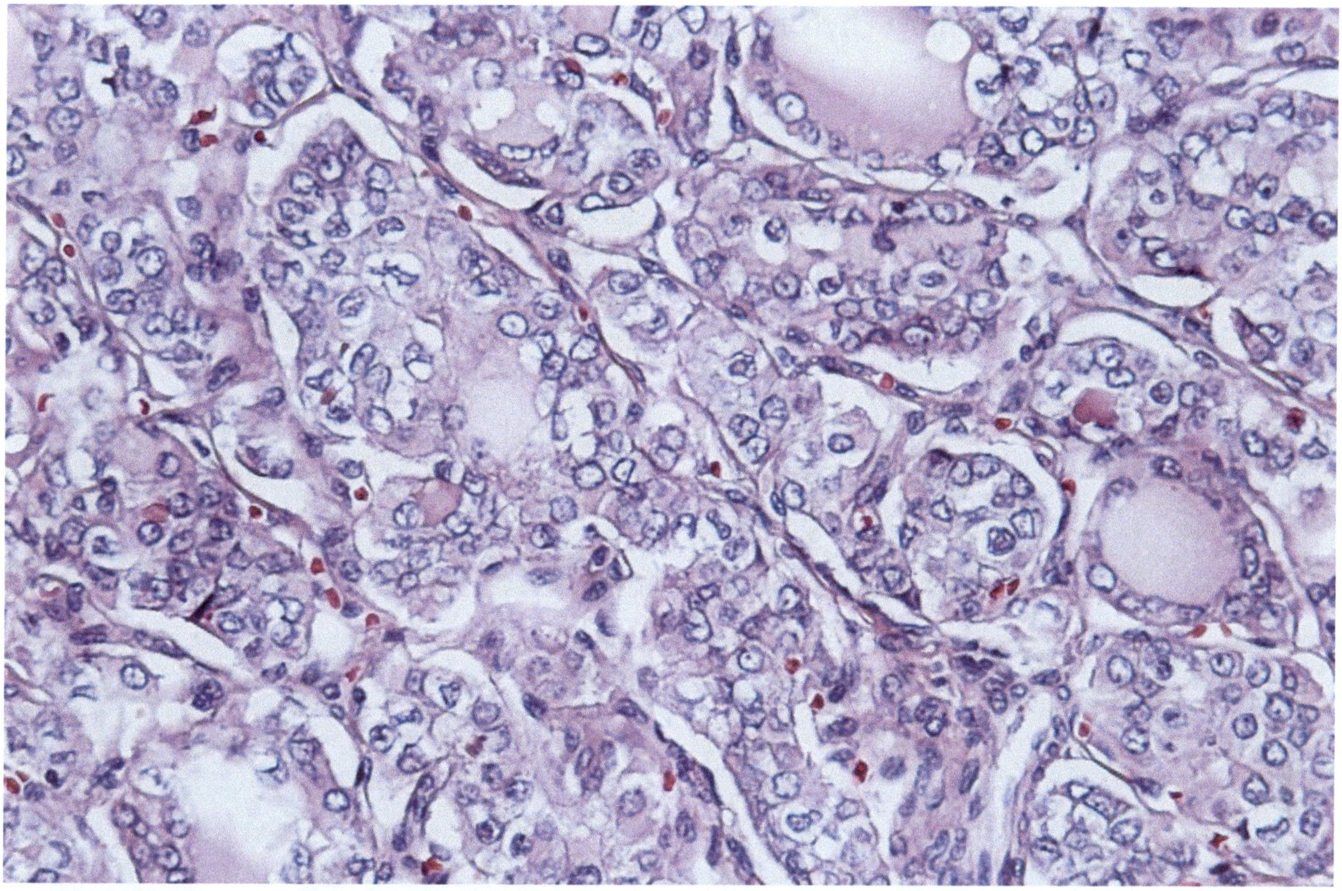

Figure 6-31. Histology: follicular growth pattern with nuclear features of papillary thyroid carcinoma.

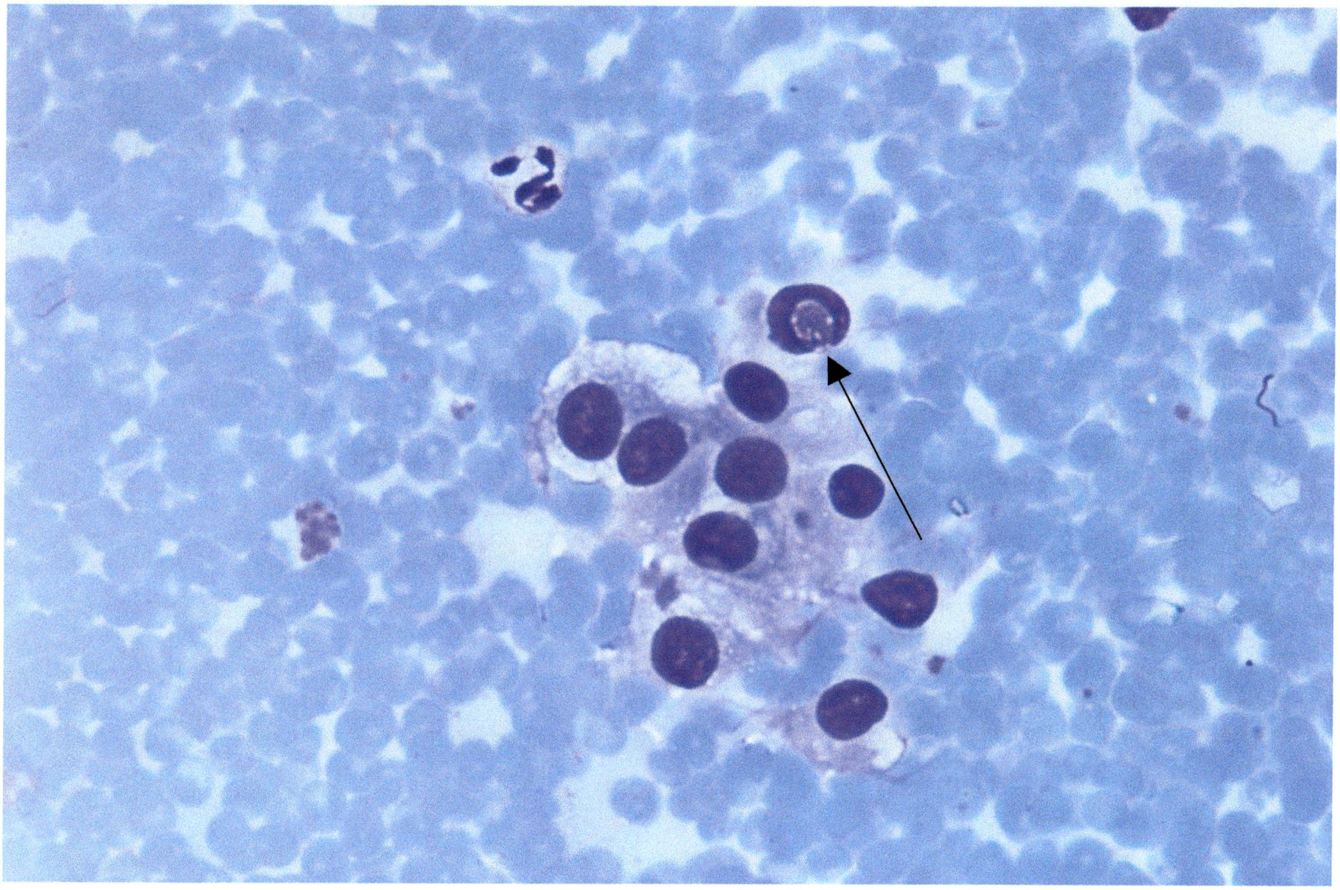

Figure 6-32. Cytology: nuclear inclusion (*arrow*).

Follicular Variant of Papillary Thyroid Carcinoma Right Lobe

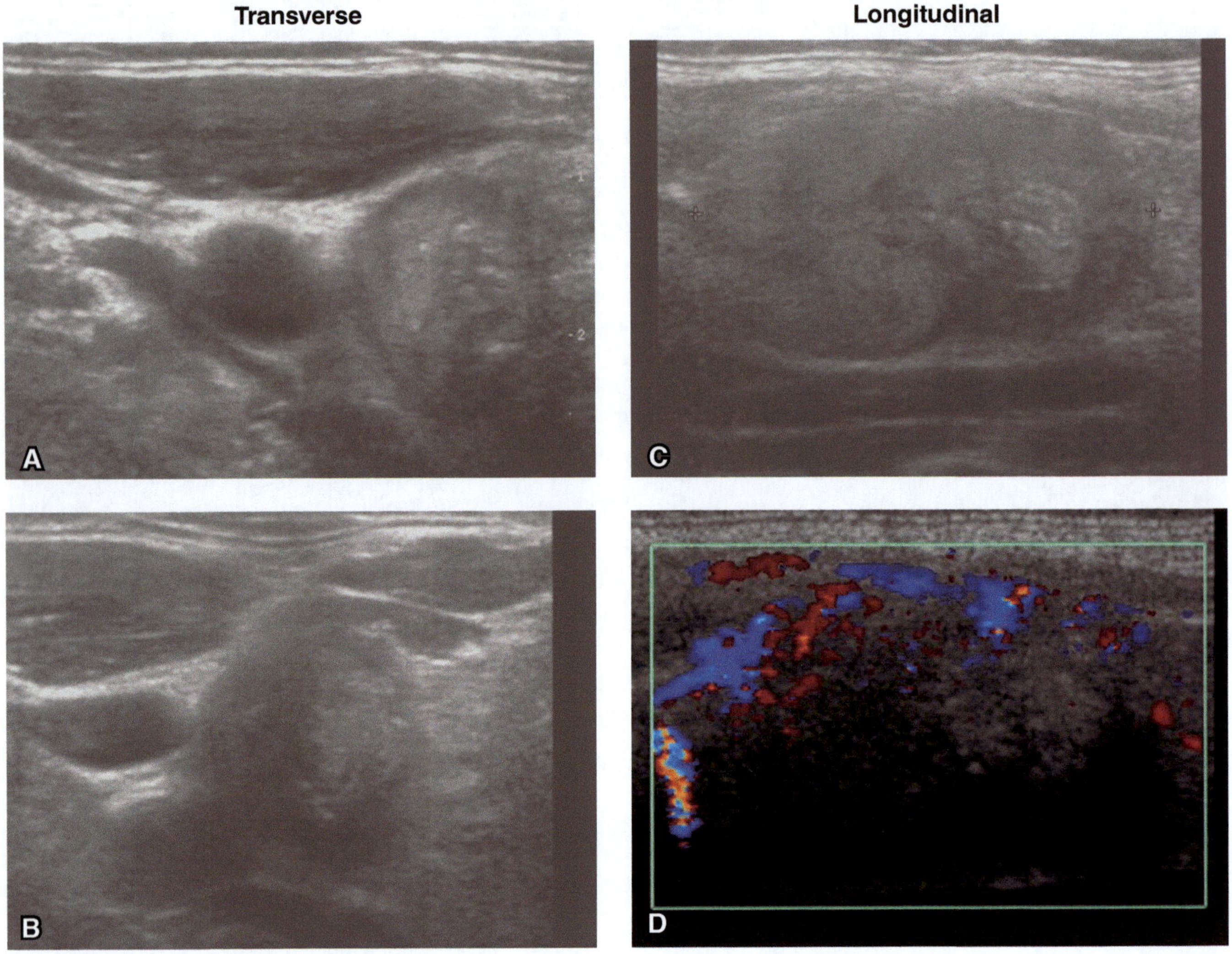

Figure 6-33. Ultrasound of follicular variant of papillary thyroid carcinoma in the right lobe. **A**, Transverse, 18 x 16 mm. **B**, Transverse. **C**, Longitudinal. **D**, Color Doppler, longitudinal.

50-Year-old man

- **Clinical history:** Neck tumor in right segment 4.
- **Ultrasound:** Papillary thyroid carcinoma (PTC) with metastasis.
- **Cytology right lobe:** No diagnostic material.
- **Cytology lymph node (LN):** Epithelial cells suspicious for PTC.
- **18-Gauge histologic needle biopsy right lobe:** Epithelial cells suspicious for PTC.
- **18-Gauge histologic needle biopsy LN:** Epithelial cells suspicious for PTC.
- **Thyroidectomy + LN resection:** Follicular variant of PTC. LN with metastasis from PTC.

Features

Mixed echogenicity
Inhomogeneous echo pattern
Partially blurred margins
Not encapsulated
Microcalcifications
Scant peripheral vascularity

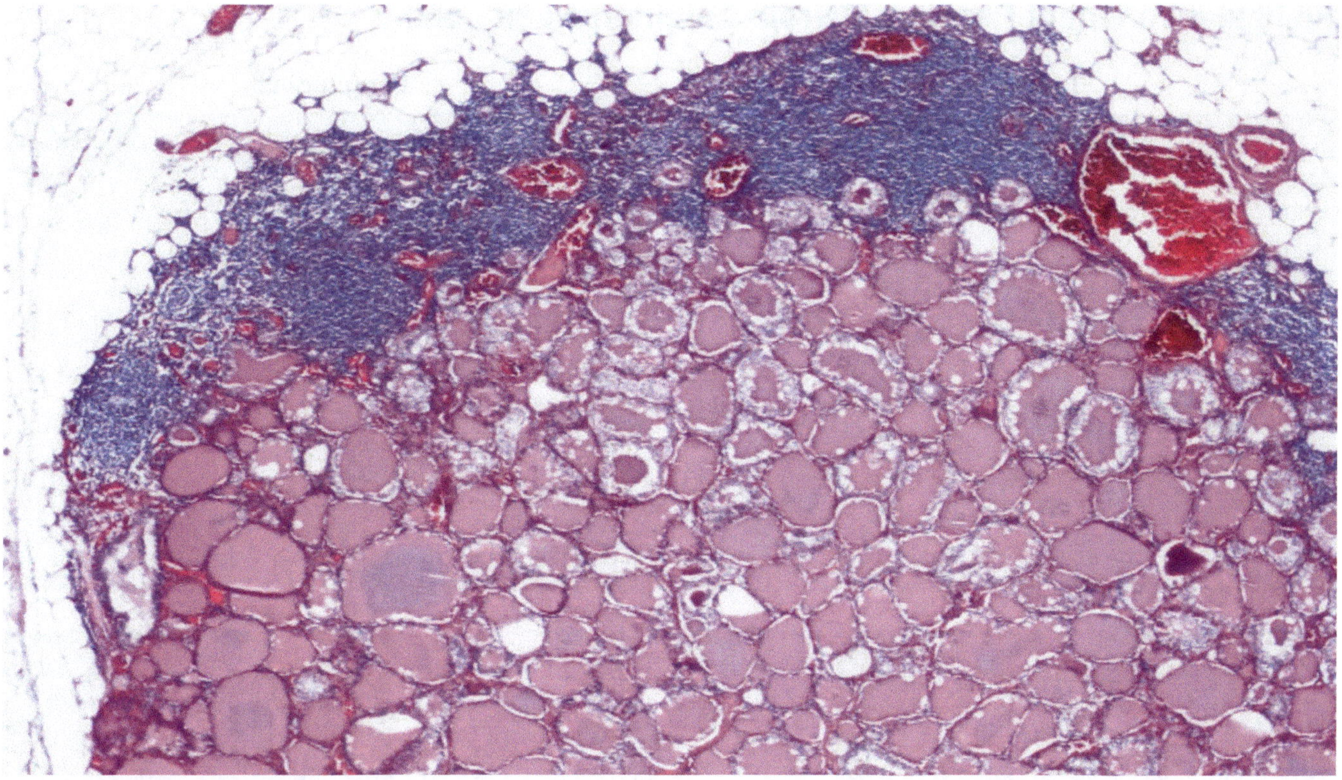

Figure 6-34. Histology: lymph node metastasis.

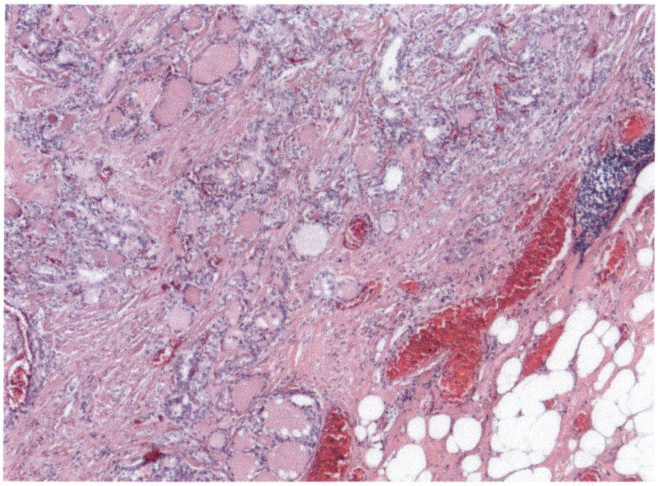

Figure 6-35. Histology: diffuse infiltration into the surrounding tissue.

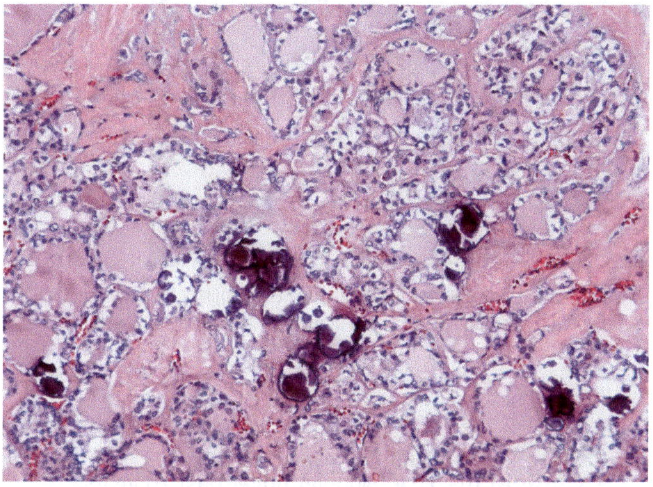

Figure 6-36. Histology: microcalcifications.

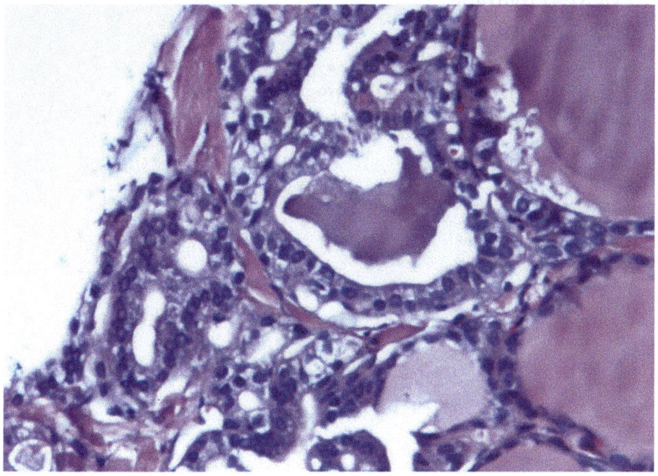

Figure 6-37. Histologic needle biopsy: nuclei suspicious for papillary thyroid carcinoma.

Follicular Variant of Papillary Thyroid Carcinoma Left Lobe

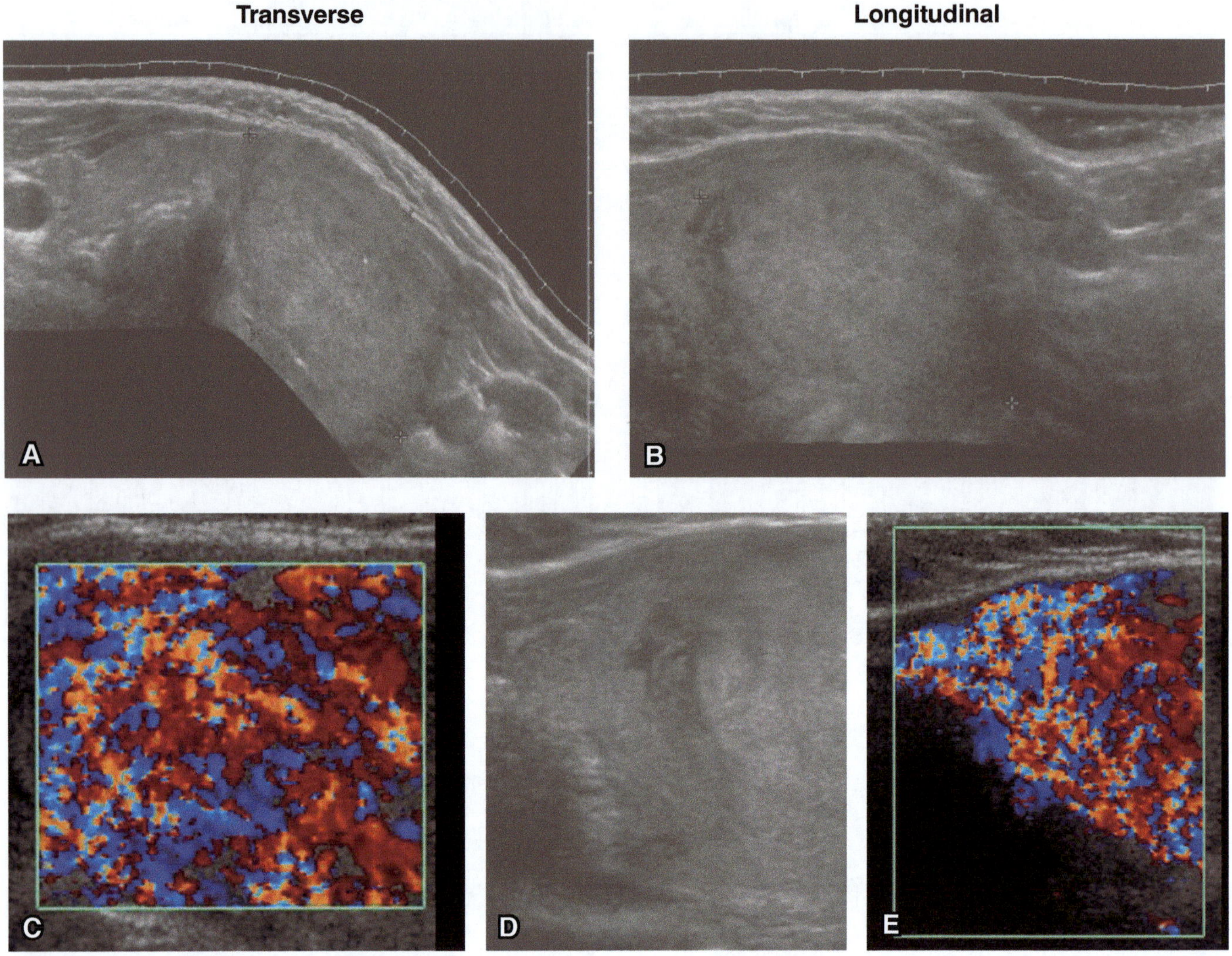

Figure 6-38. Ultrasound of follicular variant of papillary thyroid carcinoma in the left lobe. **A**, Transverse, 28 x 48 mm. **B**, Longitudinal, sagittal diameter: 46 mm. **C**, Color Doppler, transverse. **D**, Longitudinal. **E**, Color Doppler, longitudinal.

39-Year-old woman

- **Clinical history:** Nodular goiter past 20 years. No actual new symptoms.
- **Ultrasound:** Colloid nodule in left lobe + thyroiditis.
- **Cytology:** Follicular neoplasia. Follicular variant of papillary thyroid carcinoma (FVPTC) has to be excluded.
- **Left hemithyroidectomy:** FVPTC. Hashimoto's thyroiditis.

Features

Slightly hypoechoic
Inhomogeneous echo pattern
Blurred margins
Not encapsulated
One microcalcification
Both tumor and glandular tissue extremely hypervascular, "thyroid inferno"

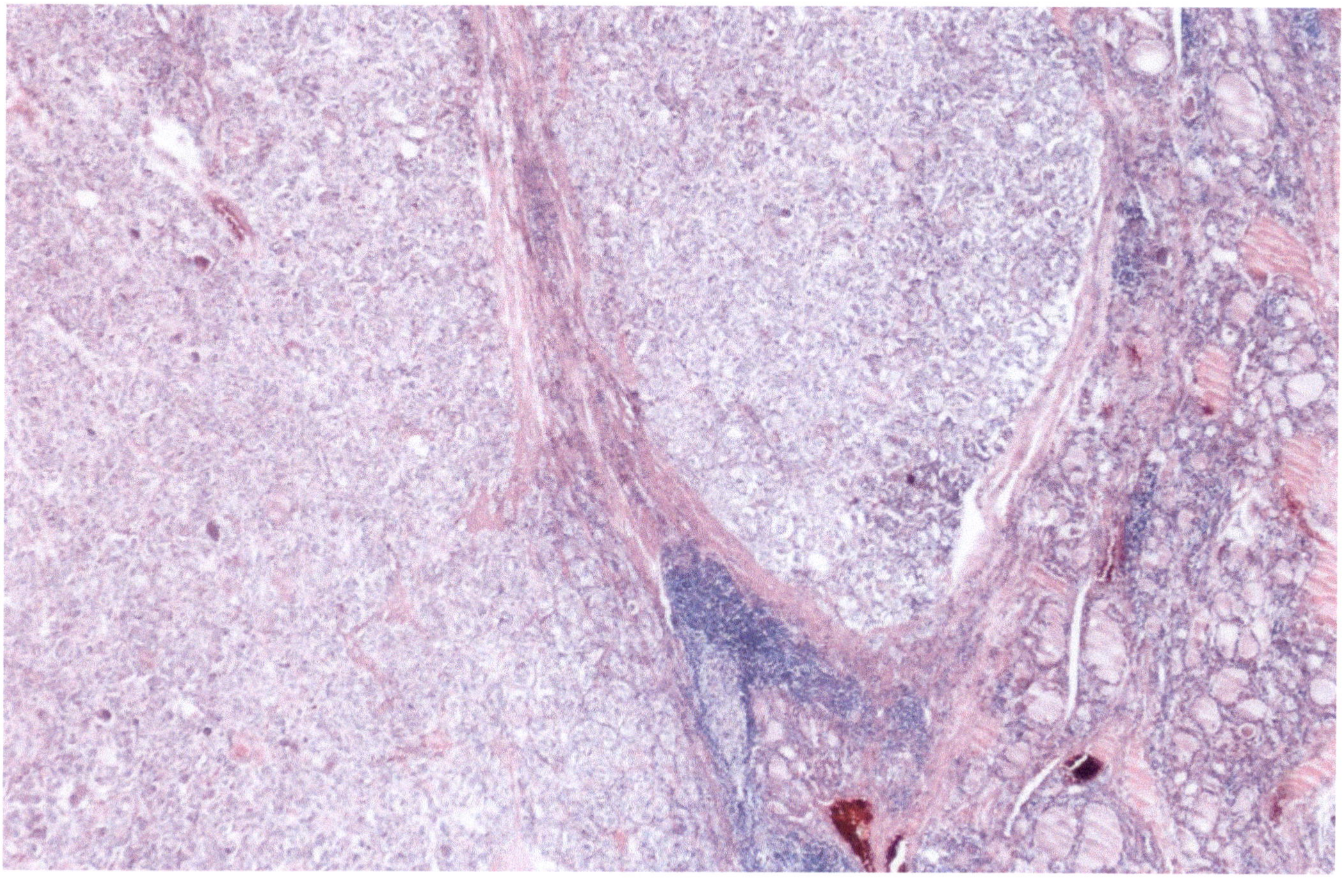

Figure 6-39. Histology: infiltration through the capsule. Follicular variant of papillary thyroid carcinoma.

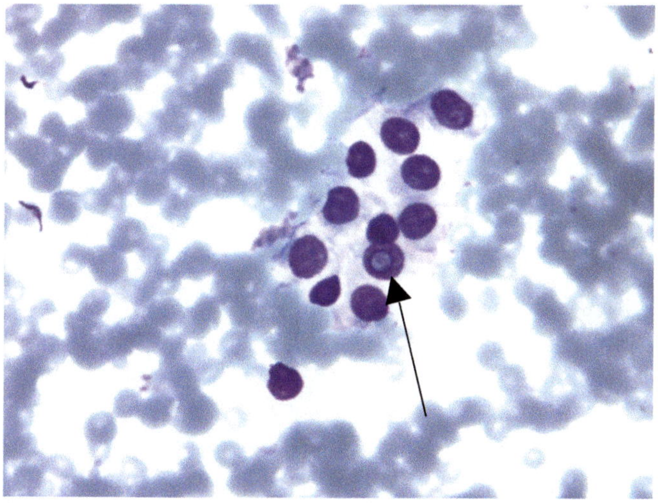

Figure 6-40. Cytology: nuclear inclusion (*arrow*).

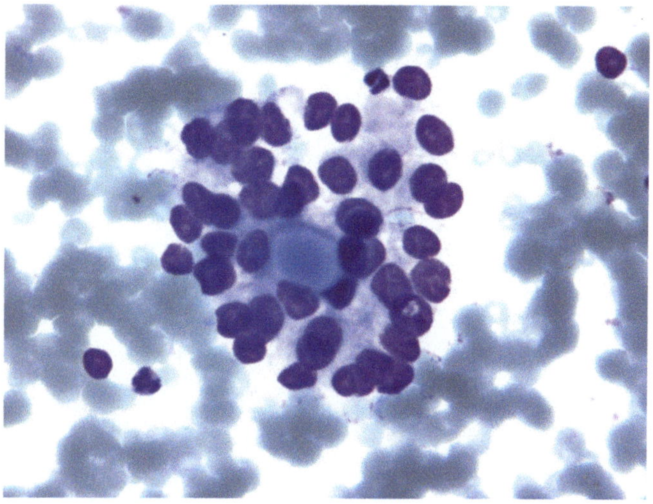

Figure 6-41. Cytology: follicular structure with central colloid.

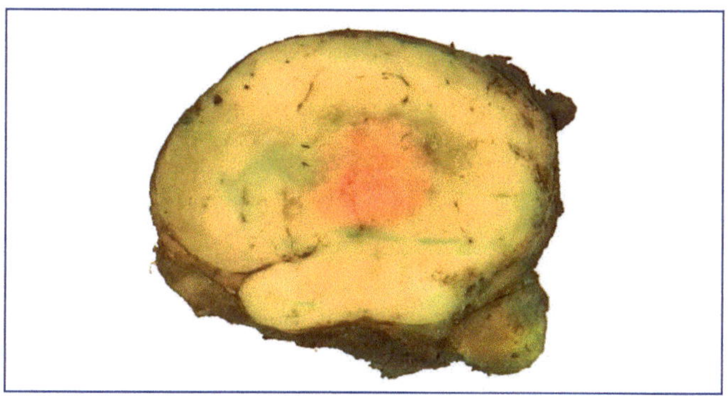

Figure 6-42. Gross section: penetration of the tumor through the capsule.

7 Papillary Thyroid Carcinoma

Papillary thyroid carcinomas (PTCs) are solid, usually hypoechoic tumors with inhomogeneous echo structure. They usually have irregular margins and often contain discrete echogenic foci, *ie*, microcalcifications. They may be solitary or multifocal. In our experience the vascularity varies from avascular to strongly vascularized. In our opinion, the ultrasound findings with highest accuracy for PTC show low echogenicity, microcalcifications, irregular margins, and neck lymph node metastases [4,6–10]. Uncommon features include hyperechoic or mixed echo texture, cysts, hypovascularity, and coarse or peripheral calcifications [18].

Common Features

Hypoechogenicity
Inhomogeneous echo pattern
Microcalcifications
Absence of peripheral halo
Irregular borders, blurred margins
Often intranodular hypervascularity
Regional lymphadenopathy

Cytologic Morphology

The material from PTC is usually abundant and consists of papillary groups of epithelium with some of the cells showing characteristic nuclear grooves or cytoplasmic inclusions. The criteria for finding these specific nuclear features is absolute and when these nuclear changes are not found, a definite diagnosis of PTC should not be made, because extensive epithelial hyperplasia with papillary formations may mimic the picture found in PTC.

Papillary Thyroid Carcinoma Right Lobe and Isthmus

Transverse

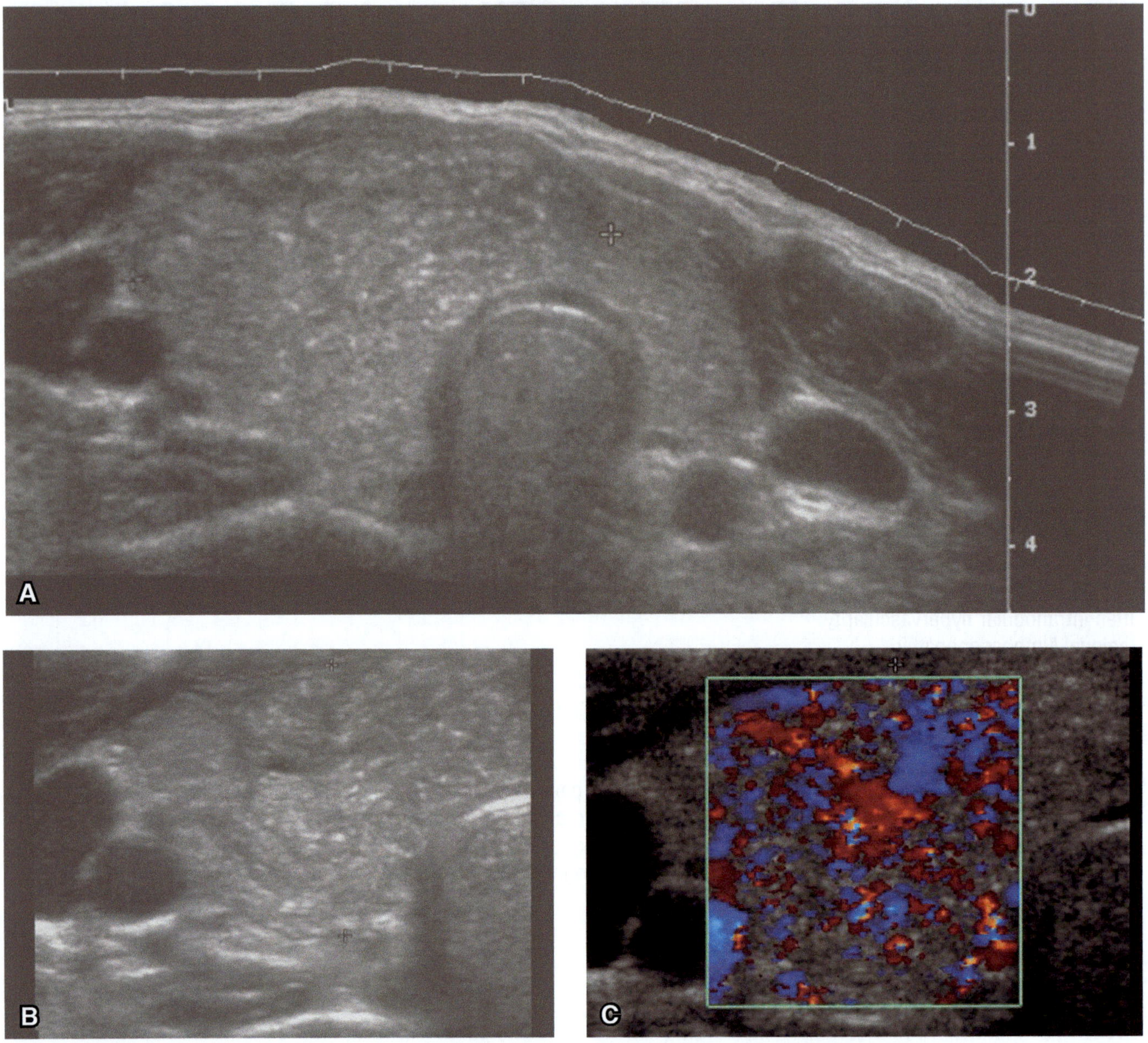

Figure 7-1. Ultrasound of papillary thyroid carcinoma in the right lobe and isthmus. **A** and **B**, Transverse. **C**, Color Doppler, transverse.

28-Year-old man

- **Clinical history:** Rapidly growing nodule in right lobe. Autoimmune thyroiditis. Anti-thyroid peroxidase > 30.
- **Ultrasound:** Papillary thyroid carcinoma (PTC) in right lobe and isthmus + metastases.
- **Cytology:** PTC + metastases.
- **Thyroidectomy:** PTC + metastases.

Features

Isoechoic

Lobulated inhomogeneous echo pattern

Quite well circumscribed

Innumerable microcalcifications

Hypervascularity

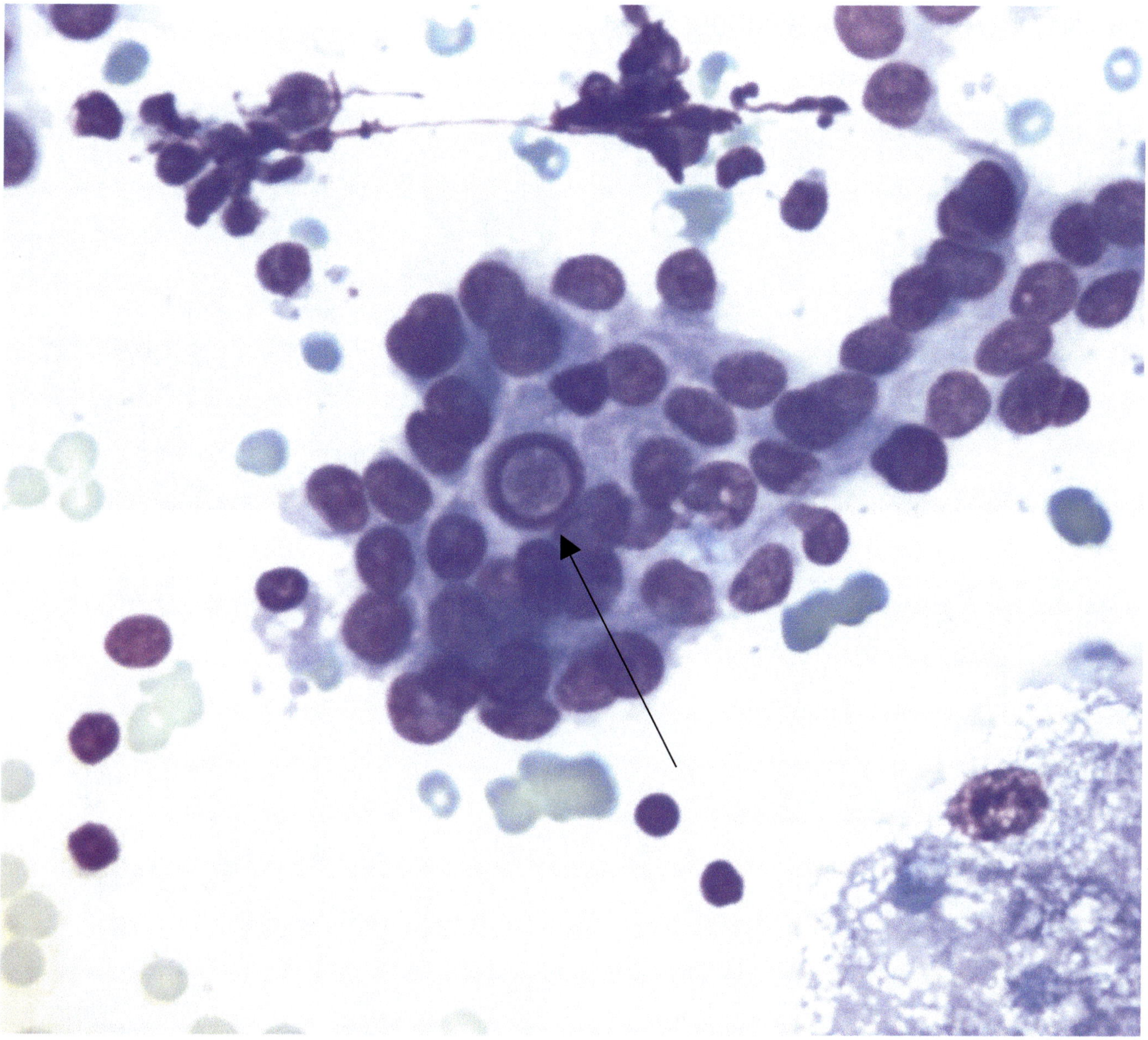

Figure 7-2. Cytology: papillary thyroid carcinoma. Nuclear inclusion (*arrow*).

Papillary Thyroid Carcinoma Right Lobe

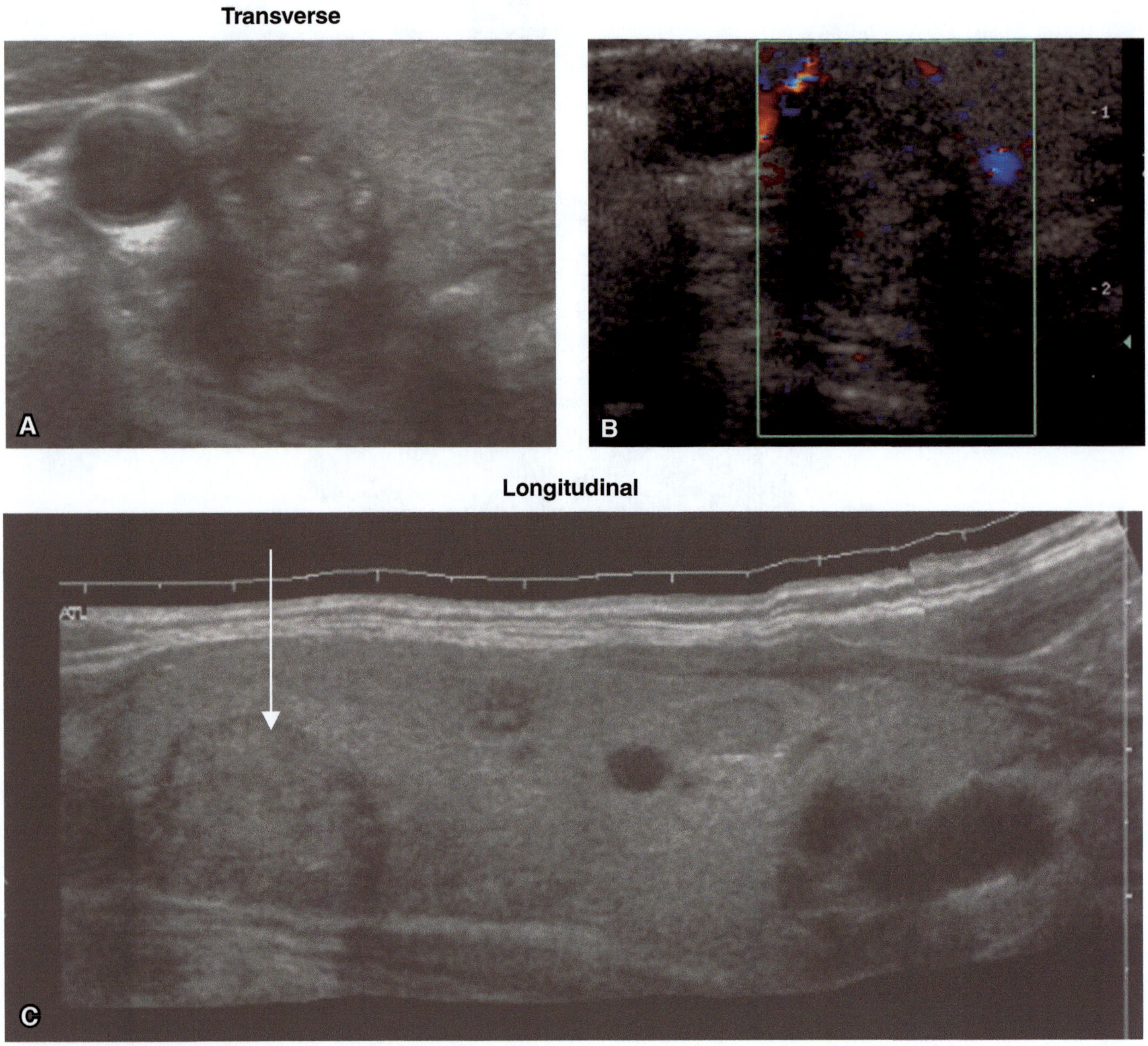

FIGURE 7-3. Ultrasound of papillary thyroid carcinoma in the right lobe. **A**, Transverse, anteroposterior diameter: 29 mm. **B**, Color Doppler. **C**, Longitudinal. PTC (*arrow*).

53-Year-old woman

- **Clinical history:** Breast carcinoma. CT of the thorax showed lesion in right thyroid lobe.
- **Ultrasound:** Papillary thyroid carcinoma (PTC).
- **Cytology:** PTC.
- **Thyroidectomy:** PTC.

Features

Hypoechoic
Inhomogeneous echo pattern
Quite well circumscribed
Refractive edge shadows
Microcalcifications
Scant vascularity

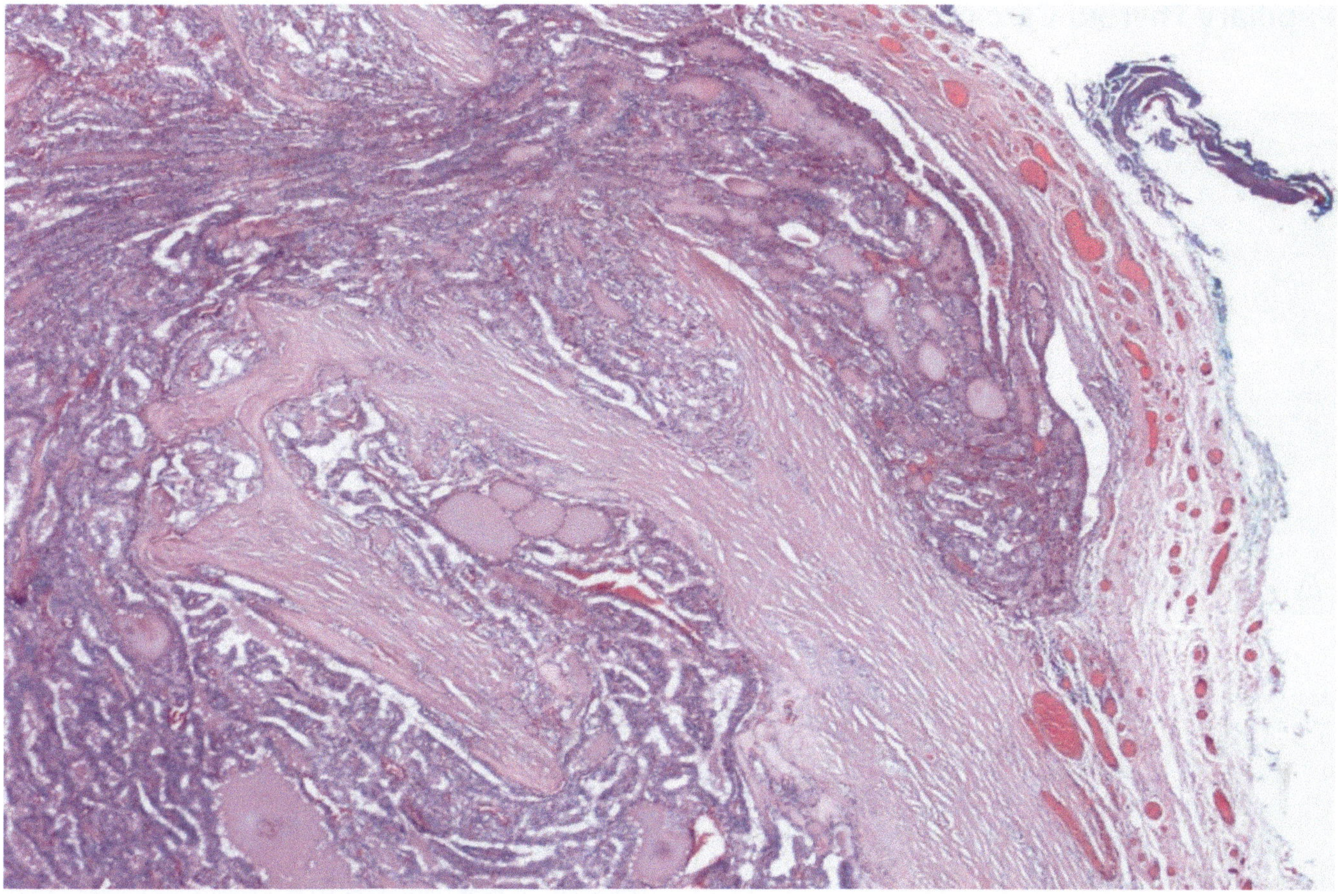

FIGURE 7-4. Histology: papillary thyroid carcinoma with fibrosis.

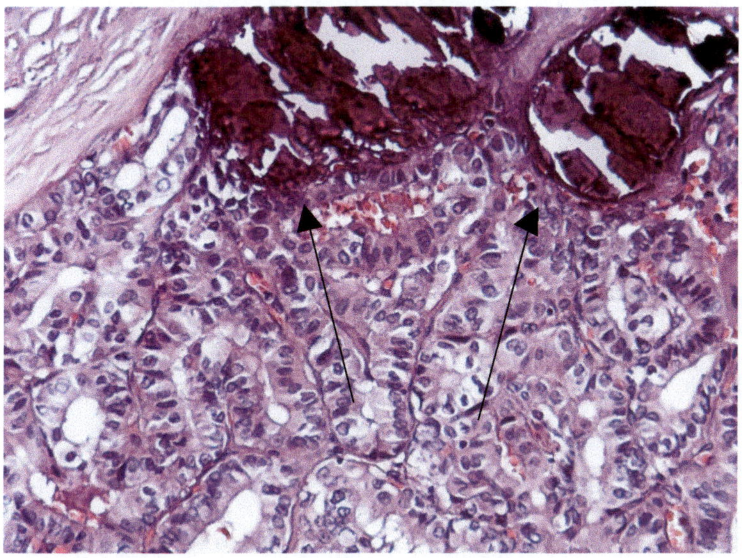

FIGURE 7-5. Histology: microcalcifications (*arrows*) in tumor.

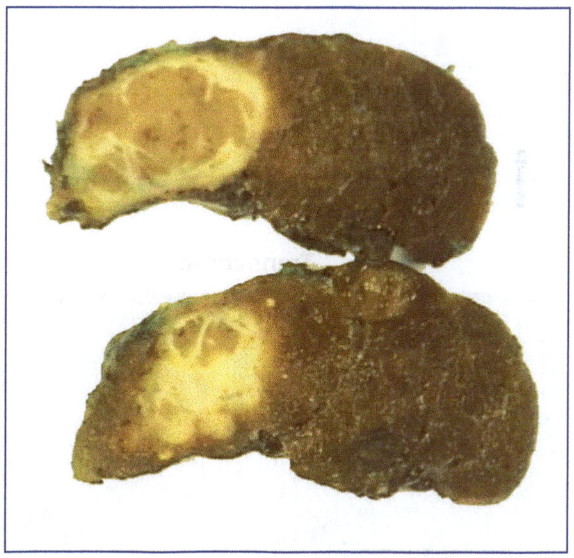

FIGURE 7-6. Gross section.

Papillary Thyroid Carcinoma: Multifocal Microcarcinoma with Metastases

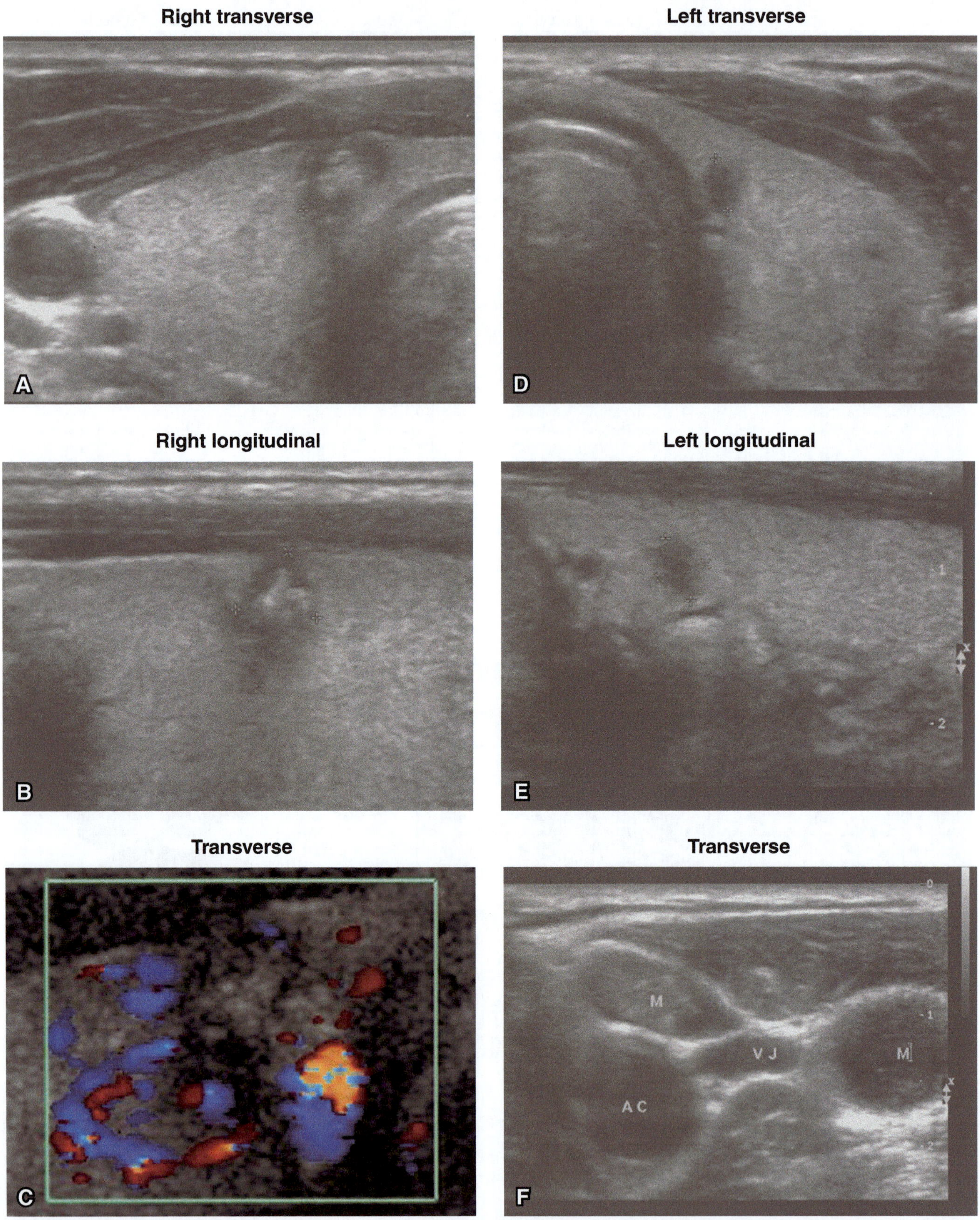

FIGURE 7-7. Ultrasound of papillary thyroid carcinoma showing multifocal microcarcinoma with metastases. **A**, Right transverse. **B**, Right longitudinal, 5 x 9 mm. **C**, Color Doppler, transverse. **D**, Left transverse. **E**, Left longitudinal. **F**, Metastases in left level IV.

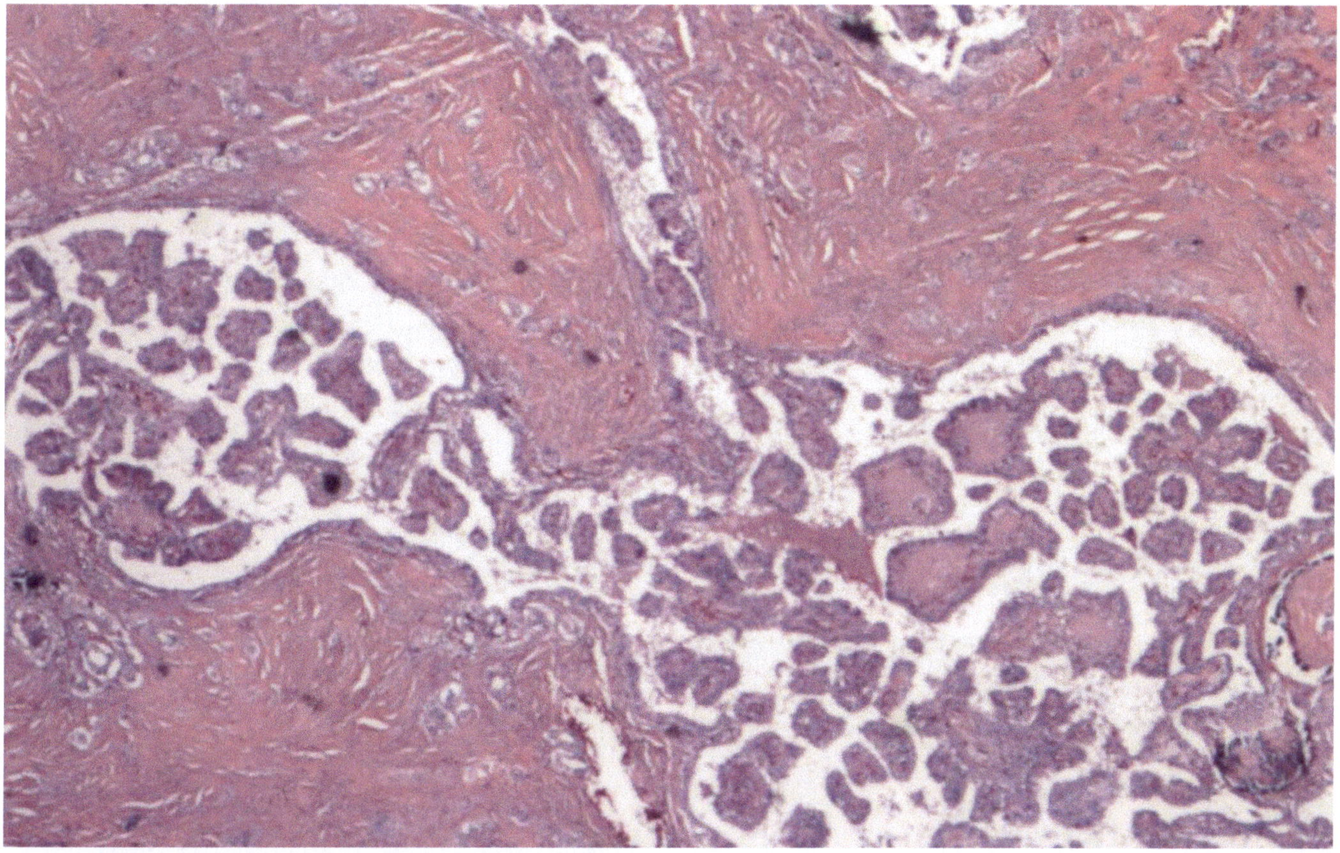

FIGURE 7-8. Histology: papillary thyroid carcinoma.

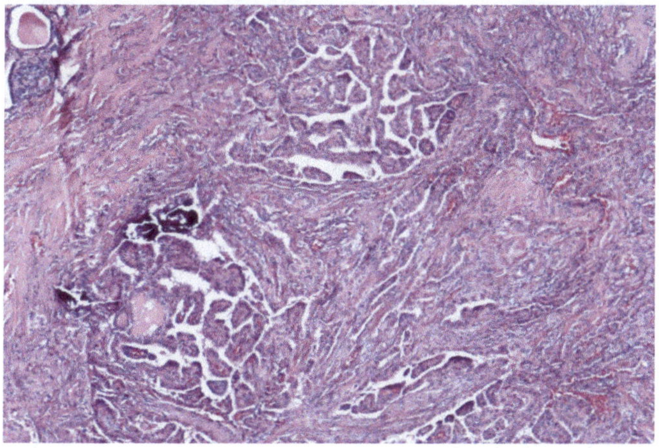

FIGURE 7-9. Histology: papillary thyroid carcinoma.

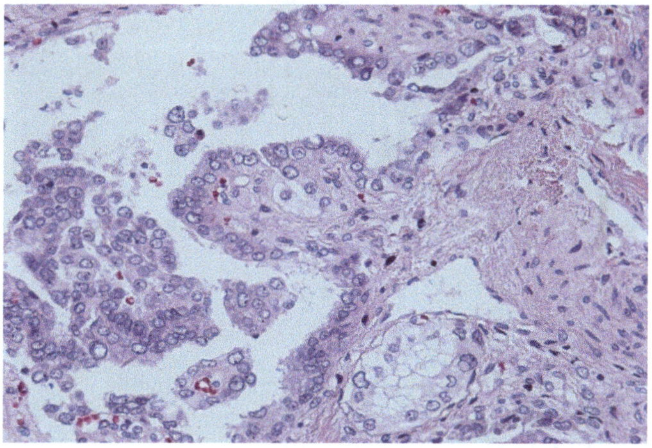

FIGURE 7-10. Histology: papillary thyroid carcinoma with characteristic optically clear nuclei.

37-Year-old man

- **Clinical history:** Enlarged neck lymph nodes.
- **Surgery:** Metastases from papillary thyroid carcinoma (PTC).
- **Ultrasound:** Multifocal PTC. Metastases both sides.
- **Cytology:** PTC in right lobe. Probably PTC in left lobe.
- **Thyroidectomy:** PTC both lobes + metastases.

Features

Hypoechoic
Blurred margins
Microcalcifications in tumor right lobe
No visible blood flow
Pathologic lymph nodes with microcalcifications
Both lesions are taller than wide

Papillary Thyroid Carcinoma Isthmus

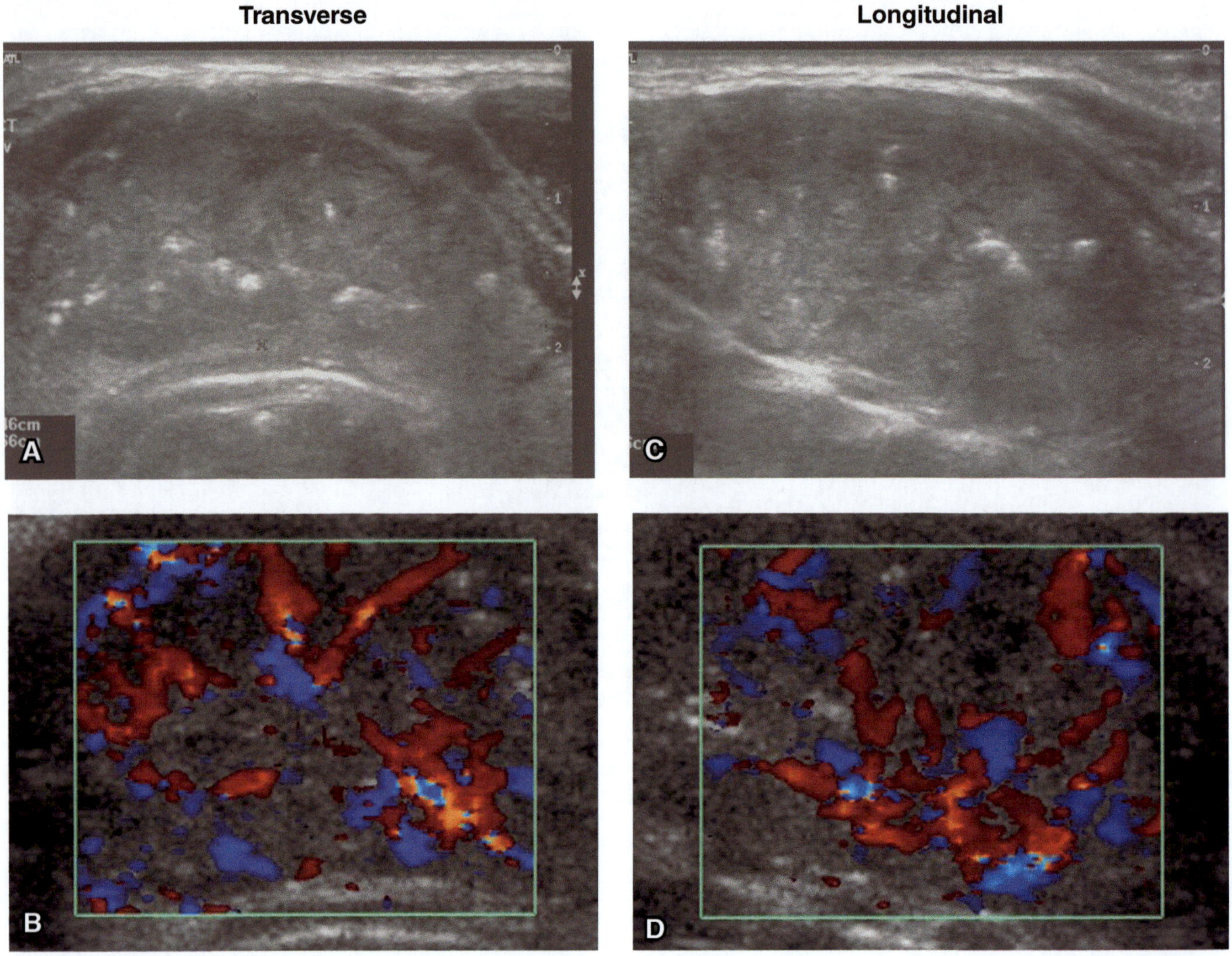

Figure 7-11. Ultrasound of papillary thyroid carcinoma in the isthmus. **A**, Transverse. **B**, Color Doppler, transverse. **C**, Longitudinal. **D**, Color Doppler, longitudinal.

42-Year-old man

- **Clinical history:** Palpable nodule in isthmus.
- **Ultrasound:** Papillary thyroid carcinoma (PTC).
- **Cytology:** Suspicious for PTC.
- **16-Gauge histologic needle biopsy:** PTC.
- **Thyroidectomy:** PTC + metastases.

Features

Hypoechoic
Inhomogeneous echo pattern
Microcalcifications
Coarse calcification
Partially blurred margins
Hypervascular

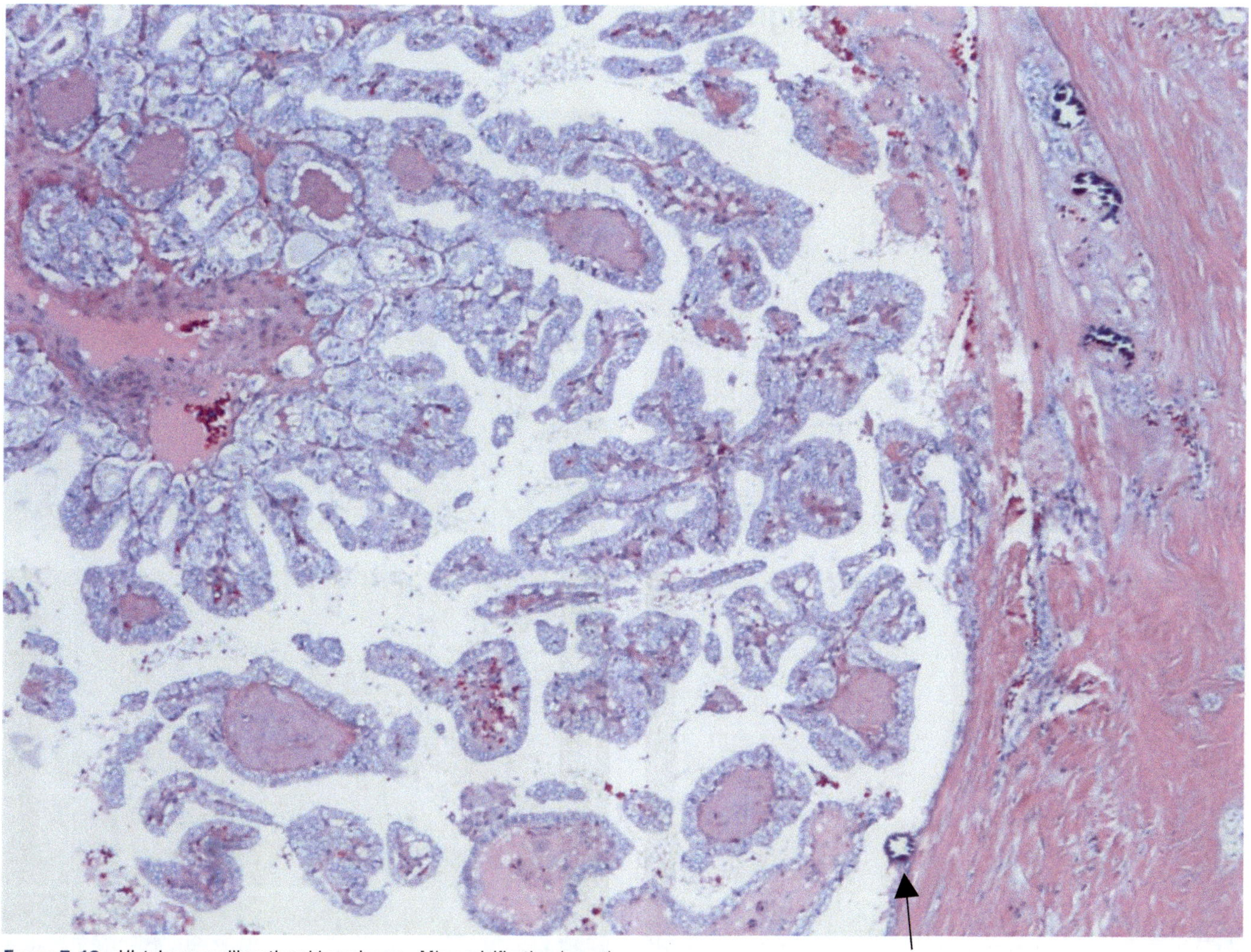

Figure 7-12. Histology: papillary thyroid carcinoma. Microcalcification (*arrow*).

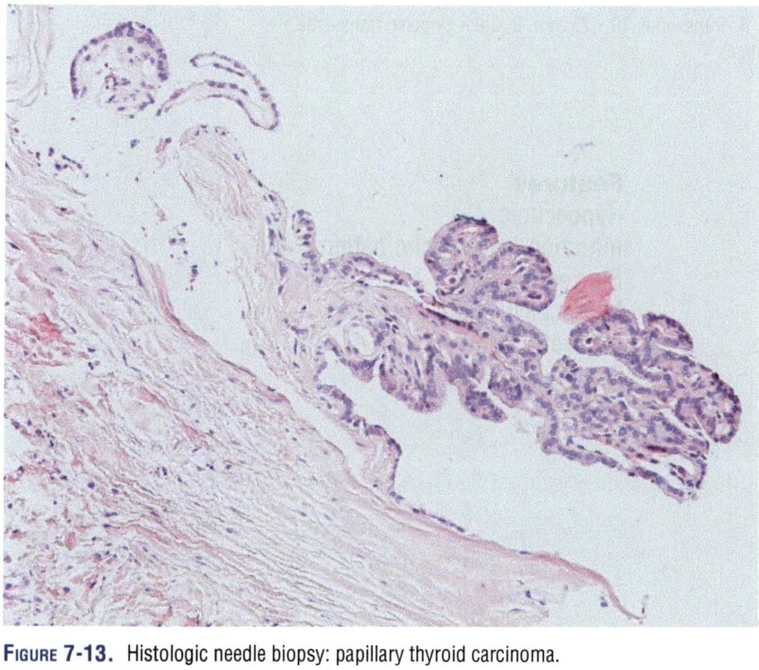

Figure 7-13. Histologic needle biopsy: papillary thyroid carcinoma.

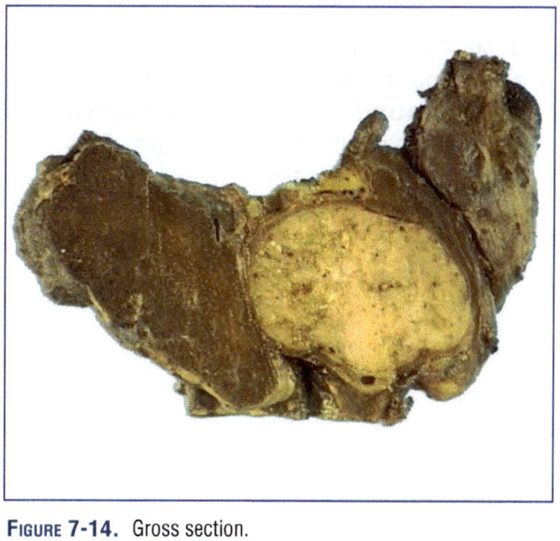

Figure 7-14. Gross section.

Papillary Thyroid Carcinoma Right Lobe

Transverse | **Longitudinal**

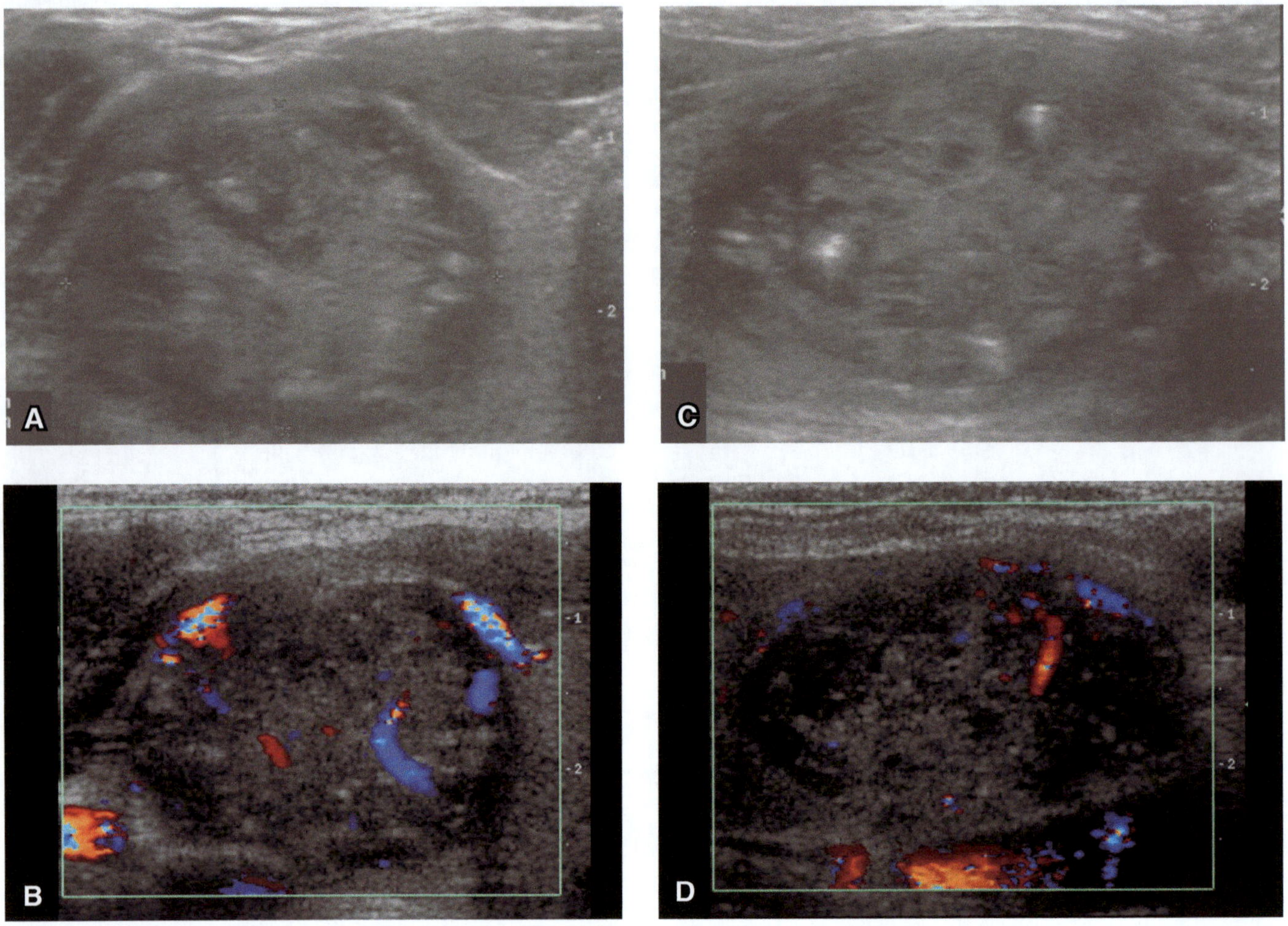

FIGURE 7-15. Ultrasound of papillary thyroid carcinoma in the right lobe. **A**, Transverse, 19 x 25 mm. **B**, Color Doppler, transverse. **C**, Longitudinal, longitudinal diameter: 30 mm. **D**, Color Doppler, longitudinal.

38-Year-old man

- **Clinical history:** Suspicious neck lymph node.
- **Ultrasound:** Papillary thyroid carcinoma (PTC) in right lobe. Normal lymph nodes.
- **Cytology:** PTC cells.
- **Thyroidectomy:** PTC + microscopic metastases.

Features

Hypoechoic
Inhomogeneous echo pattern
Blurred margins
Microcalcifications
"Comet tail" crystals
Scant vascularity

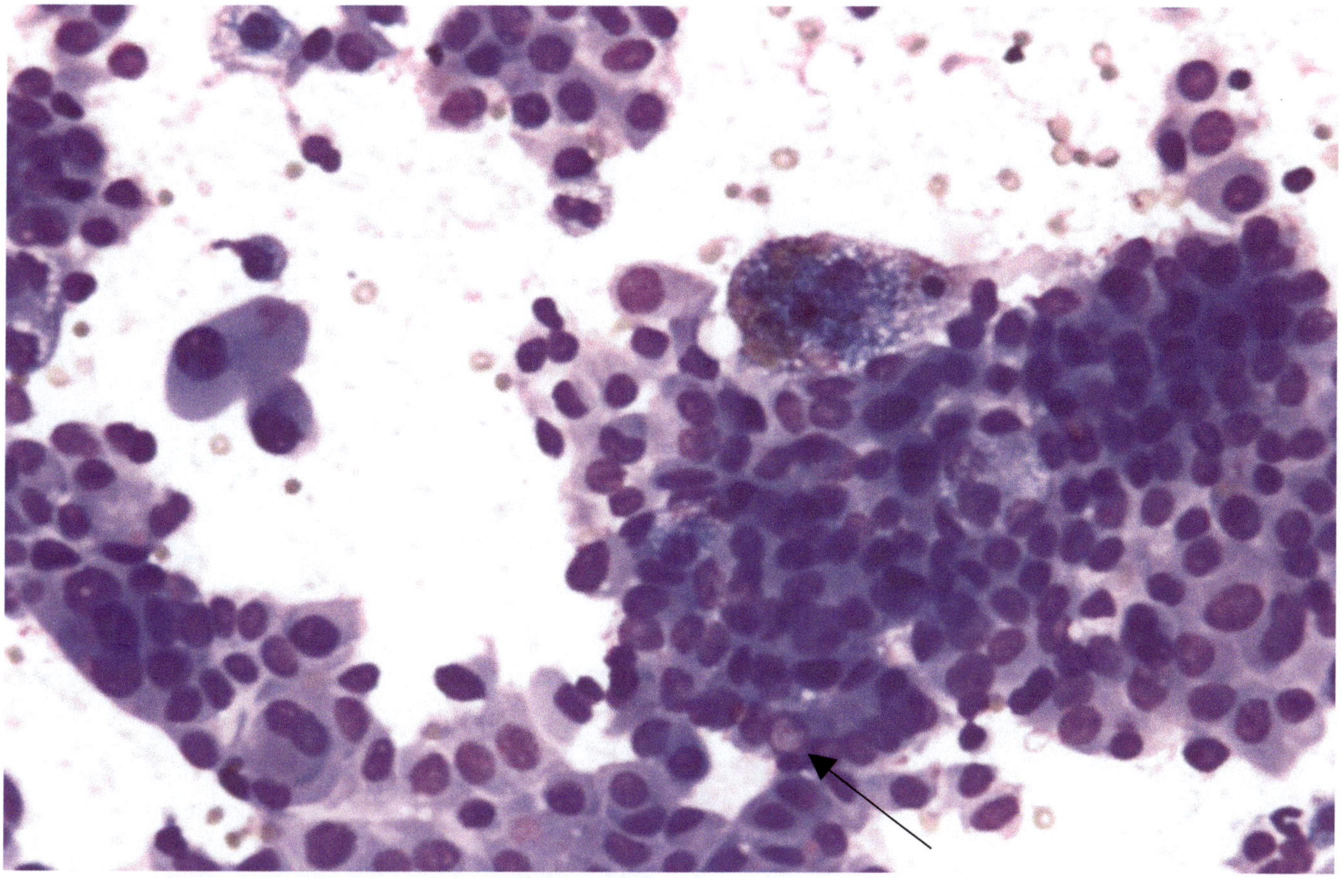

Figure 7-16. Cytology: papillary thyroid carcinoma, nuclear inclusion (*arrow*).

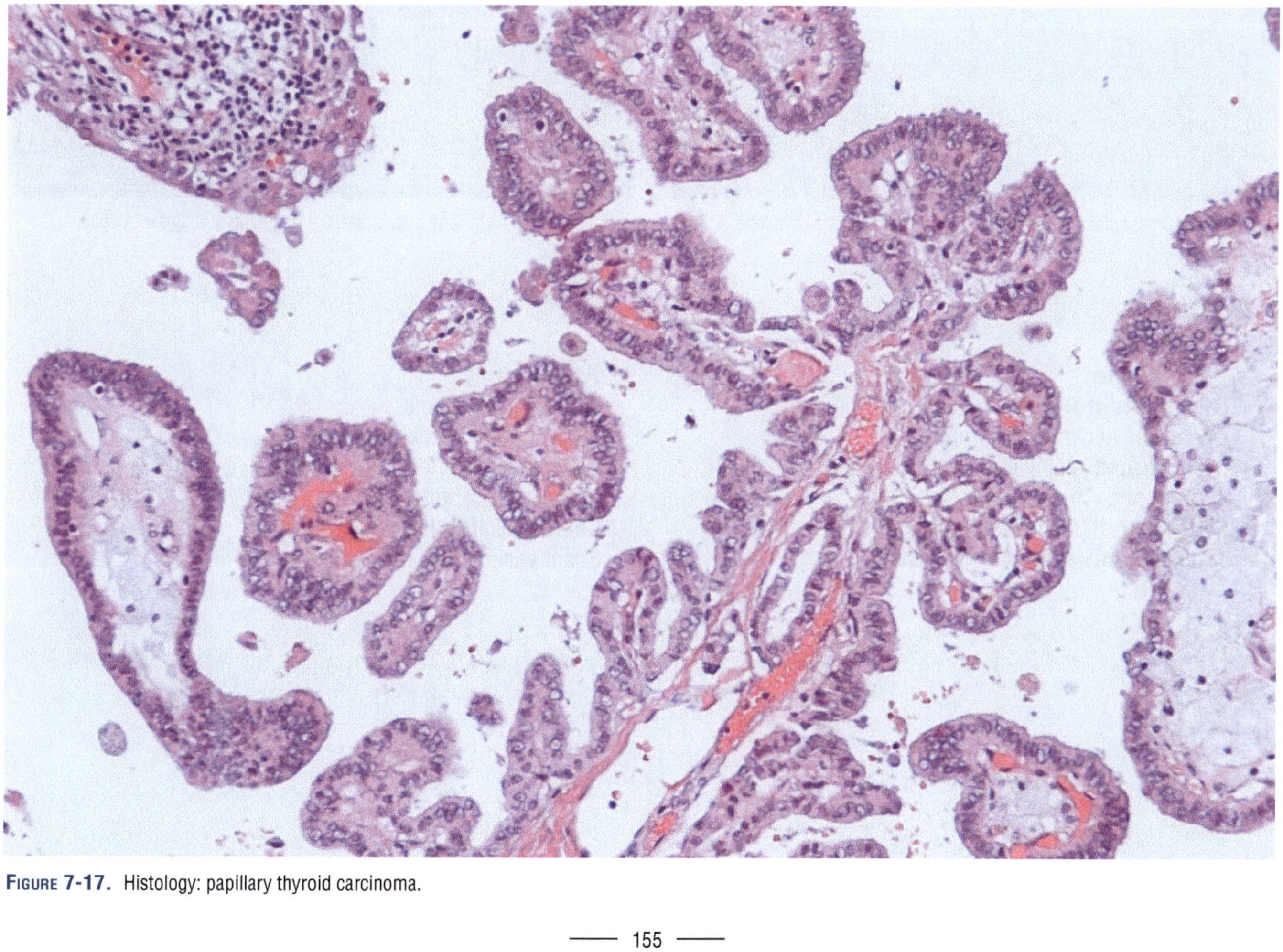

Figure 7-17. Histology: papillary thyroid carcinoma.

Papillary Thyroid Carcinoma Right Lobe

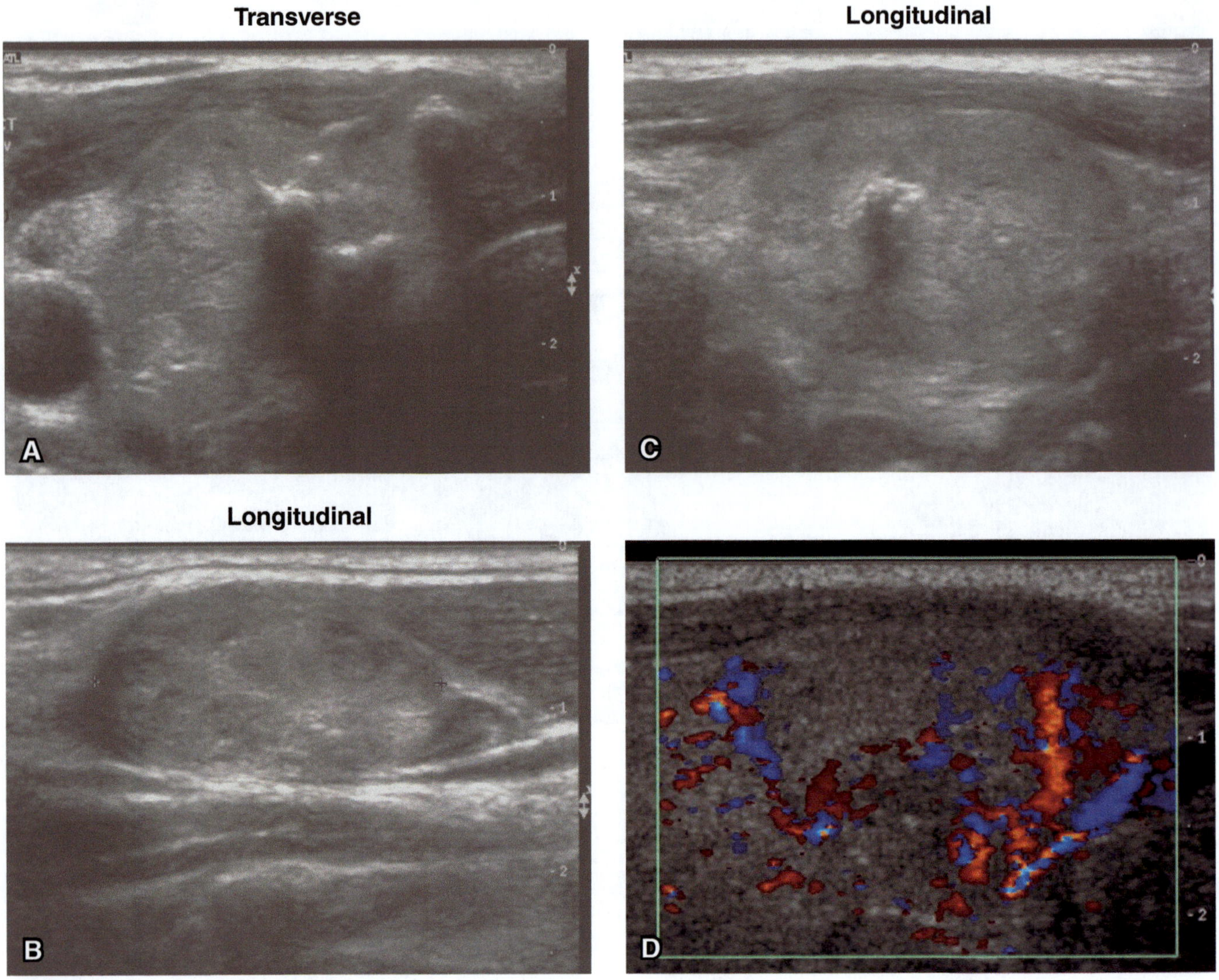

Figure 7-18. Ultrasound of papillary thyroid carcinoma in the right lobe. **A**, Transverse. **B**, Longitudinal showing metastasis. **C**, Longitudinal. **D**, Color Doppler, longitudinal.

27-Year-old man

- **Clinical history:** Enlarged lymph node right side of the neck. Lymphoma?
- **Ultrasound:** Papillary thyroid carcinoma (PTC) in right lobe + metastases.
- **Cytology:** PTC + metastases.
- **Thyroidectomy:** PTC + metastases.

Features

Slightly hypoechoic
Inhomogeneous echo pattern
Well circumscribed
Microcalcifications
Coarse calcifications
Scant vascularity

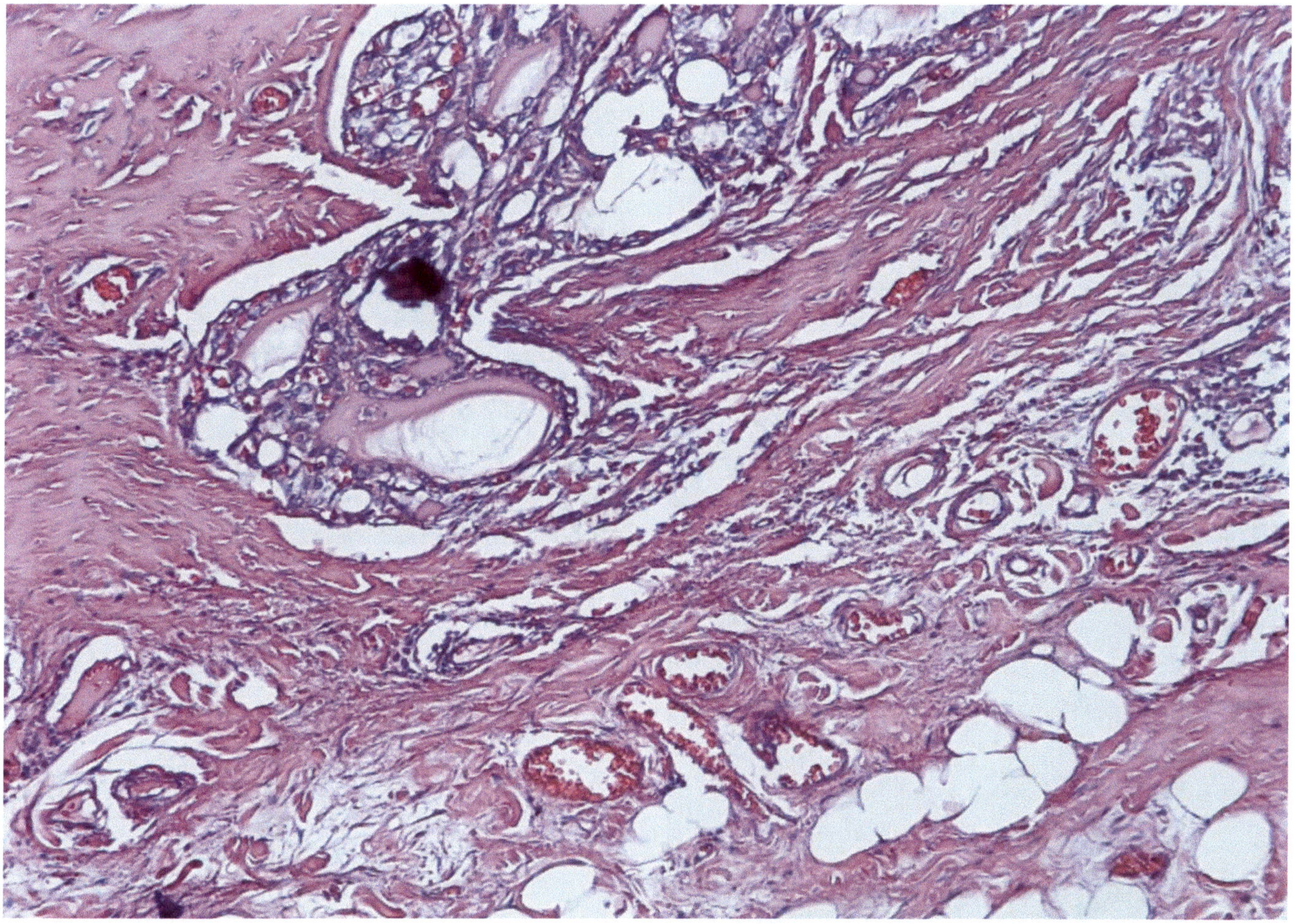

Figure 7-19. Histology: papillary thyroid carcinoma.

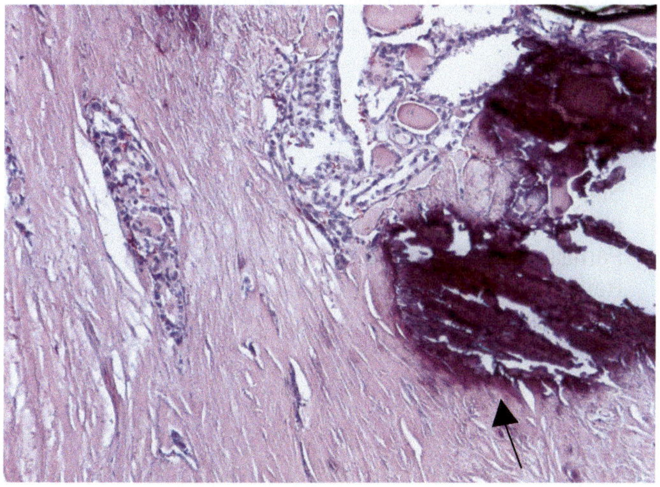

Figure 7-20. Microcalcifications (*arrow*).

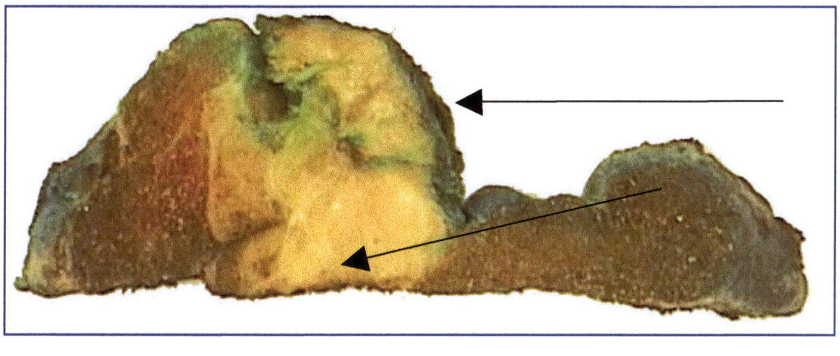

Figure 7-21. Infiltration through the whole lobe (*arrows*).

Papillary Thyroid Carcinoma Right Lobe

Transverse | **Longitudinal**

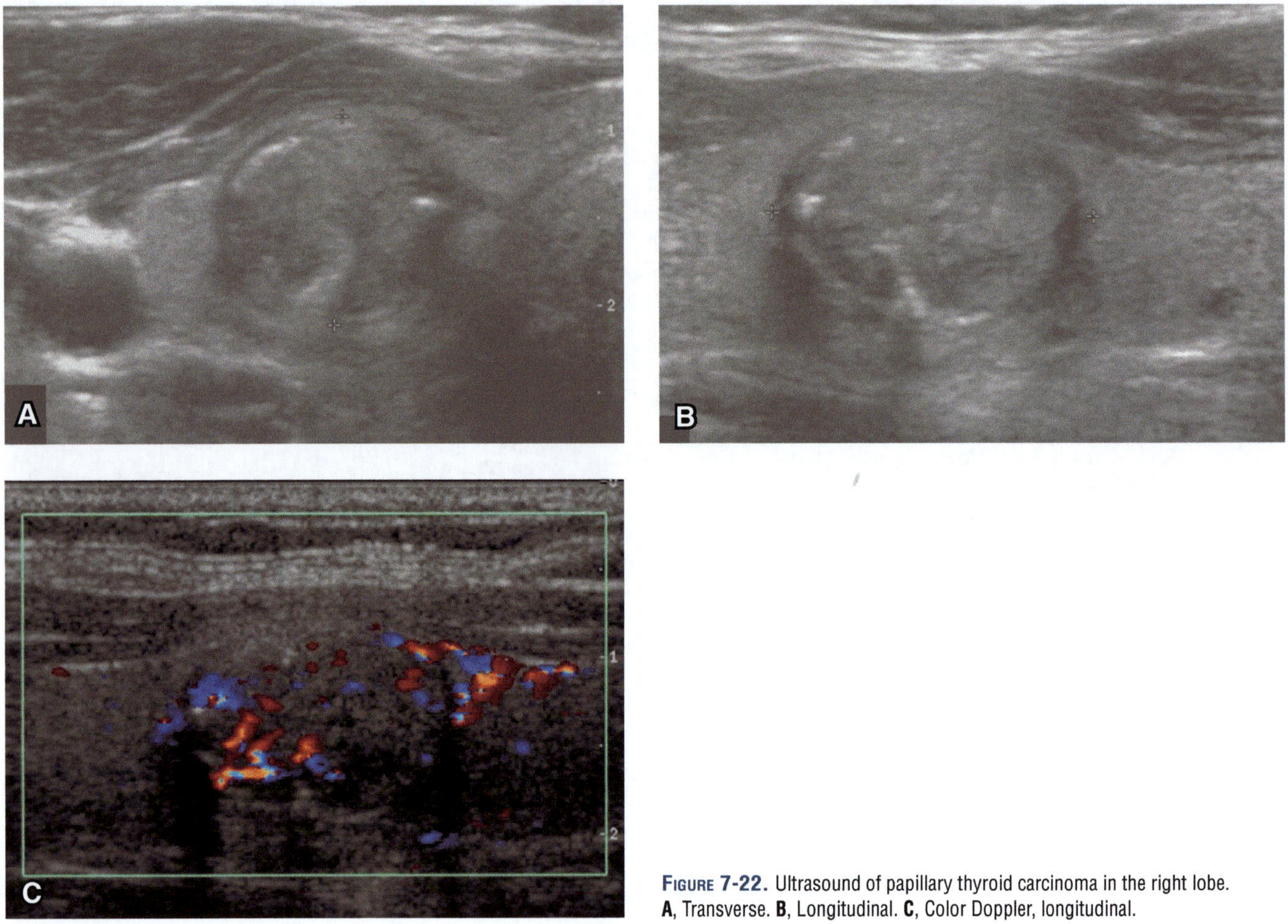

Figure 7-22. Ultrasound of papillary thyroid carcinoma in the right lobe. **A**, Transverse. **B**, Longitudinal. **C**, Color Doppler, longitudinal.

48-Year-old woman

- **Clinical history:** Ultrasound at other hospital found suspicious nodule in right thyroid lobe.
- **Ultrasound:** Suspicious for papillary thyroid carcinoma (PTC).
- **Cytology:** PTC.
- **Thyroidectomy:** PTC.

Features

Slightly hypoechoic
Inhomogeneous echo pattern
Partially well circumscribed
Refractive edge shadows
Microcalcifications
"Eggshell" calcifications
Scant vascularity

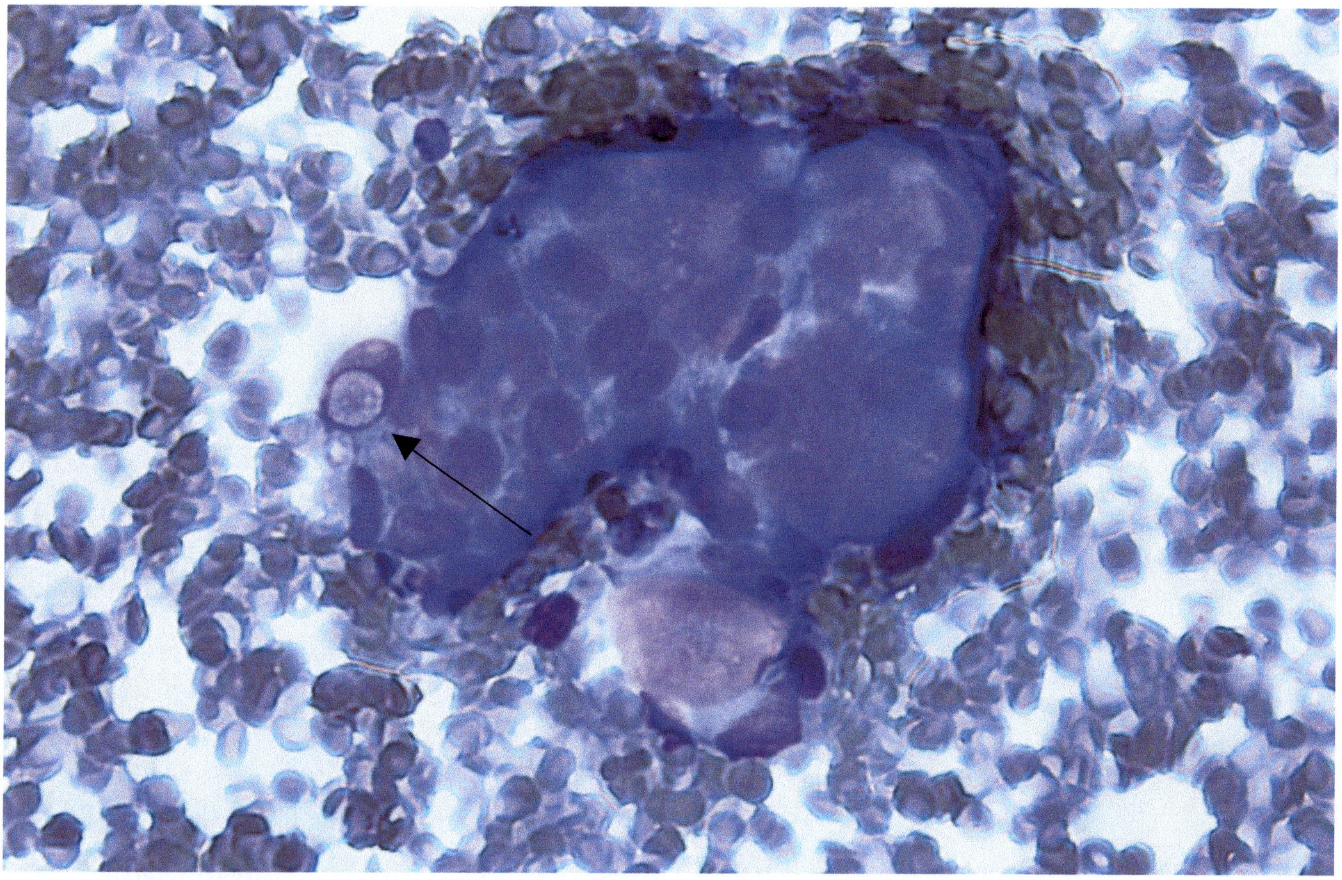

Figure 7-23. Cytology: papillary thyroid carcinoma, nuclear inclusion (*arrow*).

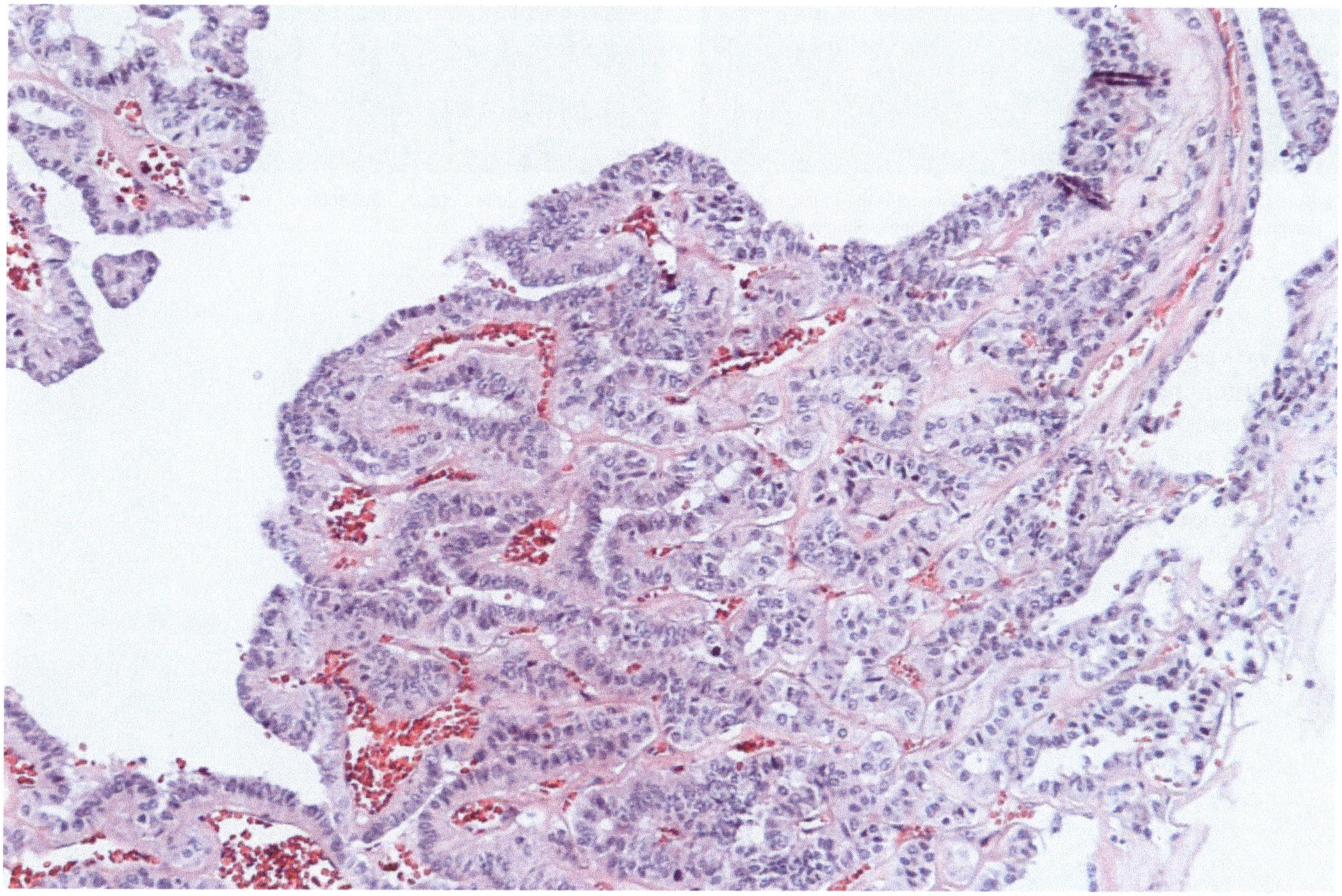

Figure 7-24. Histology: papillary thyroid carcinoma.

Papillary Thyroid Carcinoma Isthmus

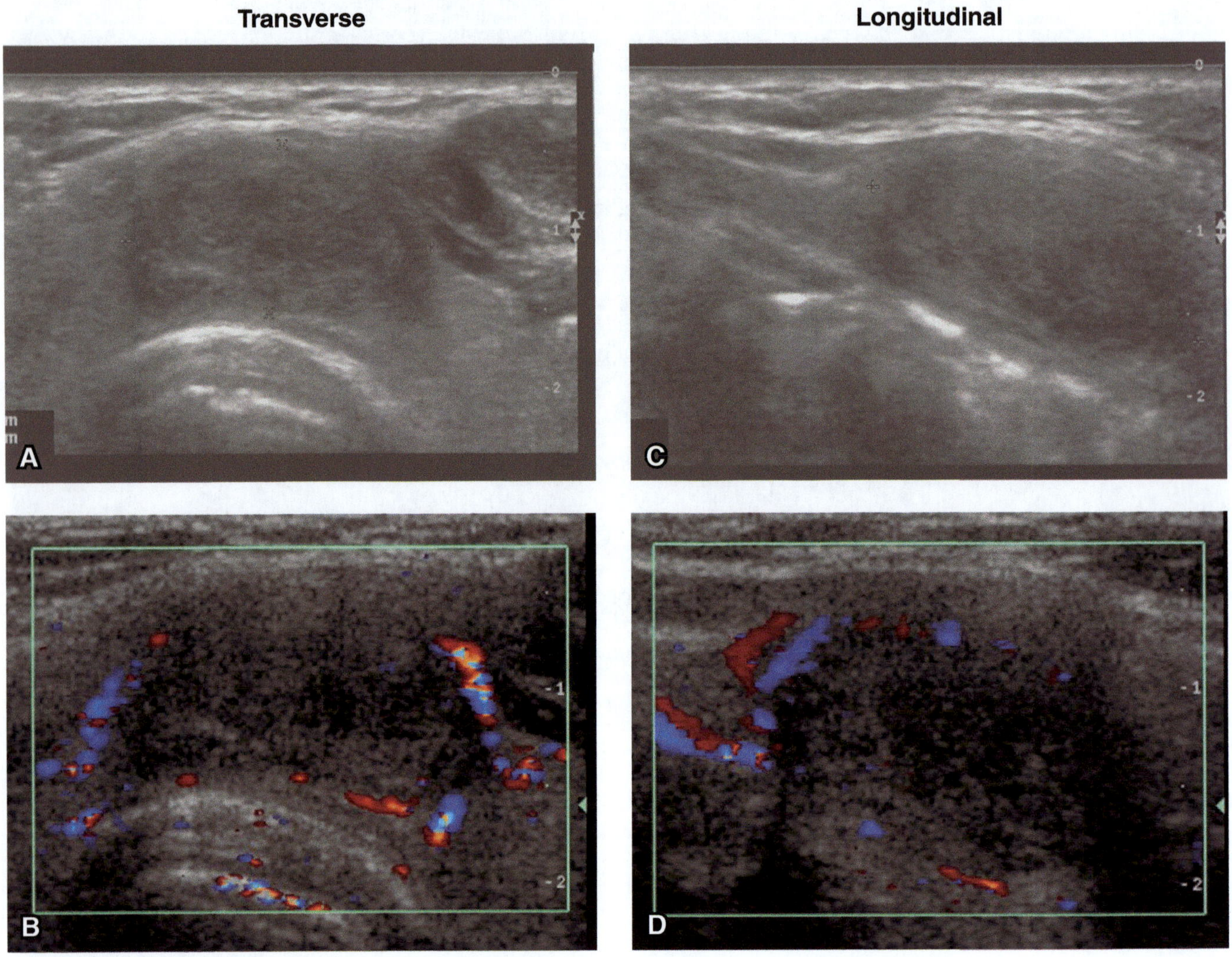

Figure 7-25. Ultrasound of papillary thyroid carcinoma in the isthmus. **A**, Transverse, 11 x 19 mm. **B**, Color Doppler, transverse. **C**, Longitudinal, sagittal diameter: 21 mm. **D**, Color Doppler, longitudinal.

56-Year-old man

- **Clinical history:** Palpable nodule in isthmus.
- **Ultrasound:** Possibly papillary thyroid carcinoma (PTC) in isthmus.
- **Cytology:** PTC.
- **Thyroidectomy:** PTC.

Features

Hypoechoic
Inhomogeneous echo pattern
Blurred margins
Scant vascularity

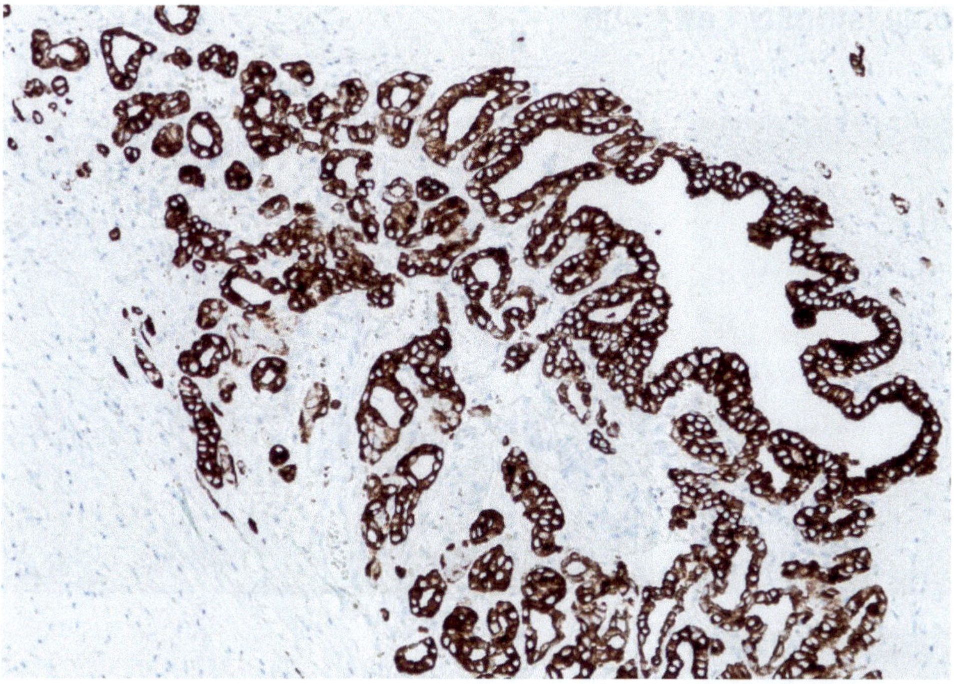

FIGURE 7-26. Immunohistochemistry: CK19 is high molecular weight cytokeratin that is usually strongly positive in papillary thyroid carcinoma.

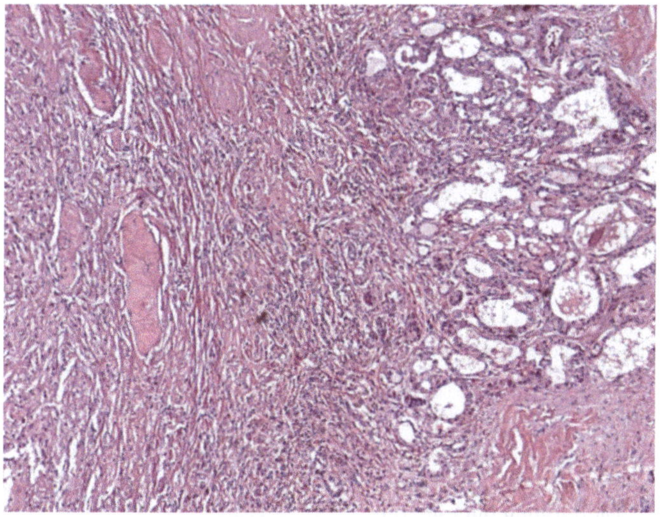

FIGURE 7-27. Histology: follicular growth.

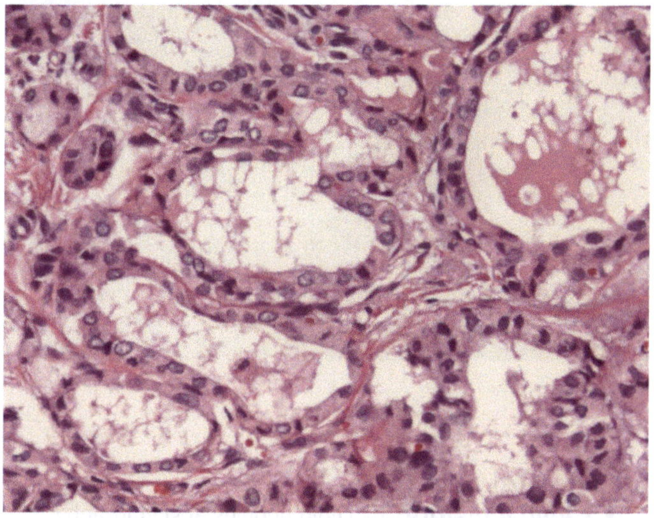

FIGURE 7-28. Histology: optically clear nuclei in papillary thyroid carcinoma.

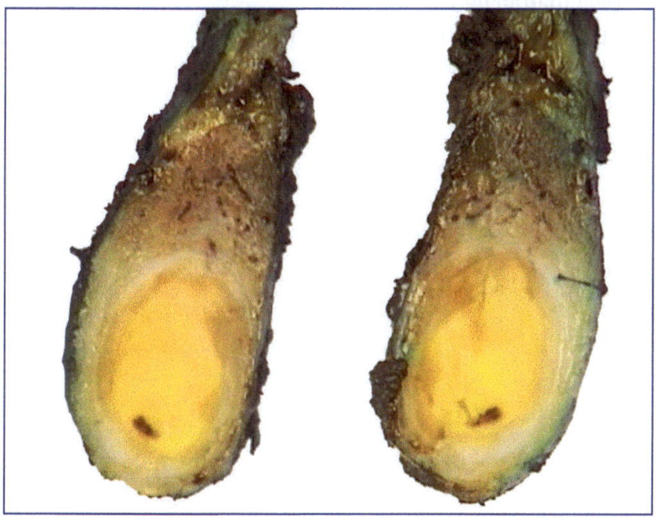

FIGURE 7-29. Gross section: well-circumscribed lesion.

Transverse

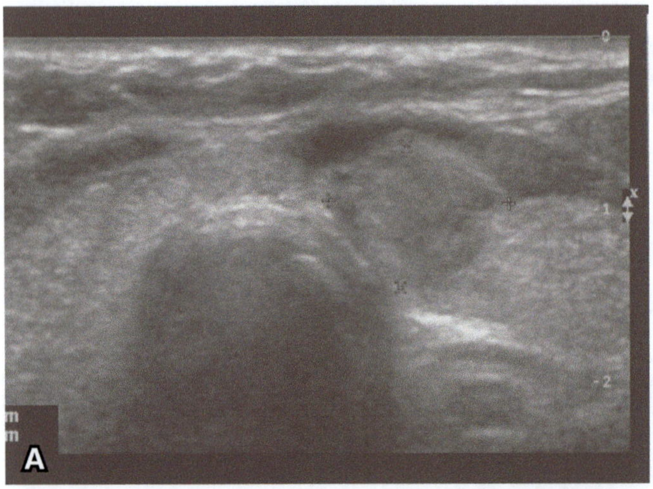

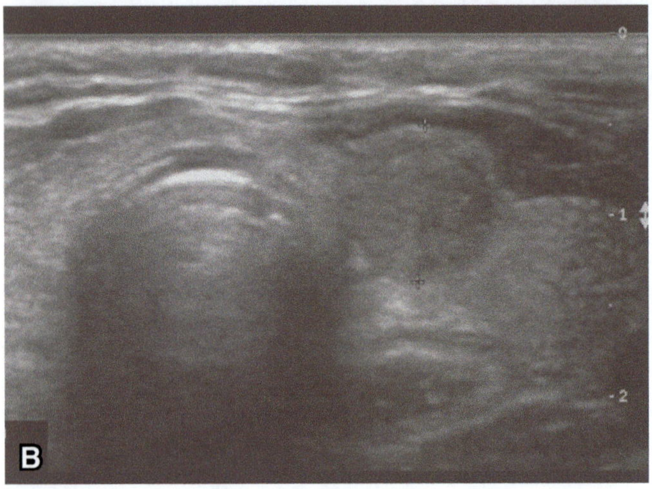

Transverse

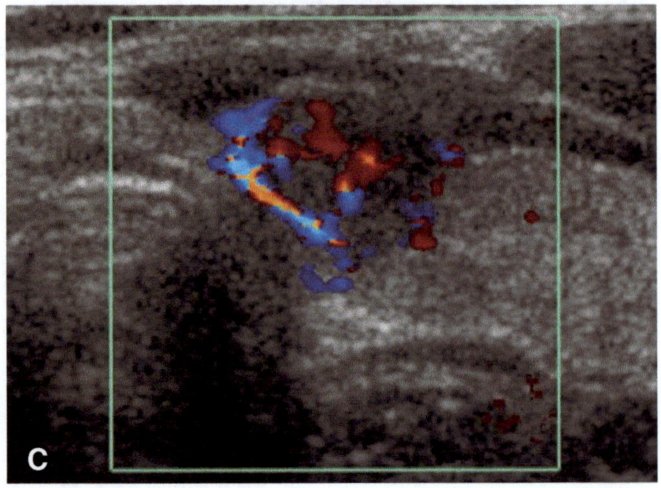

Figure 7-30. Ultrasound of papillary thyroid carcinoma in the isthmus and left lobe. **A**, Transverse, 8 x 11 mm. **B**, Transverse. **C**, Color Doppler, transverse.

37-Year-old woman

- **Clinical history:** Two cold nodules at scintigraphy.
- **Ultrasound:** Probably papillary thyroid carcinoma (PTC) in isthmus/ left lobe. No metastases.
- **Cytology:** PTC.
- **Thyroidectomy:** PTC + metastases.

See also pages 26–27

Features

Moderately hypoechoic
Inhomogeneous echo pattern
Well marginated
Suspicious disorganized vascularity

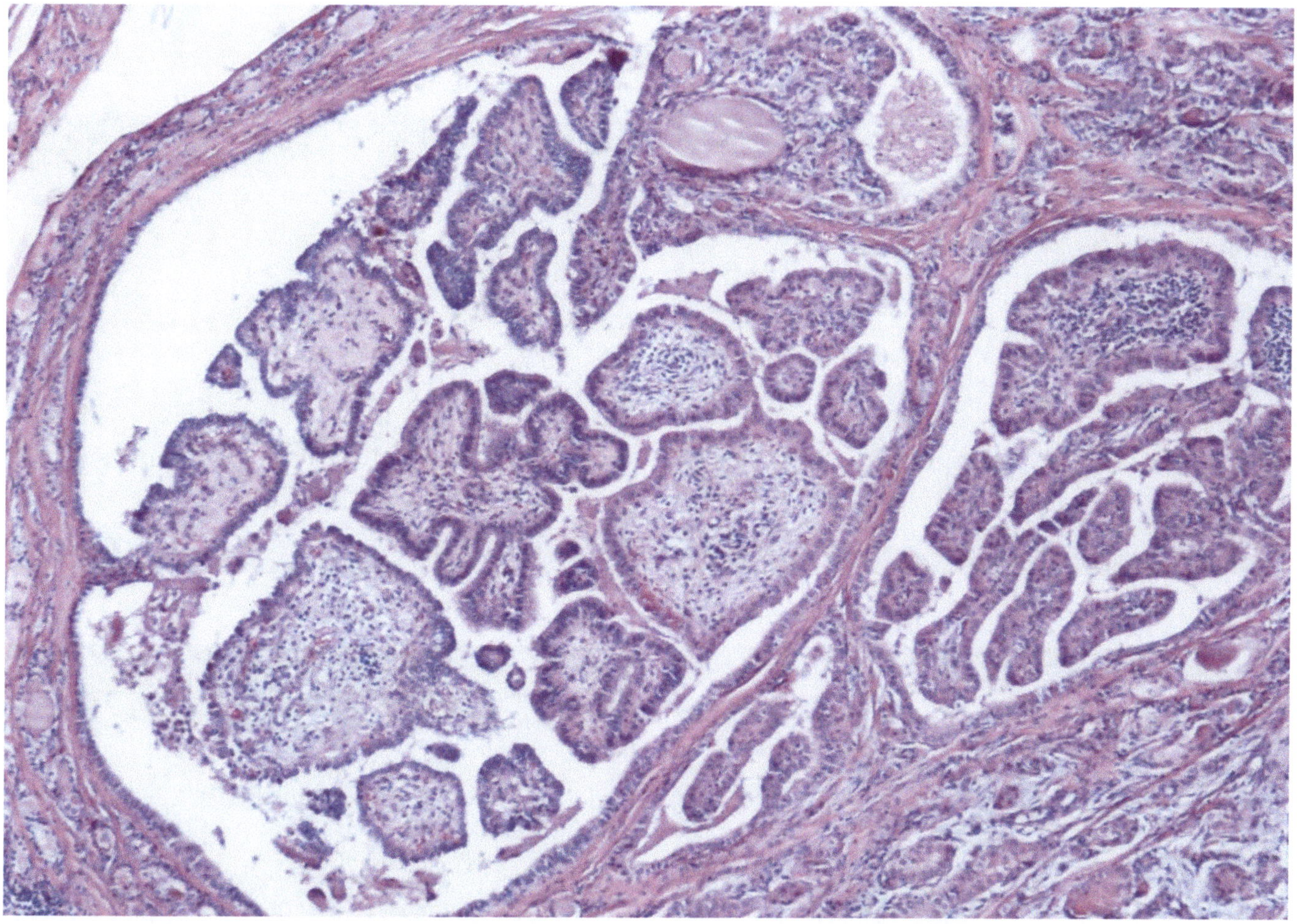

FIGURE 7-31. Histology: classical papillary growth pattern.

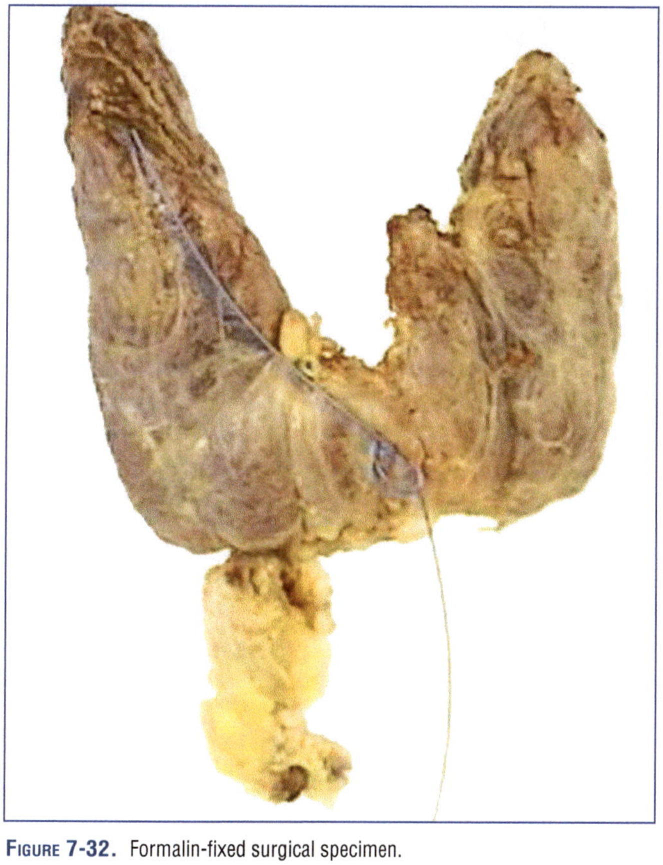

FIGURE 7-32. Formalin-fixed surgical specimen.

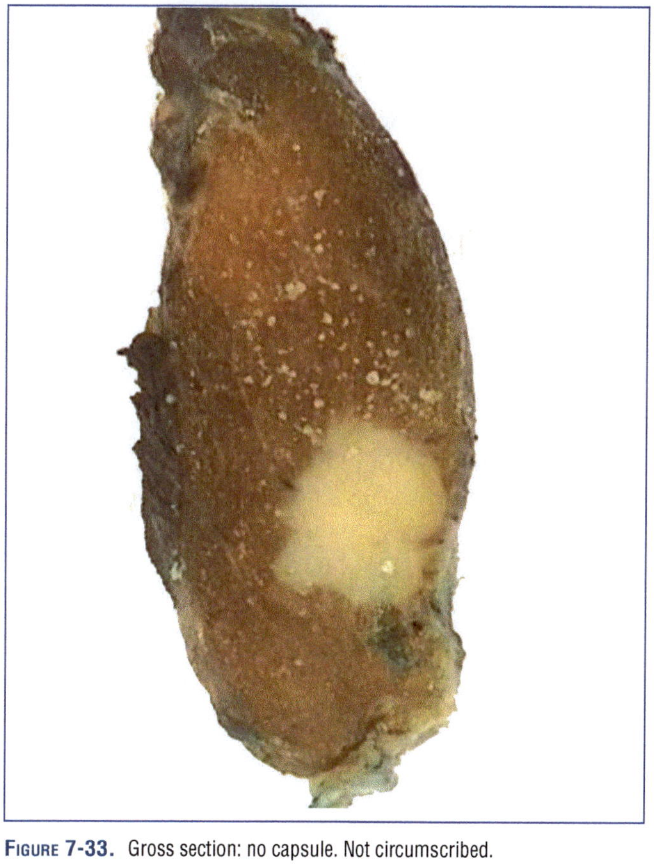

FIGURE 7-33. Gross section: no capsule. Not circumscribed.

Papillary Thyroid Carcinoma Isthmus

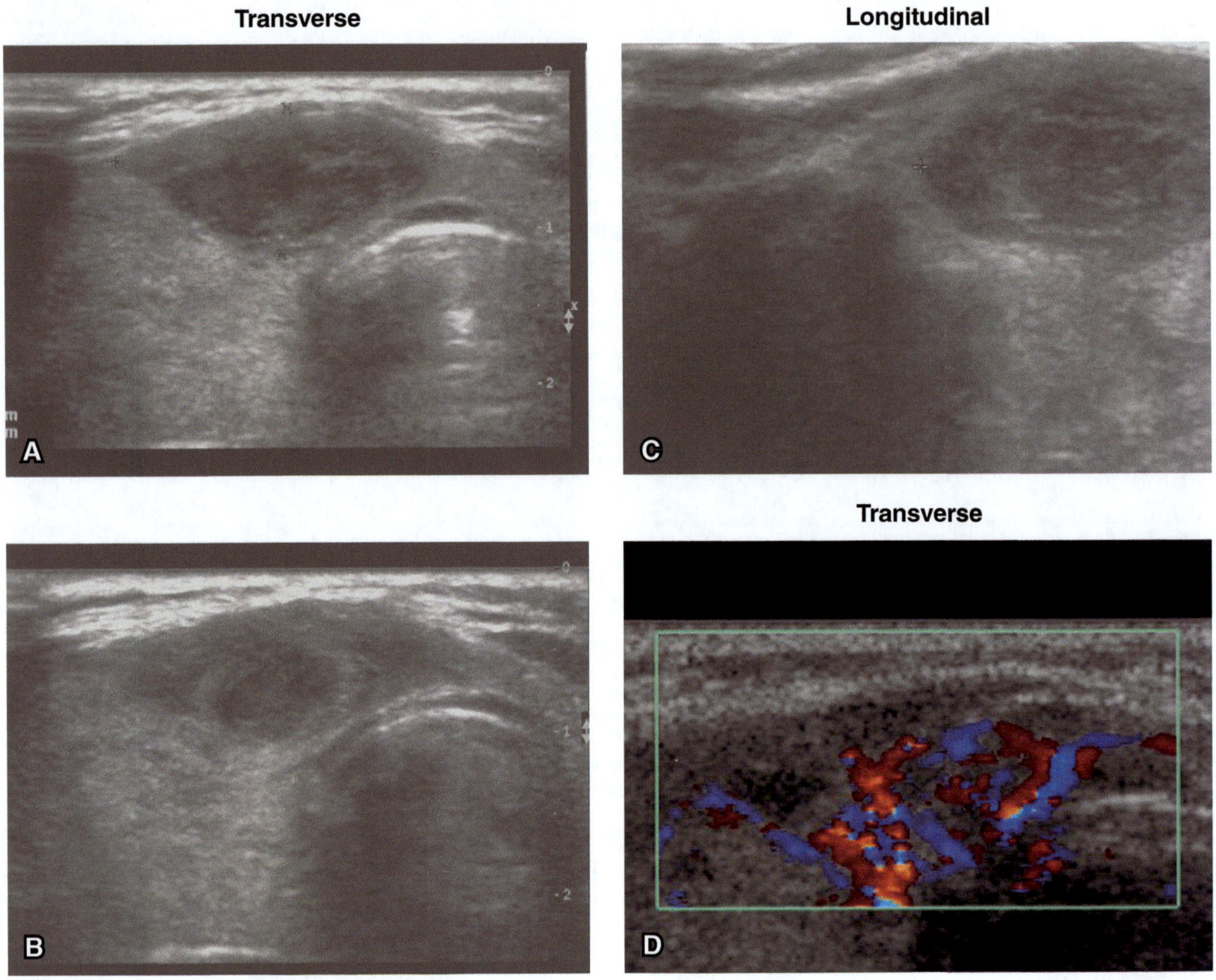

FIGURE 7-34. Ultrasound of papillary thyroid carcinoma in the isthmus. **A**, Transverse, 9 x 20 mm. **B**, Transverse. **C**, Longitudinal, 15 mm. **D**, Color Doppler, transverse.

24-Year-old woman

- **Clinical history:** Palpable nodule in isthmus.
- **Ultrasound:** Thyroiditis and possibly malignant tumor in isthmus.
- **Cytology:** Papillary thyroid carcinoma (PTC).
- **18-Gauge histologic needle biopsy:** PTC.
- **Thyroidectomy:** PTC + metastases.

Features

Hypoechoic
Inhomogeneous echo pattern
Partially blurred margins
A few microcalcifications
Hypervascular

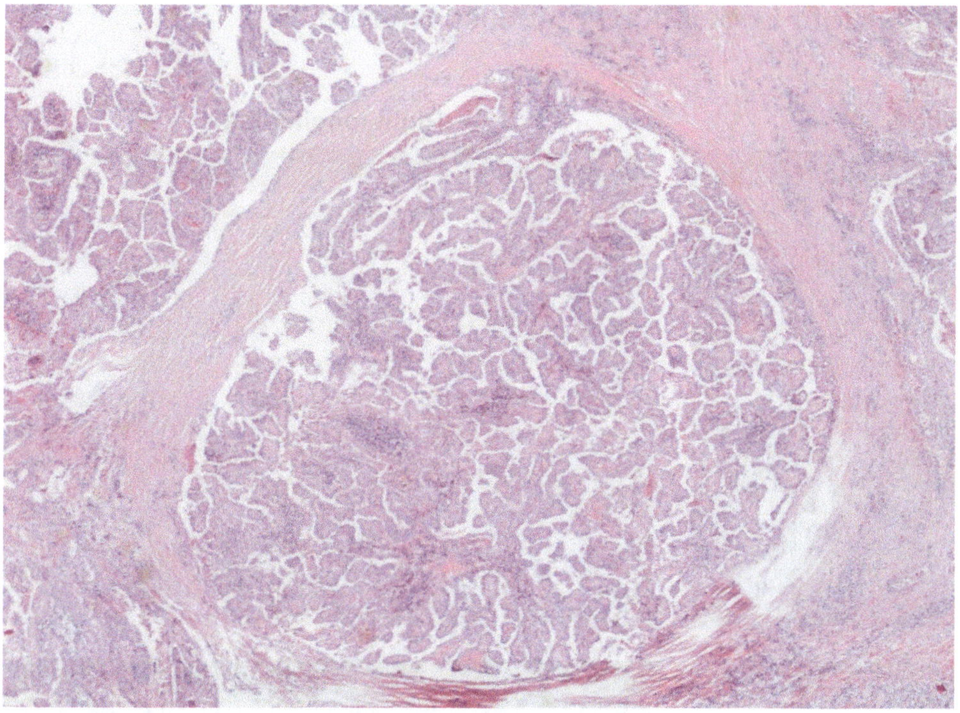

FIGURE 7-35. Histology: papillary thyroid carcinoma.

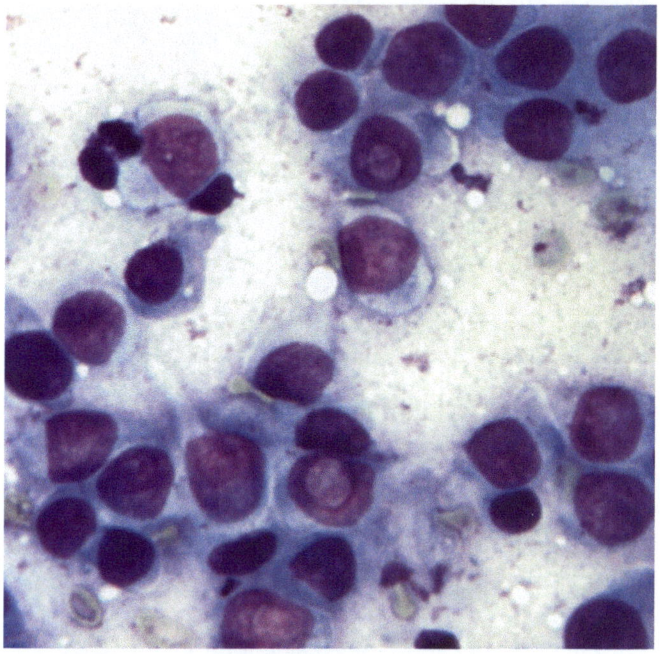

FIGURE 7-36. Cytology: nuclear inclusions.

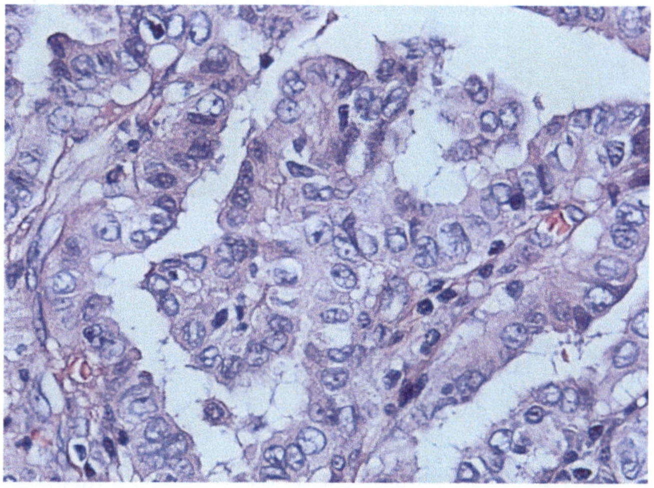

FIGURE 7-37. Histology: papillary growth in papillary thyroid carcinoma.

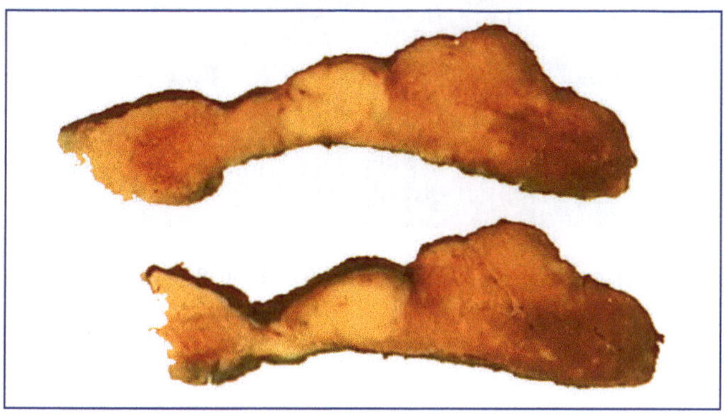

FIGURE 7-38. Gross section: ill-defined tumor margins.

Papillary Thyroid Carcinoma Right Lobe/Micro-Papillary Thyroid Carcinoma Left lobe

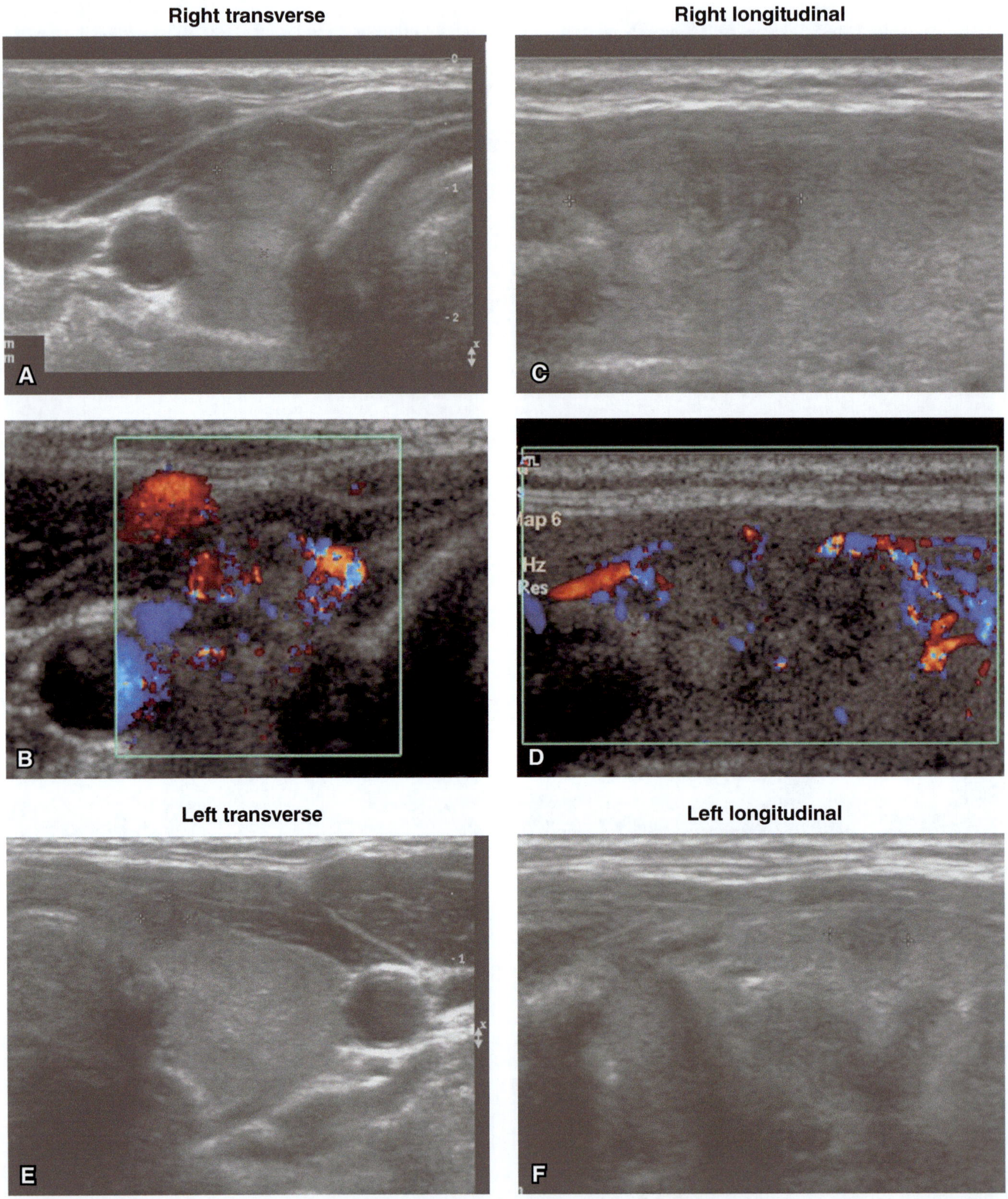

Figure 7-39. Ultrasound of papillary thyroid carcinoma (PTC) in the right lobe and micro-PTC in the left lobe. **A**, Right transverse, 9 x 10 mm. **B**, Color Doppler, right transverse. **C**, Right longitudinal, 15 mm. **D**, Color Doppler, right longitudinal. **E**, Left transverse, 4 mm. **F**, Left longitudinal.

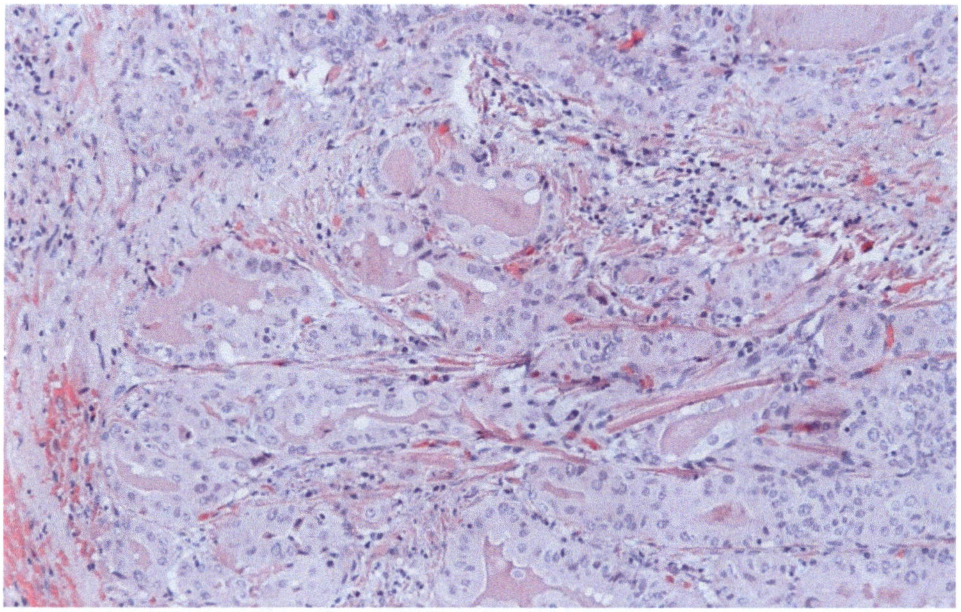

FIGURE 7-40. Histology: papillary thyroid carcinoma with cells with some oncocytic differentiations.

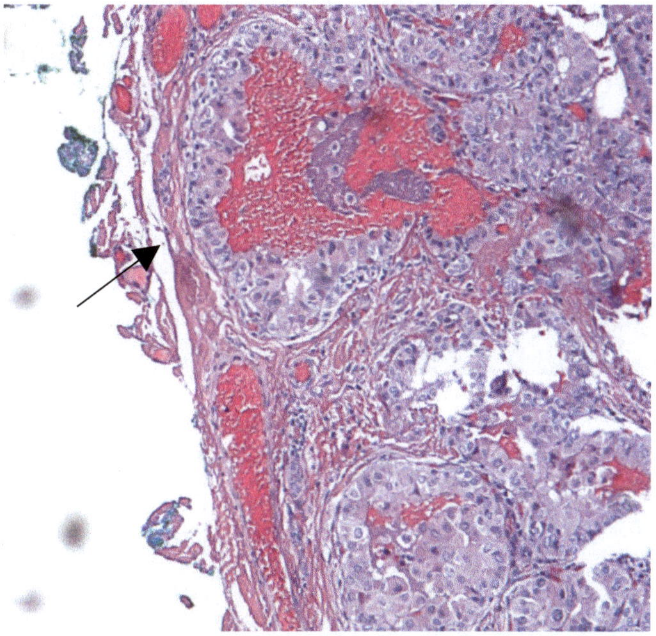

FIGURE 7-41. Histology: tumor growth close to the resection margin (*arrow*).

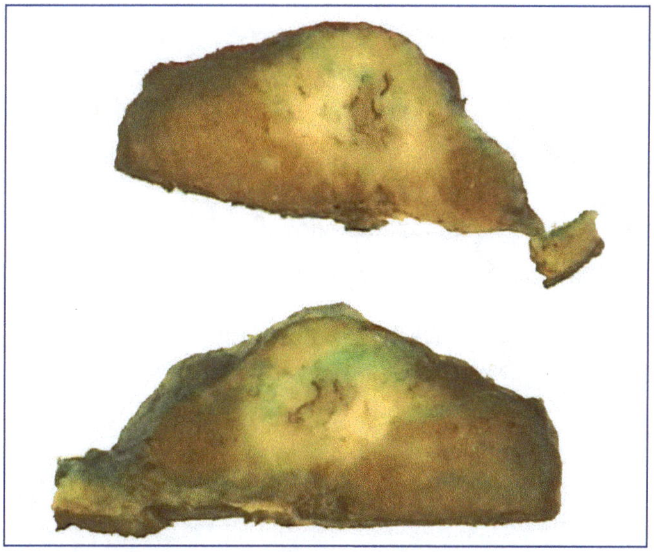

FIGURE 7-42. Gross section right lobe: tumor growth close to the resection margin.

38-Year-old woman

- **Clinical history:** Palpable nodule in right lobe.
- **Ultrasound:** Suspicious for papillary thyroid carcinoma (PTC) in right and left lobes.
- **Cytology:** PTC in right lobe. Suspicious for PTC in left lobe.
- **Thyroidectomy:** PTC in both lobes.

Features, right
Mixed echogenicity
Inhomogeneous echo pattern
Blurred margins
Scant vascularity

Features, left
Hypoechoic
Homogeneous echo pattern
Blurred margins
Taller than wide

Papillary Thyroid Carcinoma: Microcarcinomas Right Lobe and Isthmus

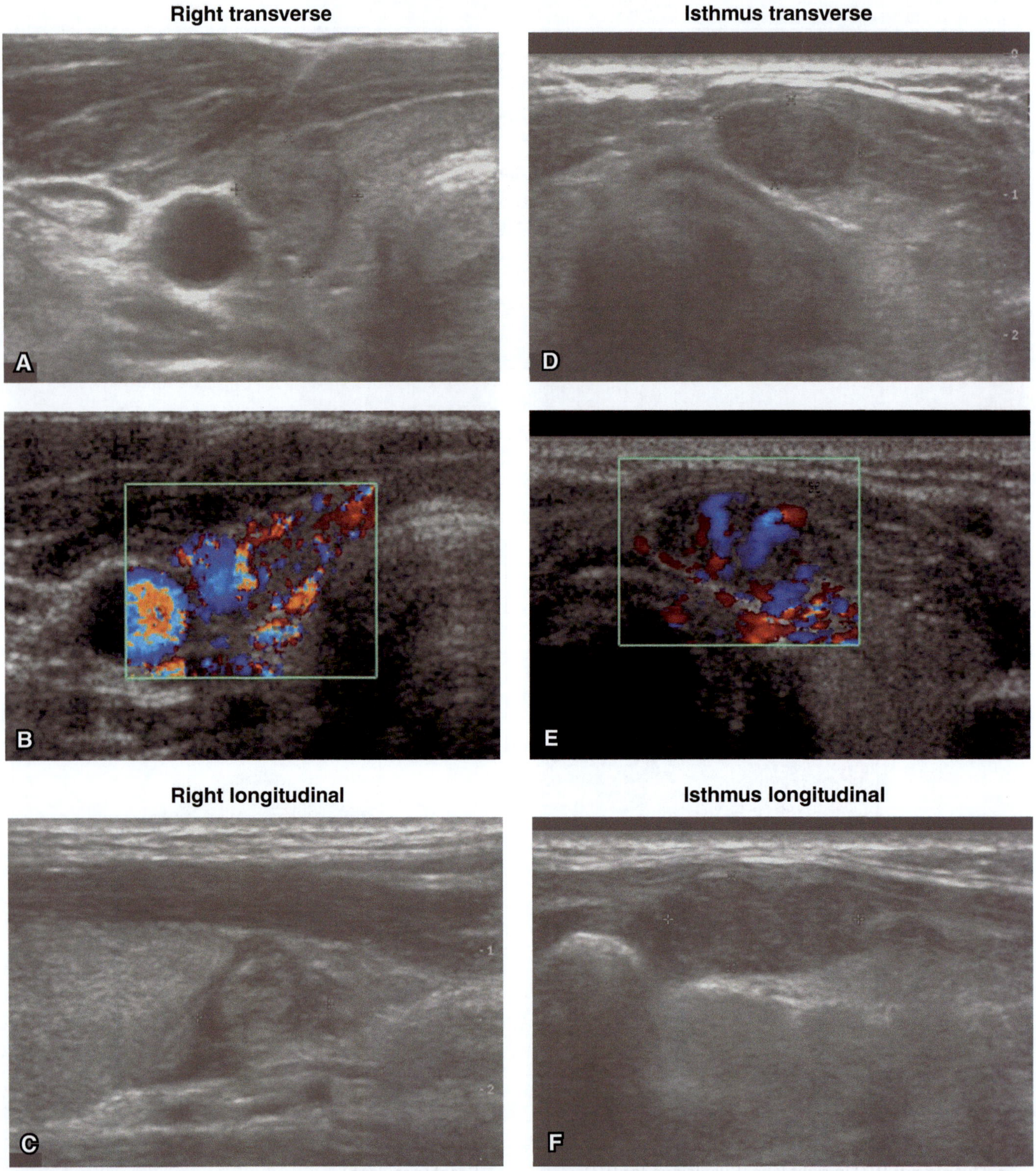

Figure 7-43. Ultrasound of papillary thyroid carcinoma with microcarcinomas in the right lobe and isthmus. **A**, Right transverse, 8 x 8 mm. **B**, Color Doppler, right transverse. **C**, Right longitudinal. **D**, Isthmus transverse, 6 x 10 mm. **E**, Color Doppler, isthmus transverse. **F**, Isthmus longitudinal, 13 mm.

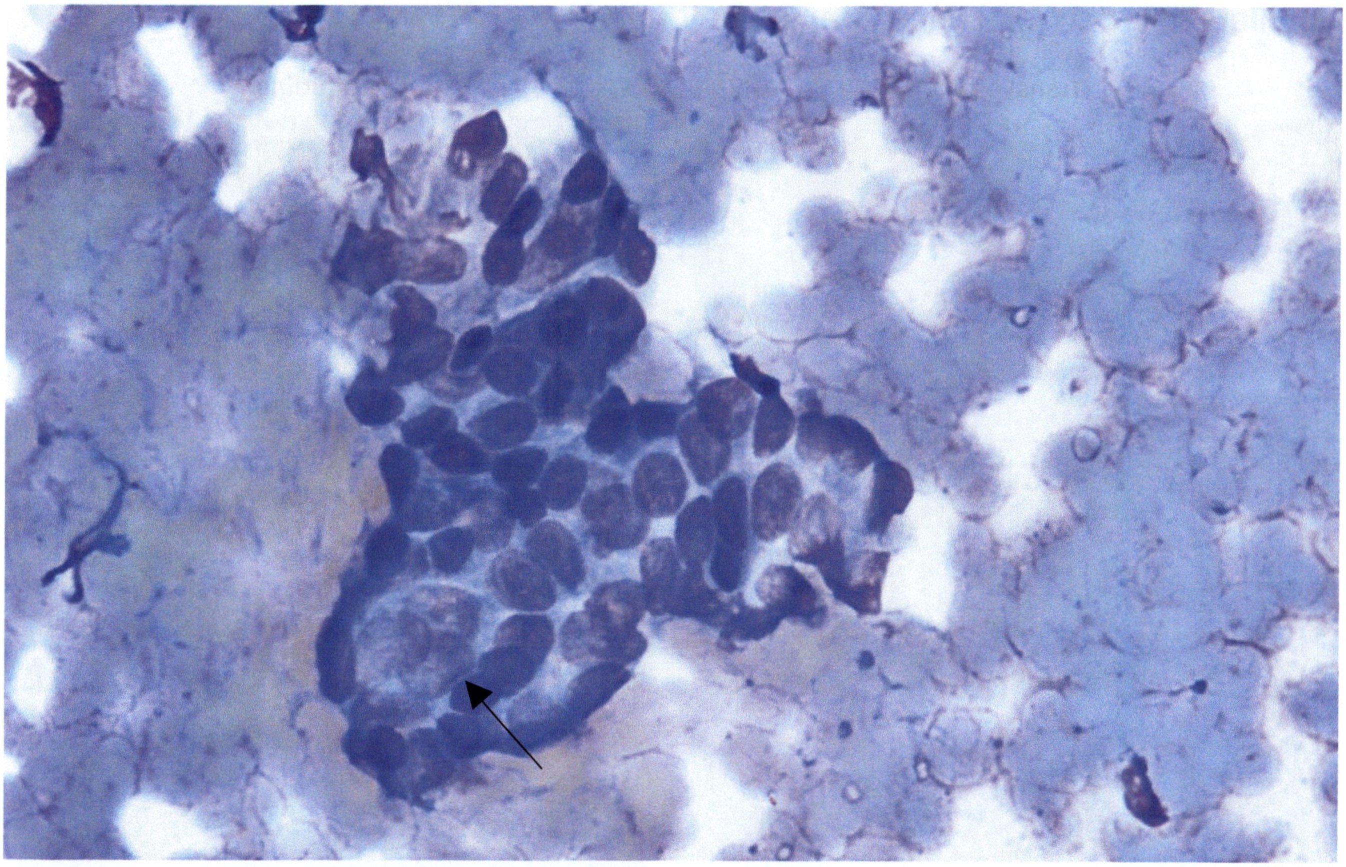

Figure 7-44. Cytology: papillary epithelial groups with atypical cells with overlapping nuclei (*arrow*).

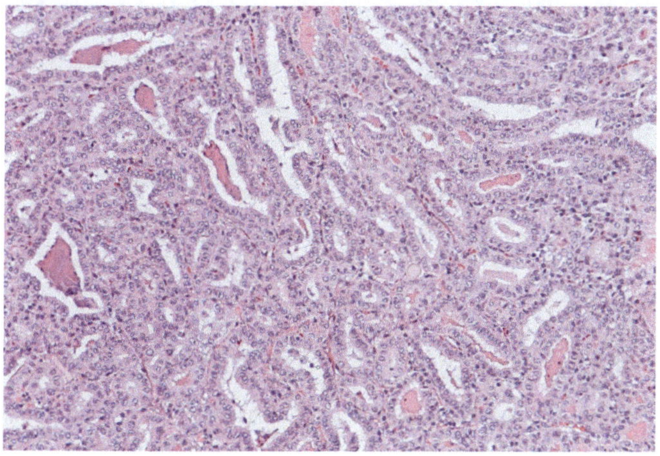

Figure 7-45. Histology: papillary thyroid carcinoma.

35-Year-old woman

- **Clinical history:** Some months with palpable nodule in isthmus.
- **Ultrasound:** Papillary thyroid carcinoma (PTC) in right lobe. Metastasis pretracheally in segment 6? 2 mm metastasis in segment 7?
- **Cytology:** PTC in right lobe and isthmus.
- **Thyroidectomy:** PTC in right lobe and isthmus. 1 mm PTC in left lobe. Metastasis in 1 of 11 lymph nodes.

Features, right
Slightly hypoechoic with hypoechoic halo
Inhomogeneous echo pattern
Partially well circumscribed
A few microcalcifications
Hypervascular

Features, isthmus
Hypoechoic
Well marginated
Homogeneous echo pattern
Moderately vascular

Papillary Thyroid Carcinoma Isthmus/Left Lobe

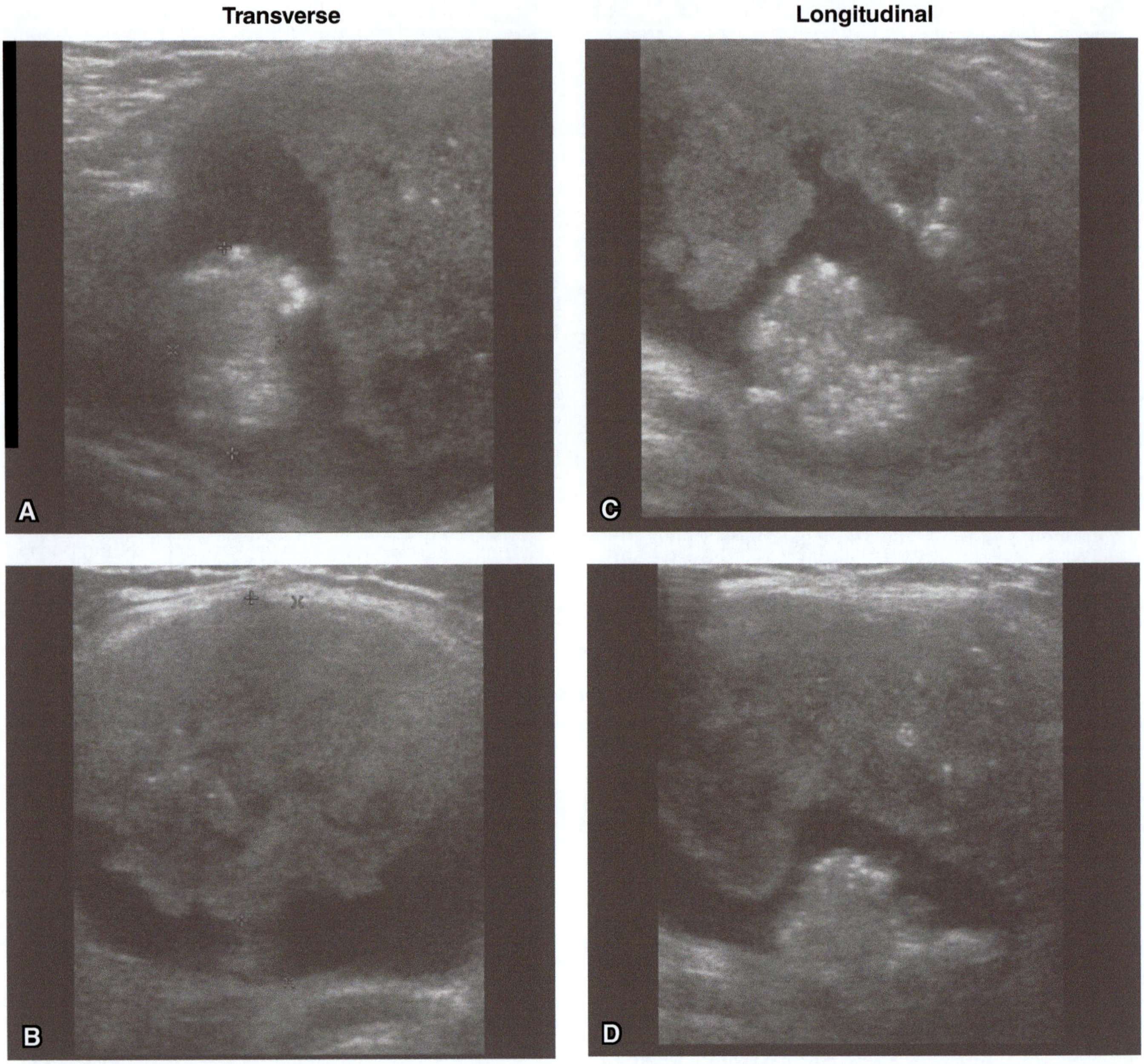

Figure 7-46. Ultrasound of partially cystic papillary thyroid carcinoma in the isthmus and left lobe. **A** and **B**, Transverse. **C** and **D**, Longitudinal.

43-Year-old man

- **Clinical history:** Aspirated 6 cm cyst in left lobe.
- **Ultrasound:** Suspicious for papillary thyroid carcinoma (PTC). No metastases.
- **Cytology:** PTC with cystic degeneration.
- **Thyroidectomy:** Partially cystic 4 cm PTC in left lobe. 5 mm PTC in right lobe. One metastasis in segment 6.

Features

Mixed echogenicity
Well circumscribed
Inhomogeneous echo pattern
Microcalcifications
Cystic degeneration

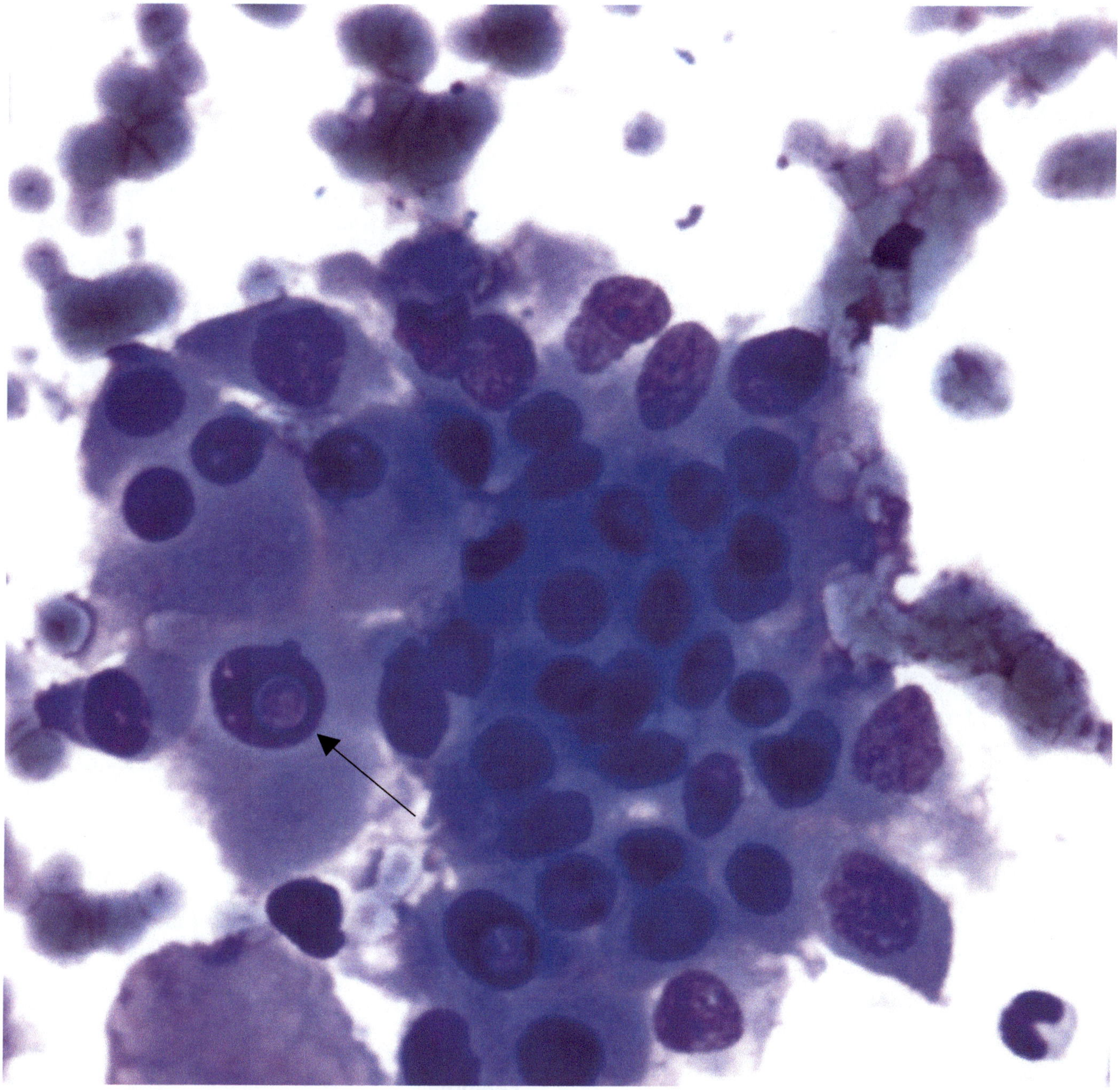

FIGURE 7-47. Cytology: papillary thyroid carcinoma, classic intranuclear inclusion (*arrow*).

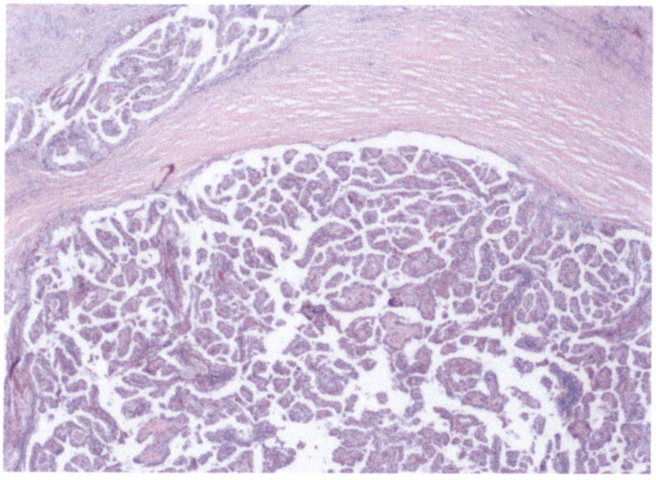

FIGURE 7-48. Histology: papillary growth pattern.

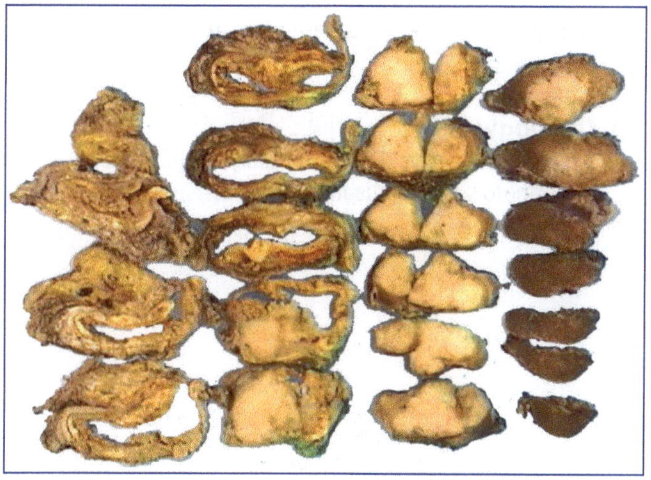

FIGURE 7-49. Gross section: solid and cystic components.

Papillary Thyroid Carcinoma Right Lobe

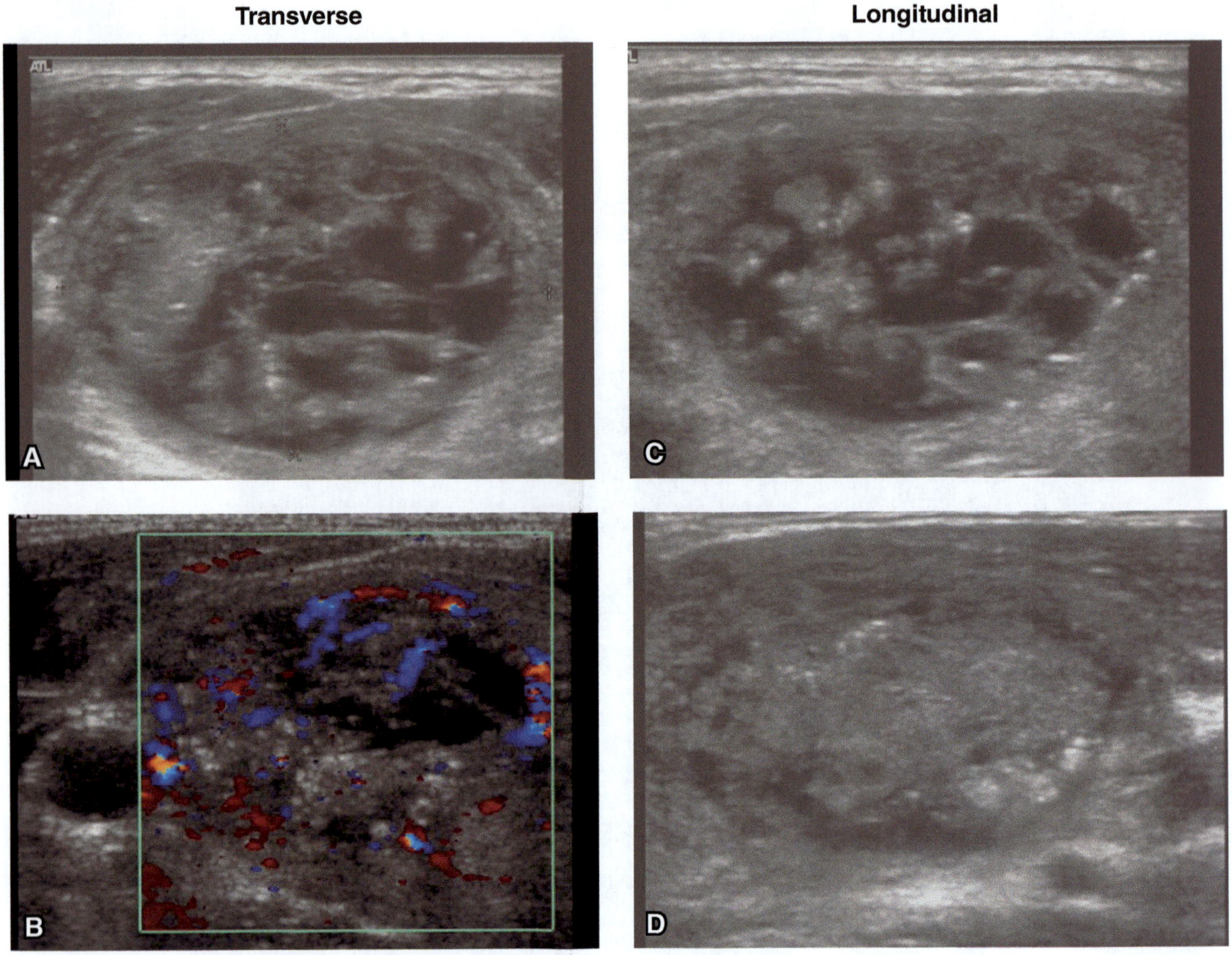

Figure 7-50. Ultrasound of papillary thyroid carcinoma in the right lobe. **A**, Transverse, 24 x 35 mm. **B**, Color Doppler, transverse. **C**, Longitudinal, 40 mm. **D**, Color Doppler, longitudinal.

52-Year-old man

- **Clinical history:** Autoimmune thyroiditis. Growing nodule in right lobe.
- **Ultrasound:** Suspicious for papillary thyroid carcinoma (PTC) in right lobe. Thyroiditis in both lobes.
- **Cytology:** PTC.
- **Thyroidectomy:** 45 mm partially cystic PTC. Hashimoto's thyroiditis in both lobes.

Features

Isoechoic solid tissue
Cystic degeneration
Well circumscribed
Microcalcifications and some colloid crystals
Scant vascularity

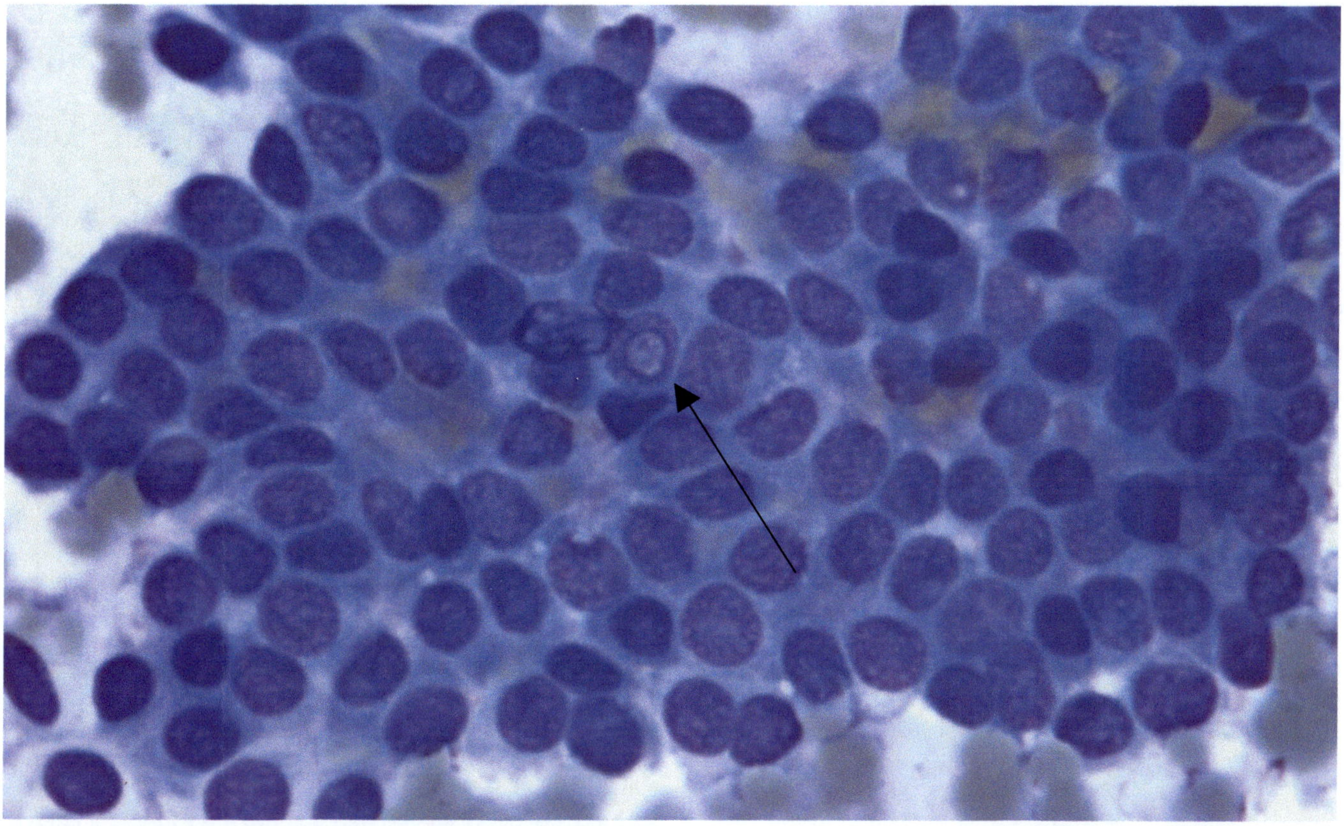

Figure 7-51. Cytology: papillary thyroid carcinoma, classic nuclear inclusion (*arrow*).

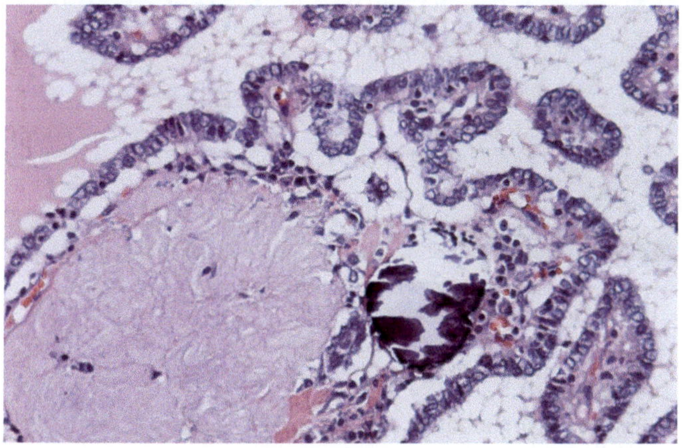

Figure 7-52. Histology: microcalcifications.

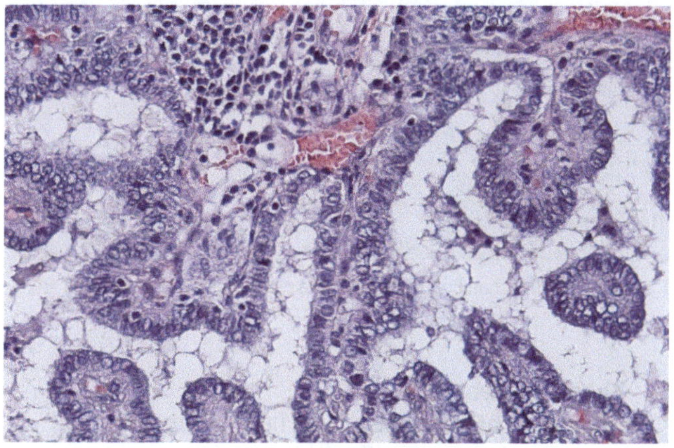

Figure 7-53. Histology: papillary structures.

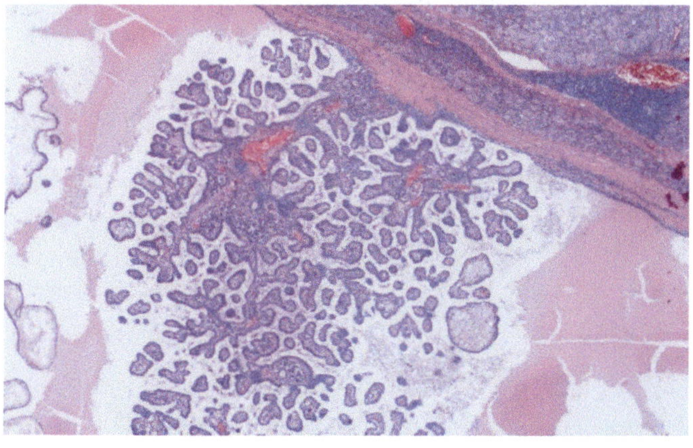

Figure 7-54. Histology: partially cystic with papillary structures, papillary thyroid carcinoma.

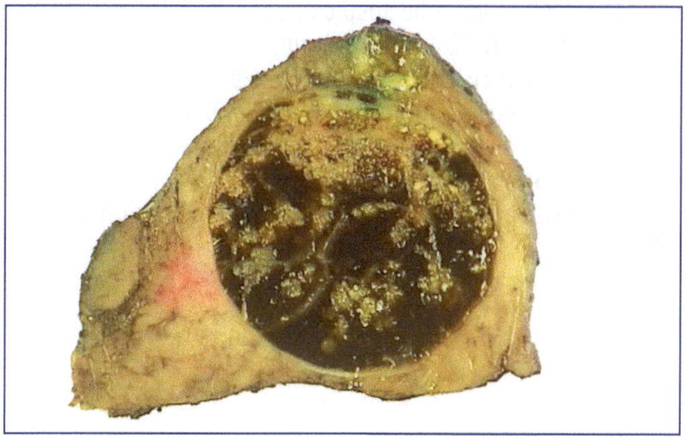

Figure 7-55. Gross section: circumscribed, well-defined lesion with papillary structures into the cystic lumen.

Papillary Thyroid Carcinoma Left Lobe

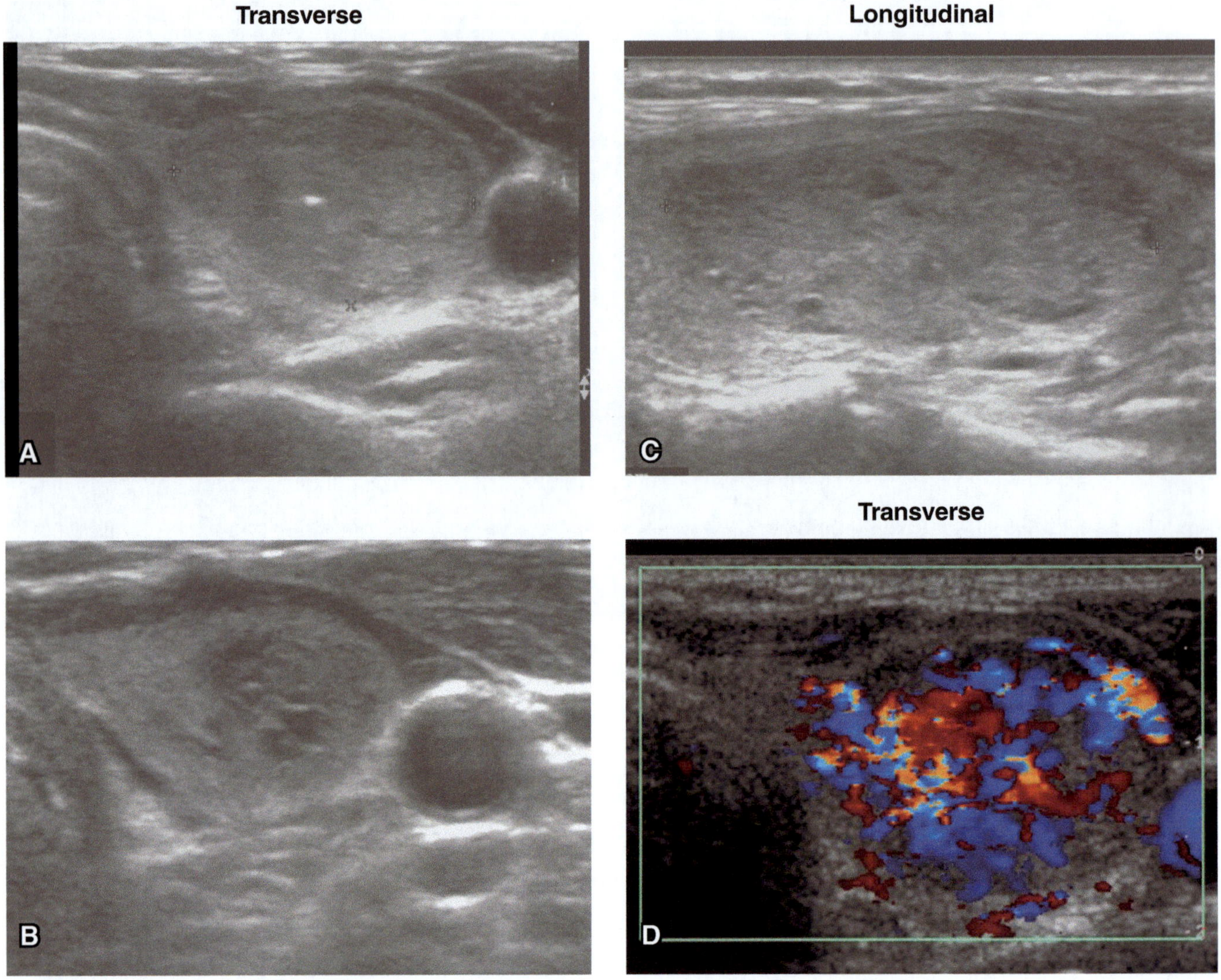

Figure 7-56. Ultrasound of papillary thyroid carcinoma in the left lobe. **A** and **B**, Transverse. **C**, Longitudinal. **D**, Color Doppler, transverse.

49-Year-old woman

- **Clinical history:** Removed benign tumor in isthmus 4 years ago. Examination of two nodules, one in each lobe 1 year ago.
  Cytology of left lobe suspicious for papillary thyroid carcinoma (PTC). No follow-up.
- **Ultrasound:** Cystic colloid nodule in right lobe. Probably colloid nodule in left lobe, but with a hypoechoic, somewhat suspicious area.
- **Cytology:** PTC in left lobe. Cyst in right lobe.
- **Thyroidectomy:** PTC in left lobe. Cyst in right lobe.

See also pages 32–33

Features

Slightly hypoechoic
Well circumscribed
Spongy echo pattern
One coarse calcification
Hypervascular

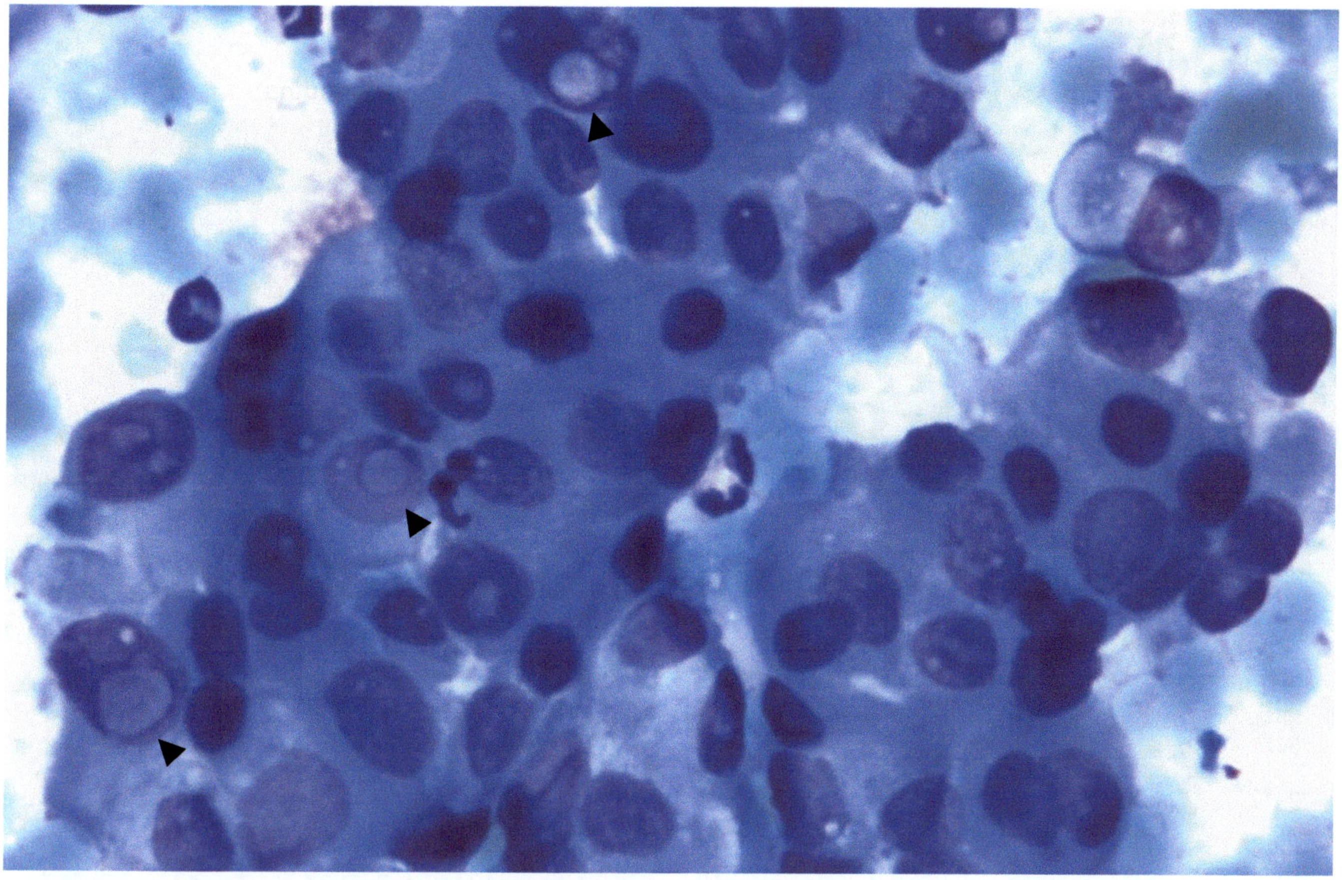

Figure 7-57. Cytology: papillary thyroid carcinoma, several intranuclear inclusions (*arrowheads*).

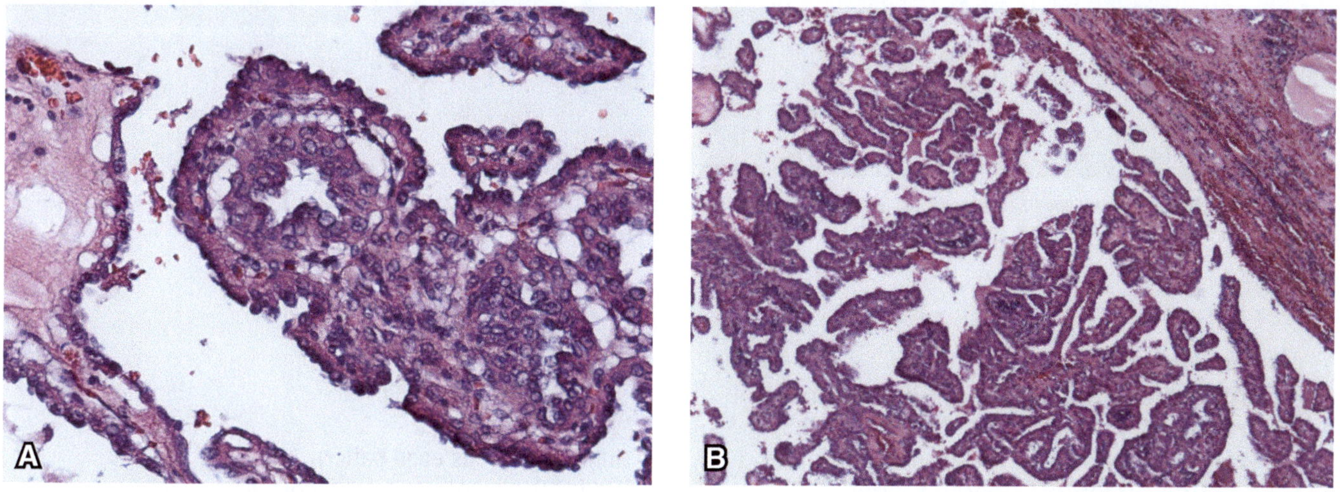

Figure 7-58. **A** and **B**. Left lobe: papillary carcinoma.

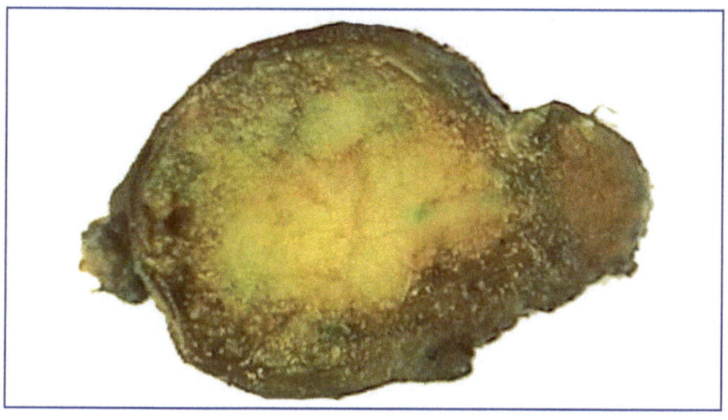

Figure 7-59. Gross section: ill-defined tumor borders. This tumor has infiltrated almost the entire lobe.

Papillary Thyroid Carcinoma Right Lobe

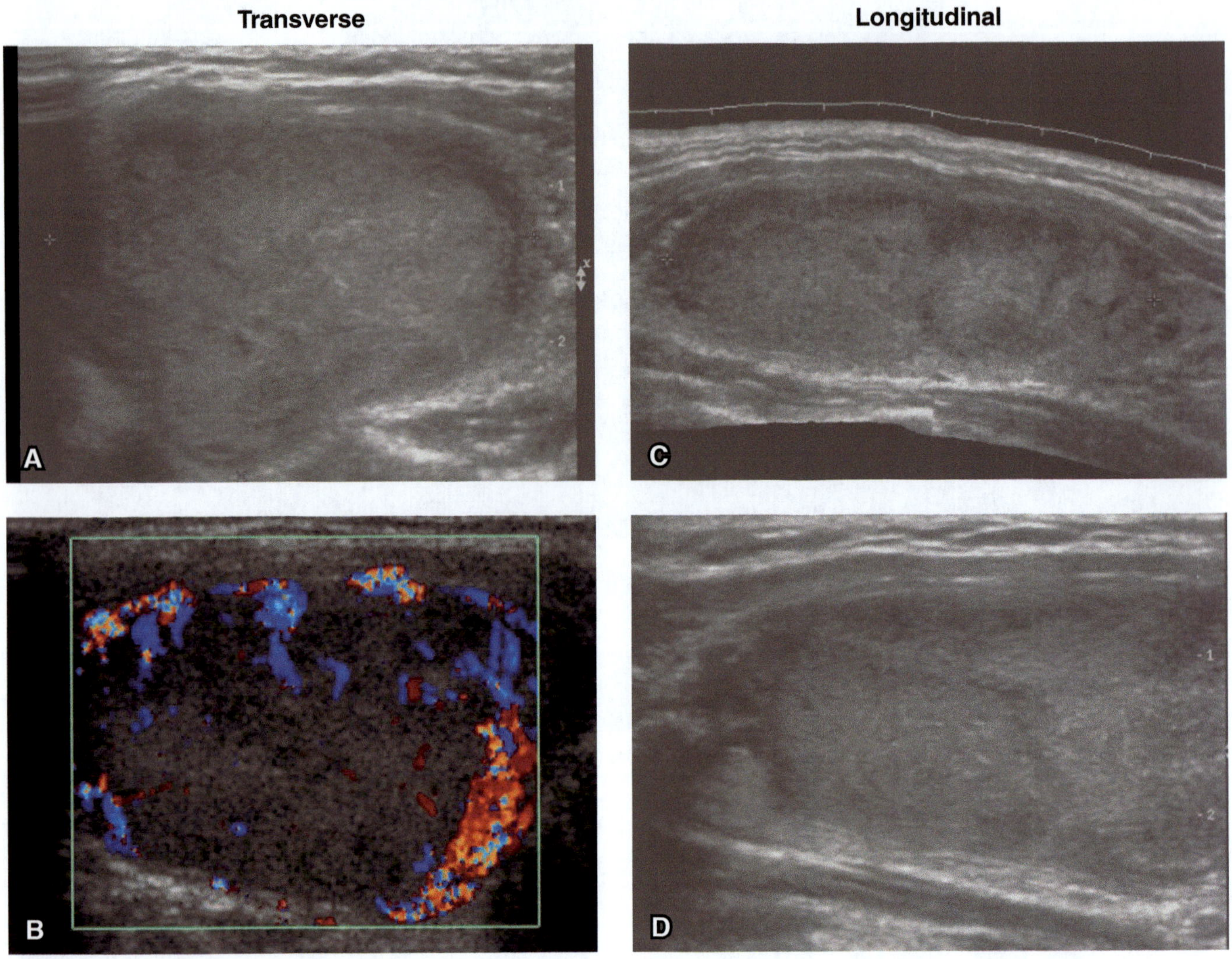

FIGURE 7-60. Ultrasound of papillary thyroid carcinoma in the right lobe. **A**, Transverse, 23 x 31 mm. **B**, Color Doppler, transverse. **C**, Longitudinal, 44 mm. **D**, Longitudinal.

46-Year-old woman

- **Clinical history:** Colloid nodule in right lobe.
- **Ultrasound:** Follicular tumor. Malignant?
- **Cytology:** Papillary thyroid carcinoma (PTC).
- **16-Gauge histologic needle biopsy:** PTC.
- **Thyroidectomy:** PTC.

Features

Moderately hypoechoic
Well circumscribed
Inhomogeneous echo pattern
Partial thick, uneven, hypoechoic halo
Suggestion of "spoke-and-wheel-like" vascularity

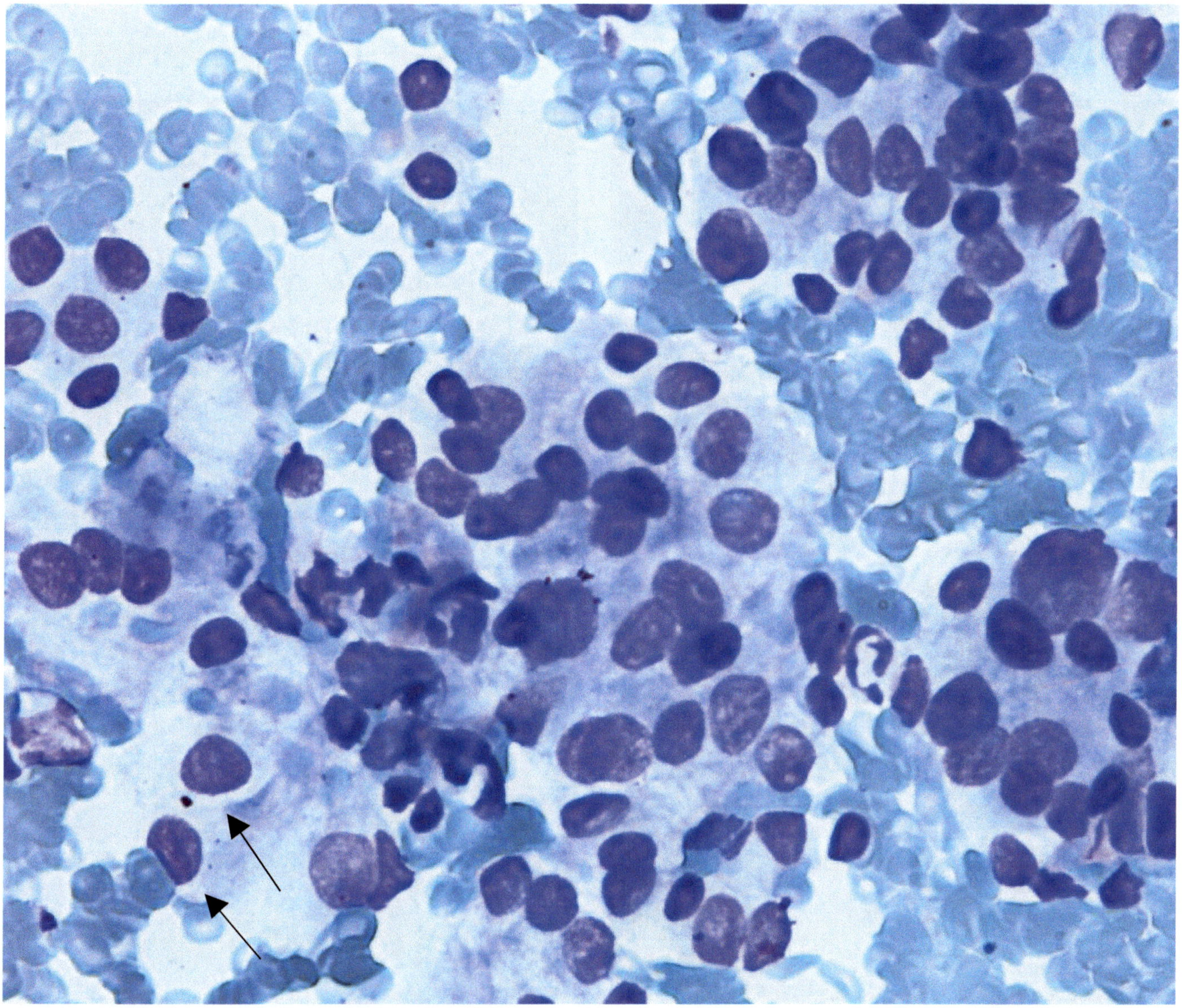

Figure 7-61. Cytology: partly overlapping nuclei with grooves (*arrows*).

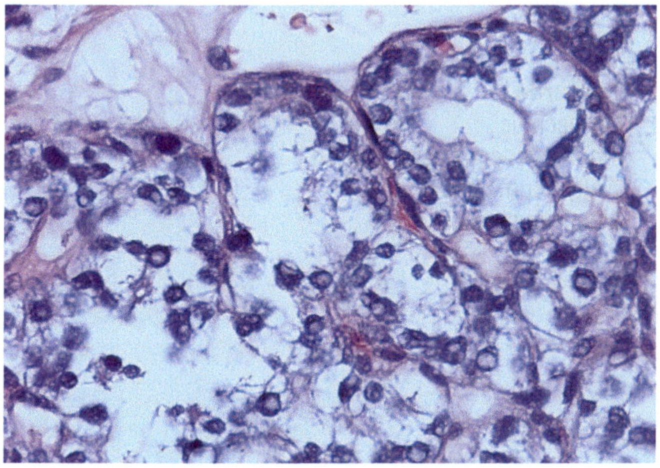

Figure 7-62. Histologic needle biopsy: trabecular and follicular growth pattern.

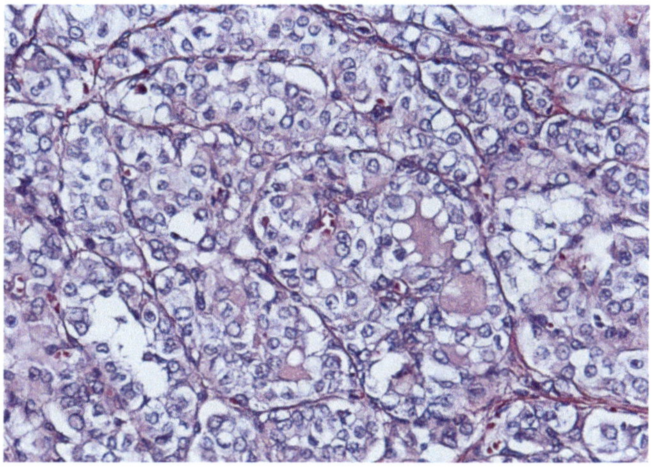

Figure 7-63. Histology: trabecular and follicular growth pattern.

Papillary Thyroid Carcinoma: Microcarcinoma Right Lobe

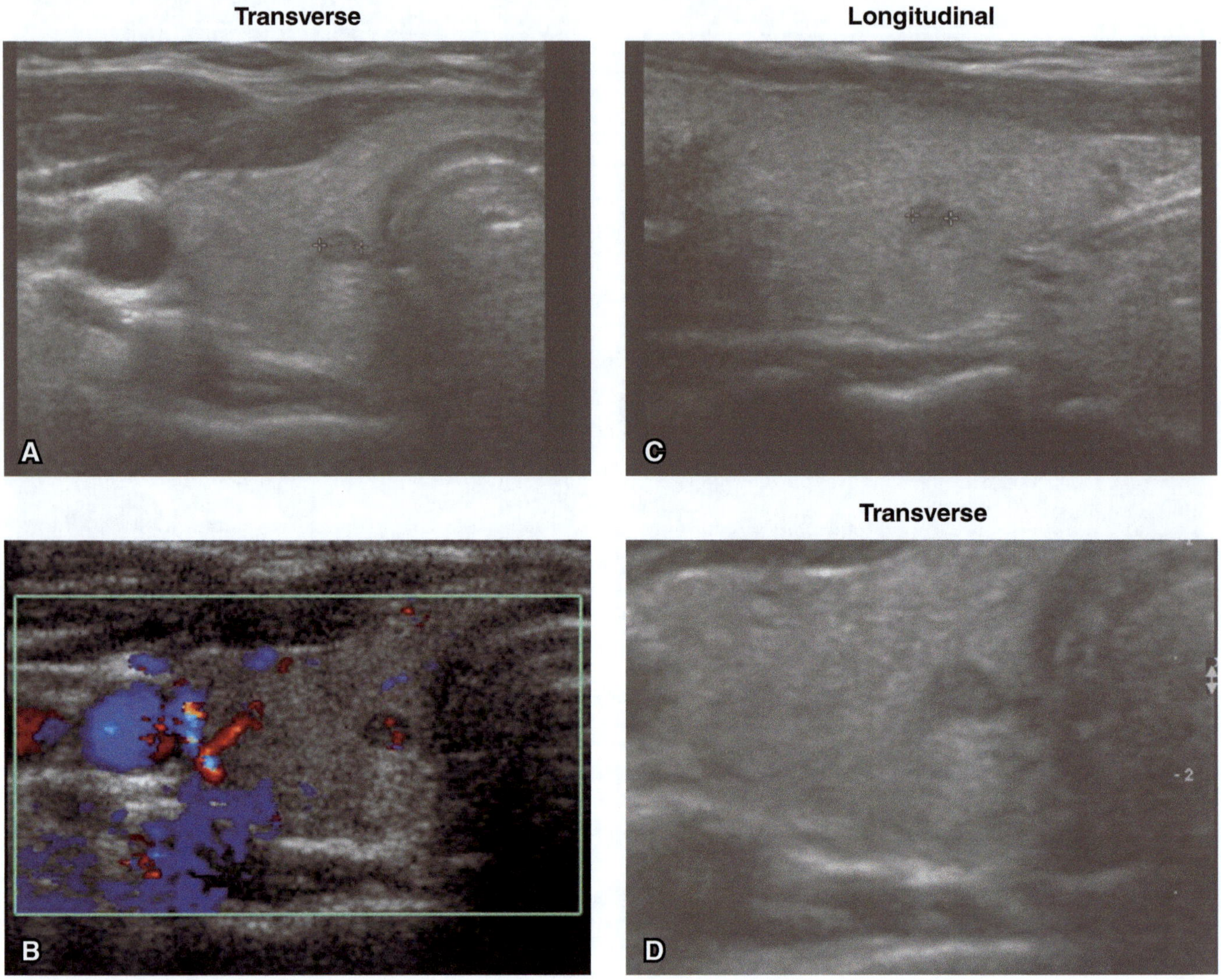

Figure 7-64. Ultrasound of papillary thyroid microcarcinoma. **A**, Transverse diameter: 3 mm. **B**, Color Doppler, transverse. **C**, Longitudinal, 3 mm. **D**, Transverse.

30-Year-old woman

- **Clinical history:** Grandmother and mother had papillary thyroid carcinoma (PTC).
- **Ultrasound:** Solitary 3 mm lesion suspicious for PTC.
- **Cytology:** PTC.
- **Thyroidectomy:** PTC.

Features

Hypoechoic
Inhomogeneous echo pattern
Well circumscribed
Suspicious vascularity

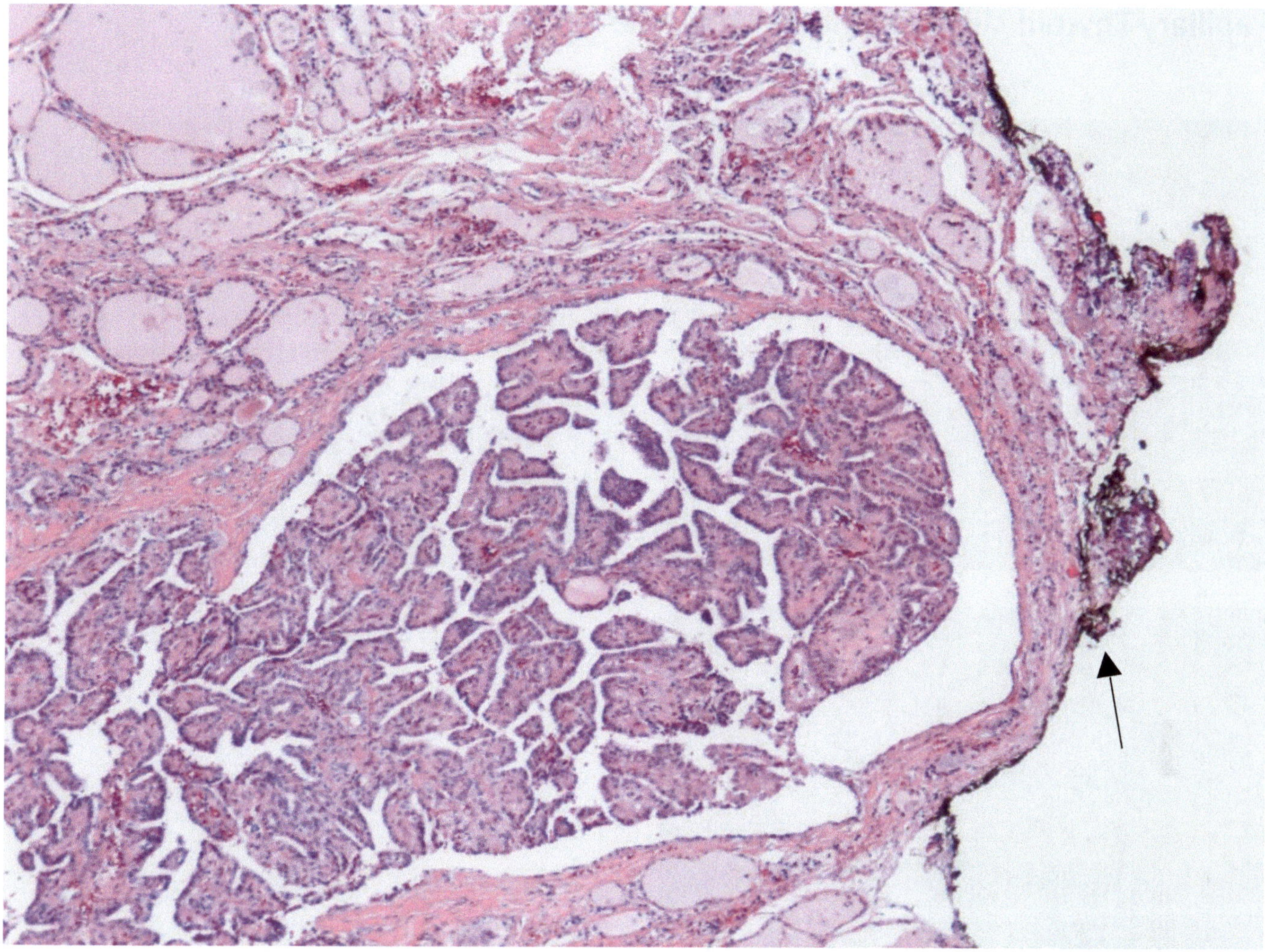

Figure 7-65. Papillary microcarcinoma 3 mm close to the resection margin (*arrow*).

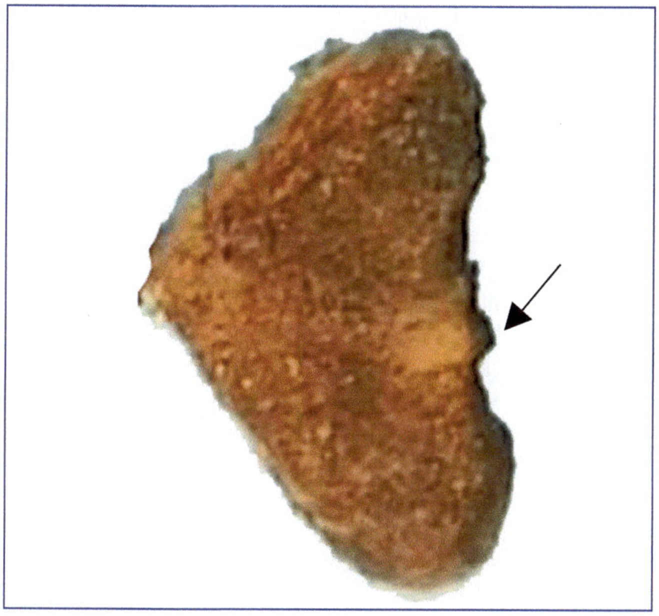

Figure 7-66. Gross section showing papillary microcarcinoma close to the resection margin (*arrow*).

Papillary Thyroid Microcarcinoma Left Lobe

Transverse

Longitudinal

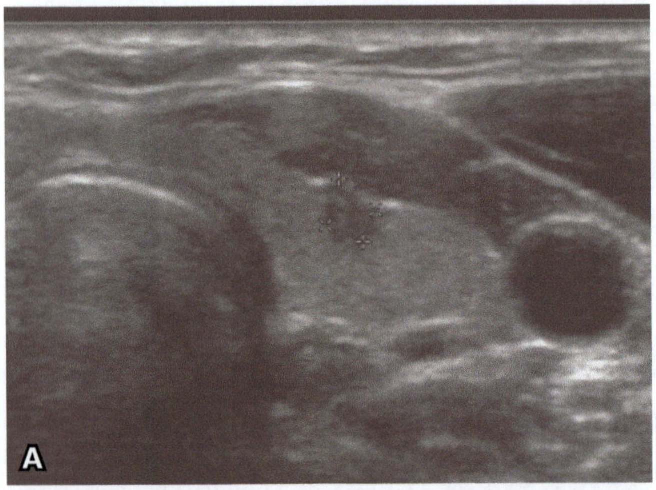

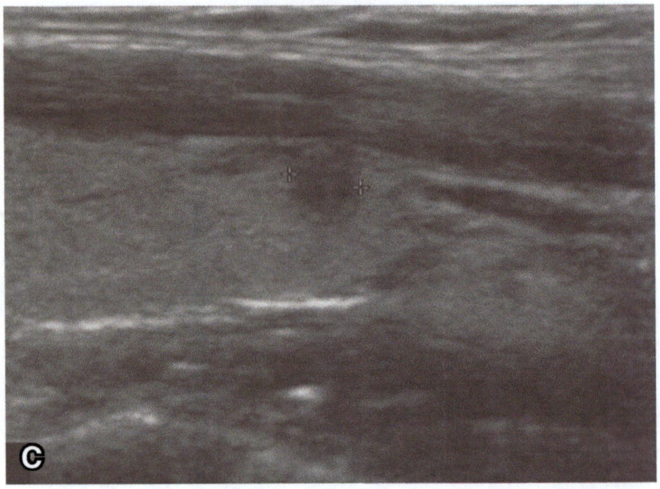

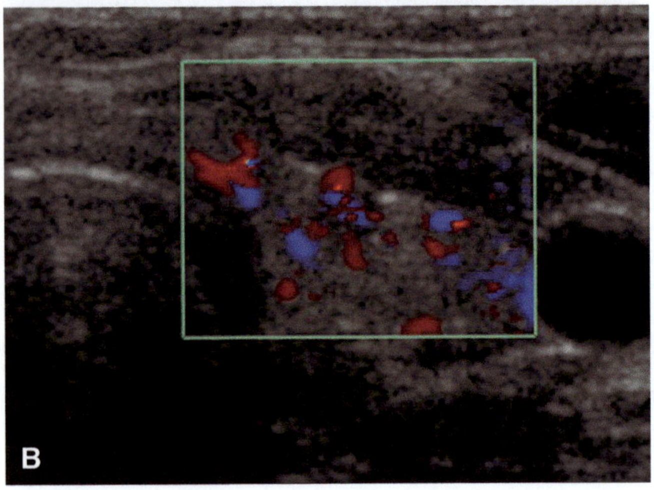

FIGURE 7-67. Ultrasound of papillary thyroid carcinoma: microcarcinoma in the left lobe. **A**, Transverse. **B**, Color Doppler, transverse. **C**, Longitudinal.

38-Year-old woman

- **Clinical history:** Many family members have papillary thyroid carcinoma (PTC). Anxious of having carcinoma herself.
- **Ultrasound:** Suspicious for PTC in left lobe.
- **Cytology:** PTC.
- **Thyroidectomy:** PTC, infiltration through thyroid capsule.

Features

Hypoechoic
Inhomogeneous echo pattern
Blurred margins
Capsular infiltration?
Hypervascular
Taller than wide

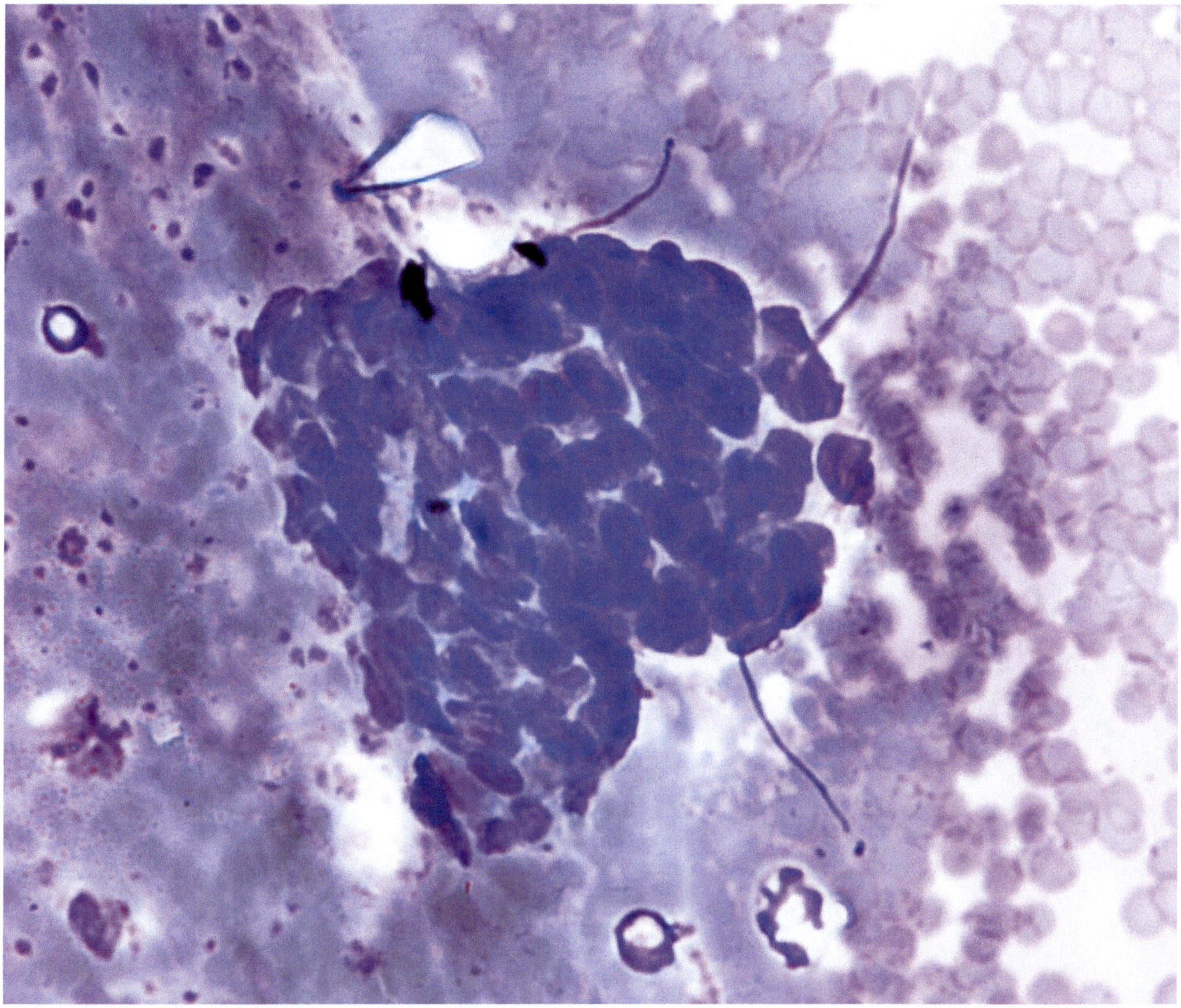

FIGURE 7-68. Cytology: classic papillary growth pattern.

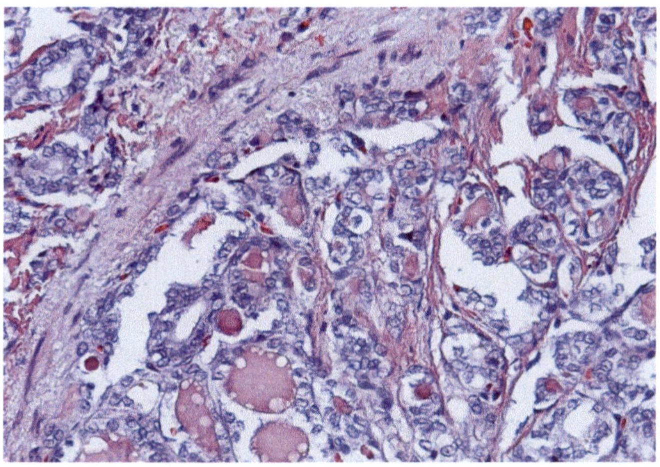

FIGURE 7-69. Histology: classic papillary growth pattern.

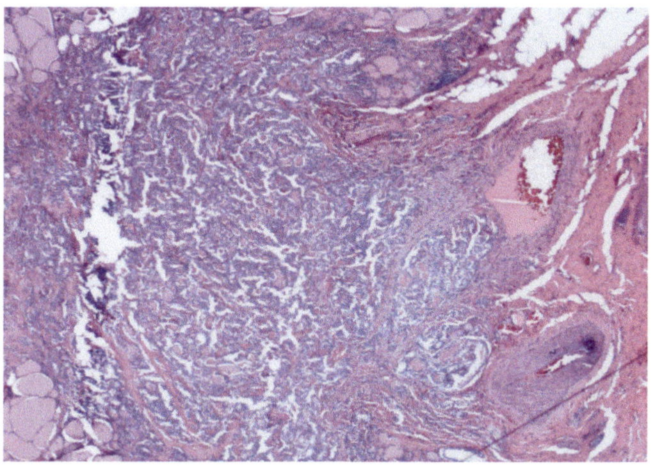

FIGURE 7-70. Histology: classic papillary growth pattern.

8 Medullary Thyroid Carcinoma

Medullary thyroid carcinoma (MTC) is typically located at the junction of the upper third and the lower two thirds of the thyroid lobes [6]. MTC consists of sheets of spindle-shaped, round or polygonal C cells separated by fibrous stroma [19]. The tumors are usually solitary, strongly hypoechoic, and sharply circumscribed with a homogeneous echo pattern, except for centrally located calcifications that may be of the micro type. They may, however, be more coarse than the calcifications found in papillary carcinomas [6,10]. The same type of calcifications are often found in regional lymph node metastases [(6,7].

Common Features

Hypoechoic
Well marginated, sharply circumscribed
Upper/mid lobe
Centrally located separate coarse or micro-calcifications
Regional lymphadenopathy

Cytologic Morphology

The morphology is often characterized by no colloid or only a sparse amount of colloid. Epithelial cells are rich in cytoplasm and form groups or nests. The staining of calcitonin will readily demonstrate positive cells. The finding of amyloid is not usual in cytologic smears.

Medullary Thyroid Carcinoma Right Lobe

Transverse | Longitudinal

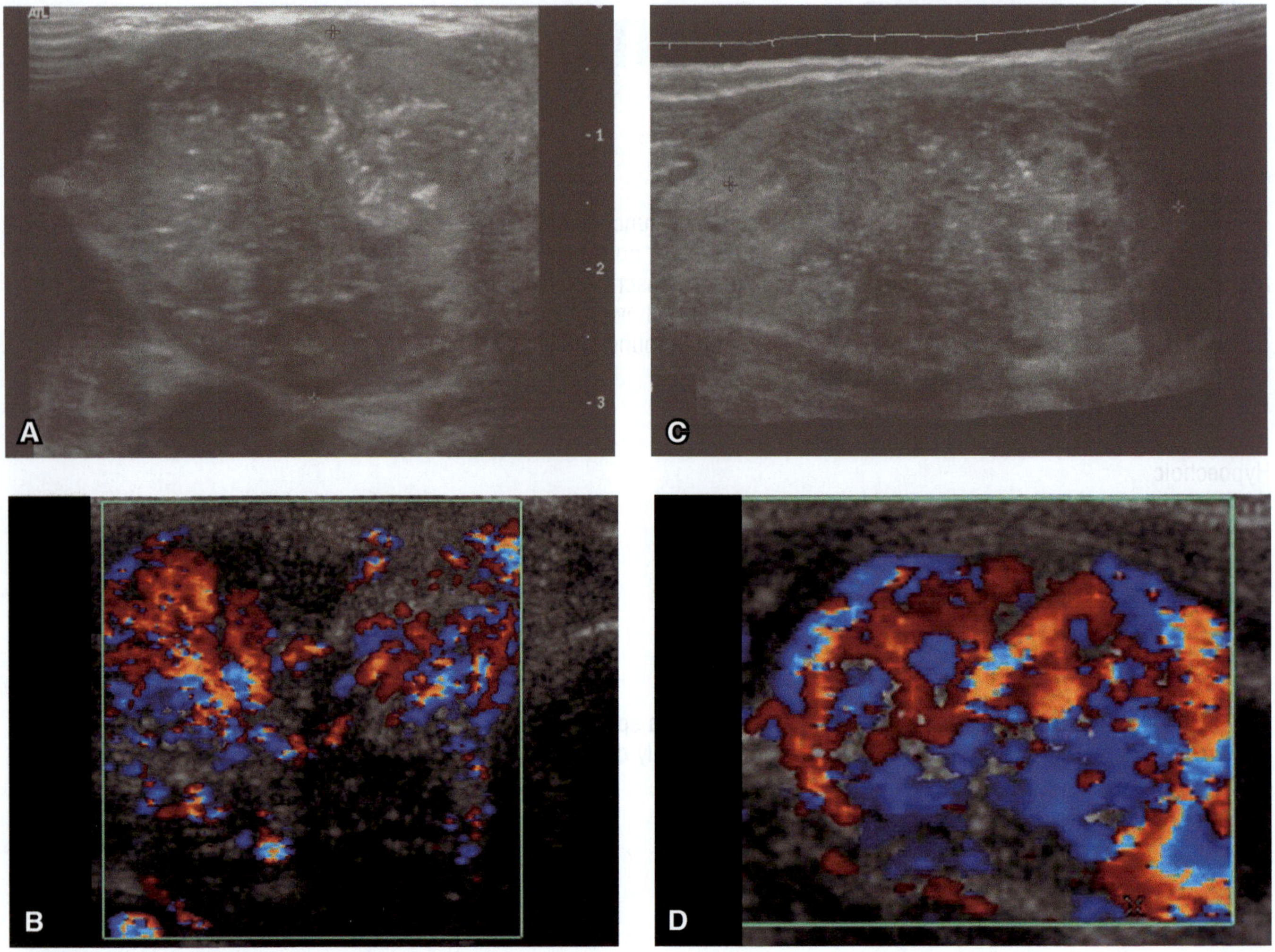

Figure 8-1. Ultrasound of medullary thyroid carcinoma in the right lobe. **A**, Transverse, 28 x 33 mm. **B**, Color Doppler, transverse. **C**, Longitudinal, sagittal diameter: 44 mm. **D**, Color Doppler, longitudinal.

83 Year-old woman

- **Clinical history:** Myelomatosis in remission. Growing tumor in right thyroid lobe.
- **Ultrasound:** Probably papillary thyroid carcinoma (PTC) in right lobe + metastases.
- **Cytology:** Medullary thyroid carcinoma (MTC) + metastases.
- **18-Gauge histologic needle biopsy:** MTC.
- **Thyroidectomy:** MTC + metastases.

Features

Mixed echogenicity
Inhomogeneous echo pattern
Partially well circumscribed
Microcalcifications
Some coarse calcifications
Hypervascularized
Hypervascular calcified lymph nodes

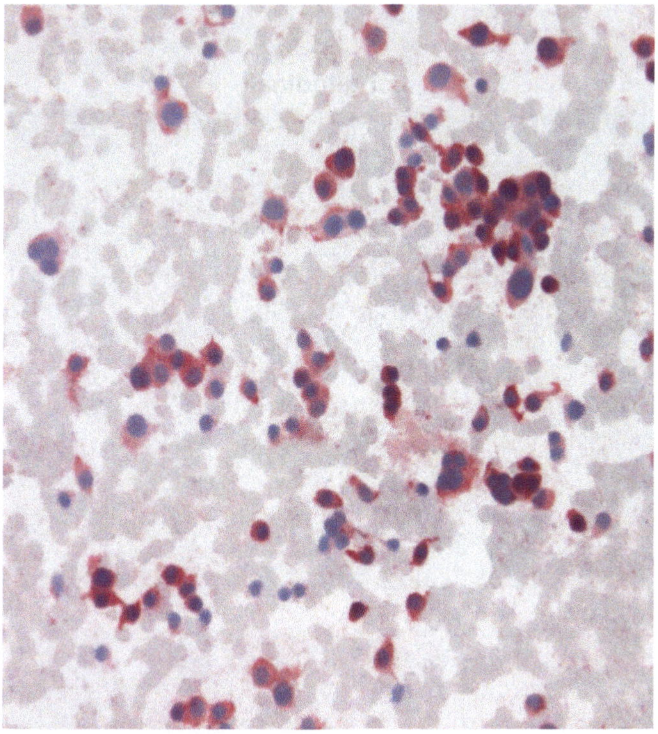

Figure 8-2. Cytology: calcitonin-positive cell.

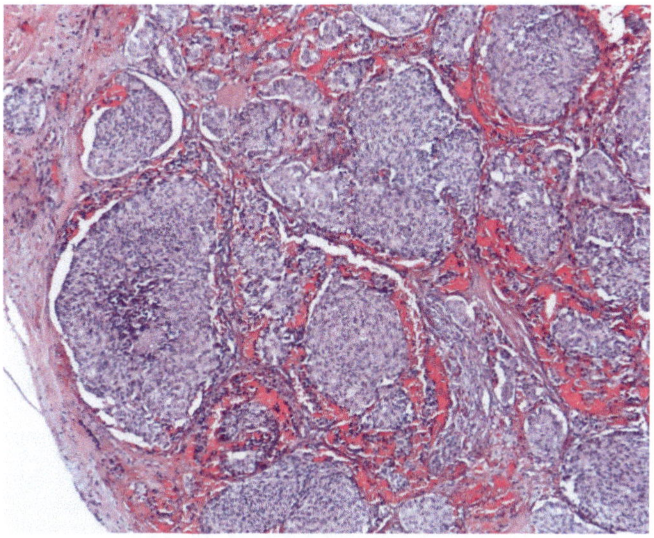

Figure 8-3. Histology: medullary thyroid carcinoma.

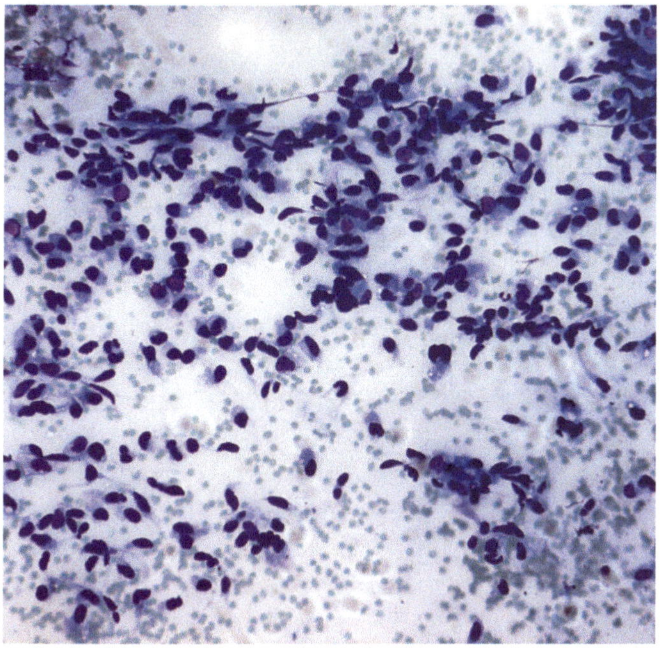

Figure 8-4. Cytology: partially spindle-shaped cells.

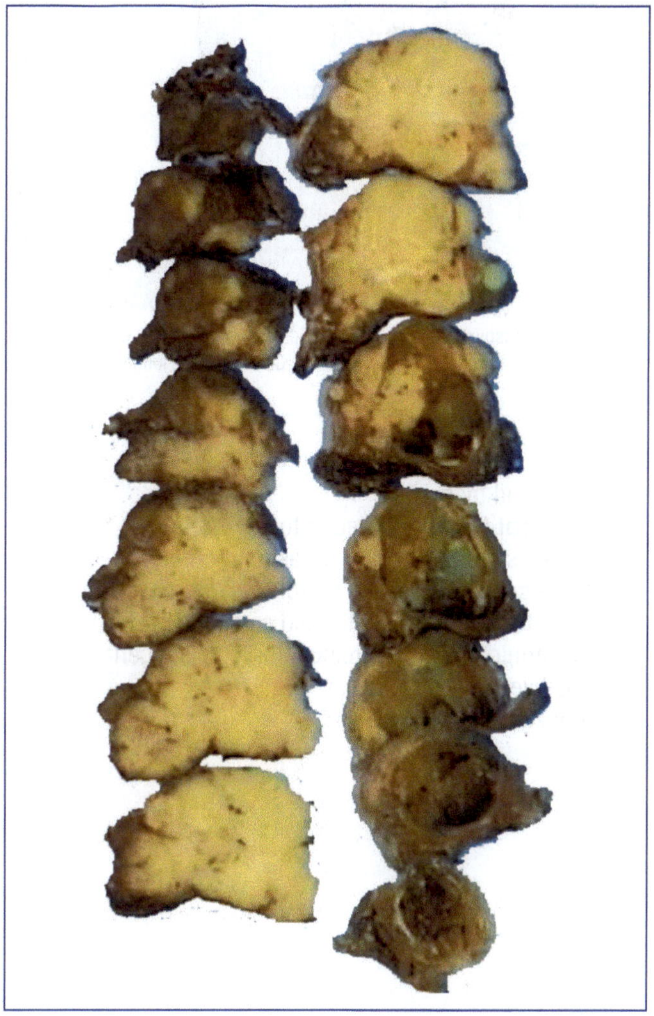

Figure 8-5. Gross section: tumor extensively involves the central part of the lobe.

Medullary Thyroid Carcinoma Right Lobe

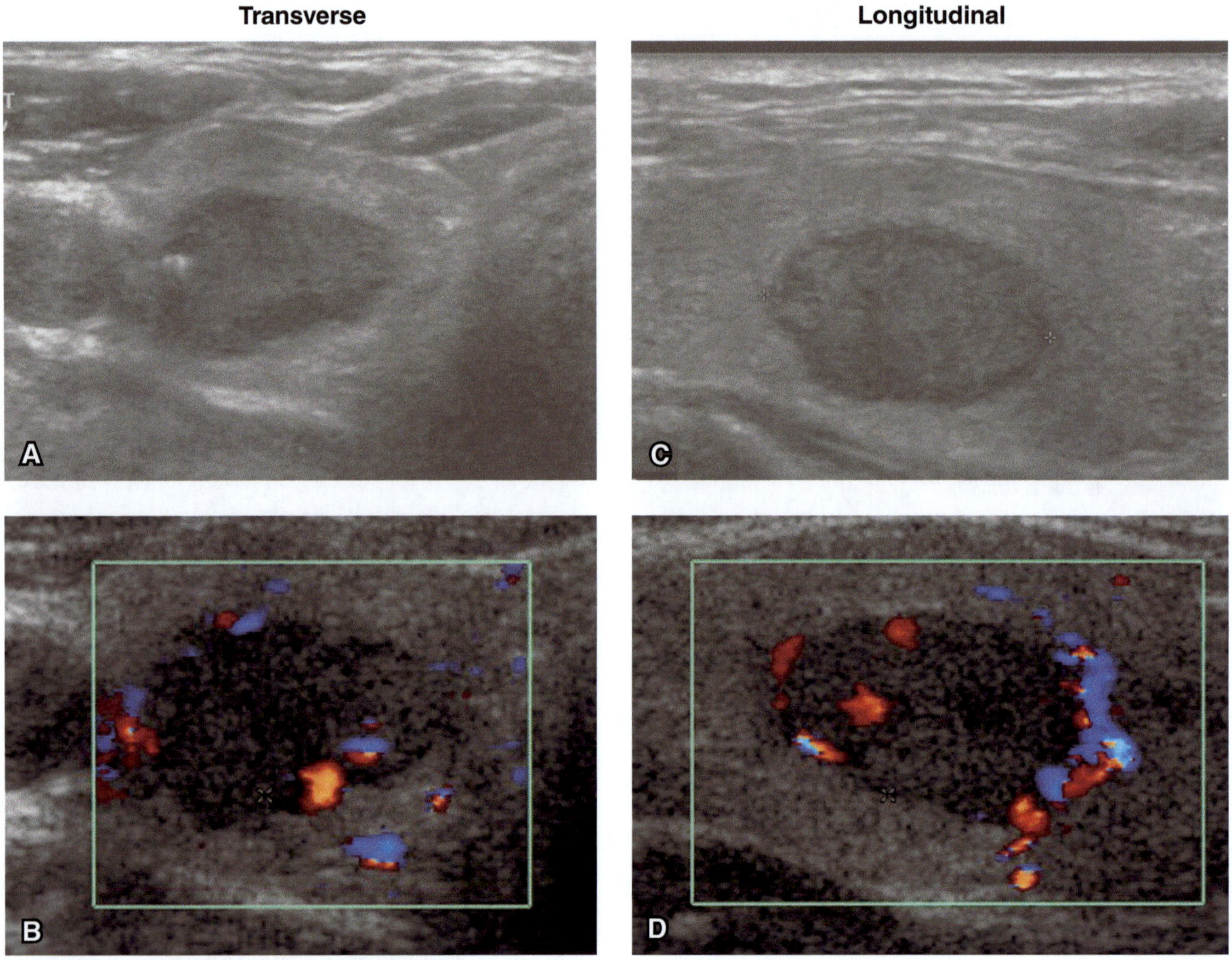

Figure 8-6. Ultrasound of medullary thyroid carcinoma in the right lobe. **A**, Transverse, 9 x 16 mm. **B**, Color Doppler, transverse. **C**, Longitudinal, sagittal diameter: 17 mm. **D**, Color Doppler, longitudinal.

51-Year-old man

- **Clinical history:** Rheumatoid arthritis. Throat symptoms. Neck ultrasound ordered.
- **Ultrasound:** Papillary thyroid carcinoma (PTC)?
- **Cytology:** Medullary thyroid carcinoma (MTC). Calcitonin positive. Carcinoembryonic antigen positive.
- **Thyroidectomy:** MTC.

Features

Strongly hypoechoic
Homogeneous echo pattern
Sharply marginated
Microcalcifications
Scant vascularity

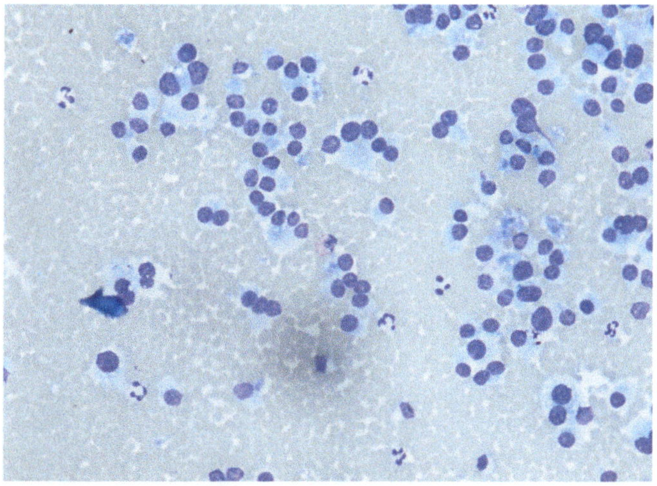

Figure 8-7. Cytology: dispersed cells, rich in cytoplasm.

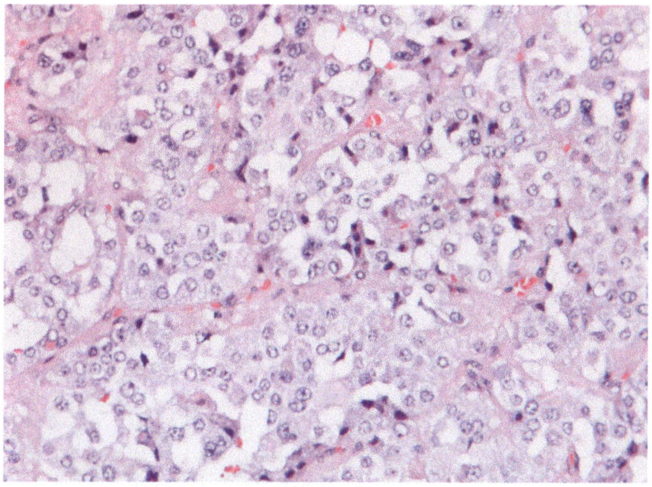

Figure 8-8. Histology: medullary thyroid carcinoma.

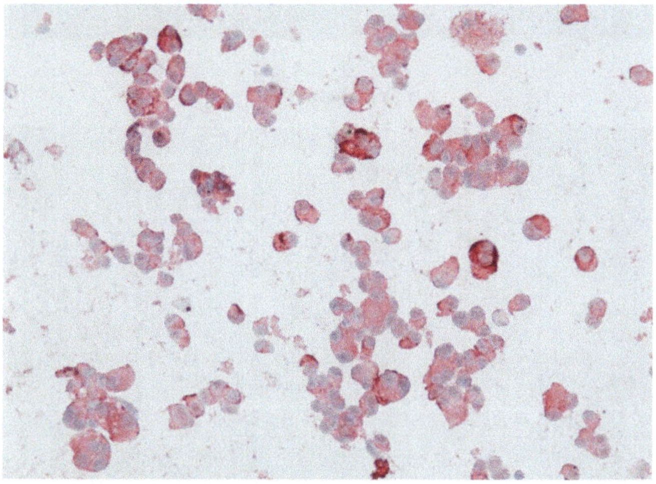

Figure 8-9. Cytology: calcitonin-positive cells.

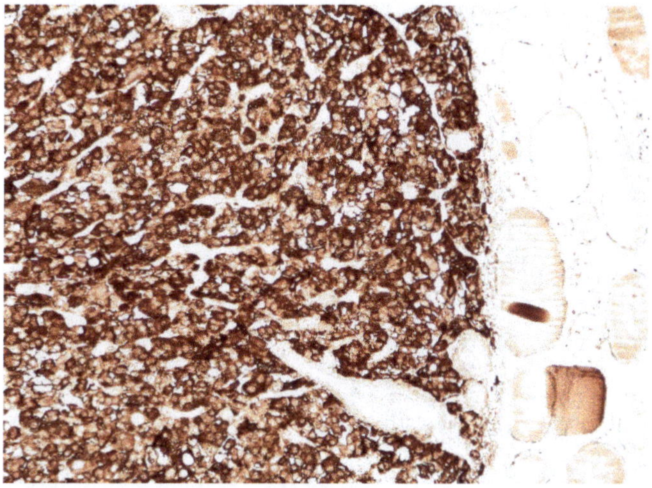

Figure 8-10. Histology: calcitonin-positive cells.

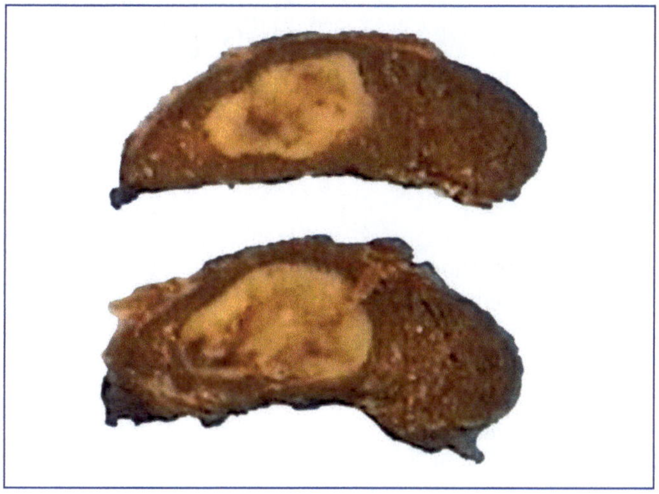

Figure 8-11. Gross section: medullary thyroid carcinoma.

Medullary Thyroid Carcinoma Right Lobe

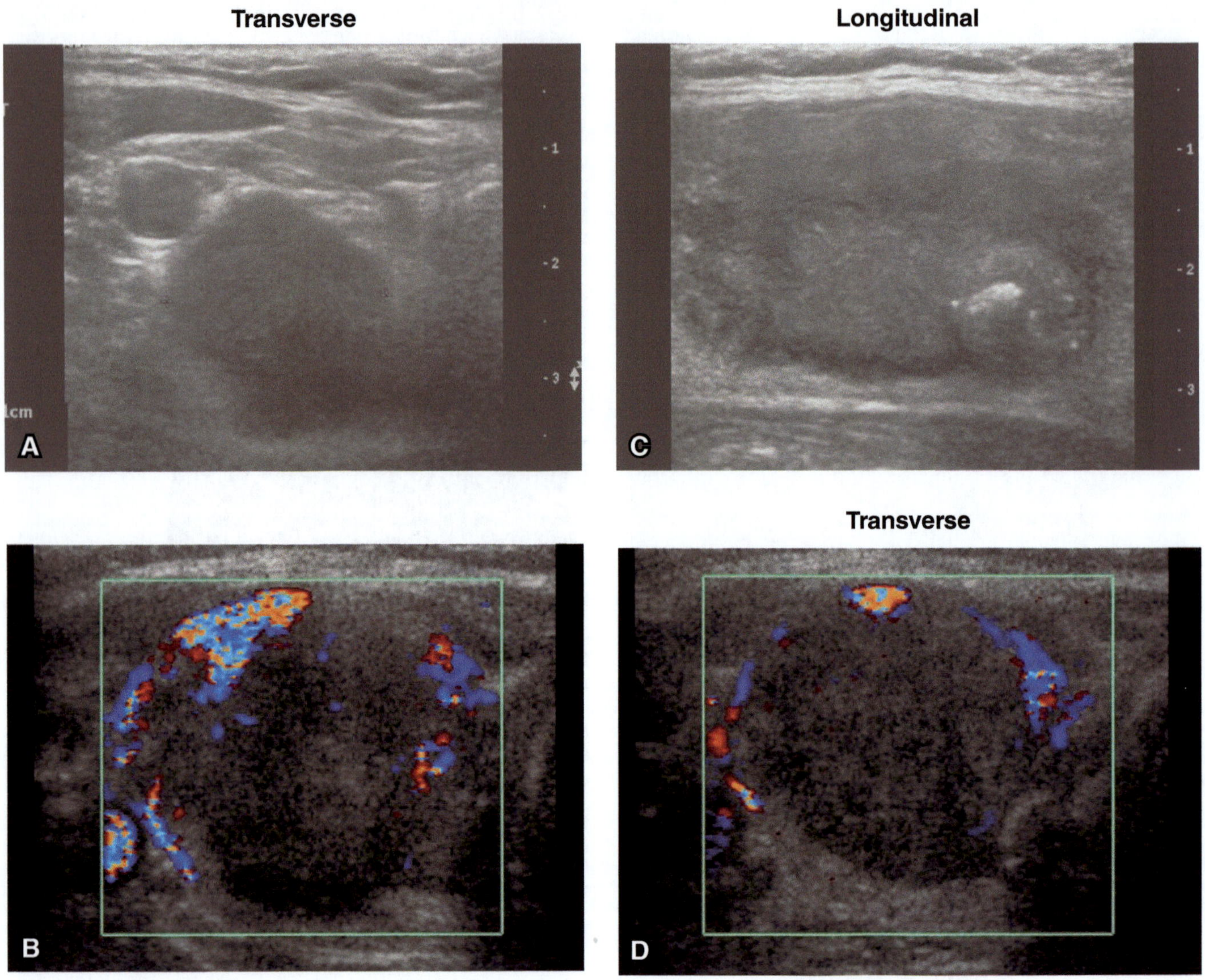

Figure 8-12. Ultrasound of medullary thyroid carcinoma in the right lobe. **A**, Transverse, 19 x 19 mm. **B**, Color Doppler, transverse. **C**, Longitudinal, sagittal diameter: 34 mm. **D**, Color Doppler, transverse.

60-Year-old woman

- **Clinical history:** Paraneoplastic cerebellar degeneration past 4 months. Lung and liver metastases.
  CT shows tumor in right thyroid lobe.
- **Ultrasound:** Malignant tumor in right lobe + metastases.
- **Cytology:** Medullary thyroid carcinoma (MTC) + metastases.
- **16-Gauge histology needle biopsy:** MTC.
- **Thyroidectomy:** MTC + metastases.

Features

Mostly hypoechoic
Inhomogeneous echo pattern
Irregular margin cranially
Coarse calcifications
Microcalcifications
Peripheral vascularity

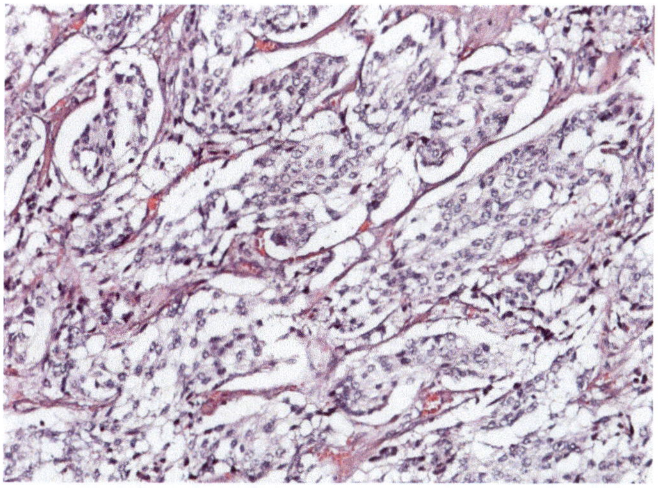

Figure 8-13. Histology: medullary thyroid carcinoma.

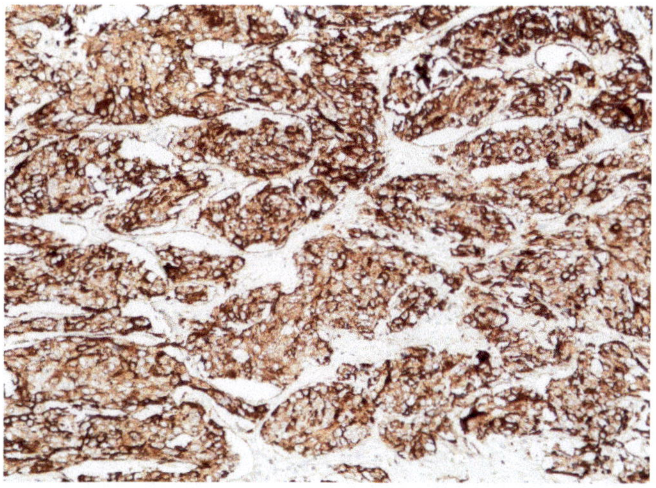

Figure 8-14. Histology: medullary thyroid carcinoma. Calcitonin-positive cells.

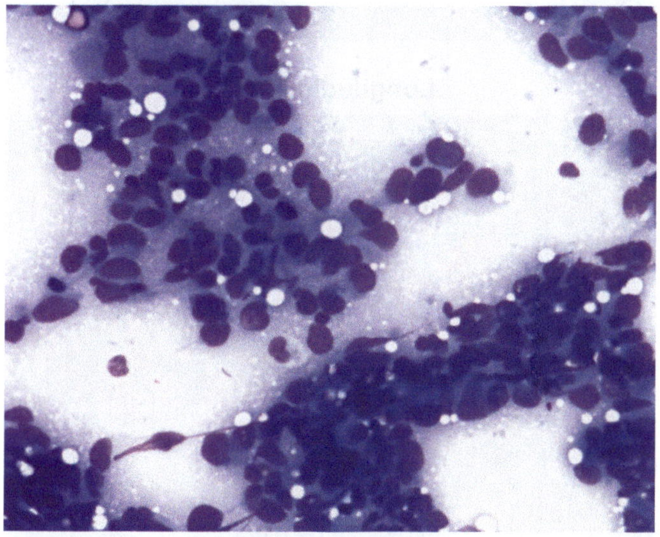

Figure 8-15. Cytology: medullary thyroid carcinoma.

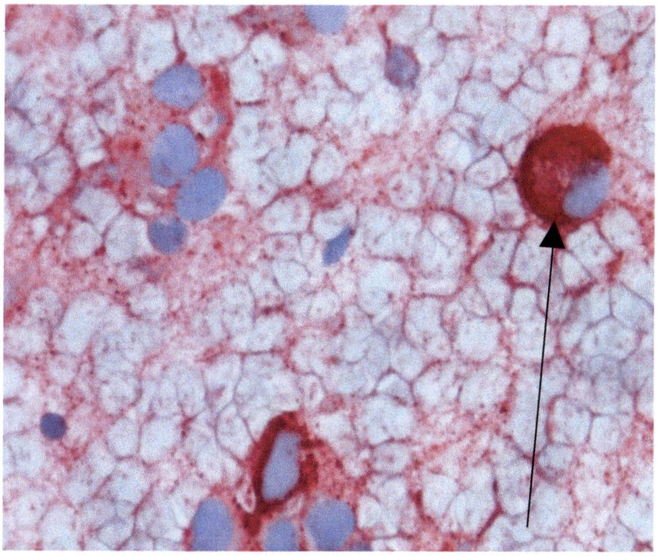

Figure 8-16. Cytology: medullary thyroid carcinoma. Calcitonin-positive tumor cells (*arrow*).

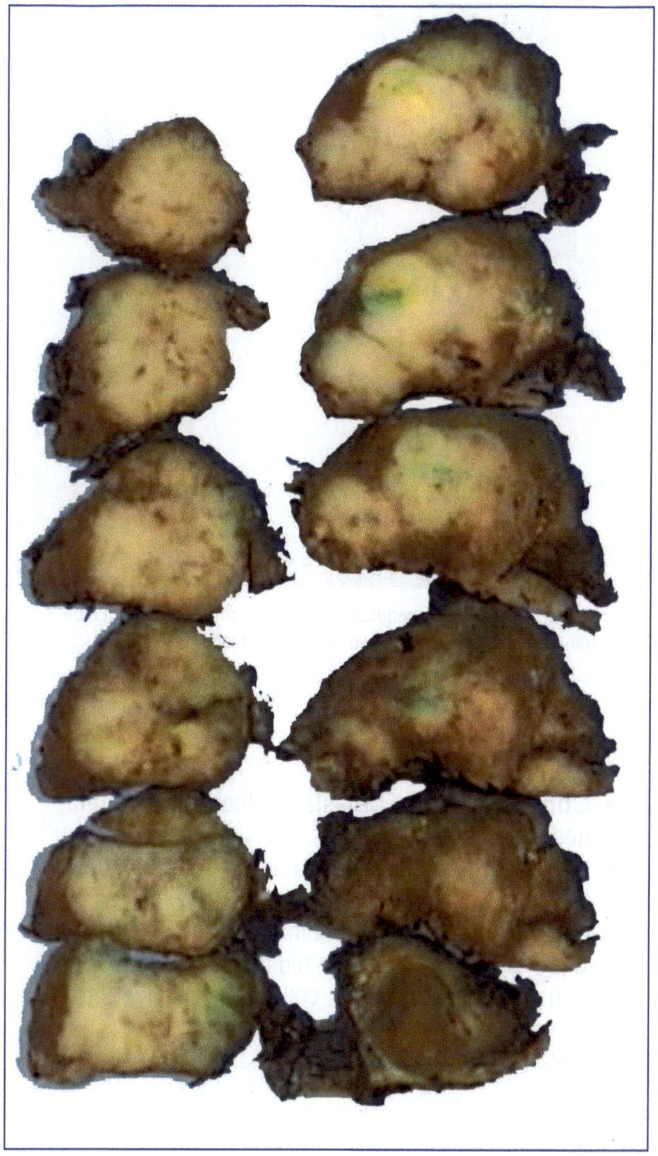

Figure 8-17. Gross section.

Medullary Thyroid Carcinoma Right Lobe

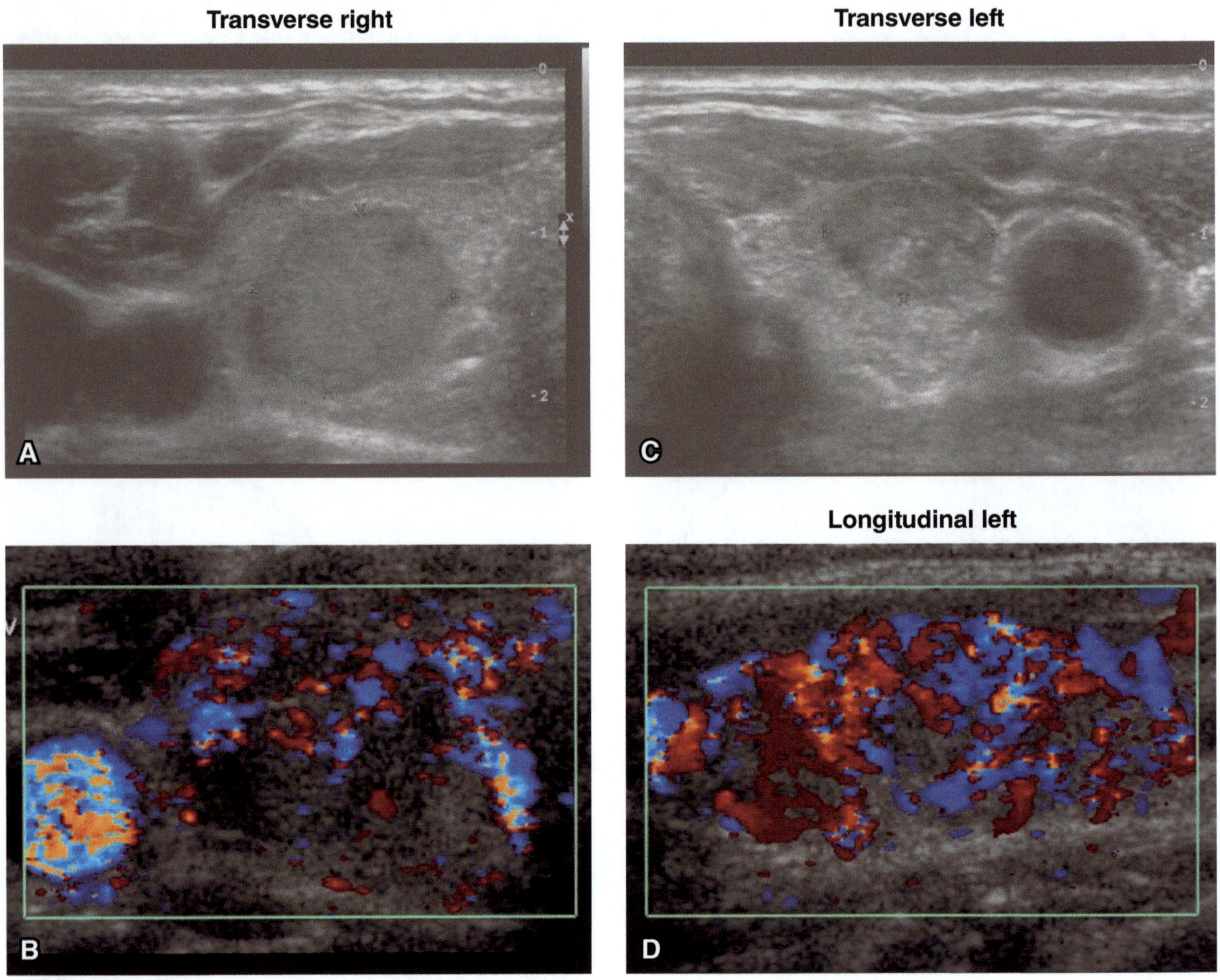

FIGURE 8-18. Ultrasound of medullary thyroid carcinoma in the right lobe. **A**, Right transverse, 10 x 12 mm. **B**, Color Doppler, right transverse. **C**, Left transverse, 7 x 10 mm. **D**, Color Doppler, left longitudinal.

67-Year-old woman

- **Clinical history:** Metastases. Incidentally found nodules in both lobes.
- **Ultrasound:** Suspicious tumor in both right and left lobe. Colloid nodules. General hypervascularity due to thyroiditis ("thyroid inferno").
- **Cytology:** Medullary thyroid carcinoma (MTC) in right lobe. Partially cystic colloid nodule in left lobe.
- **Thyroidectomy:** MTC in right lobe, colloid nodules, and Hashimoto's thyroiditis.

Features

Hypoechoic
Homogeneous echo pattern
Well circumscribed
Scant vascularity

Other findings

Suspicious tumor with microcalcifications in left lobe
Colloid nodule in right lobe
General hypervascularity

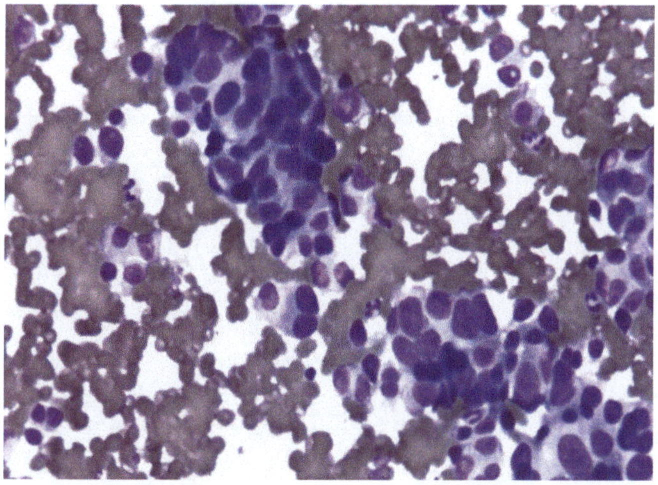

Figure 8-19. Cytology: carcinoma cells partly dispersed, partly in clusters.

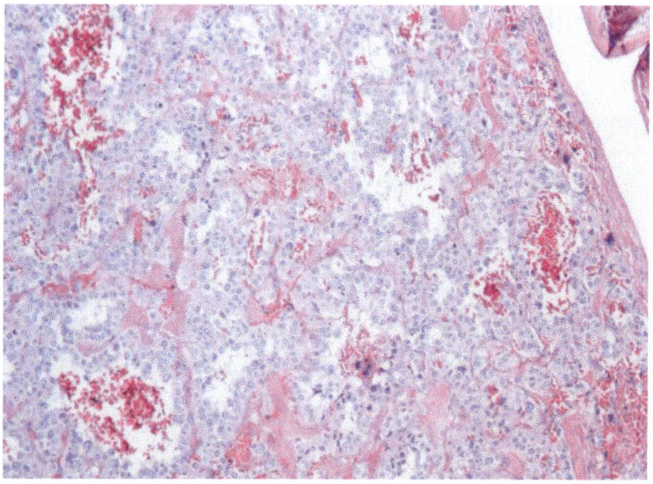

Figure 8-20. Histology: Hürtle-like atypical cells in nests and diffusely infiltrating.

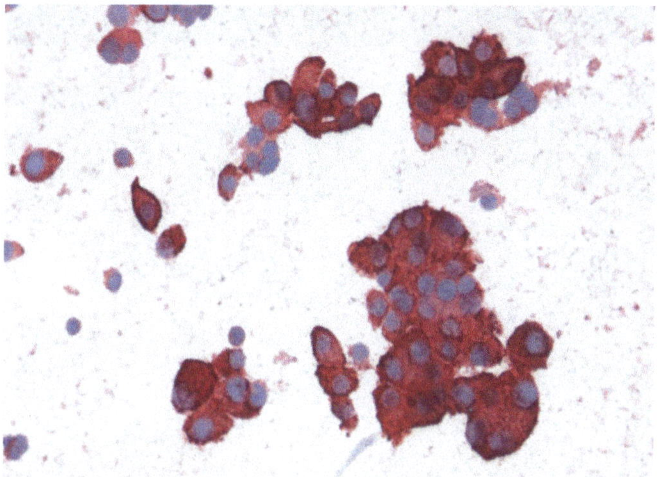

Figure 8-21. Cytology: calcitonin-positive cells.

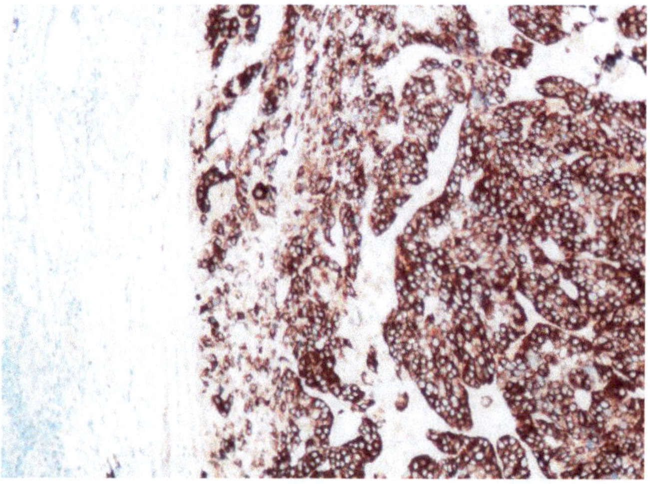

Figure 8-22. Histology: calcitonin-positive cells.

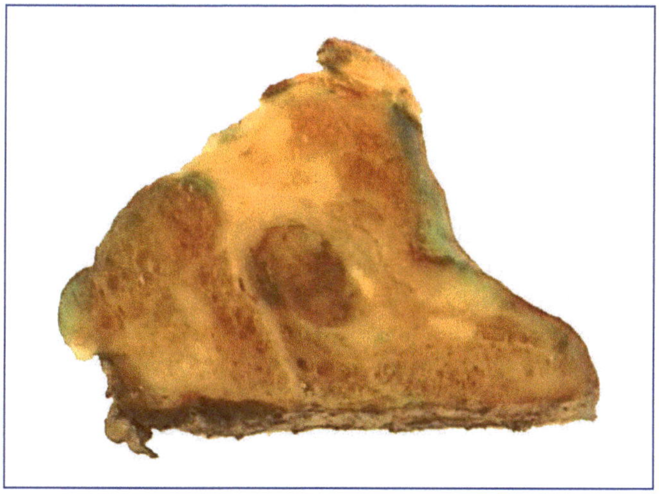

Figure 8-23. Gross section: diffuse infiltration.

Medullary Thyroid Carcinoma Right Lobe

Transverse | **Longitudinal**

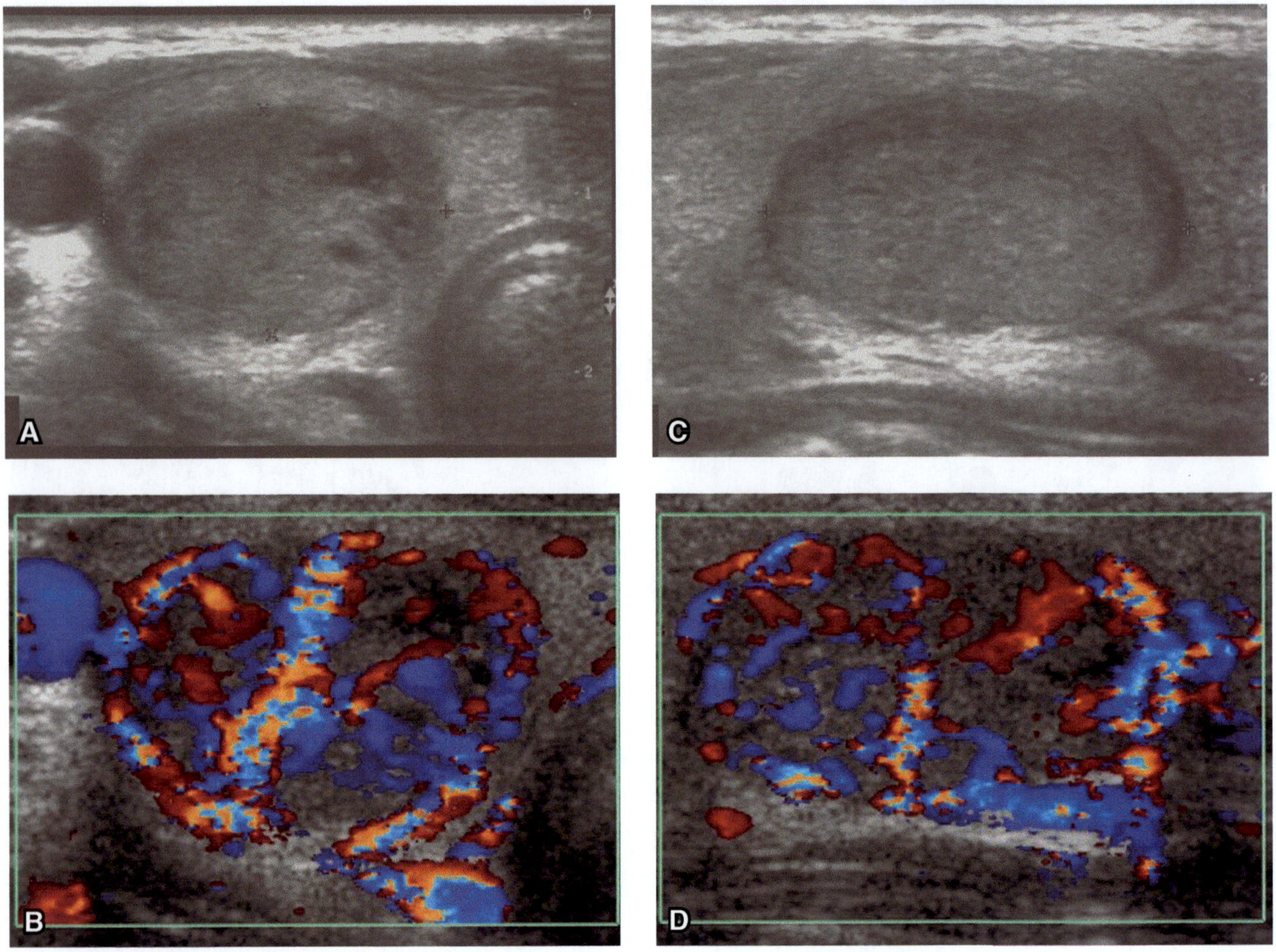

Figure 8-24. Ultrasound of medullary thyroid carcinoma in the right lobe. **A**, Transverse, 13 x 19 mm. **B**, Color Doppler, transverse. **C**, Longitudinal, sagittal diameter: 22 mm. **D**, Color Doppler, longitudinal.

39-Year-old woman

- **Clinical history:** Patient palpates nodule on right side of the neck past 2 months. No symptoms.
- **Ultrasound:** Colloid nodule? Papillary thyroid carcinoma (PTC)?
- **Cytology:** Medullary thyroid carcinoma (MTC), calcitonin positive.
- **18-Gauge histologic needle biopsy:** MTC.
- **Thyroidectomy:** MTC.

Features

Slightly hypoechoic
Inhomogeneous echo pattern
Small cysts
Well circumscribed
Partially thin hypoechoic halo
A few microcalcifcations
Suggestion of "spoke-and-wheel-like" hypervascularity

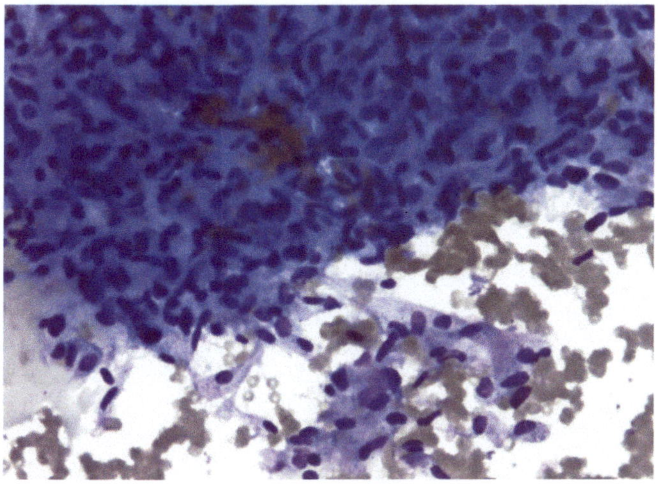

Figure 8-25. Cytology: medullary thyroid carcinoma.

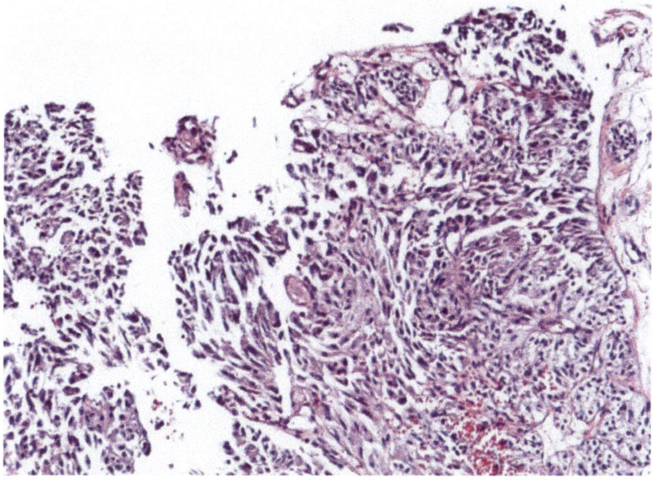

Figure 8-26. Histology: medullary thyroid carcinoma.

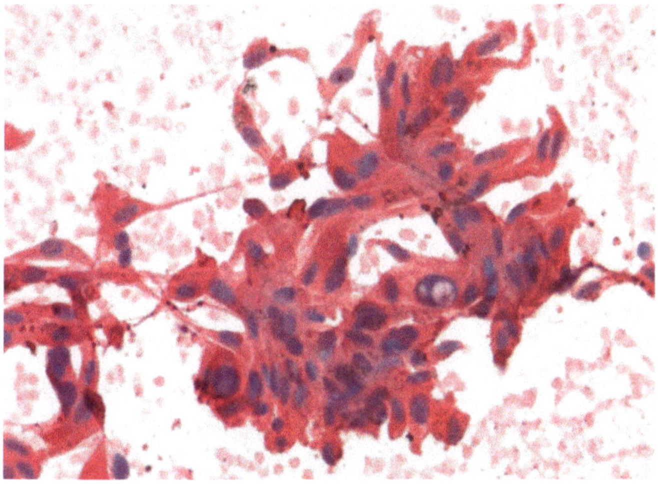

Figure 8-27. Cytology: calcitonin-positive cells, note different shapes of the cells.

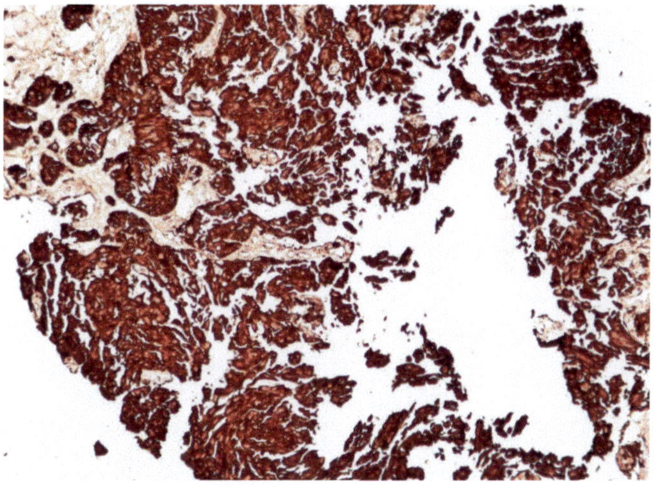

Figure 8-28. Histologic needle biopsy: medullary thyroid carcinoma. Calcitonin-positive cells.

9 Anaplastic Carcinoma

Anaplastic thyroid carcinoma is most frequently seen in elderly patients. It is often rapidly growing and therefore large when diagnosed, giving the patients different symptoms [6,7]. At the time of presentation anaplastic carcinoma is often infiltrating and inoperable. The tumors are often derived from papillary or follicular carcinomas, and may contain both papillary and anaplastic carcinoma cells [6]. Therefore, it may be impossible to distinguish between these tumors in the ultrasound examination. Clinical history, symptoms, and signs are of utmost importance. It is usually necessary to perform a computed tomography examination to assess the extension of the tumor.

Common Features

Large size
Hypoechoic
Inhomogeneous
Multilobular
Rapid growth
Clinical symptoms
Elderly patient

Cytologic Morphology

Microscopy of the smears demonstrates highly atypical cells, often difficult to classify on morphology. The cells may show a wide range of variation in size and form. Immunocytochemistry may be of some help in excluding lymphoma, sarcoma, and metastasis. The tumor is often partially necrotic, and several punctures are frequently needed before vital atypical cells are found in the specimen. The finding of differentiated papillary carcinoma in the same lesion may be of help when deciding whether the tumor is of thyroidal origin or a metastasis. The diagnosis of anaplastic carcinoma will always be the result of clinical findings and information, radiologic findings, and morphology.

Anaplastic Carcinoma Right Lobe

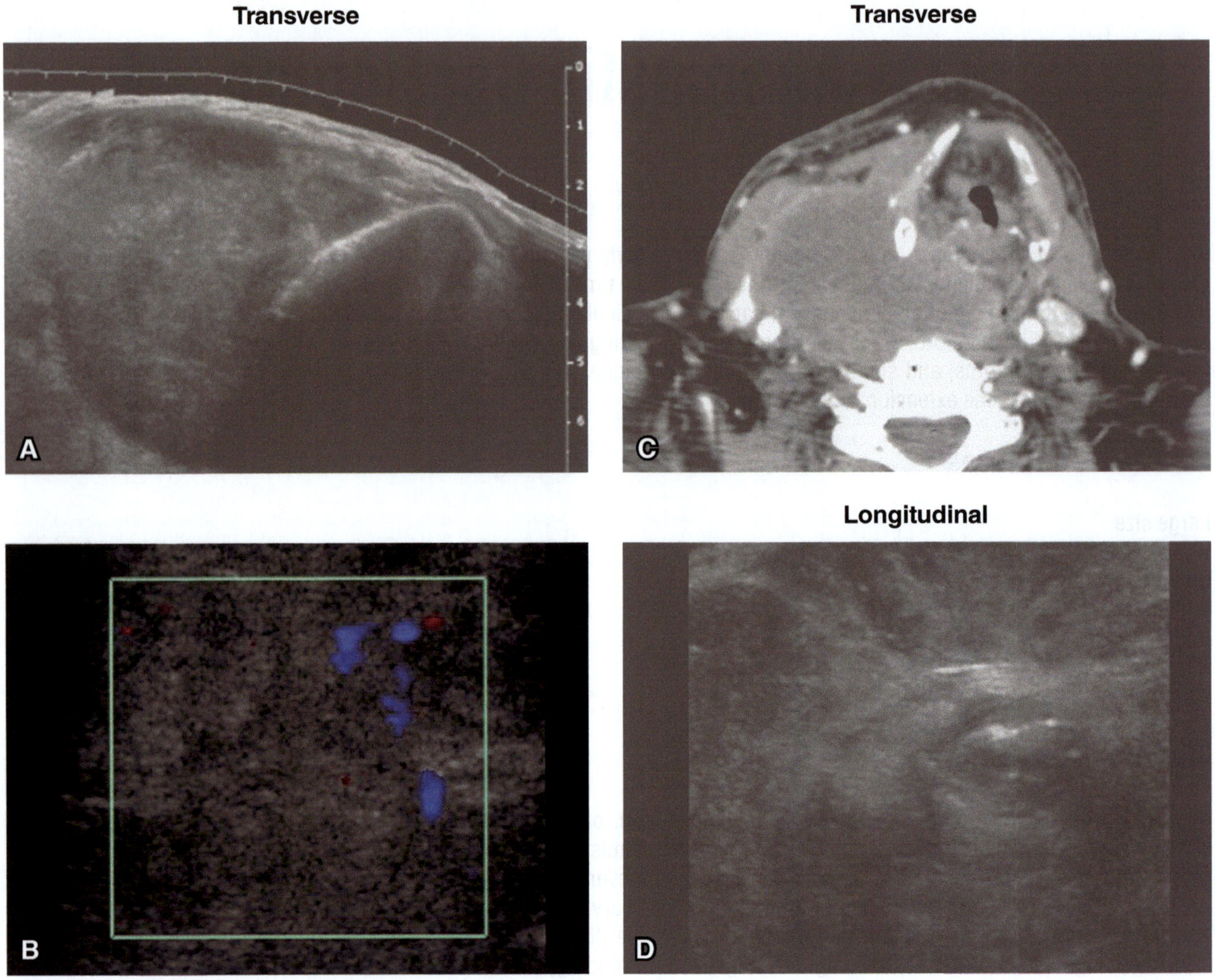

Figure 9-1. Ultrasound of anaplastic carcinoma in the right lobe. **A**, Transverse. **B**, Color Doppler, transverse. **C**, CT transverse. **D**, Longitudinal.

83-Year-old man

- **Clinical history:** Rapidly growing tumor with stridor. Swallowing problems.
- **Ultrasound:** Huge malignant tumor in right lobe with infiltration in trachea. Incomplete overview.
- **Cytology:** Highly malignant tumor.
- **16-Gauge histologic needle biopsy:** Anaplastic carcinoma.

Features

Huge
Hypoechoic
Inhomogeneous echo pattern
Partially well defined
Infiltrating trachea
A few microcalcifications
Scantly vascularized

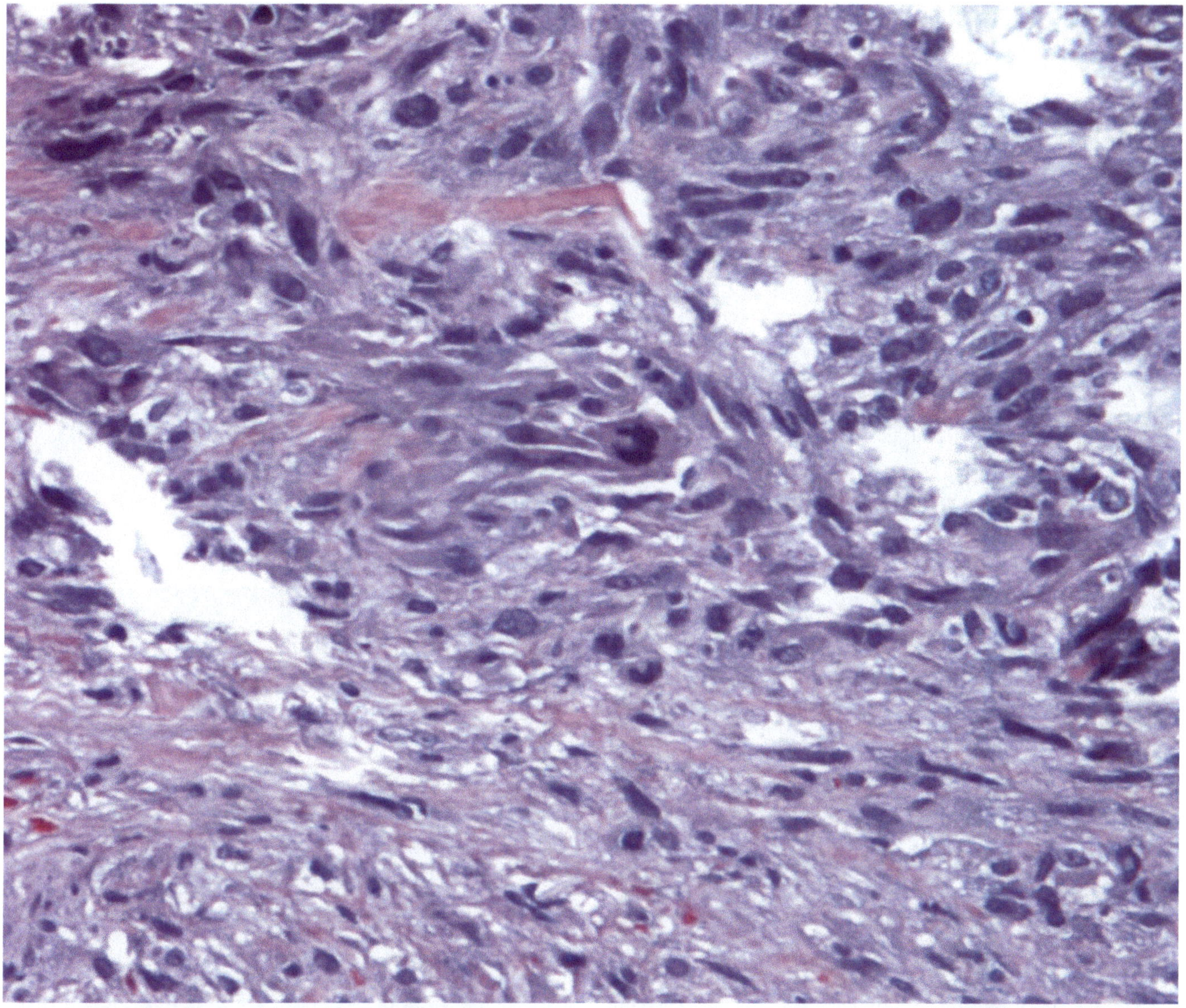

FIGURE 9-2. Histologic needle biopsy: malignant, spindle-formed cells.

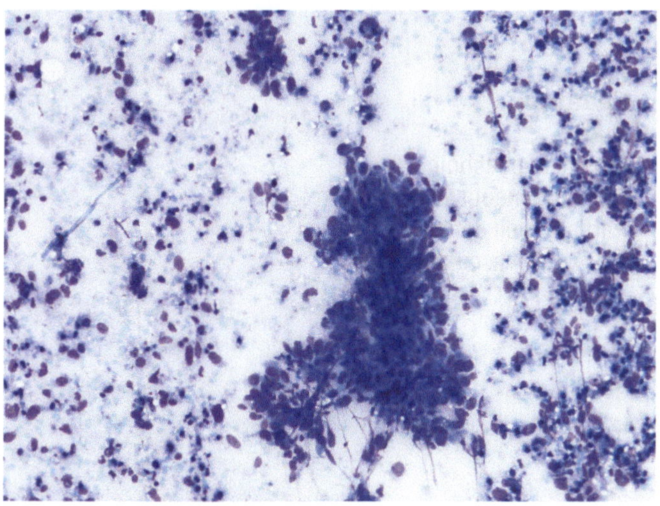

FIGURE 9-3. Cytology: spindle-shaped malignant cells.

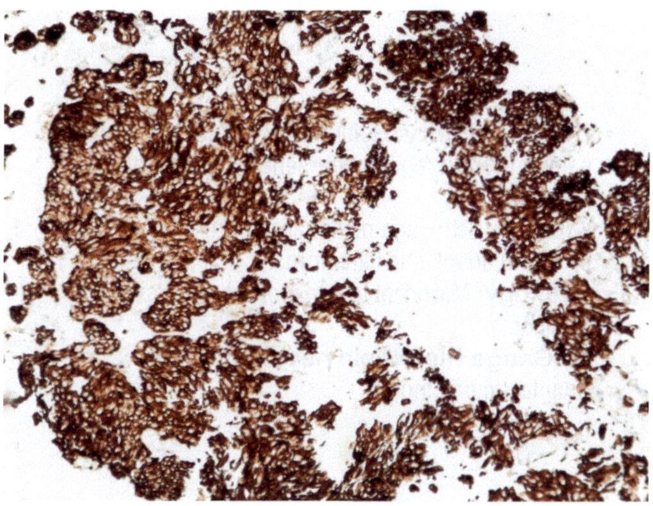

FIGURE 9-4. Immunohistochemistry: cytokeratin-positive cells indicating carcinoma.

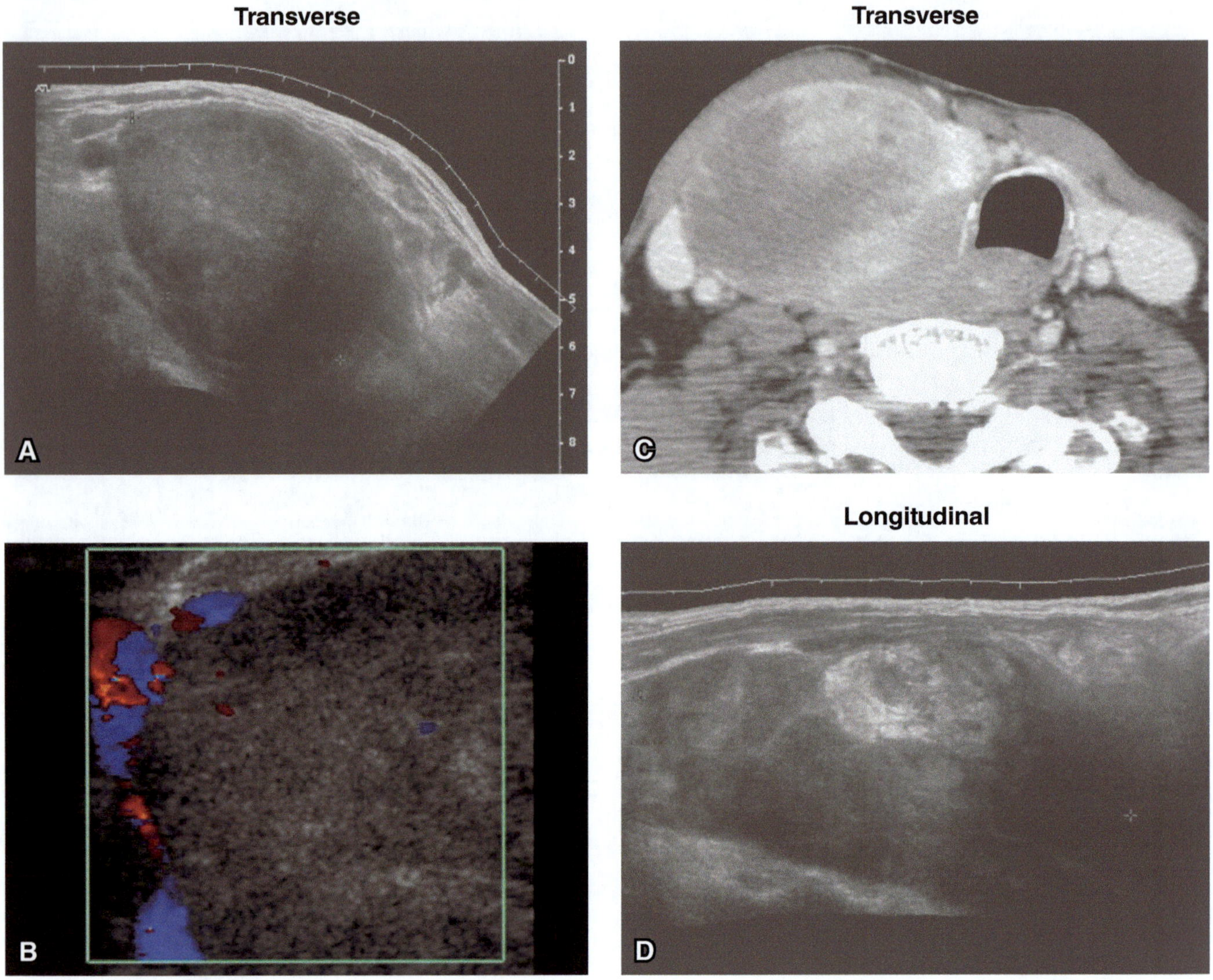

FIGURE 9-5. Ultrasound of anaplastic carcinoma in the right lobe. **A**, Transverse, 46 x 67 mm. **B**, Color Doppler, transverse. **C**, CT transverse. **D**, Longitudinal.

88-Year-old man

- **Clinical history:** Goiter past 5 years. Last 2 with pain in thyroid region, hoarseness, and breathing problems.
- **Ultrasound:** Huge malignant tumor in right lobe, probably anaplastic carcinoma.
- **Cytology:** Malignant tumor, probably anaplastic carcinoma.
- **18-Gauge histologic needle biopsy:** Anaplastic carcinoma.

Features

Huge
Mostly hypoechoic
Inhomogeneous echo pattern
Partially well defined
No visible vascularity

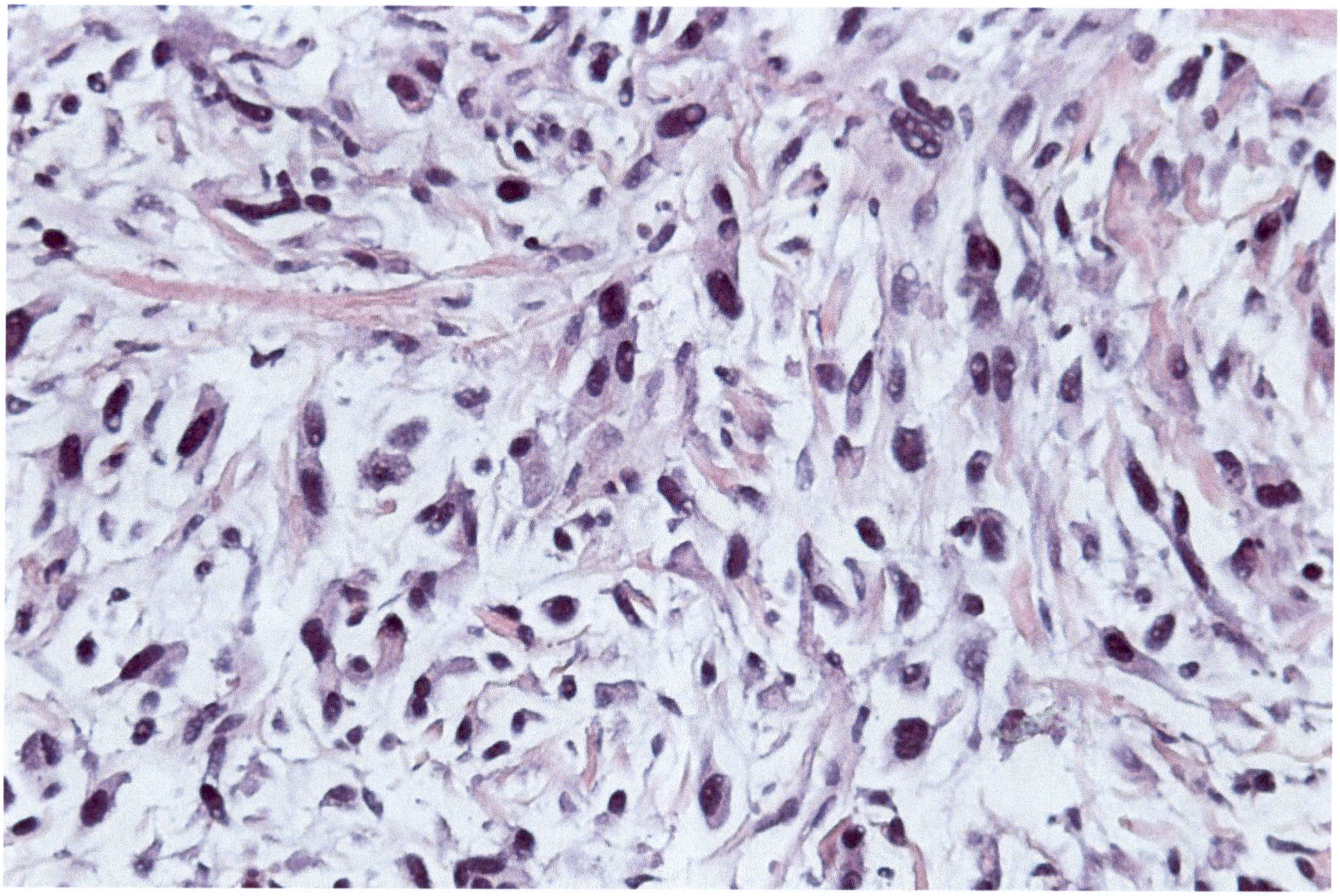

FIGURE 9-6. Histologic needle biopsy: pleomorphic malignant tumor.

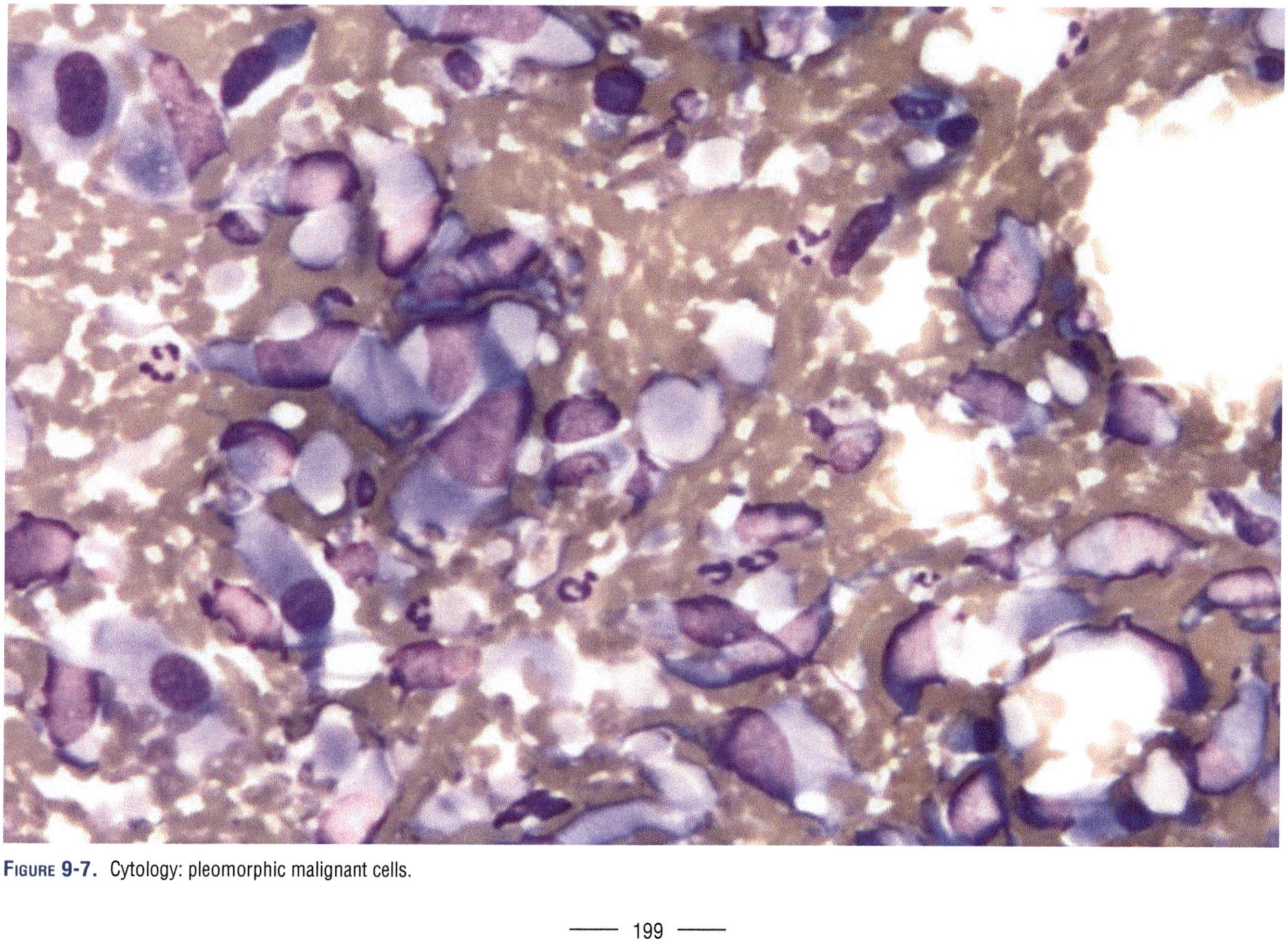

FIGURE 9-7. Cytology: pleomorphic malignant cells.

Anaplastic Carcinoma Left Lobe

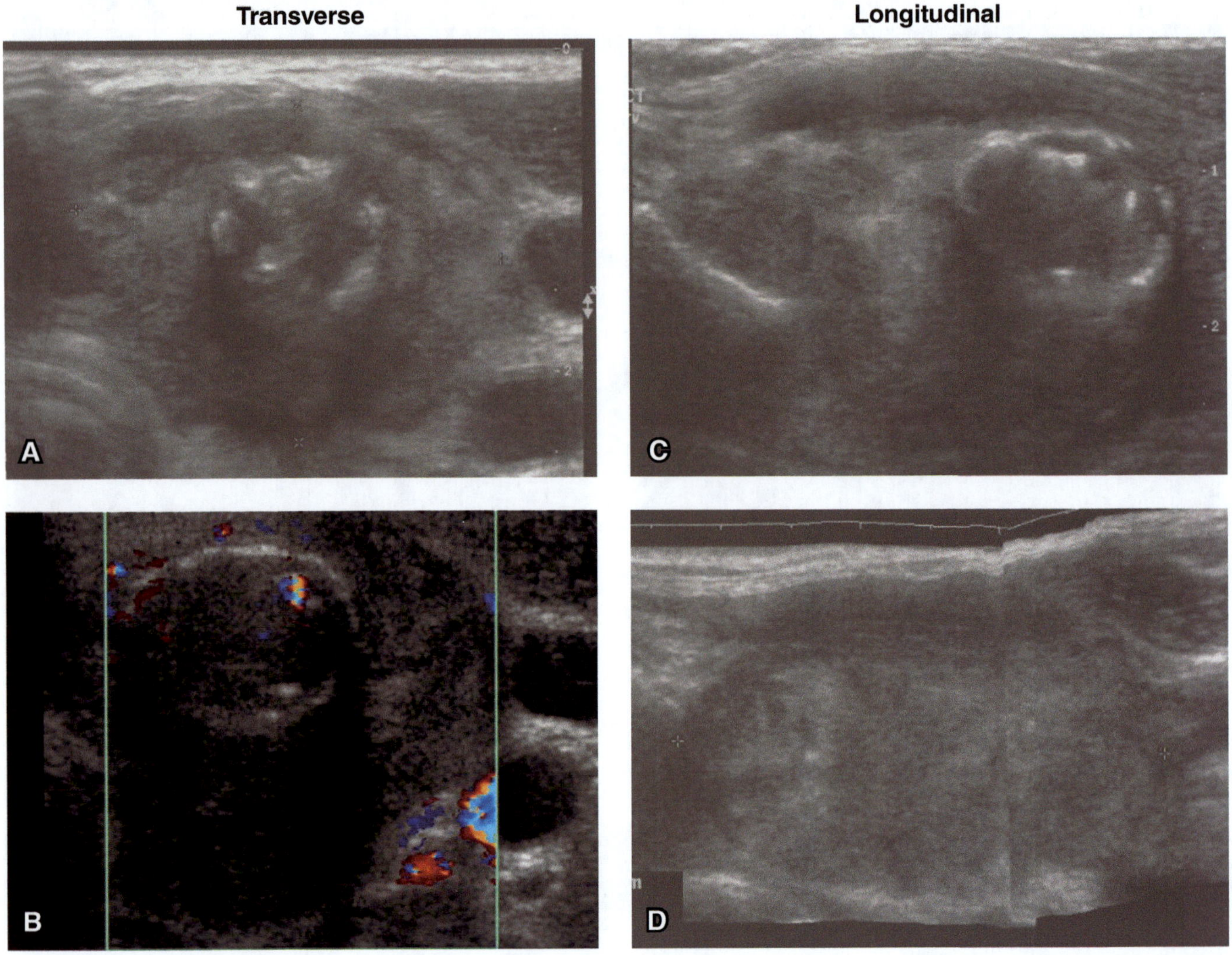

Figure 9-8. Ultrasound of anaplastic carcinoma in the left lobe. **A**, Transverse, 21 x 27 mm. **B**, Color Doppler, transverse. **C**, Longitudinal. **D**, Longitudinal, sagittal diameter: 35 mm.

72-Year-old woman

- **Clinical history:** Hypothyroidism past 14 years. Past 5 months increasing swallowing problems. Palpable tumor in left lobe.
- **Ultrasound:** Malignant tumor in left lobe.
- **Cytology:** Malignant tumor in left lobe.
- **18-Gauge histologic needle biopsy:** Anaplastic carcinoma.

Features

Mostly hypoechoic
Inhomogeneous echo pattern
Not well defined
Coarse and "eggshell" calcifications
Scantly vascularized

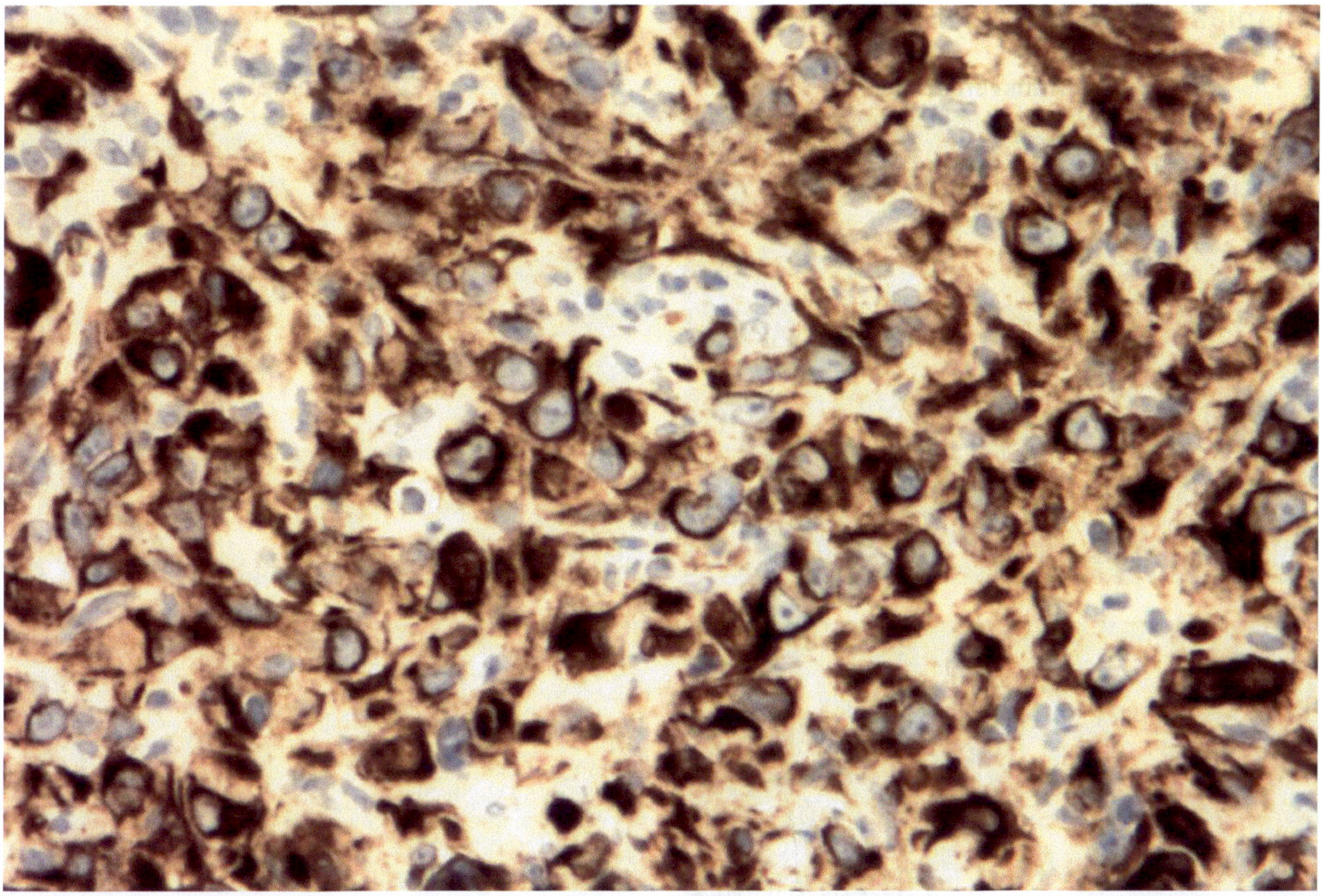

Figure 9-9. Histologic needle biopsy. Immunohistochemistry: cytokeratin-positive cells indicating carcinoma.

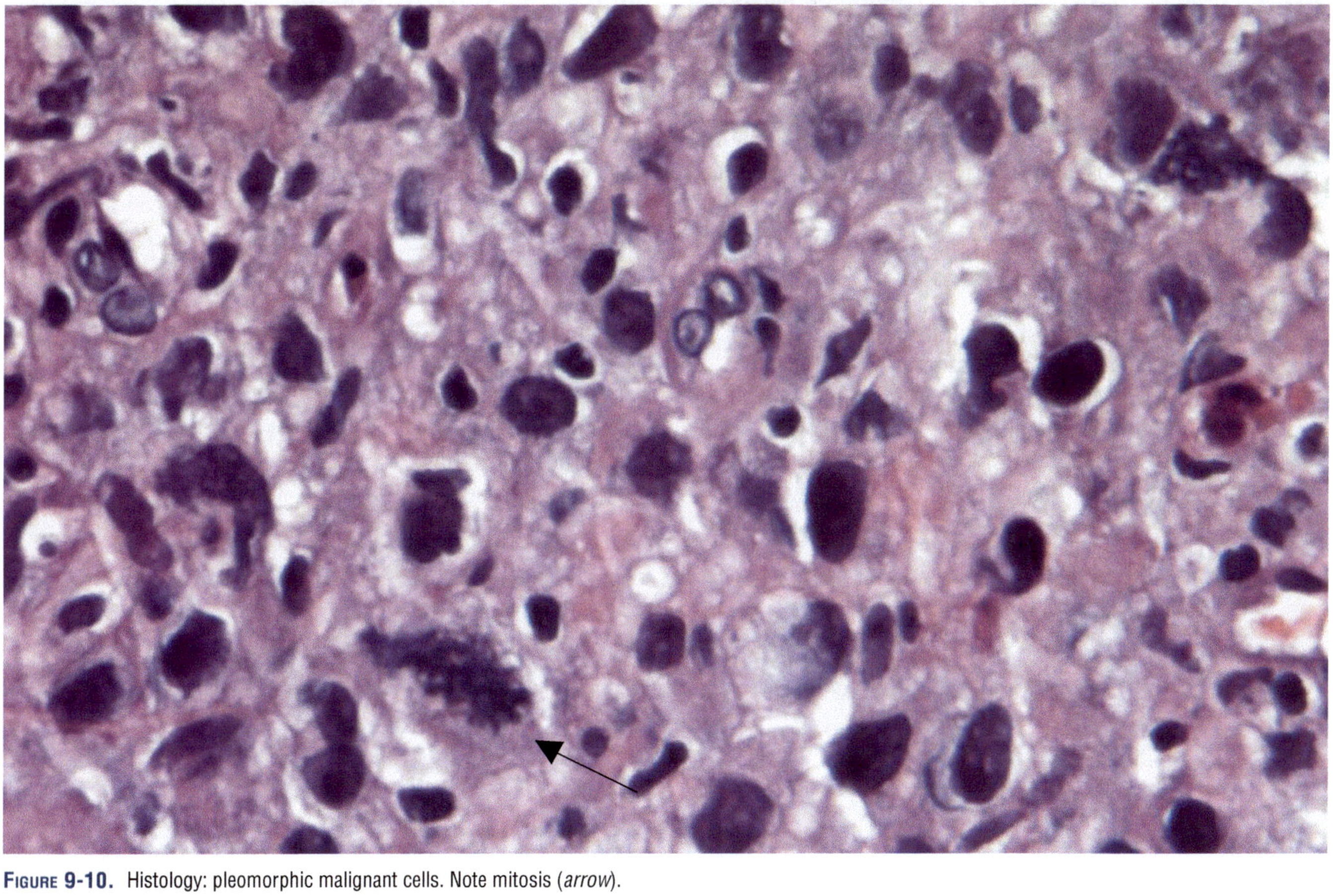

Figure 9-10. Histology: pleomorphic malignant cells. Note mitosis (*arrow*).

Anaplastic Carcinoma Right Lobe

Transverse   Transverse

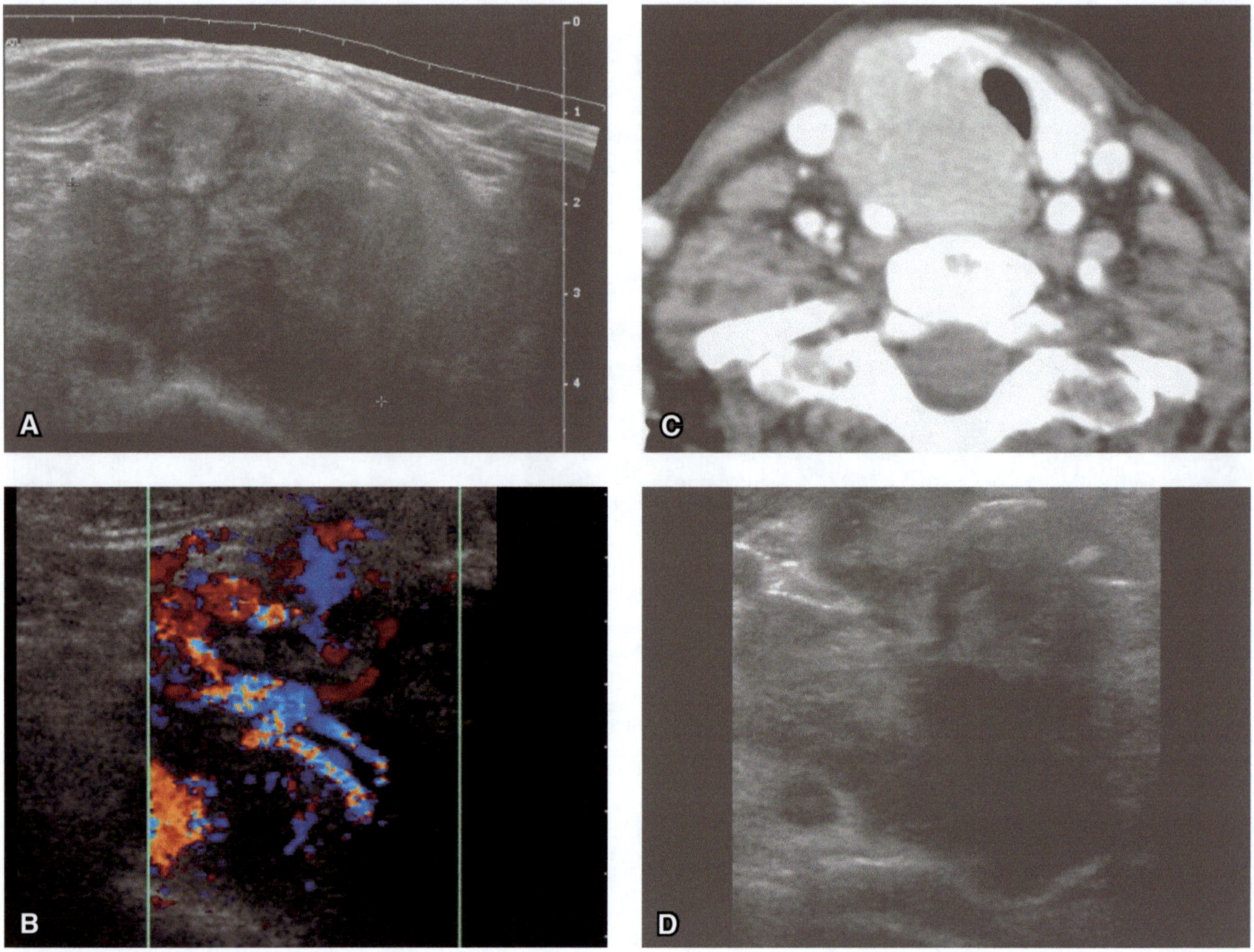

FIGURE 9-11. Ultrasound (US) of anaplastic carcinoma in the right lobe. **A**, Transverse, 32 x 42 mm. **B**, Color Doppler, transverse. **C**, CT transverse. **D**, Transverse.

78-Year-old woman

- **Clinical history:** Past 6 months increasing dyspnea. CT showed large tumor.
- **Ultrasound:** Malignant tumor in right lobe with suspicion of tracheal infiltration.
- **Cytology:** Papillary thyroid carcinoma (PTC).
- **Thyroidectomy:** Anaplastic carcinoma derived from PTC.

Features

Hypoechoic
Inhomogeneous echo pattern
Partially well defined
Hypervascular
Microcalcifications
Infiltrating trachea

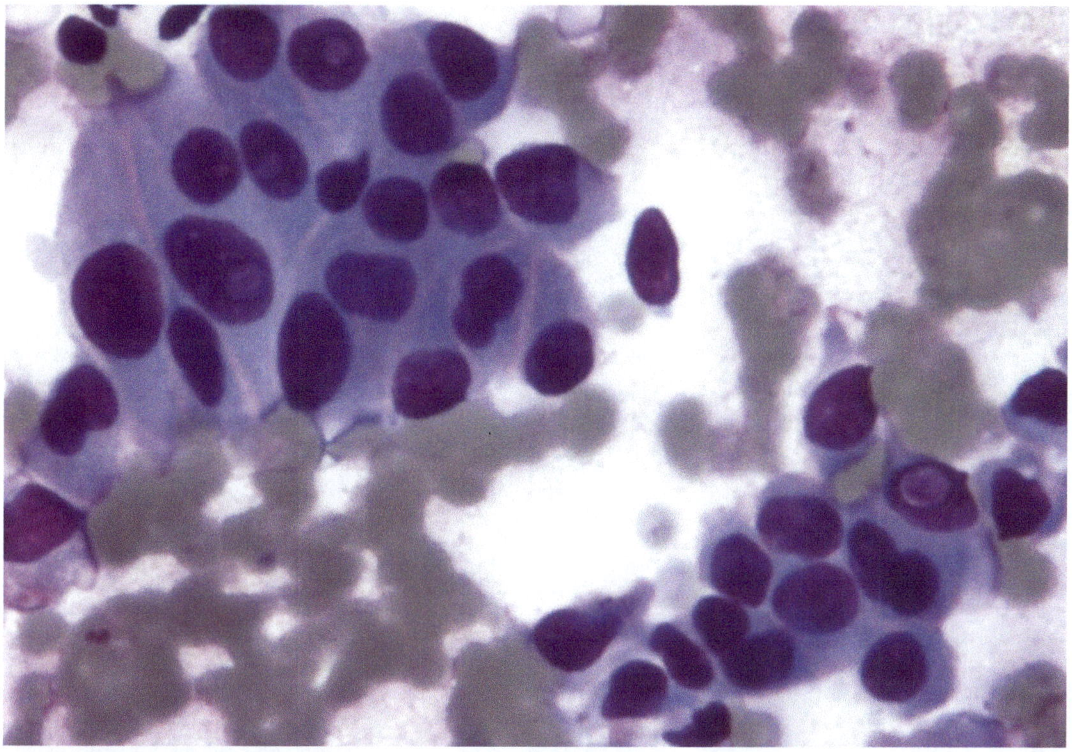

Figure 9-12. Cytology: only papillary thyroid carcinoma cells are present.

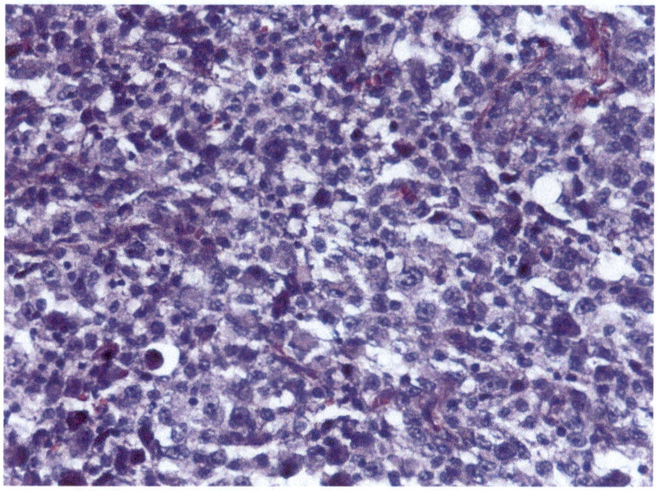

Figure 9-13. Histology: area with anaplastic carcinoma.

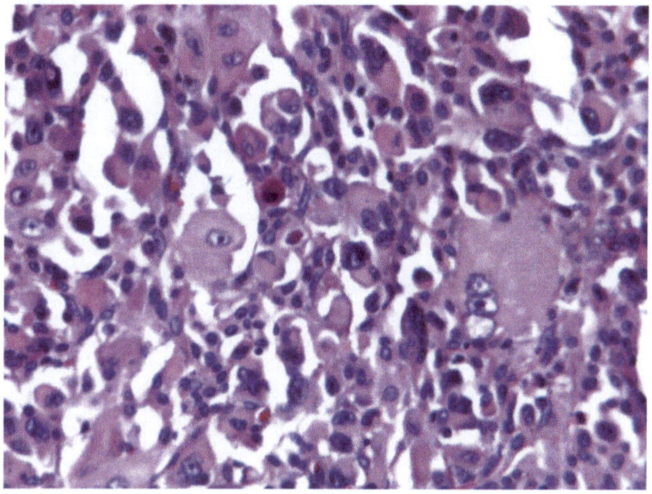

Figure 9-14. Histology: pleomorphic cells.

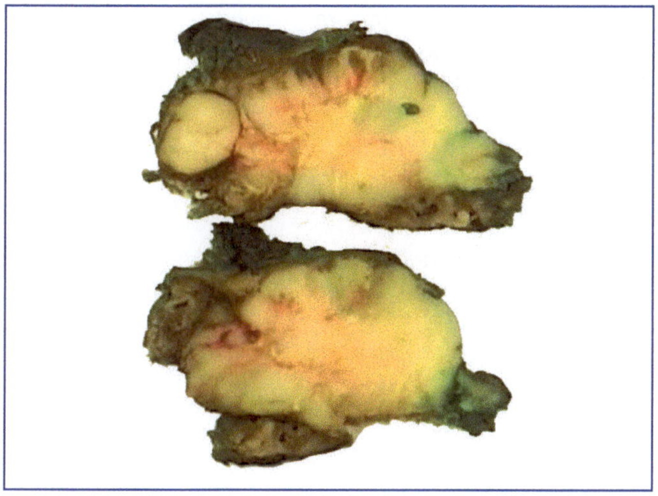

Figure 9-15. Gross section.

Anaplastic Carcinoma Right Lobe

Transverse | Longitudinal

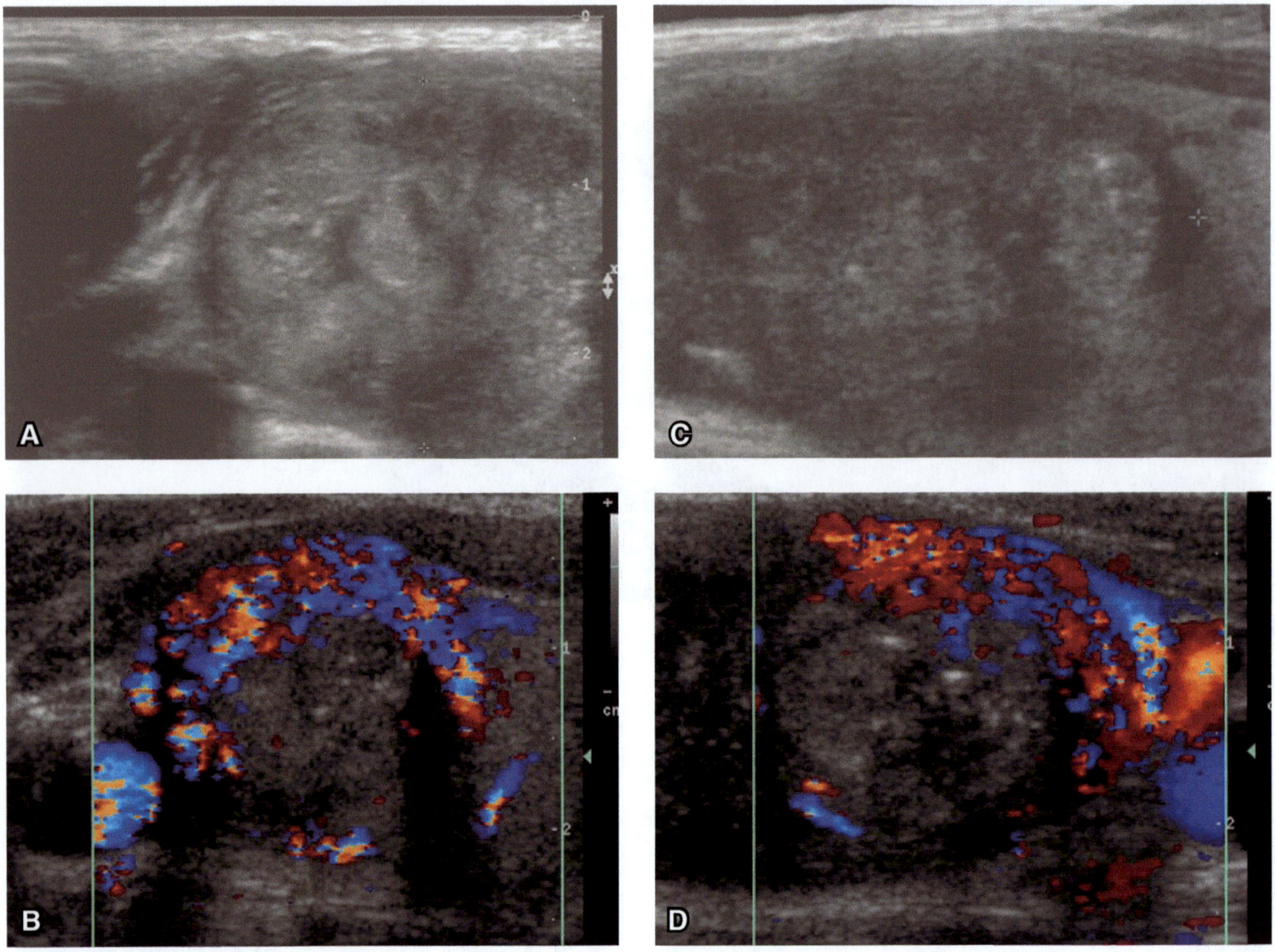

Figure 9-16. Ultrasound of anaplastic carcinoma in the right lobe. **A**, Transverse, 24 x 25 mm. **B**, Color Doppler, transverse. **C**, Longitudinal, sagittal diameter: 36 mm. **D**, Color Doppler, longitudinal.

66-Year-old woman

- **Clinical history:** Growing nodule in right lobe for past 10 months.
- **Ultrasound:** Papillary thyroid carcinoma (PTC) in right lobe + metastases.
- **Cytology:** PTC + metastases.
- **Thyroidectomy:** Anaplastic carcinoma derived from PTC.

Features

Mostly hypoechoic
Quite well defined
Inhomogeneous echo pattern
Peripheral hypervascularity
Microcalcifications

Other findings

Hypervascular pathologic lymph node consistent with metastasis

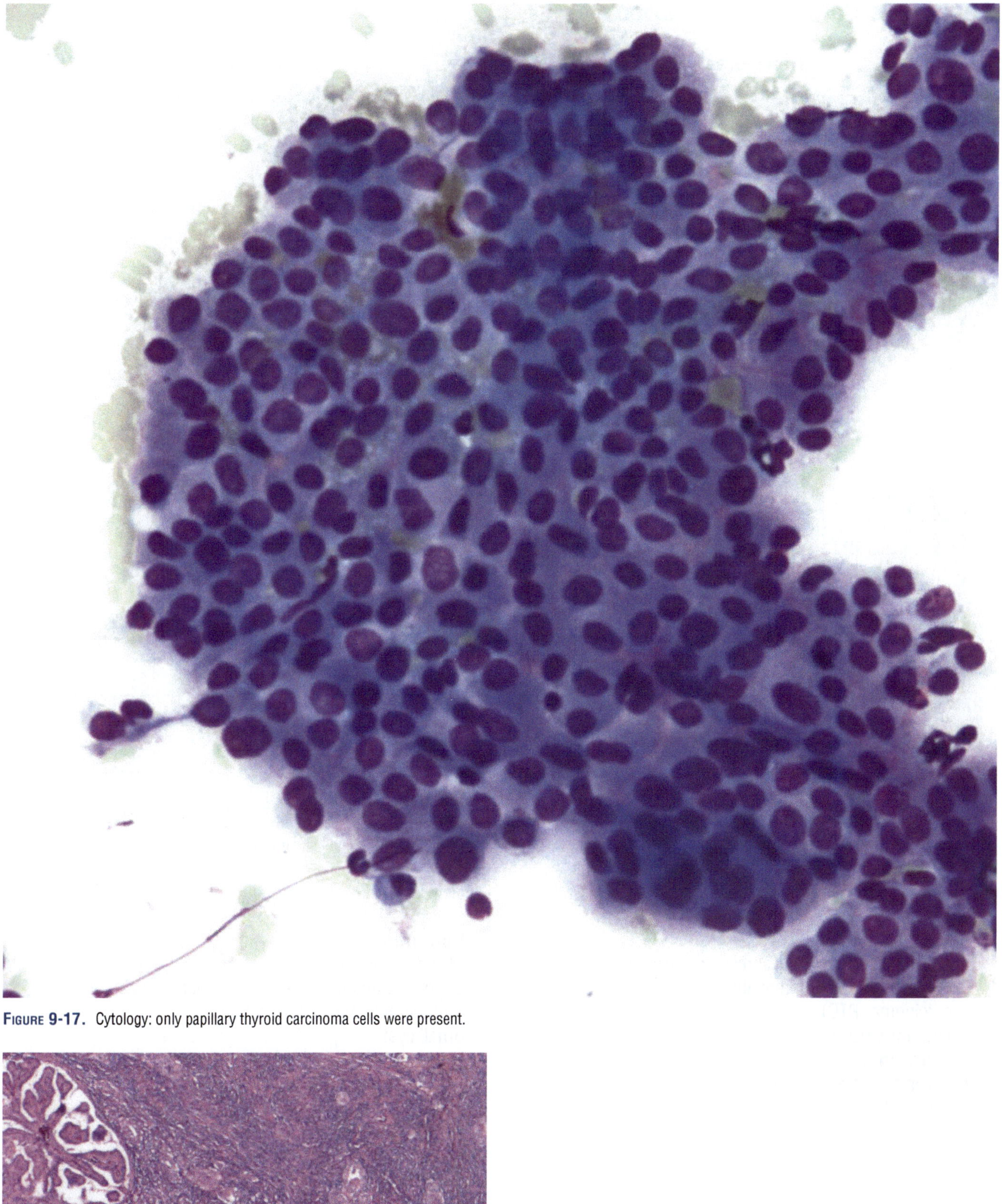

Figure 9-17. Cytology: only papillary thyroid carcinoma cells were present.

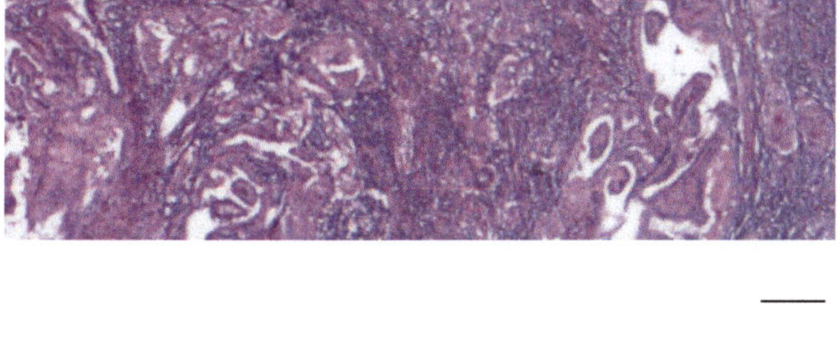

Figure 9-18. Histology: rest of papillary carcinoma on the *left* side, anaplastic carcinoma on the *right* side.

Anaplastic Carcinoma Left Lobe

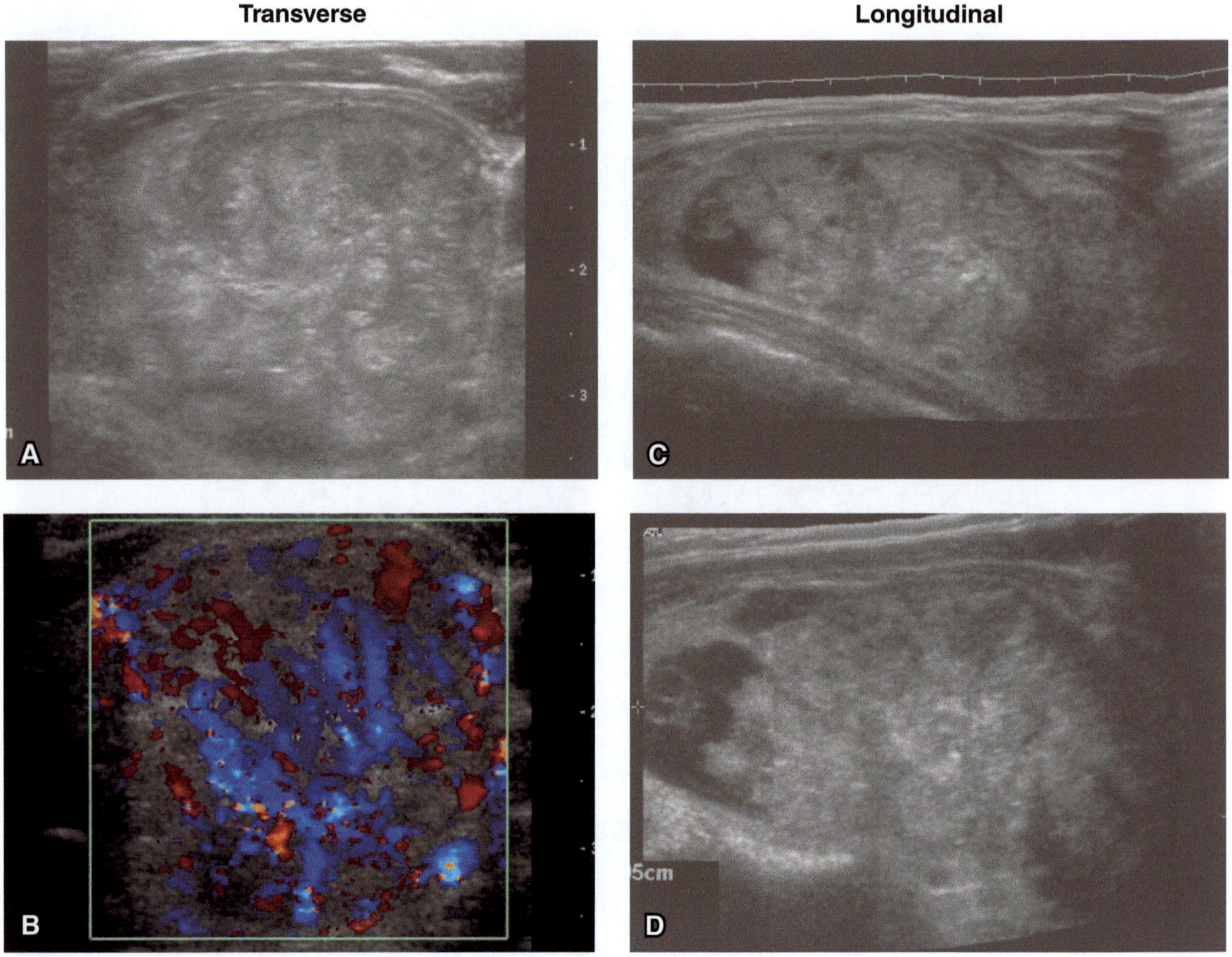

FIGURE 9-19. Ultrasound of anaplastic carcinoma in the left lobe. **A**, Transverse, anteroposterior diameter: 29 mm. **B**, Color Doppler, transverse. **C** and **D**, Longitudinal.

60-Year-old woman

- **Clinical history:** Local relapse from previously operated poorly differentiated papillary thyroid carcinoma (PTC).
- **Ultrasound:** PTC.
- **Cytology:** PTC.
- **Reoperation:** Anaplastic carcinoma derived from PTC.

Features

Mixed echogenicity
Lobulated inhomogeneous echo pattern
Innumerable microcalcifications
Small cyst
Hypervascularity

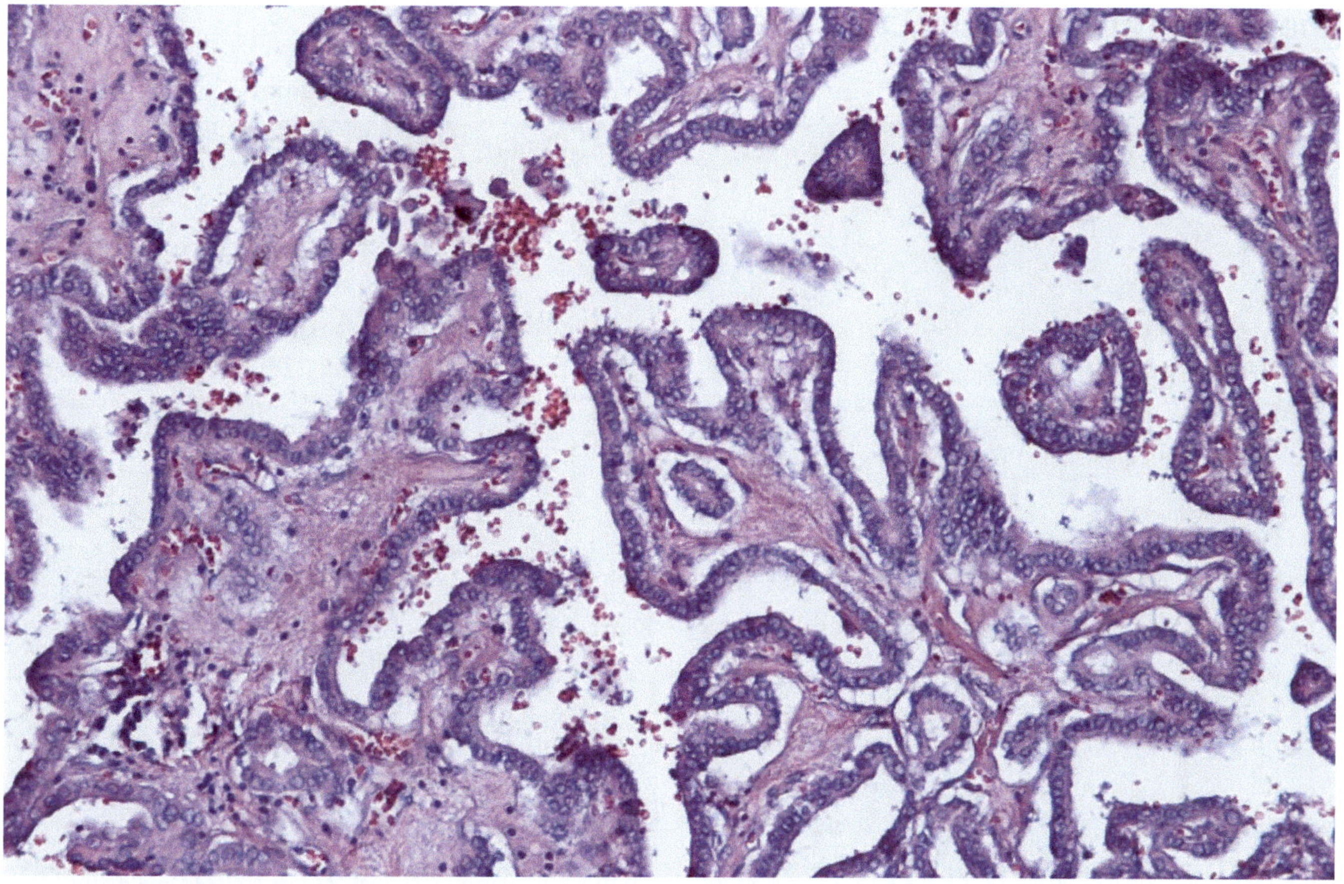

Figure 9-20. Histology: classic papillary growth/extensions into the lumen. Classic atypical cells: nuclear inclusions and overlapping nuclei.

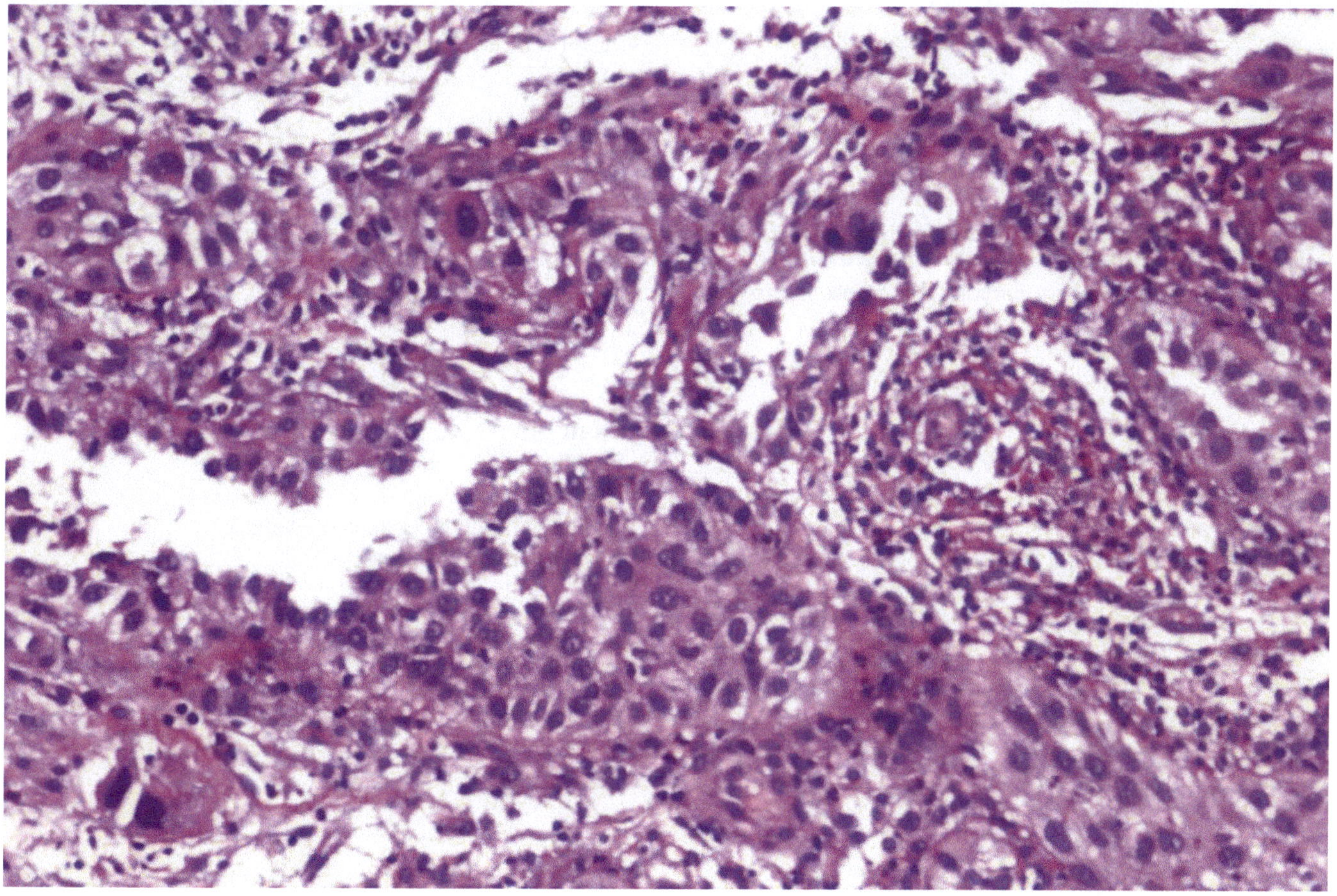

Figure 9-21. Histology: foci of anaplastic differentiation.

Anaplastic Carcinoma Left Lobe

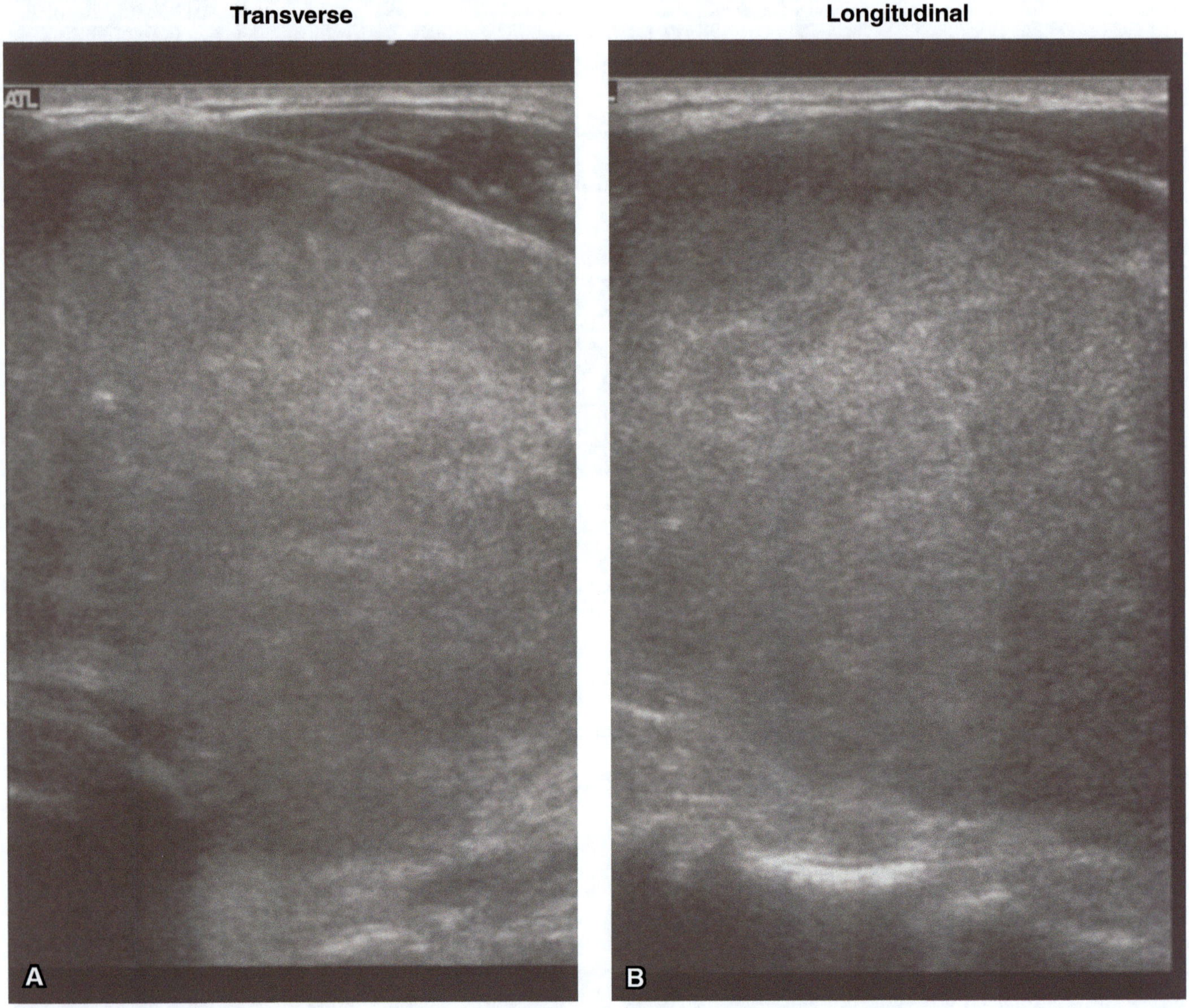

FIGURE 9-22. Ultrasound of anaplastic carcinoma in the left lobe. **A**, Transverse, anteroposterior diameter: 48 mm. **B**, Longitudinal.

52-Year-old man

- **Clinical history:** Not known.
- **Ultrasound:** Large tumor in right lobe. Benign? Malignant?
- **Cytology:** Polymorphic cells. Anaplastic carcinoma.
- **16-Gauge histologic needle biopsy:** Anaplastic carcinoma.

Features

Slightly hypoechoic
Well defined
Slightly inhomogeneous echo pattern
A few microcalcifications

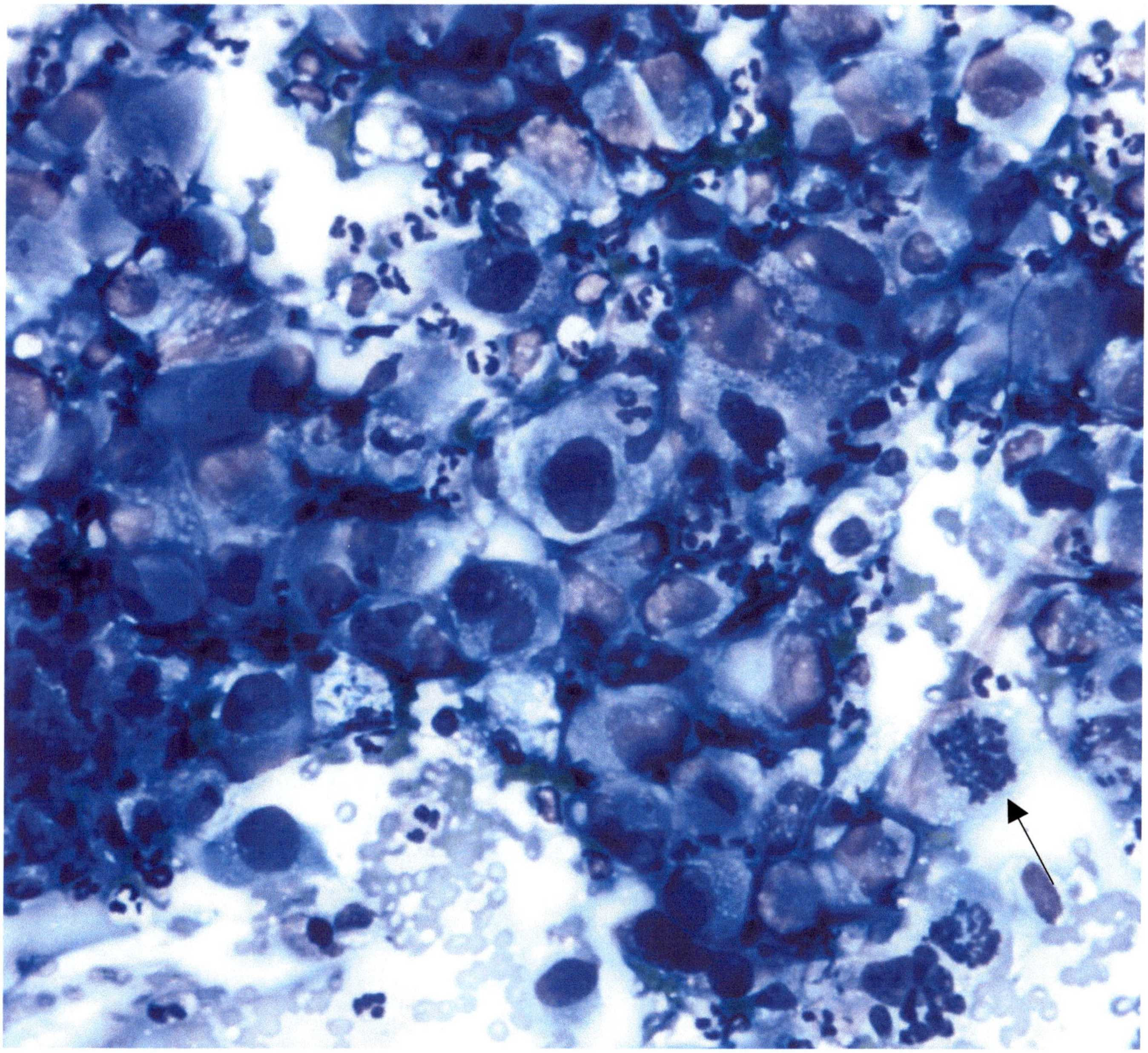

Figure 9-23. Cytology: pleomorphic malignant cells. Note mitosis (*arrow*).

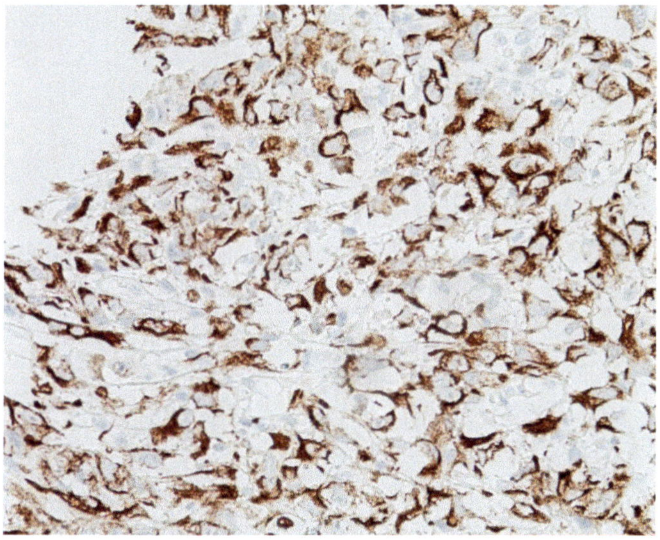

Figure 9-24. Histologic needle biopsy: cytokeratin-positive malignant tumor.

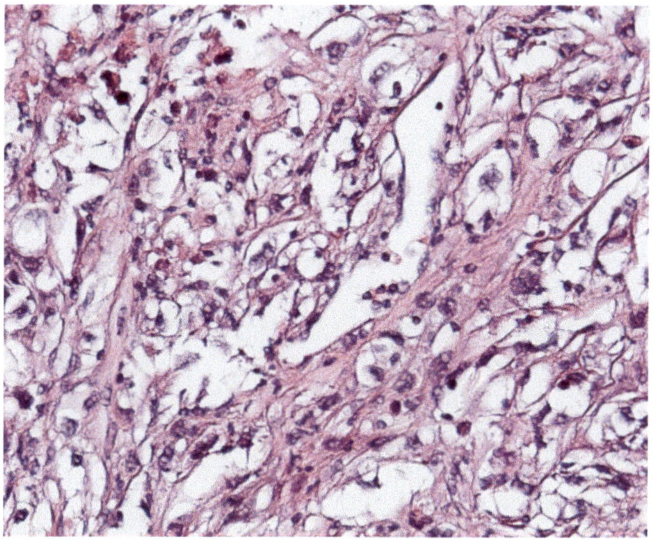

Figure 9-25. Histology: pleomorphic malignant cells.

10 Lymphoma and Plasmacytoma

A lymphoma may affect the whole gland, but is often found only on one side. The regional lymph nodes are often affected as well. In about 70% of cases lymphoma arises from a preexisting chronic lymphocytic thyroiditis (Hashimoto's thyroiditis) [6,7,20]. The tumor is strongly hypoechoic, often well marginated, but usually causes enlargement of the affected lobe. The echo pattern varies from micronodular to homogeneous. Thyroid lymphomas are usually poorly vascularized, but may also show blood vessels with chaotic distribution [6]. The micronodular lymphomas may resemble Hashimoto's thyroiditis, and may also be surrounded by thyroiditis.

Common Features of Lymphoma

Hypoechoic
Homogeneous or nodular echo pattern
Well marginated
Regional lymph node affection

Cytologic Morphology of Lymphoma

The cytopathologist should always consider the possible presence and amount of lymphoid cells, even when the clinical or radiologic findings show no indication of thyroiditis or lymphoma. In specimens rich in blood, one may find some scattered leukocytes, but distinguising a smear with lymphoid cells due to other reasons is seldom challenging. The finding of lymphoid cells together with oncocytic cells is usually consistent with Hashimoto's thyroiditis. The variation in the size of the nuclei in the oncocytes may be extensive (anisocytosis). In smears with an abundant amount of lymphocytes, but depleted of oncocytes, the possibility of a lymphoid neoplasm must be investigated. An extra cytologic biopsy for flow cytometric immunophenotyping preferably should be taken. This is especially important in elderly patients (over 60 years of age), because lymphoid lesions in these patients are often found to be lymphoma.

Features of Plasmacytoma

In the thyroid gland, plasma cell neoplasms usually appear in the form of extraosseous plasmacytoma, which is extremely rare [21]. In our ultrasound practice we have only one case. At ultrasound the actual tumor appears less hypoechoic and with larger nodules compared with what is usually found in a lymphoma. Nobody knows if these features could be significant.

Histologic and Cytologic Morphology of Plasmacytoma

The neoplasm consists of a tumorous mass of usually mature, or more seldom, immature plasma cells. Mature plasma cells demonstrate the characteristic features with eccentric nuclei and abundant basophilic cytoplasm. Immature plasma cells demonstrate a high nuclear–cytoplasmic ratio and prominent nucleoli. Flow cytometric immunophenotyping demonstrating a population of lymphoid cells monoclonal for intracytoplasmic light chain immunoglobulin is of crucial importance when making the diagnosis of plasmacytoma.

Lymphoma Both Lobes

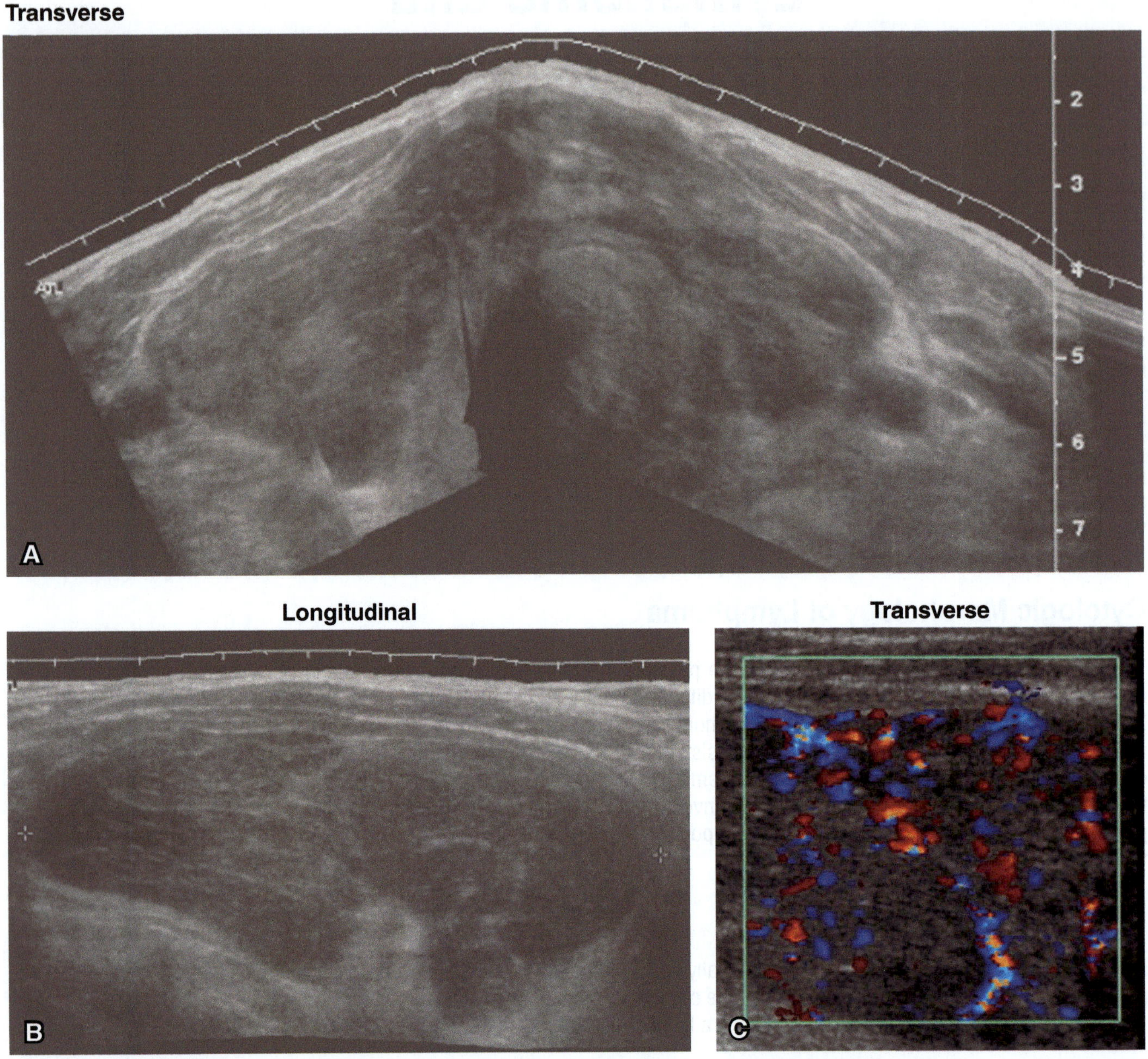

FIGURE 10-1. Ultrasound of lymphoma in both lobes. **A**, Transverse. **B**, Longitudinal, sagittal diameter: 75 mm. **C**, Color Doppler, transverse.

75-Year-old man

- **Clinical history:** Enlarged, hard thyroid, highly suspicious for malignancy at CT.
- **Ultrasound:** Lymphoma. Also thyroiditis in right lobe?
- **Cytology left lobe:** Non-Hodgkin B-cell lymphoma.
- **18-Gauge histologic needle biopsy left lobe:** Diffuse large cell B-cell lymphoma.

Features

Lobulated nodular, affecting both lobes
Hypoechoic
Inhomogeneous echo pattern
Coarse septations
Scant vascularity

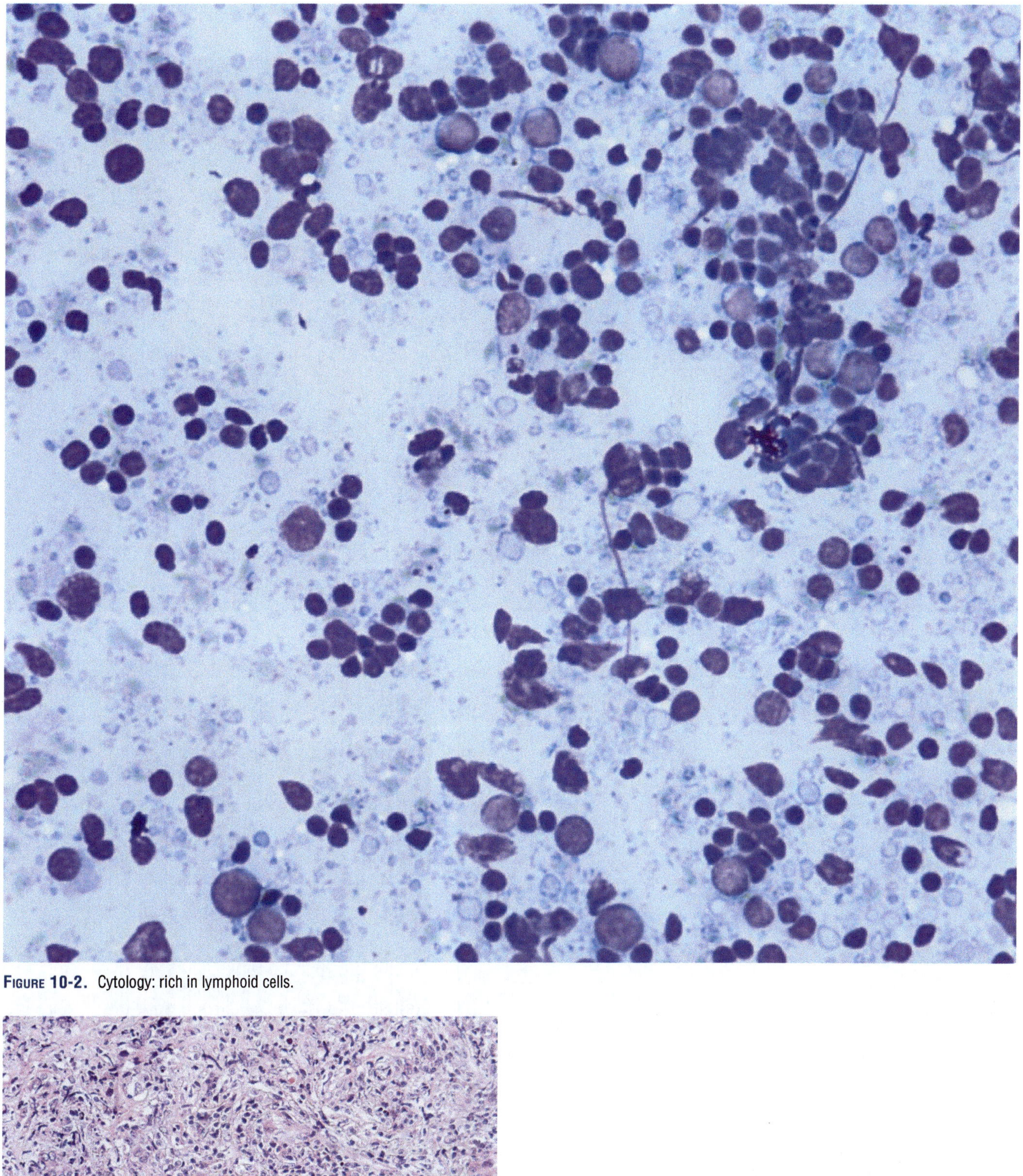

Figure 10-2. Cytology: rich in lymphoid cells.

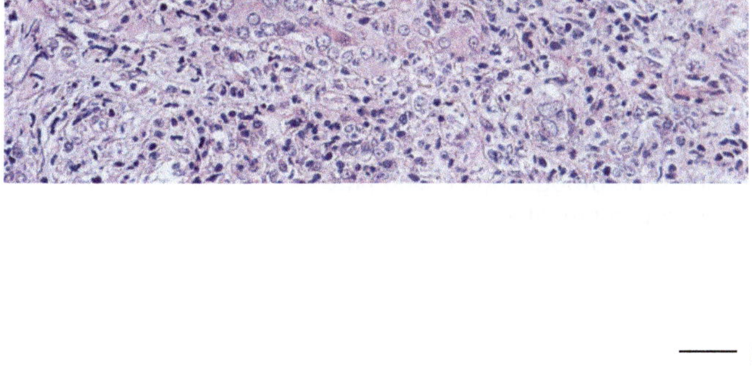

Figure 10-3. Histologic needle biopsy.

Lymphoma Left Lobe

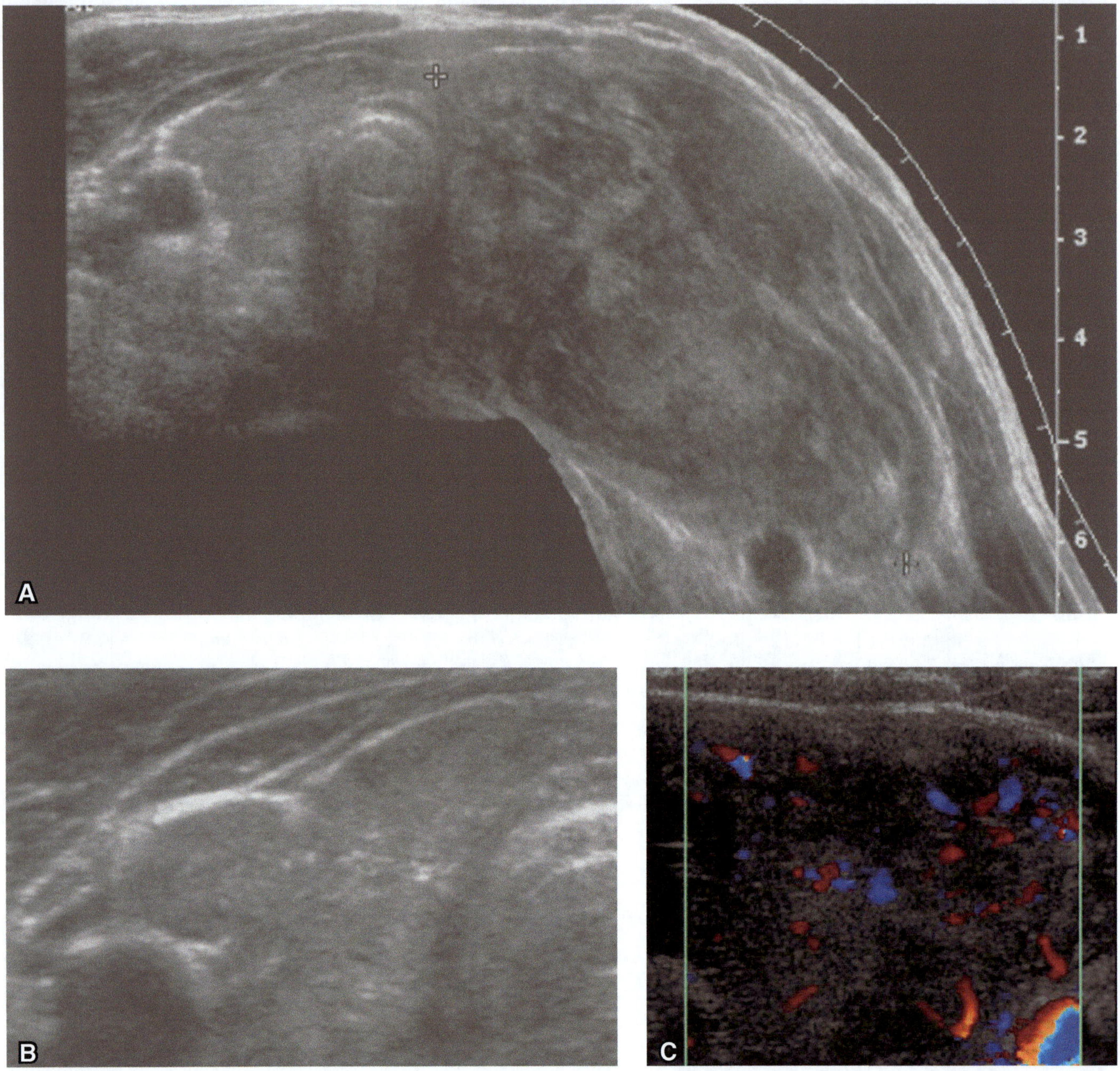

Figure 10-4. **A** and **C**, Ultrasound of lymphoma in the left lobe. **B**, Thyroiditis in the right lobe.

43-Year-old woman

- **Clinical history:** Lymphoma in uterus, vagina, and neck lymph nodes. Large left thyroid lobe.
- **Ultrasound:** Lymphoma in left lobe. Thyroiditis in right lobe.
- **Cytology left lobe:** Burkitt's lymphoma.

Features, left lobe
Hypoechoic
Inhomogeneous nodular echo pattern
Affecting whole lobe and strap muscles
Scant vascularity

Features, right lobe
Hypoechoic
Less inhomogeneous echo pattern
A few microcalcifications

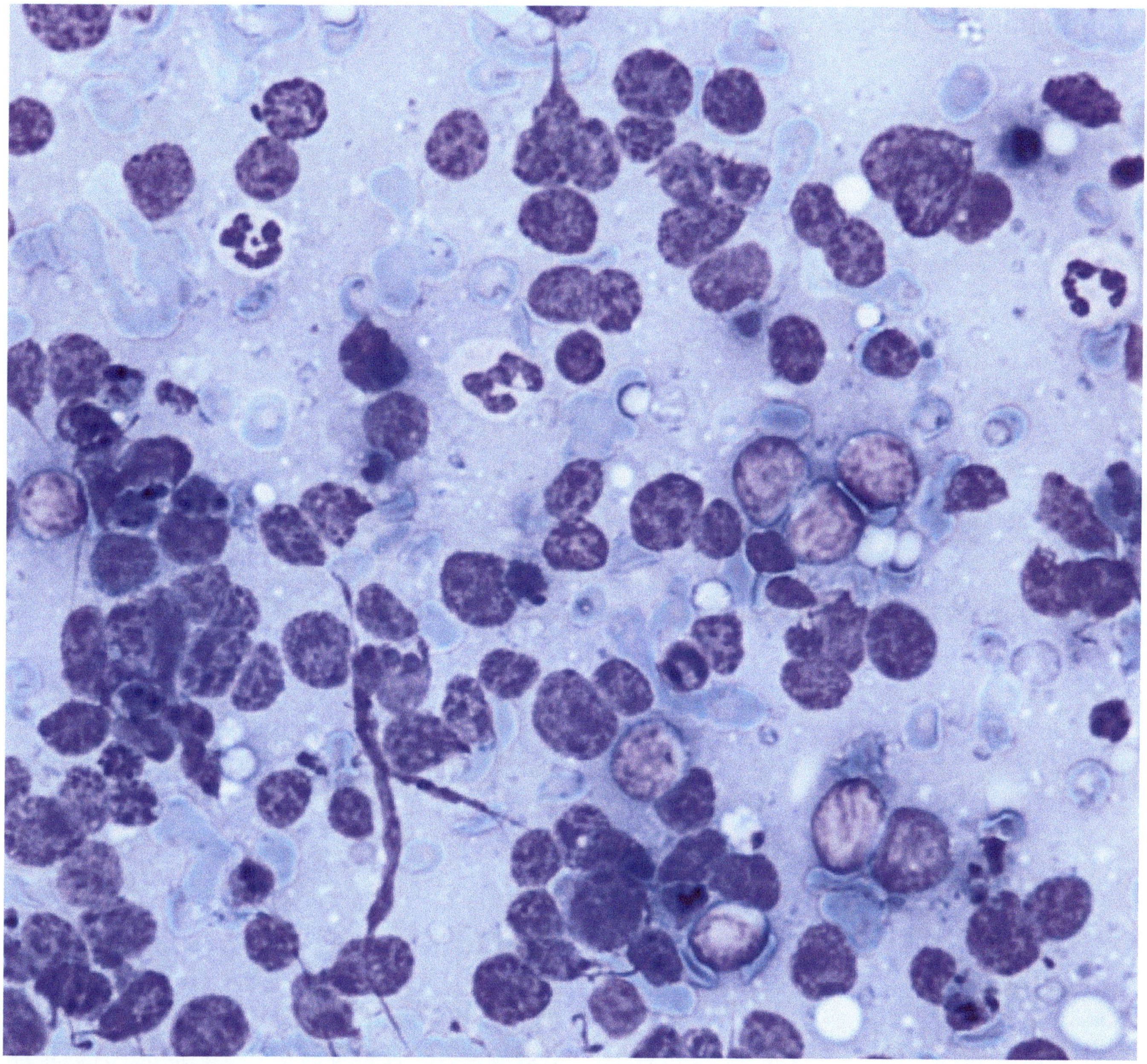

Figure 10-5. Cytology: large, atypical lymphoid cells with basophilic cytoplasm.

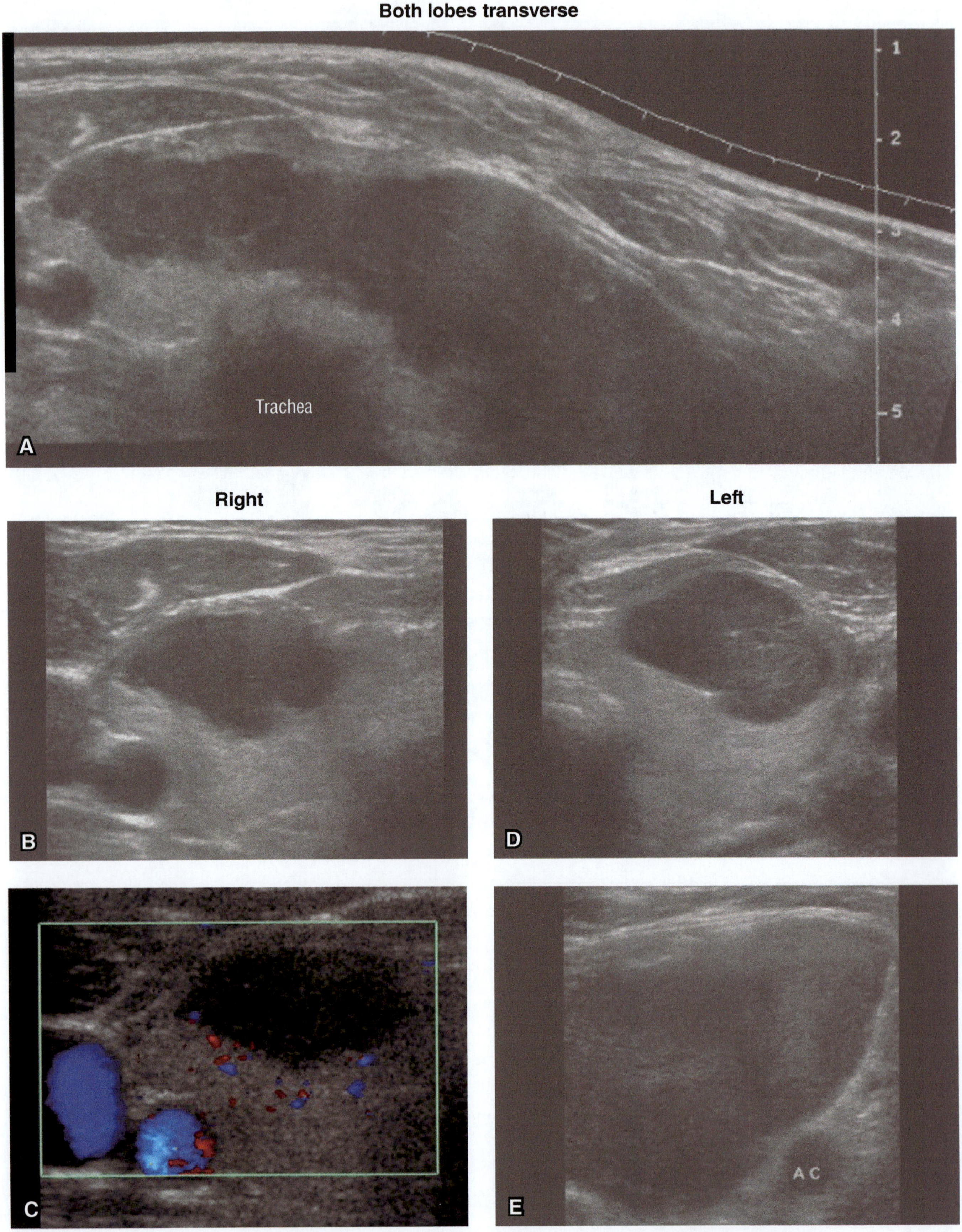

Figure 10-6. Ultrasound of lymphoma in both lobes. **A**, Both lobes transverse. **B**, Right lobe. **C**, Color Doppler, right lobe. **D** and **E**, Left lobe.

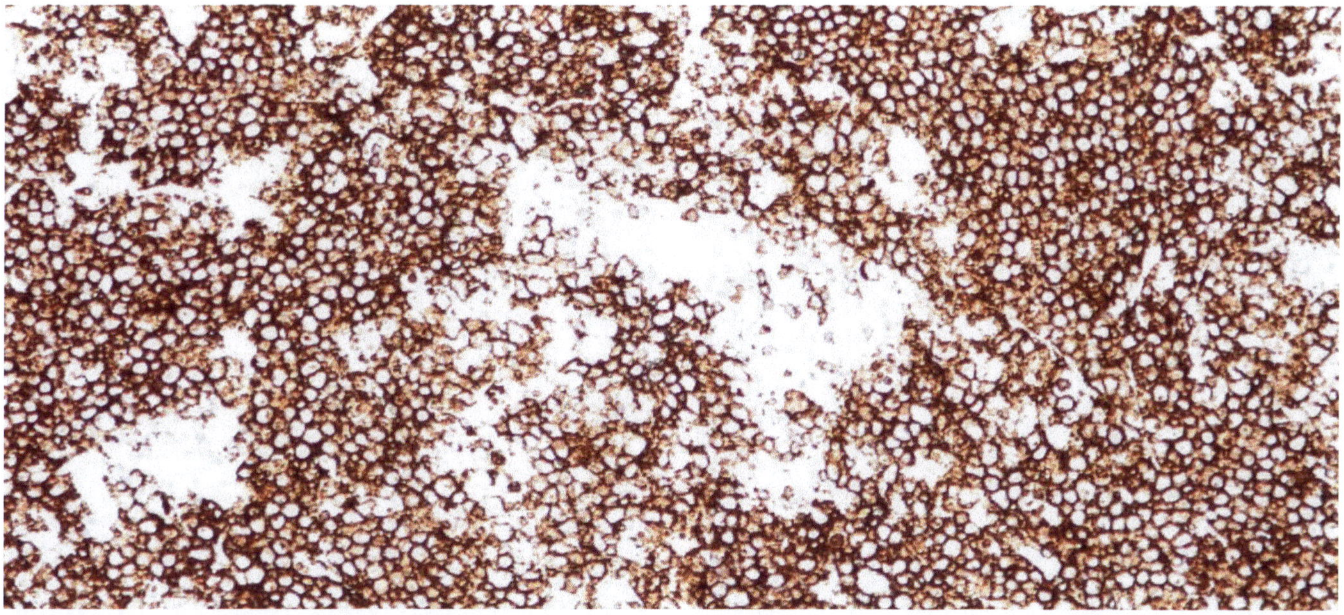

Figure 10-7. Immunoreactivity for CD 20, a pan B-cell marker.

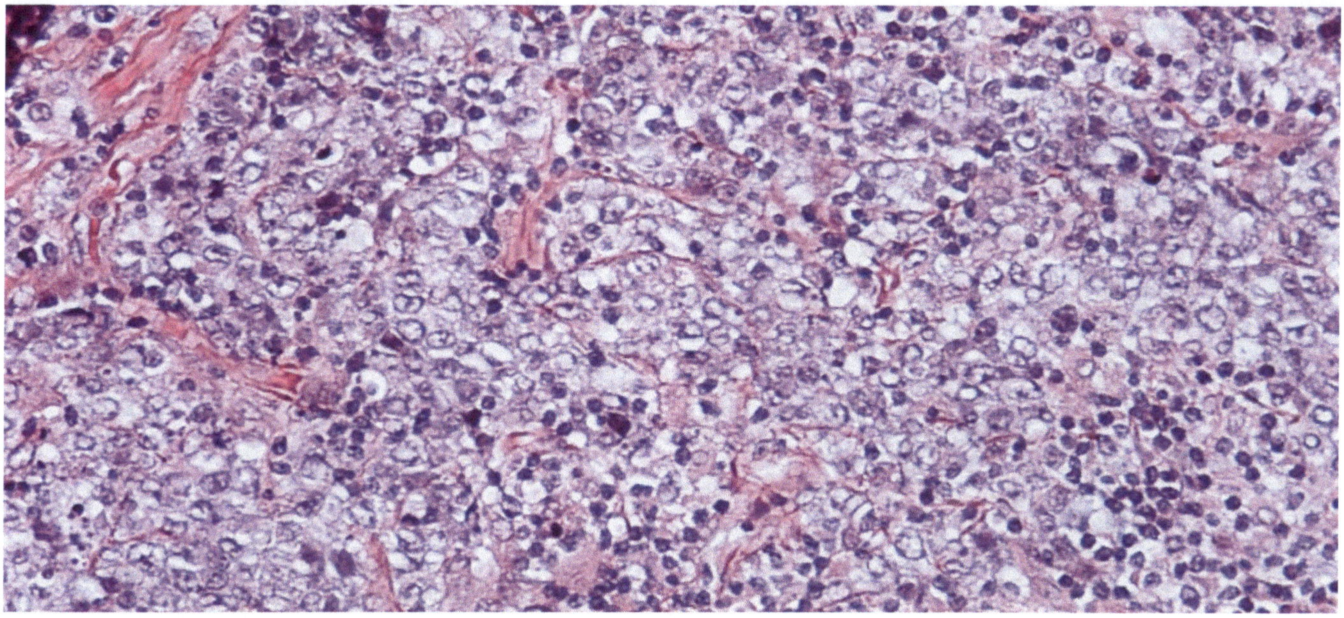

Figure 10-8. Histology: diffuse large B-cell lymphoma.

55-Year-old woman

- **Clinical history:** Large neck tumor evaluated with CT. Surgical histology shows diffuse large B-cell lymphoma.
- **Ultrasound:** Multiple intrathyroidal tumors consistent with lymphoma.
- **Thyroidectomy:** B-cell lymphoma.

Features

Multifocal
Strongly hypoechoic
Homogeneous echo pattern
Well circumscribed
No visualized vascularity
Microcalcifications?

Lymphoma Right Lobe

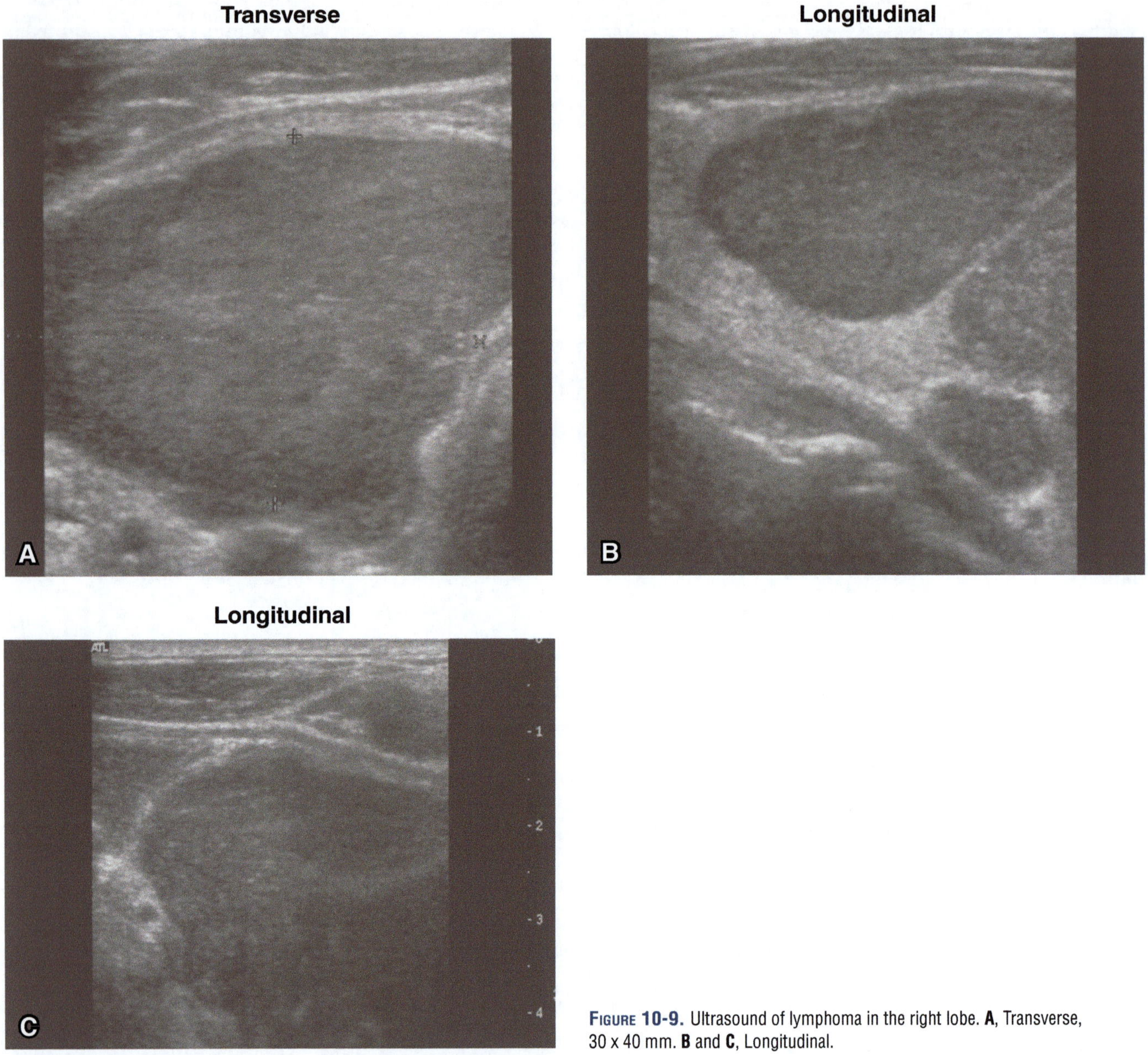

Figure 10-9. Ultrasound of lymphoma in the right lobe. **A**, Transverse, 30 x 40 mm. **B** and **C**, Longitudinal.

77-Year-old man

- **Clinical history:** Pathologic neck lymph nodes, probably lymphoma.
- **Ultrasound:** Multiple intrathyroidal tumors with no visible vascularity, probably lymphoma.
- **Cytology:** Non-Hodgkin B-cell lymphoma.
- **18-Gauge histologic needle biopsy:** Diffuse large B-cell lymphoma.

Features

Multifocal
Strongly hypoechoic
Homogeneous granular echo pattern
Well circumscribed

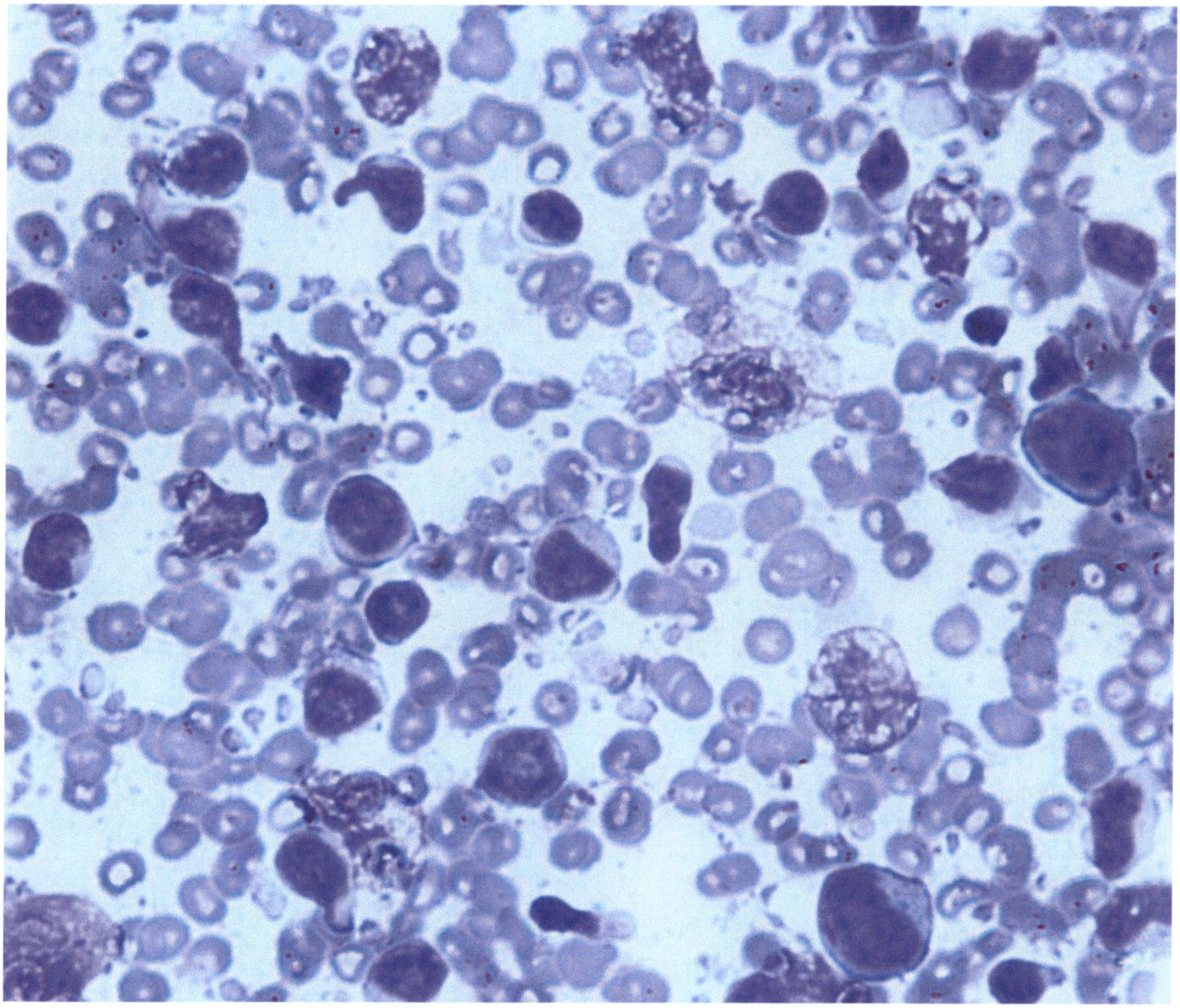

Figure 10-10. Cytology: atypical lymphoid cells consistent with diffuse large B-cell lymphoma.

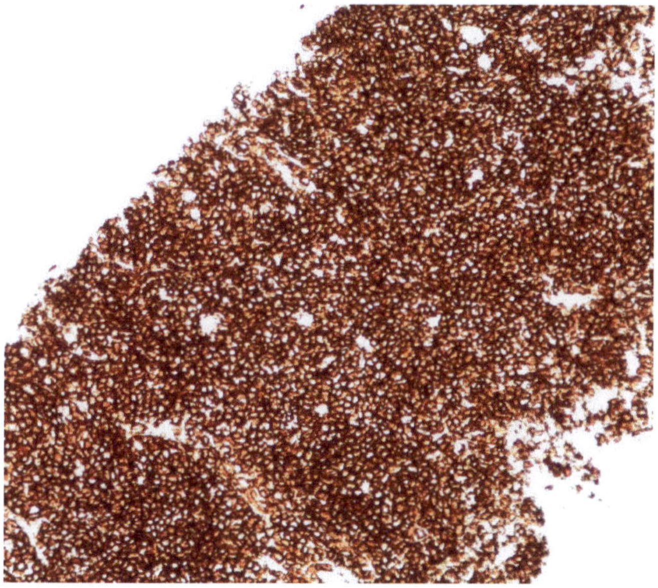

Figure 10-11. Immunohistochemistry: CD 45 (common leukocytic antigen).

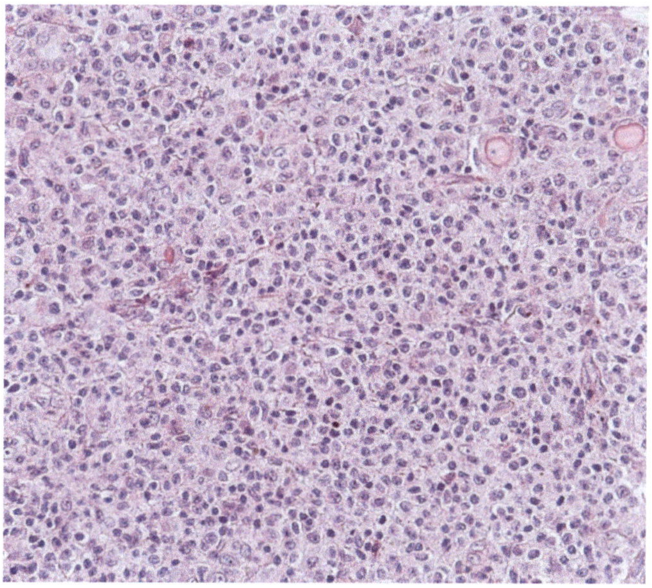

Figure 10-12. Histologic needle biopsy: diffuse large B-cell lymphoma.

Plasmacytoma Right Lobe

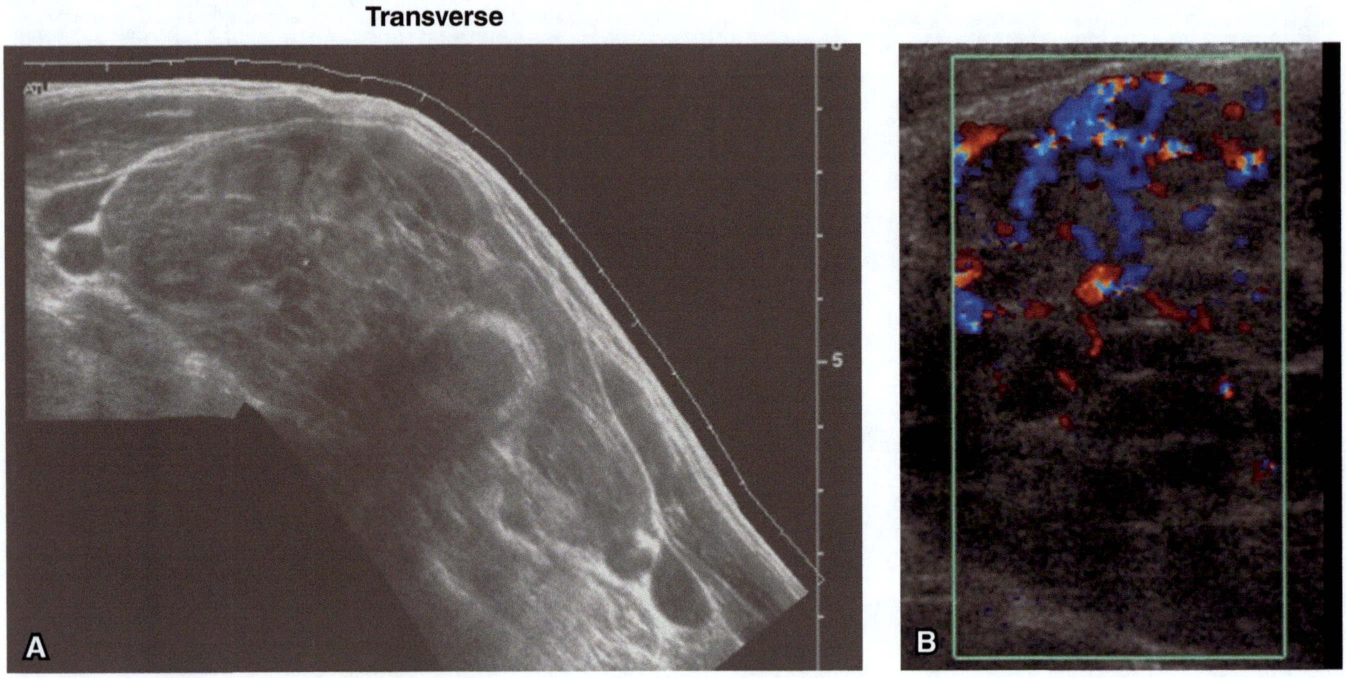

Figure 10-13. Ultrasound of plasmacytoma in the right lobe. **A**, Transverse. **B**, Color Doppler, transverse.

53-Year-old man

- **Clinical history:** Large tumor in right thyroid lobe.
- **Ultrasound:** Possibly lymphoma, but not typical.
- **Cytology:** Atypical plasmacytoid cells. Plasmacytoma?
- **18-Gauge histologic needle biopsy:** Plasmacytoma.

Features

Lobulated nodular
Mixed echogenicity
Inhomogeneous echo pattern
Moderately vascularized

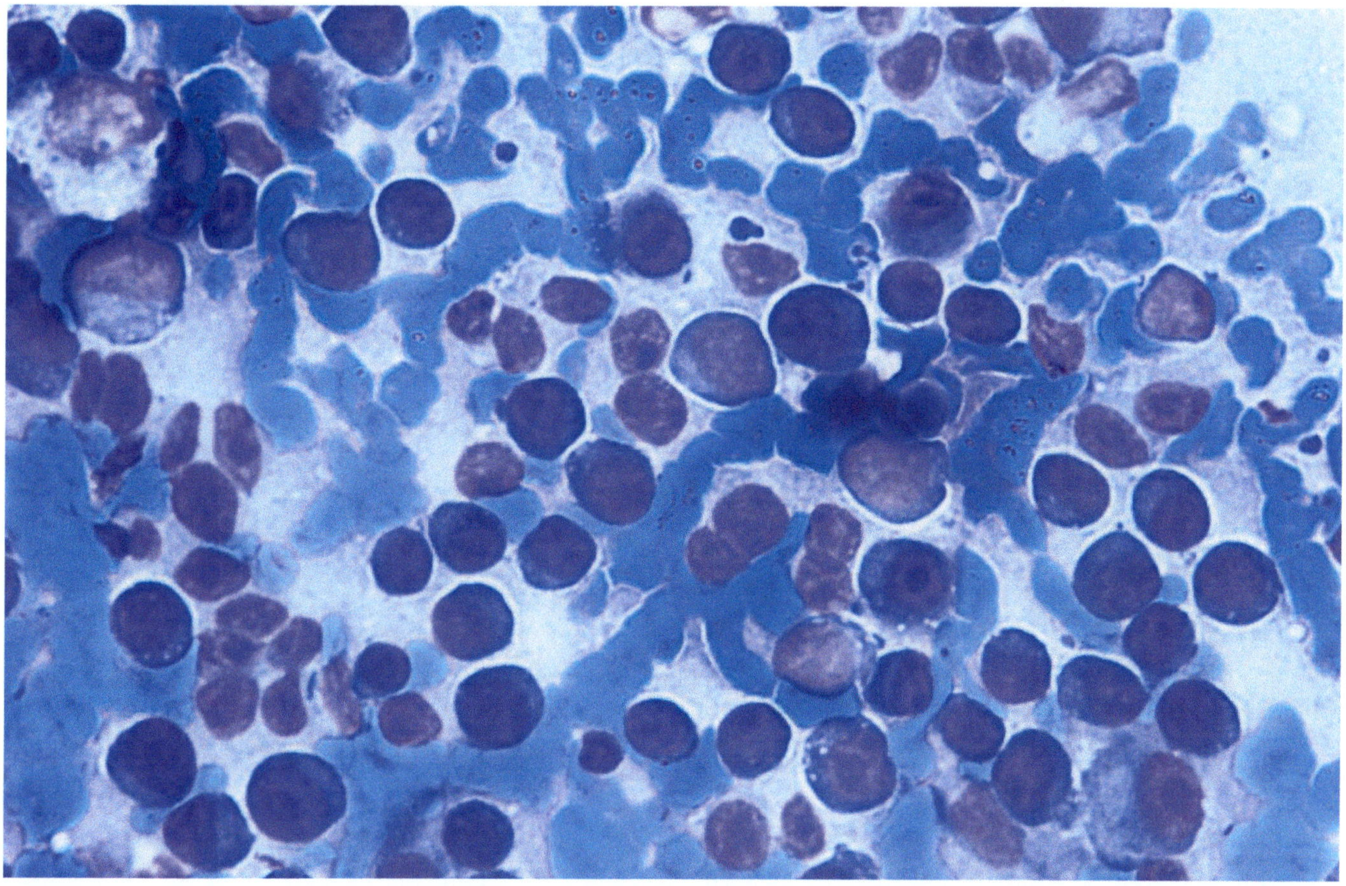

Figure 10-14. Cytology: dispersed cells with characteristic eccentric nuclei and basophilic cytoplasm. (Almost only neoplastic cells and eryhrocytes in this image).

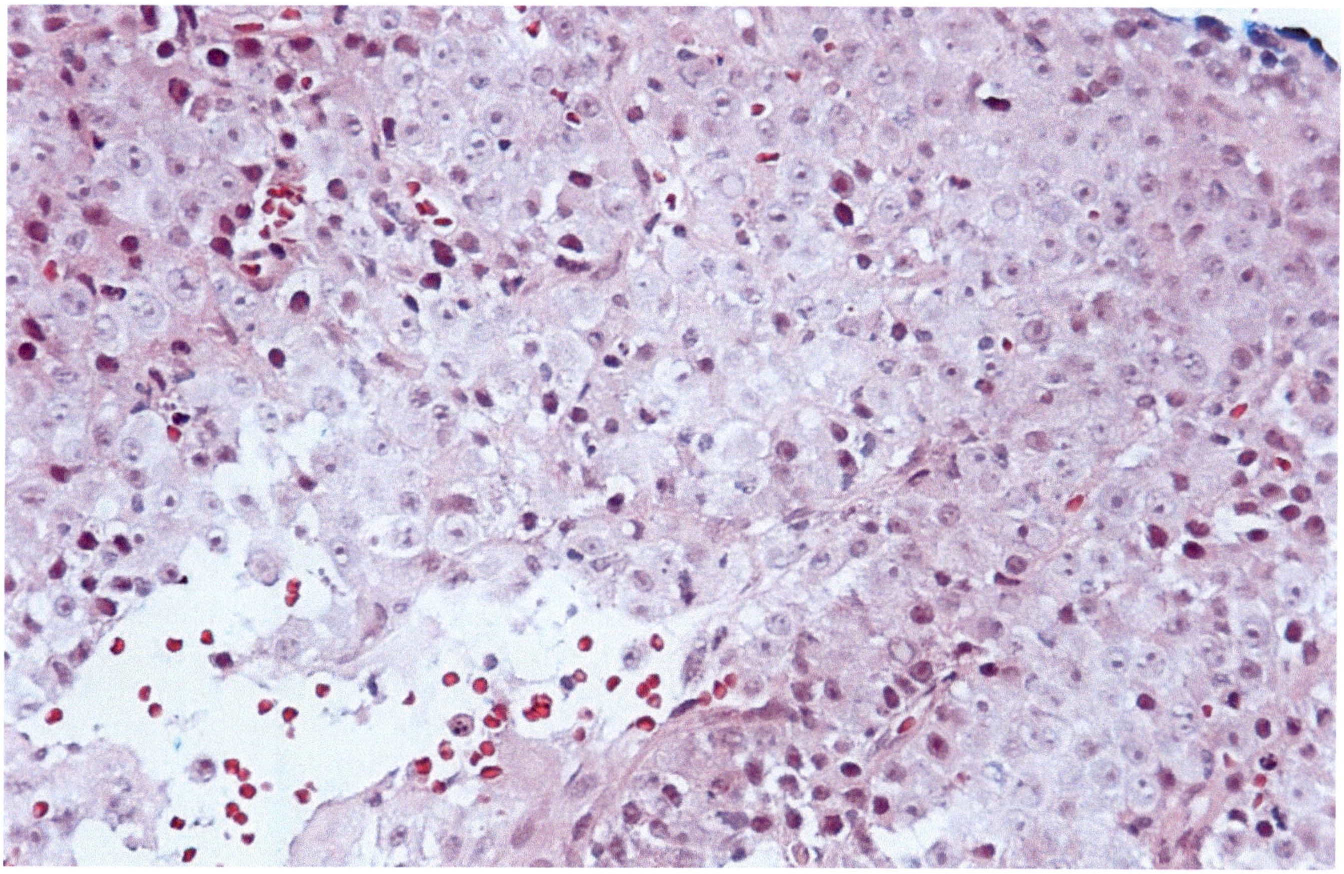

Figure 10-15. Histologic needle biopsy: plasmacytoma.

11 Thyroiditis

Among the inflammatory diseases of the thyroid, Hashimoto's thyroiditis is the most common [4,6,10,22]. Patients frequently have no symptoms when it is found on ultrasound examination. Usually the whole gland is affected, or the changes are found in parts of the gland where there are no nodules. The thyroid gland may be enlarged, but often the size is normal. The tissue is usually strongly hypoechoic with a micronodular pattern. The micronodules range in size from about 1 to 6 mm. The vascularity in Hashimoto's thyroiditis varies from scant to rich, but occasionally is extremely rich, the so-called "thyroid inferno," which is often seen in Grave's disease (see page 142) [6]. Sometimes a cytologic biopsy is somewhat painful.

Common Features

General hypoechogenicity
Micronodular echo pattern
General affection
Septations

Cytologic Morphology

The cytologic picture in smears from thyroiditis displays a wide range of patterns, from just a few lymphoid cells to more florid inflammation with a heterogeneous presentation of lymphoid cells. In smears rich in blood, the relative number of lymphoid cells must be considered. When the number of lymphoid cells seems to exceed the number of leukocytes in blood, additional punctures should be performed in different areas of the gland.

Oncocytic cells may indicate Hashimoto's thyroiditis, but lack of them does not exclude this diagnosis. In elderly people in particular (over 60 years of age), one should always exclude the diagnosis of low-grade lymphoma. One extra cytologic biopsy should routinely be taken for flow cytometric immunophenotyping. The finding of cells indicating thyroiditis in a patient with no earlier diagnosis of thyroiditis implies that the patient must undergo a laboratory investigation, including parameters such as TRAS and thyroid-stimulating hormone.

Thyroiditis Both Lobes

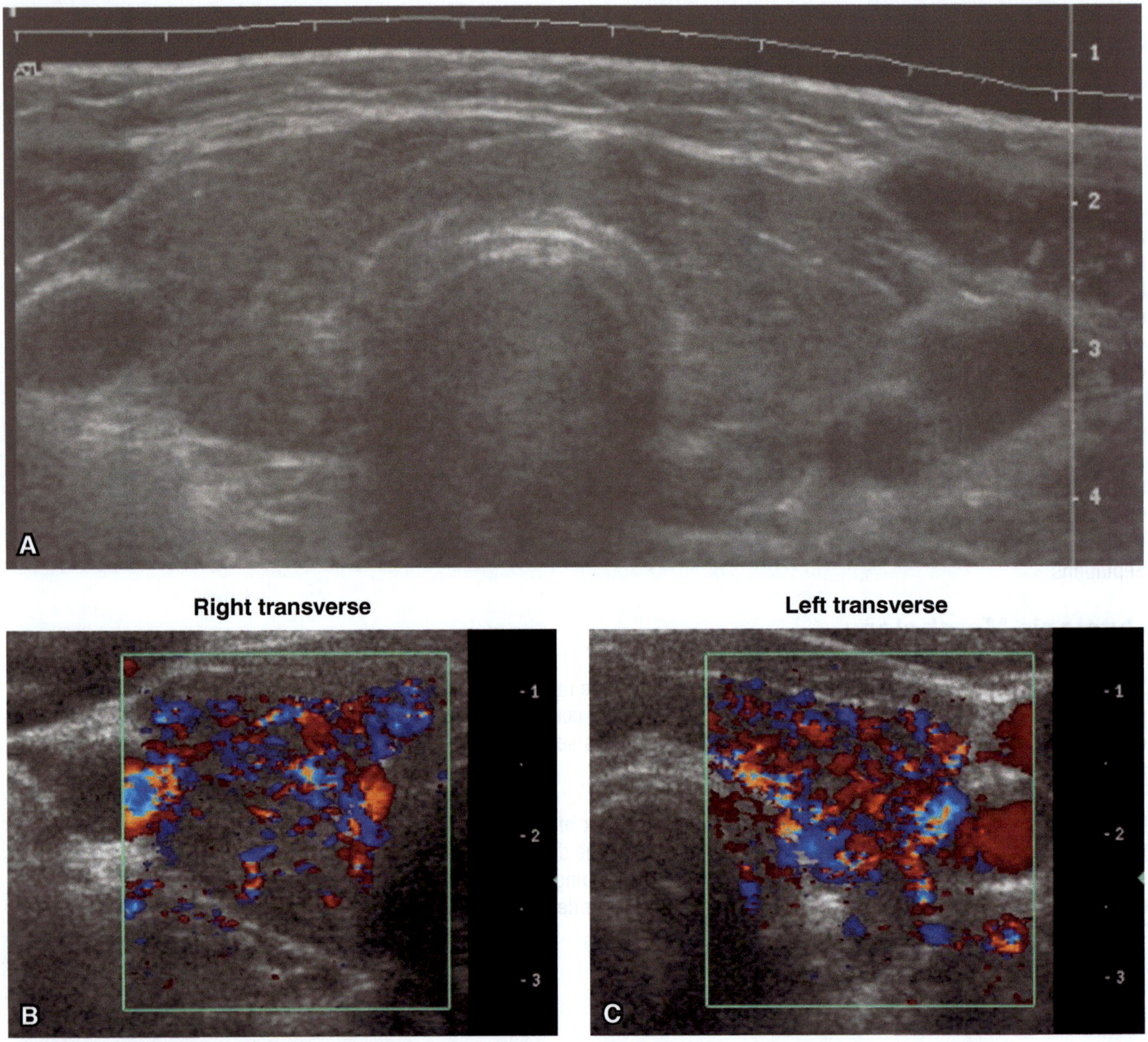

Figure 11-1. Ultrasound of thyroiditis in both lobes. **A**, Both lobes. **B**, Color Doppler, right lobe transverse. **C**, Color Doppler, left lobe transverse.

58-Year-old woman

- **Clinical history:** Cervical cancer. Enlarged thyroid gland.
- **Ultrasound:** Thyroiditis.
- **Cytology:** Hashimoto's thyroiditis.

Features

Hypoechoic
Moderately enlarged
Whole gland affected
Granular echo pattern
Coarse septations
Hypervascular

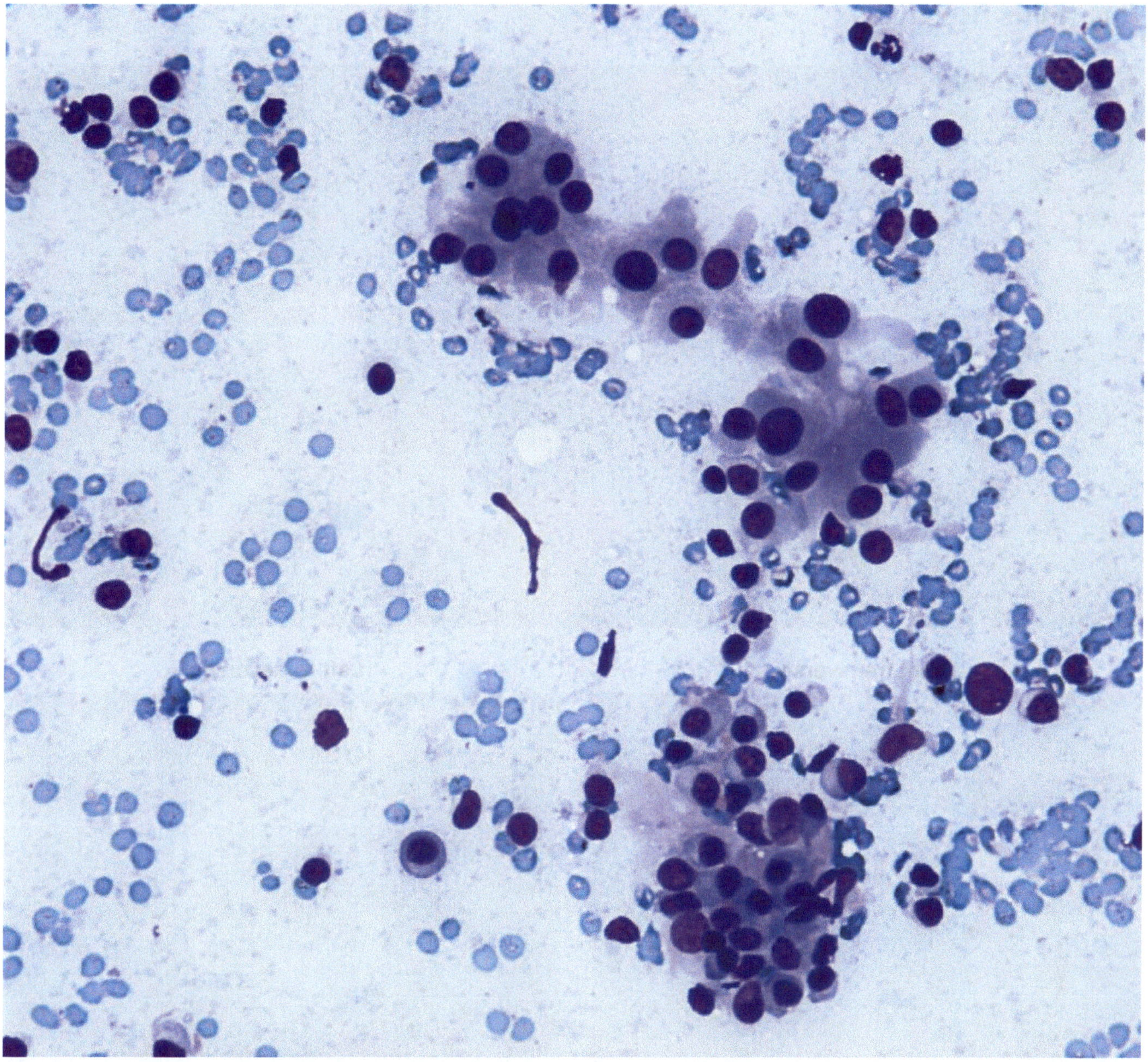

Figure 11-2. Cytology: mixed cell population; lymphoid cells and follicular cells with oncocytic features.

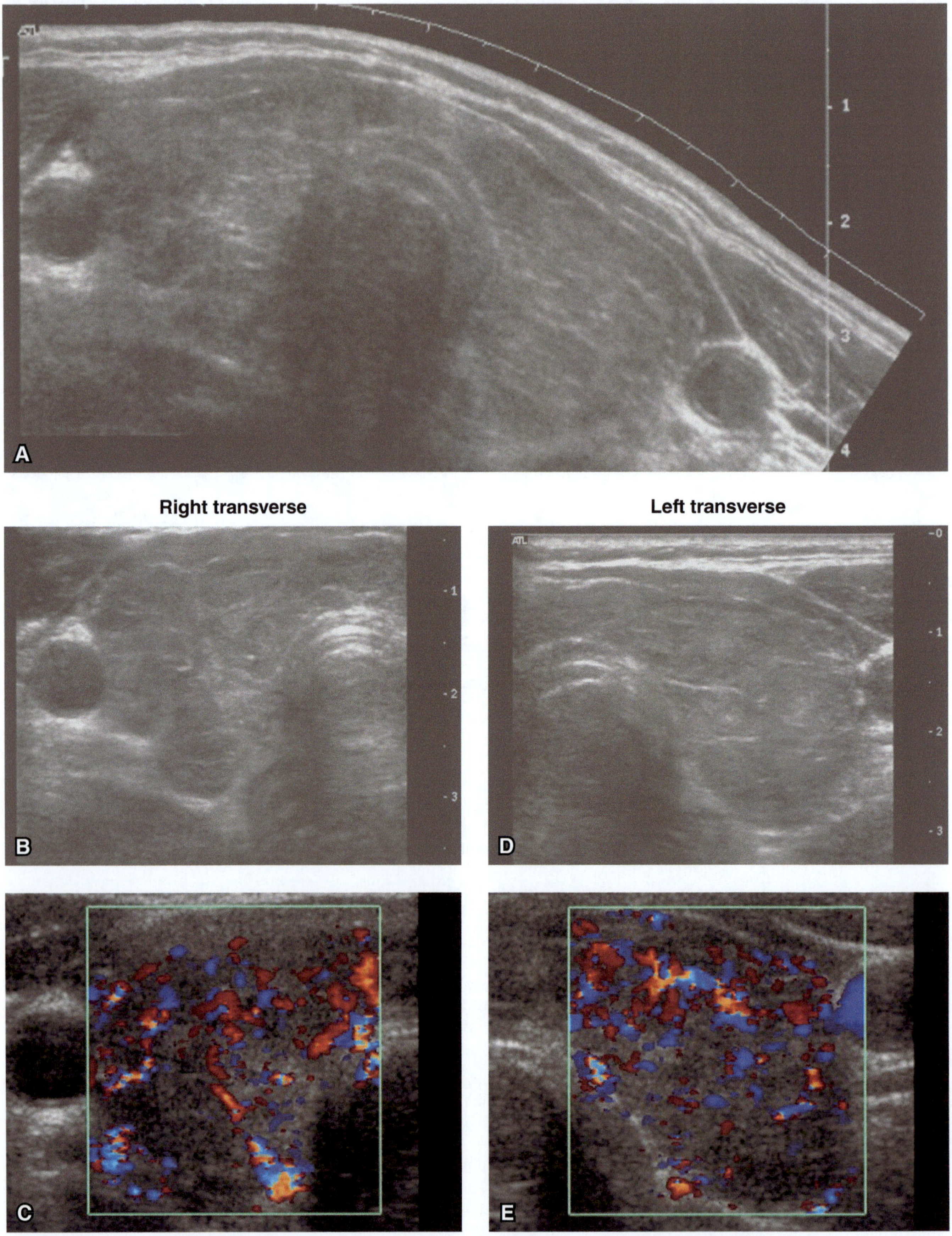

Figure 11-3. Ultrasound of thyroiditis in both lobes. **A**, Both lobes. **B**, Right lobe transverse. **C**, Color Doppler, right lobe transverse. **D**, Left lobe transverse. **E**, Color Doppler, left lobe transverse.

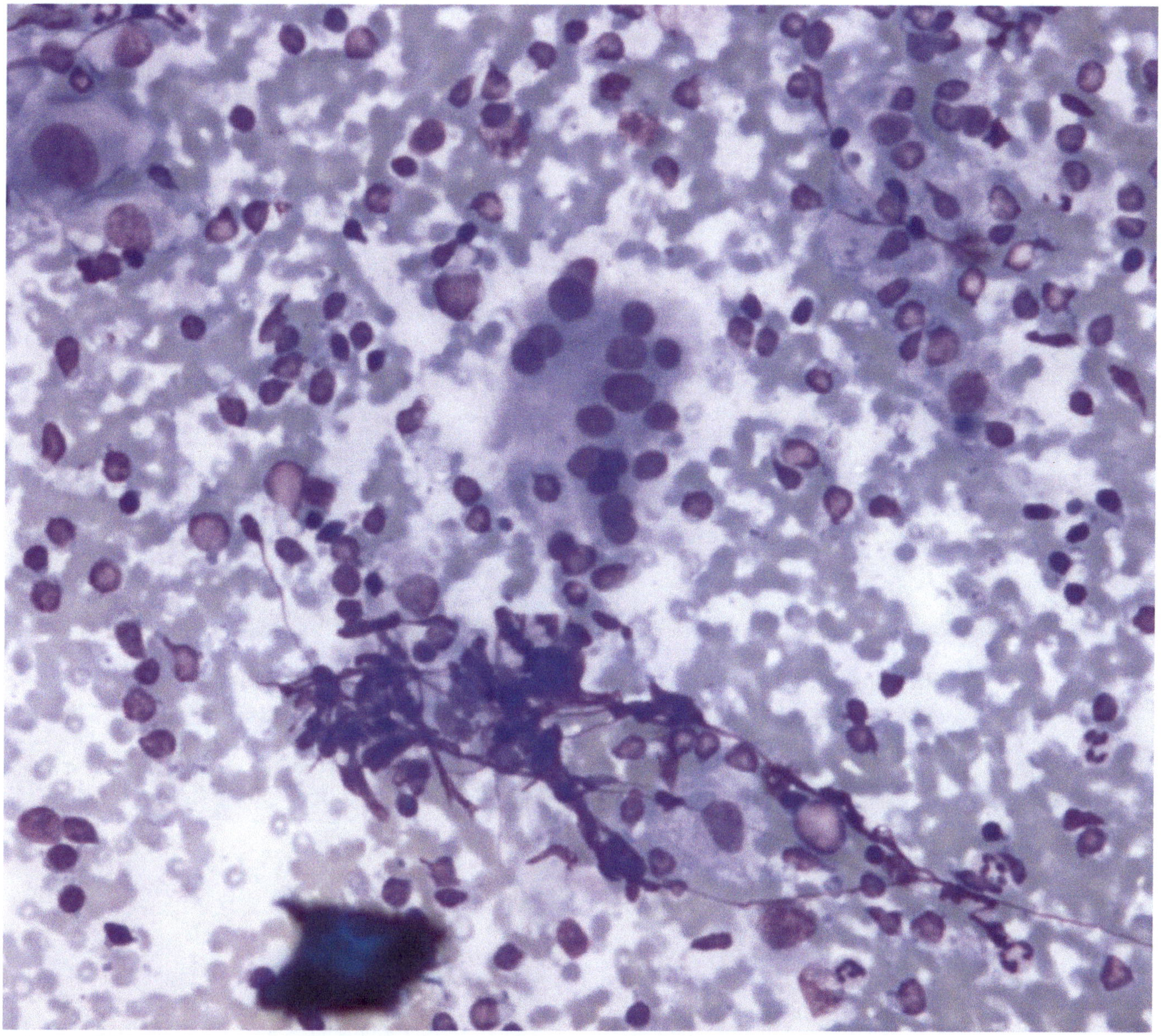

Figure 11-4. Cytology: mixed cell population; lymphoid cells and follicular cells with oncocytic features.

61-Year-old woman

- **Clinical history:** Liver metastasis. Adenocarcinoma. Origo incerta.
- **Ultrasound:** Thyroiditis.
- **Cytology:** Hashimoto's thyroiditis.

Features

Moderately hypoechoic
Whole gland affected
Granular, lobulated, inhomogeneous echo pattern with a few septations
Moderate vascularity

Thyroiditis Both Lobes

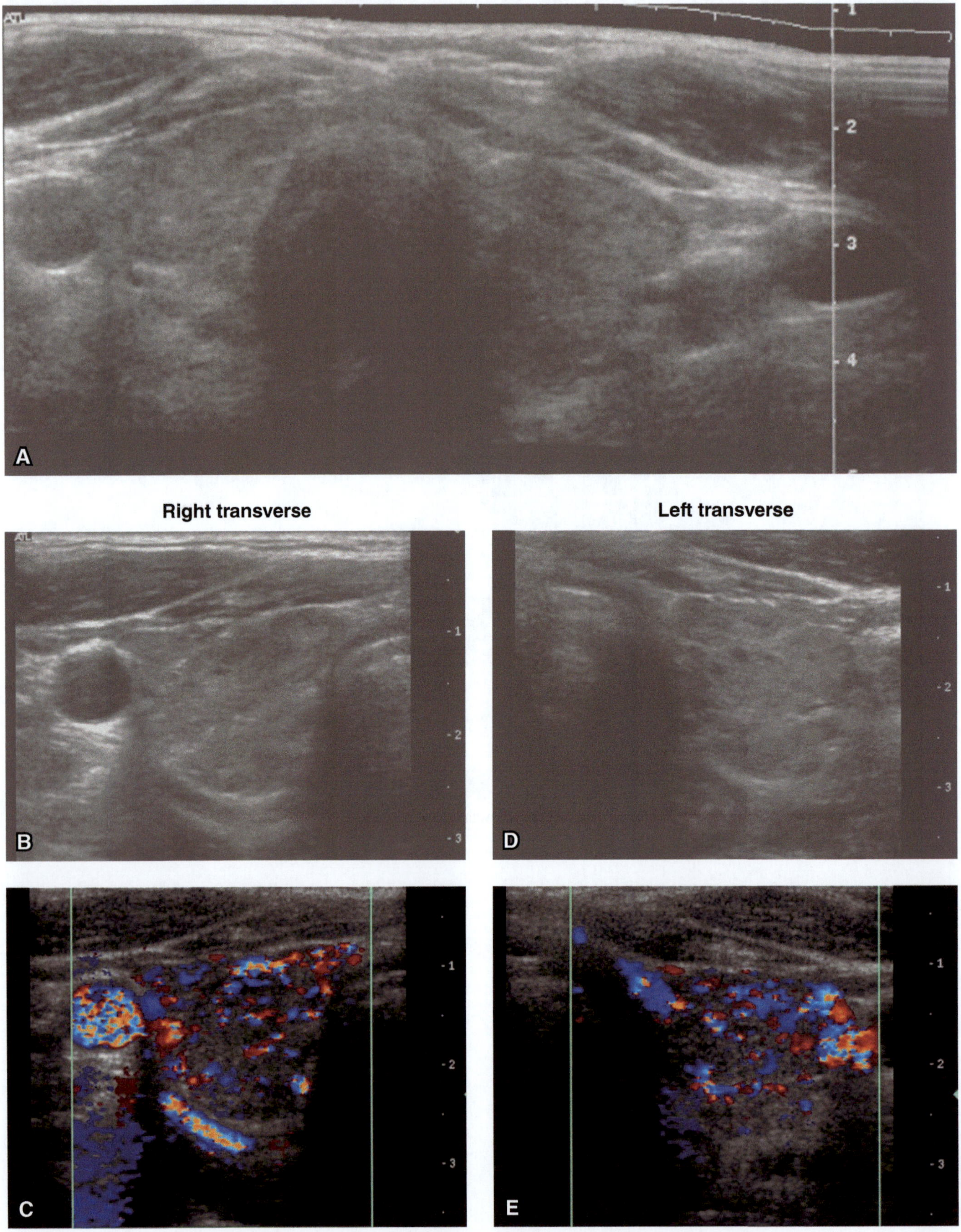

Figure 11-5. Ultrasound of thyroiditis in both lobes. **A**, Both lobes. **B**, Right lobe transverse. **C**, Color Doppler, right lobe transverse. **D**, Left lobe transverse. **E**, Color Doppler, left lobe transverse.

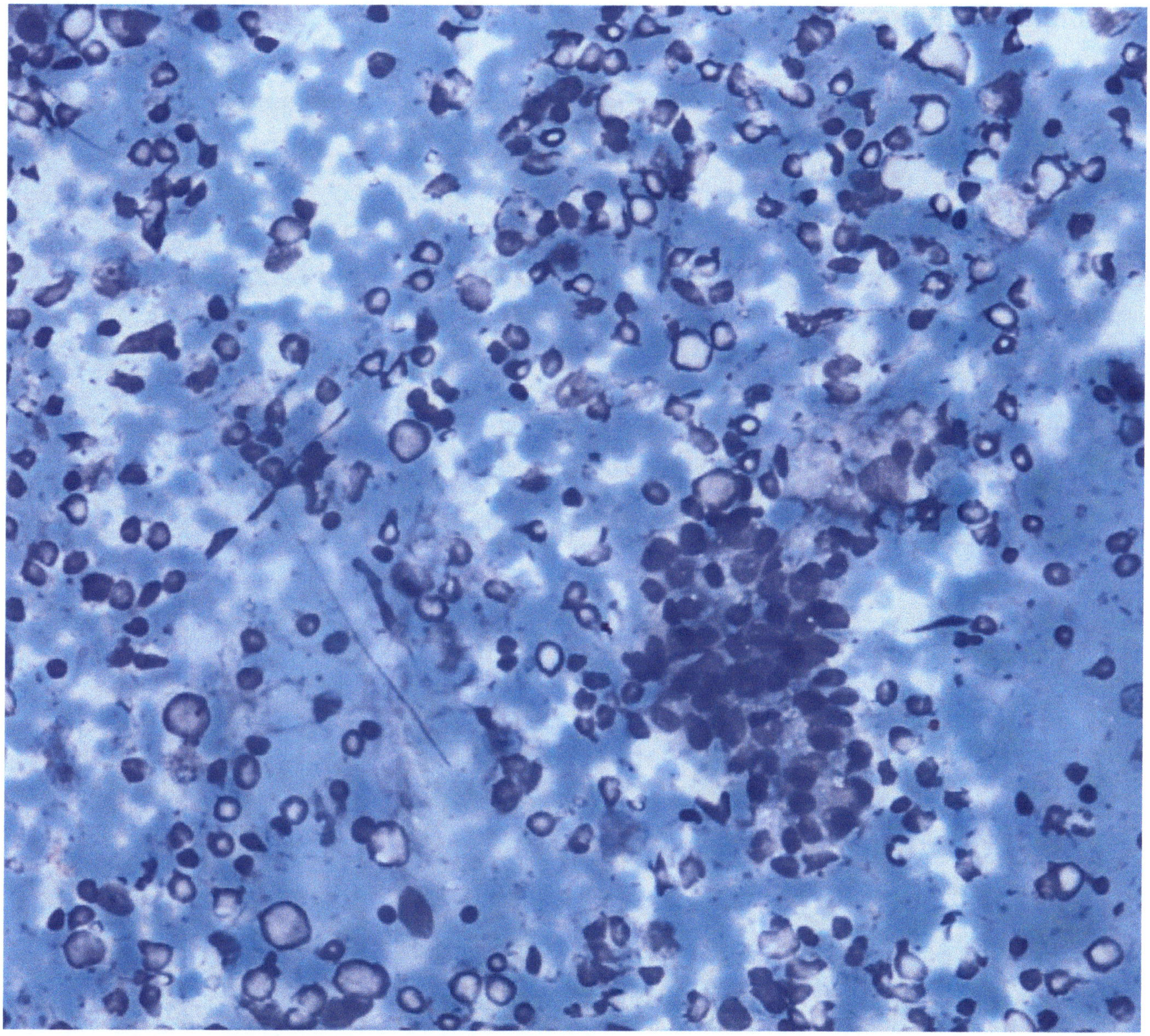

Figure 11-6. Cytology: rich in lymphoid cells. One group of benign, follicular epithelium.

58-Year-old man

- **Clinical history:** Severe hypothyroidism.
- **Ultrasound:** Thyroiditis.
- **Cytology:** Lymphocytic thyroiditis.

Features

Hypoechoic
Whole gland affected
Inhomogeneous, granular echo pattern
Moderate vascularity

Thyroiditis Both Lobes

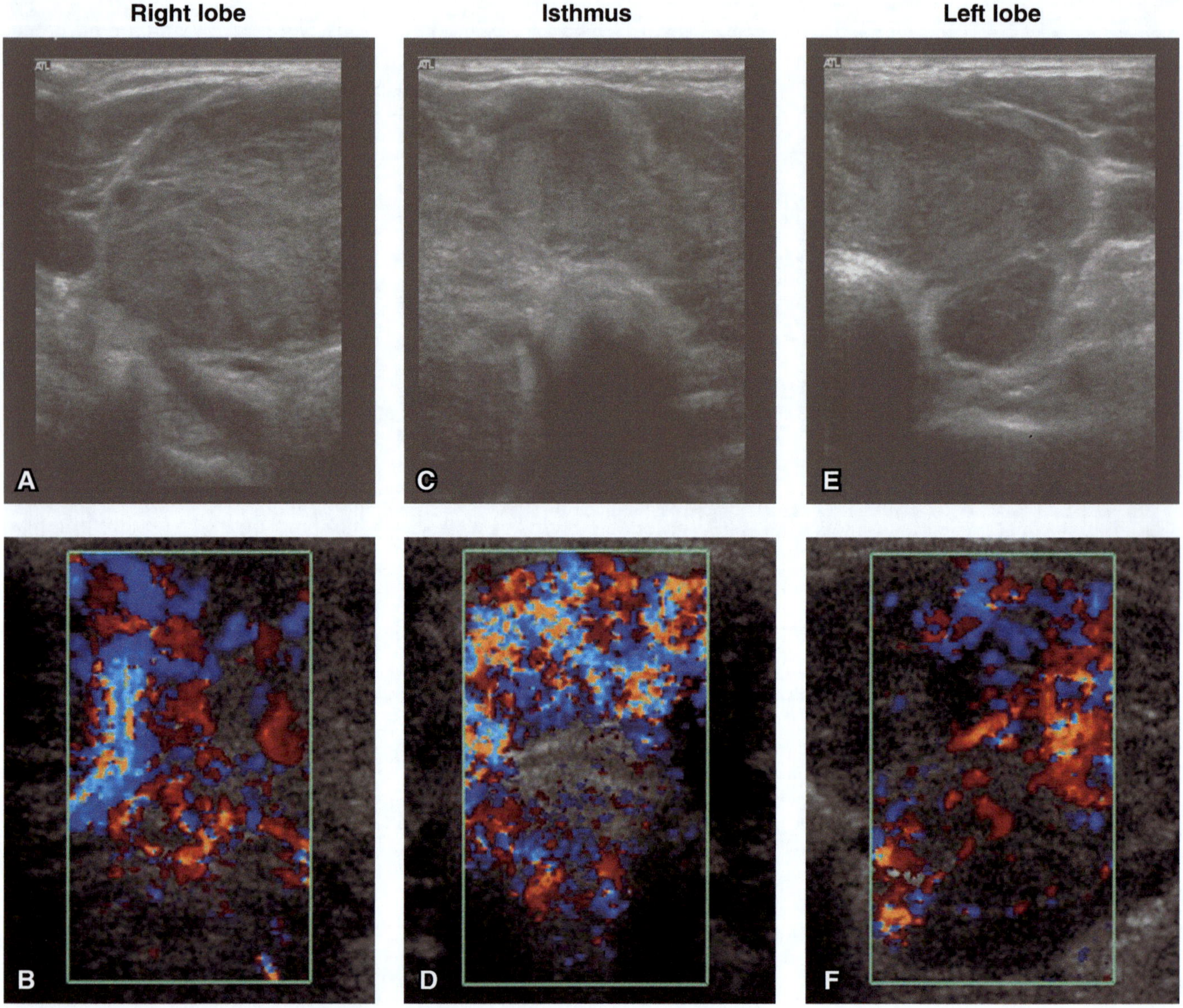

Figure 11-7. Ultrasound of thyroiditis in both lobes. **A**, Right lobe. **B**, Color Doppler, right lobe. **C**, Isthmus. **D**, Color Doppler, isthmus. **E**, Left lobe. **F**, Color Doppler, left lobe.

74-Year-old woman

- **Clinical history:** Rapidly growing thyroid. Anaplastic carcinoma? Lymphoma?
- **Ultrasound:** Probably Hashimoto's thyroiditis.
- **Cytology:** Oxyphilic metaplasia and lymphoid cells.
- **16-Gauge histologic needle biopsy:** Hashimoto's thyroiditis.

Features

Hypoechoic
Whole gland affected
Inhomogeneous, granular echo pattern
Coarse septations
Hypervascular

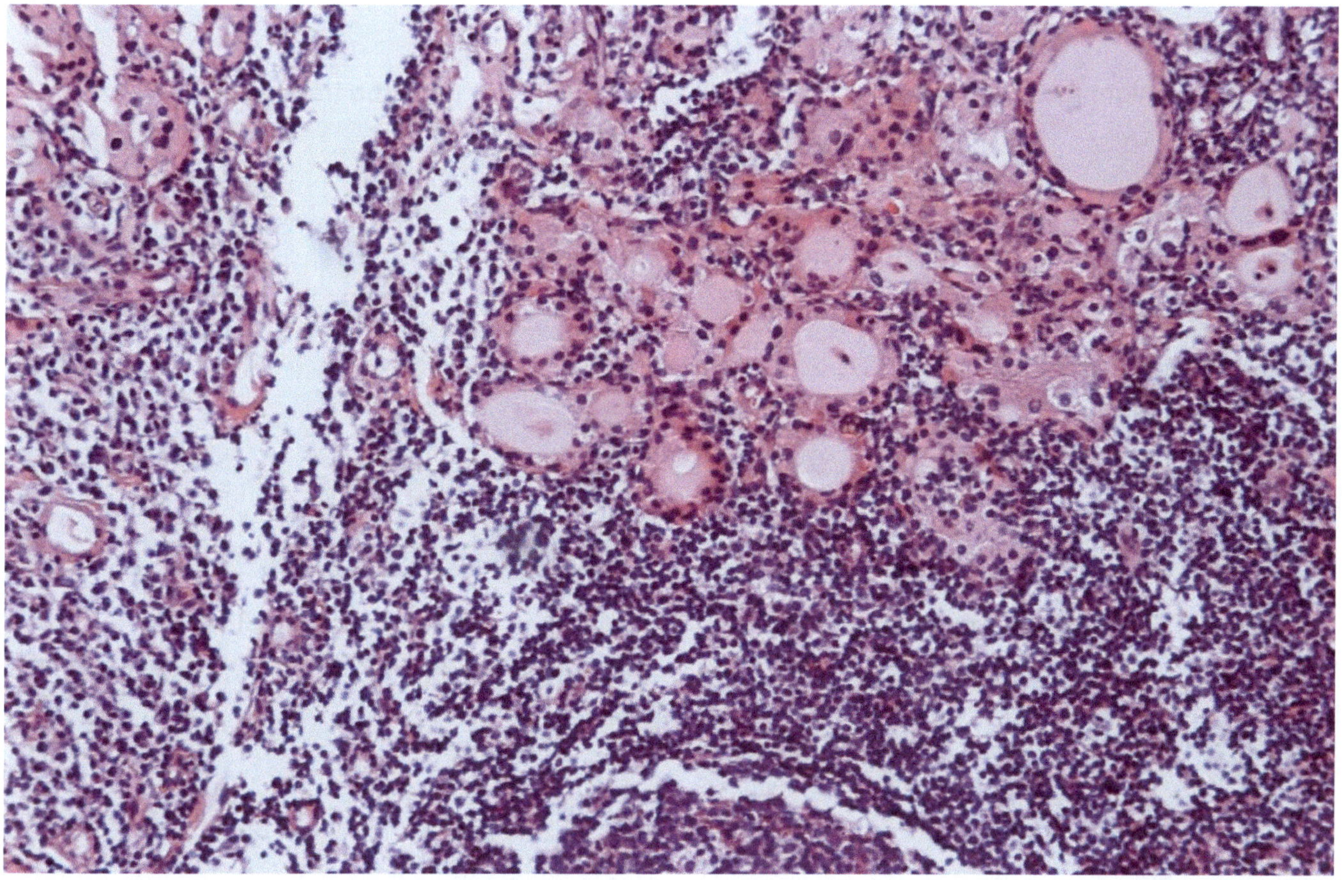

Figure 11-8. Histologic needle biopsies: Hashimoto's thyroiditis.

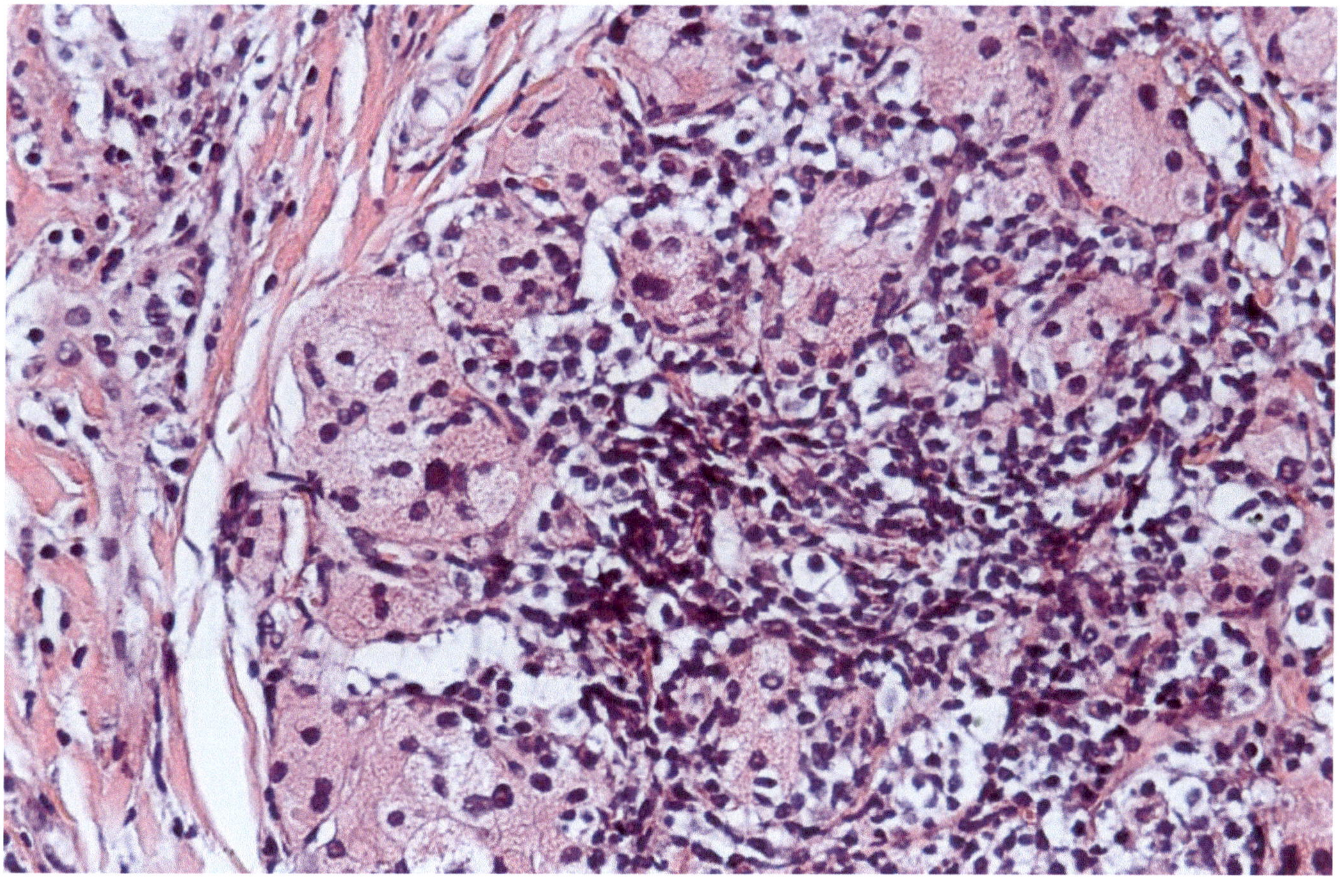

Figure 11-9. Histologic needle biopsies: Hashimoto's thyroiditis.

Thyroiditis Both Lobes

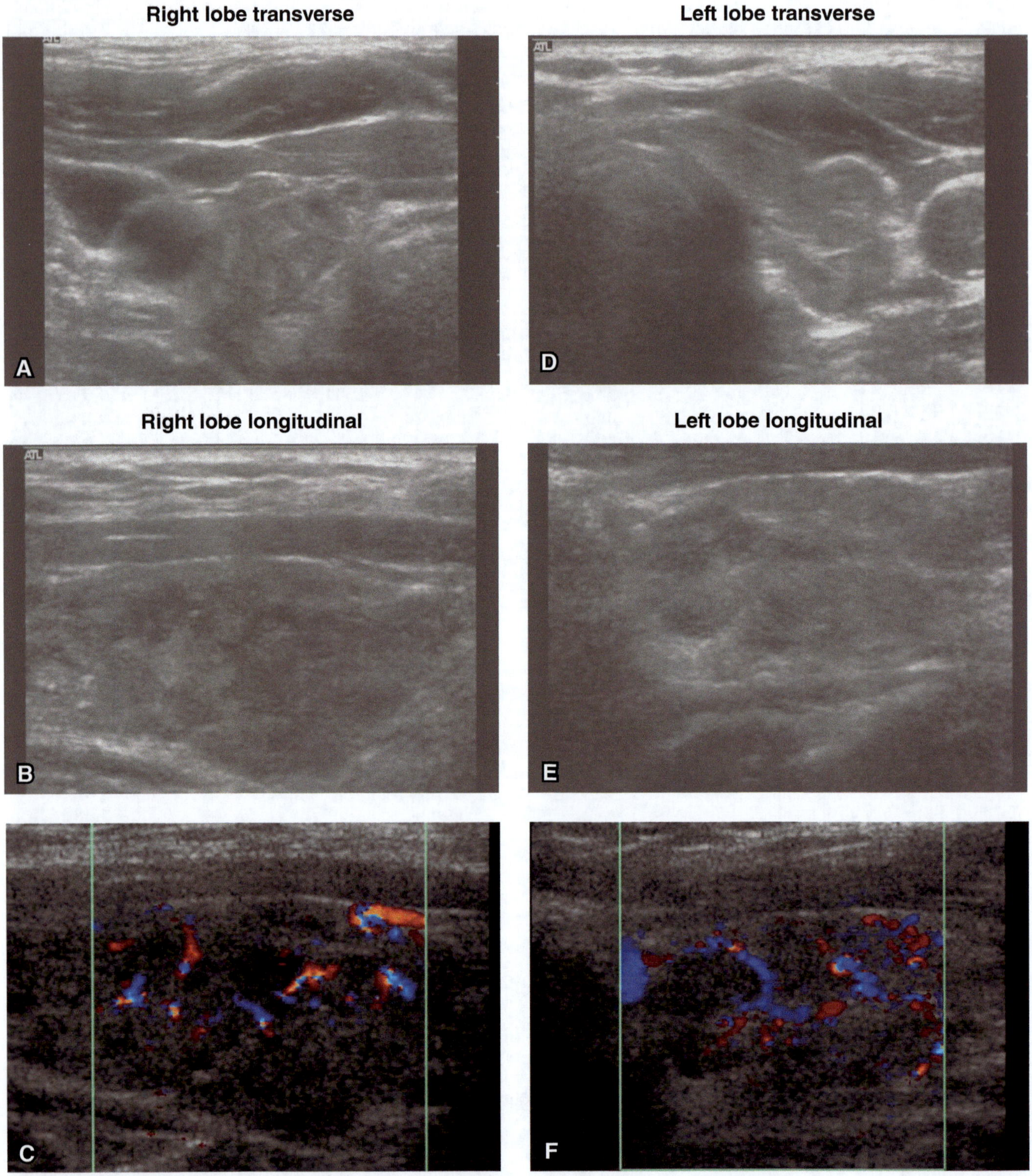

Figure 11-10. Ultrasound of thyroiditis in both lobes. **A**, Right lobe transverse. **B**, Right lobe longitudinal. **C**, Color Doppler, right lobe. **D**, Left lobe transverse. **E**, Left lobe longitudinal. **F**, Color Doppler, left lobe.

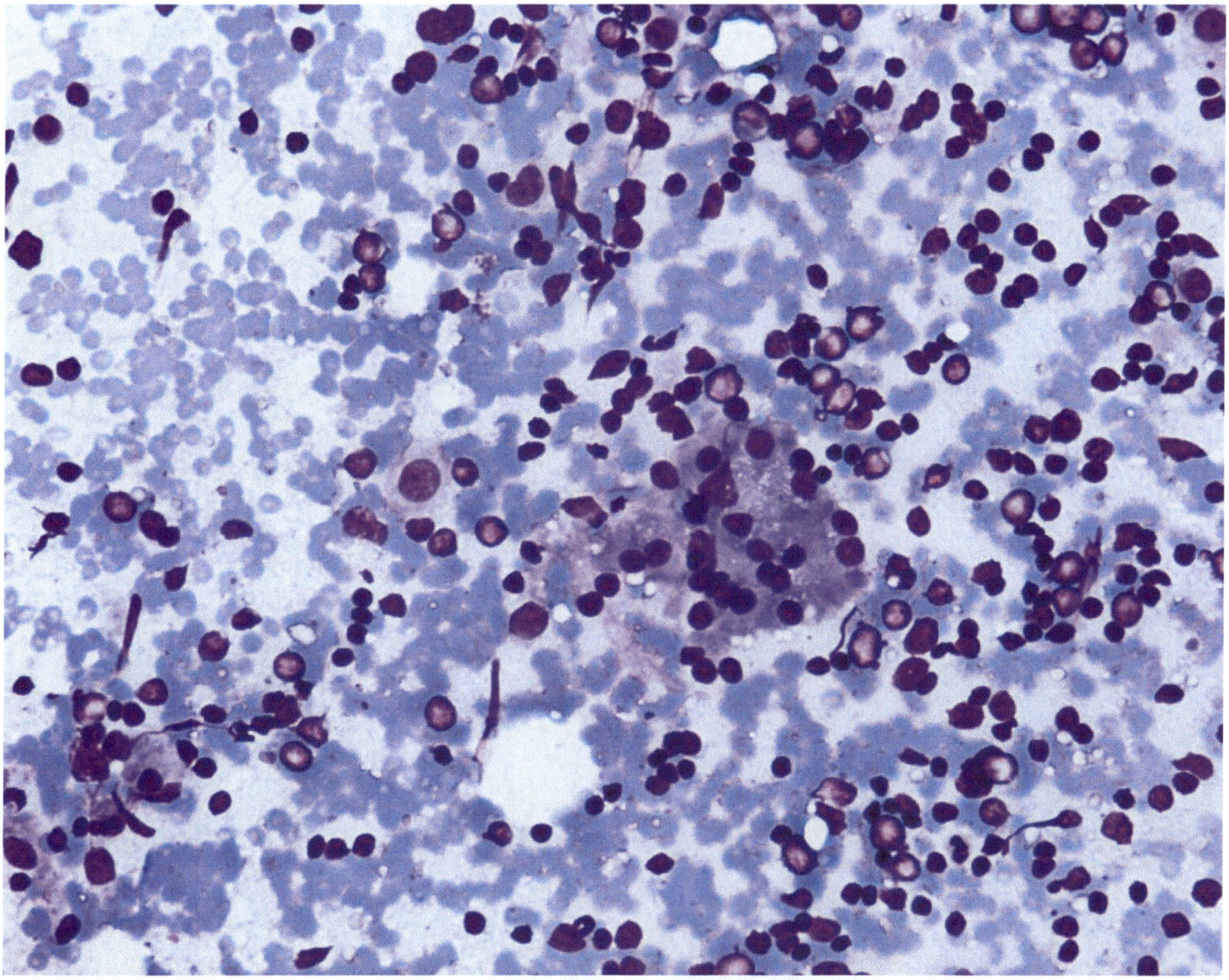

Figure 11-11. Cytology: mixed cell population; lymphoid cells and follicular cells with oncocytic features.

66-Year-old man

- **Clinical history:** Hypothyreosis.
- **Ultrasound:** Hashimoto's thyroiditis.
- **Cytology:** Hashimoto's thyroiditis.

Features

Slightly hypoechoic

Inhomogeneous nodular echo pattern

Whole gland affected

Scant vascularity

Thyroiditis Both Lobes

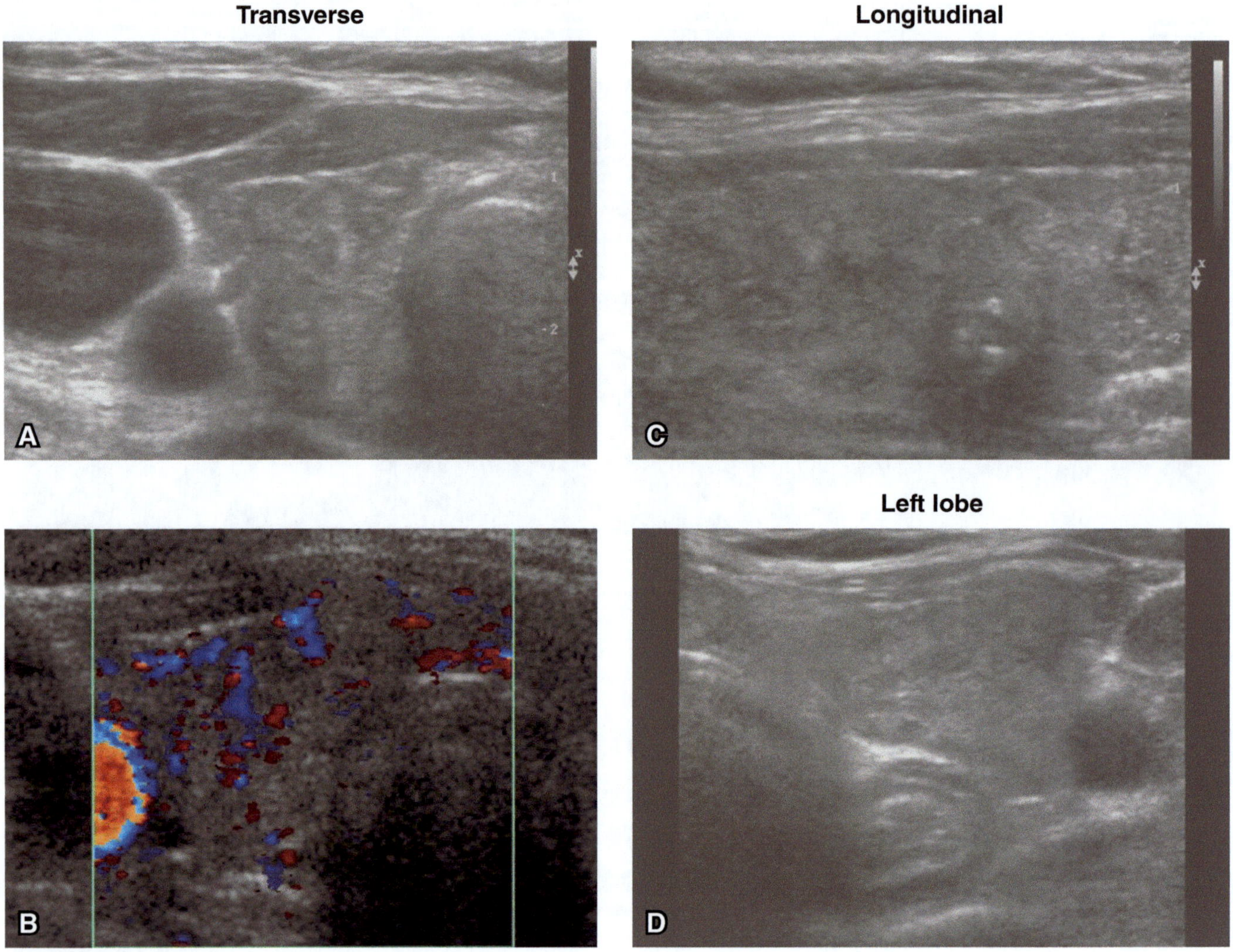

Figure 11-12. Ultrasound of thyroiditis in both lobes. **A**, Transverse. **B**, Color Doppler, transverse. **C**, Longitudinal. **D**, Left lobe longitudinal.

62-Year-old woman

- **Clinical history:** Paraneoplastic cerebellar degeneration past 4 months. Lung and liver metastasis. CT shows tumor in right thyroid lobe.
- **Ultrasound:** 8 mm papillary thyroid carcinoma (PTC) inferiorly in right lobe. Thyroiditis.
- **Cytology:** Nondiagnostic material.
- **Thyroidectomy:** Thyroiditis. 1 mm PTC centrally in right lobe. Hyalin node with calcifications inferiorly in right lobe.

Features

Slightly hypoechoic
Inhomogeneous, nodular echo pattern
Microcalcifications in fibrotic lesion in right lobe
Scant vascularity

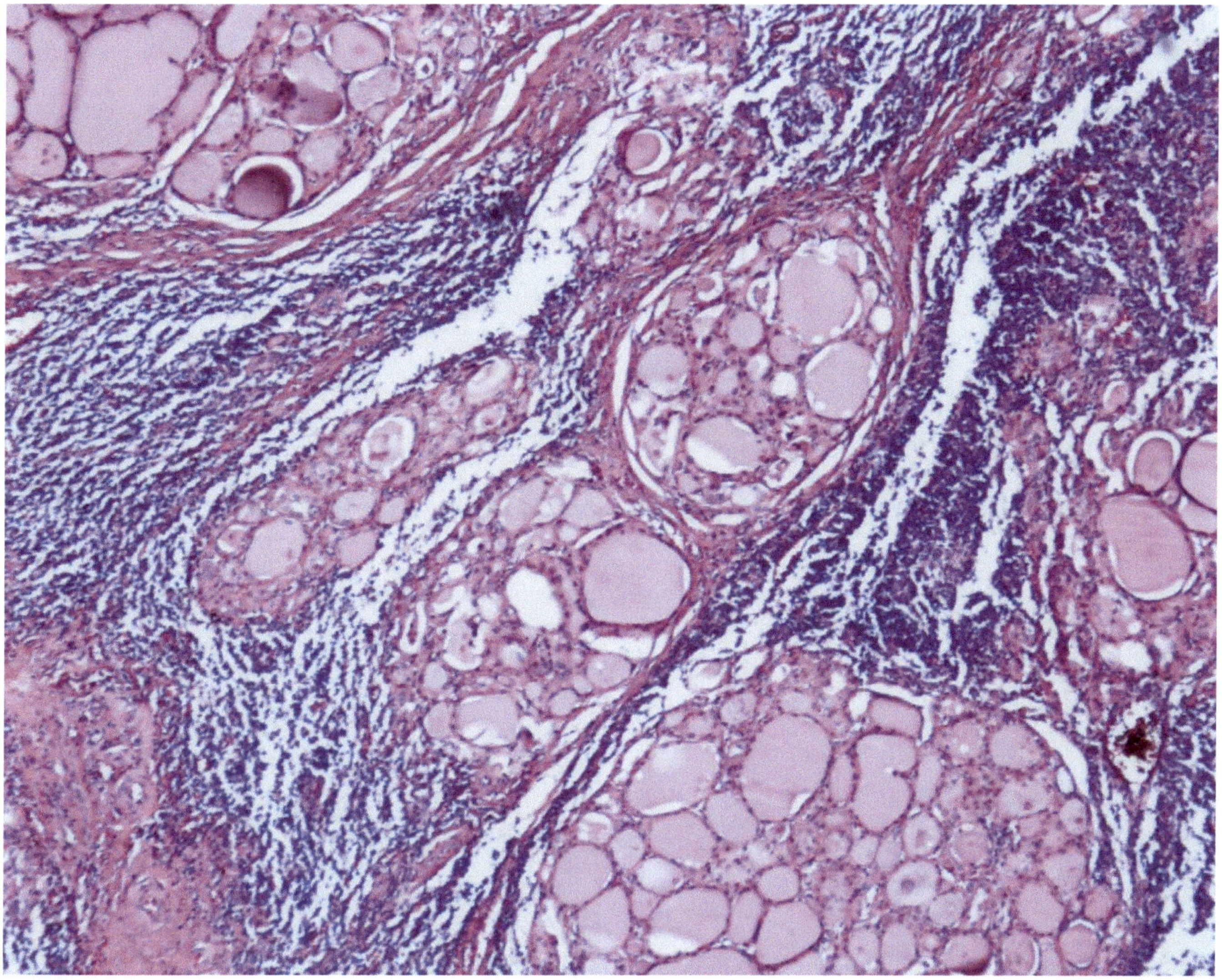

Figure 11-13. Histology: thyroiditis.

Thyroiditis Both Lobes

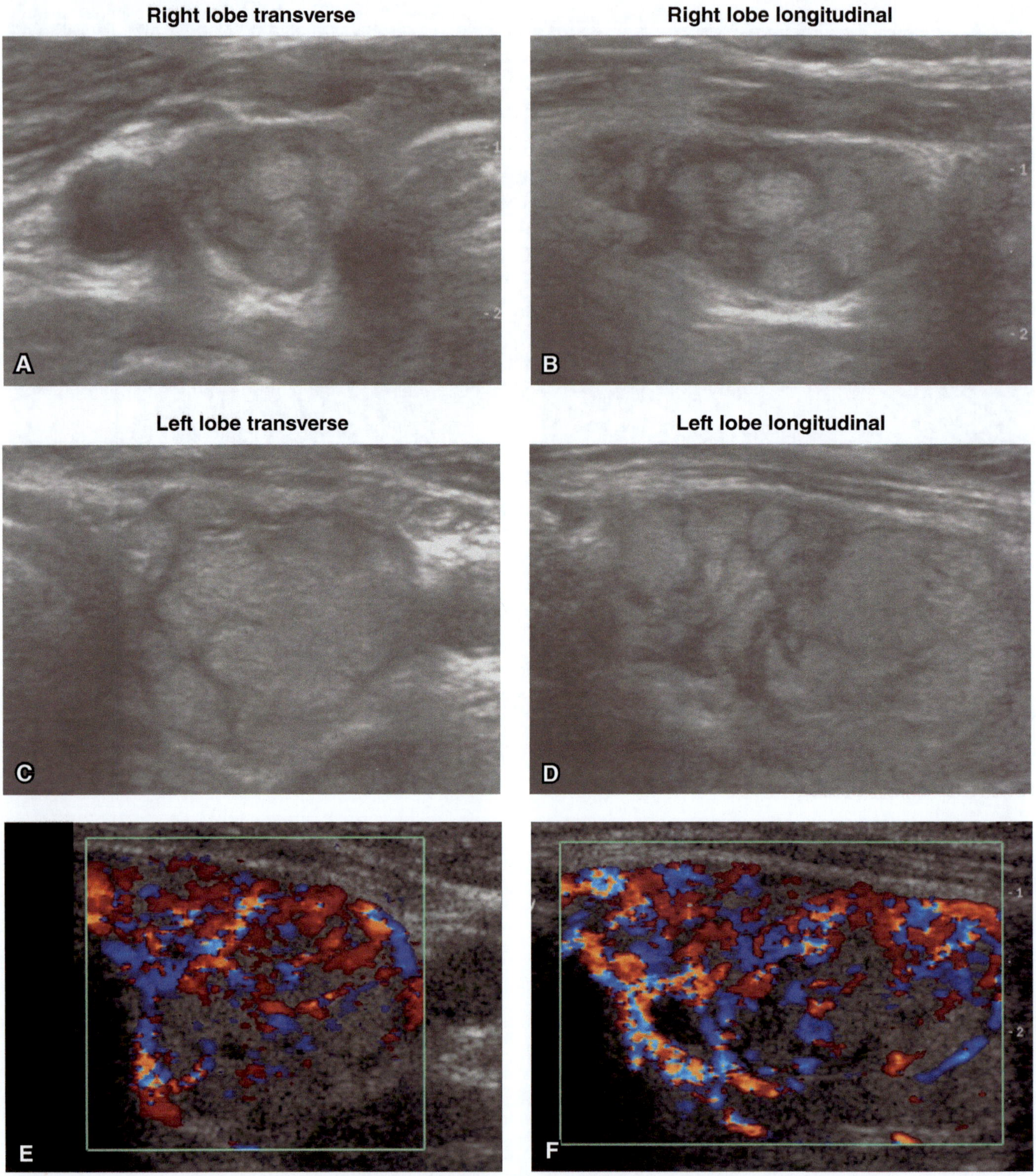

Figure 11-14. Ultrasound of thyroiditis in both lobes. **A**, Right lobe transverse. **B**, Right lobe longitudinal. **C**, Left lobe transverse. **D**, Left lobe longitudinal. **E**, Color Doppler, left lobe transverse. **F**, Color Doppler, left lobe longitudinal.

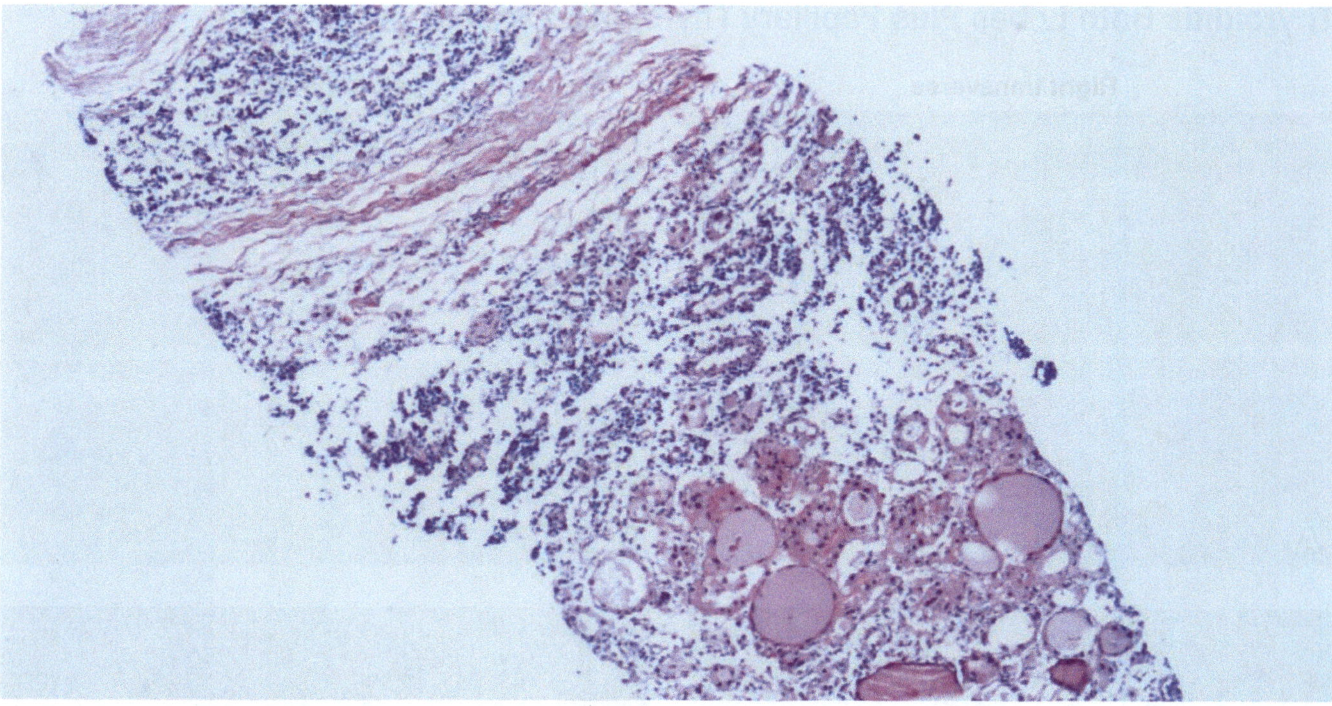

Figure 11-15. Histologic needle biopsy: lymphocytic thyroiditis, Hashimoto's type.

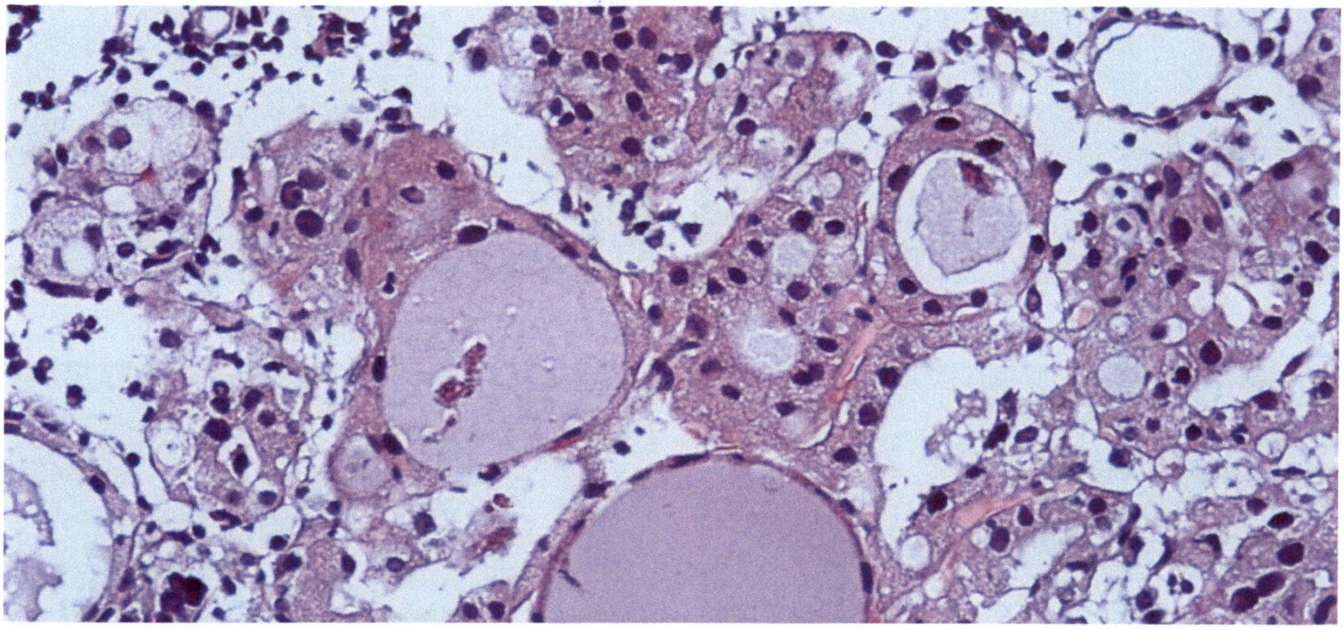

Figure 11-16. Histologic needle biopsy: Hashimoto's thyroiditis.

59-Year-old woman

- **Clinical history:** Thyroxine treatment past 20 years. 8 years ago surgery due to thyrotoxicosis. Last year enlarged left lobe.
- **Ultrasound:** Nodular tissue. Follicular tumors?
- **Cytology:** Follicular cells with oncocytic features.
- **18-Gauge histologic needle biopsy:** Hashimoto's thyroiditis.

Features

Mixed echogenicity
Quite homogeneous echo pattern within well-circumscribed nodules
Whole gland affected
Hypervascular

Thyroiditis Both Lobes Plus Papillary Thyroid Carcinoma

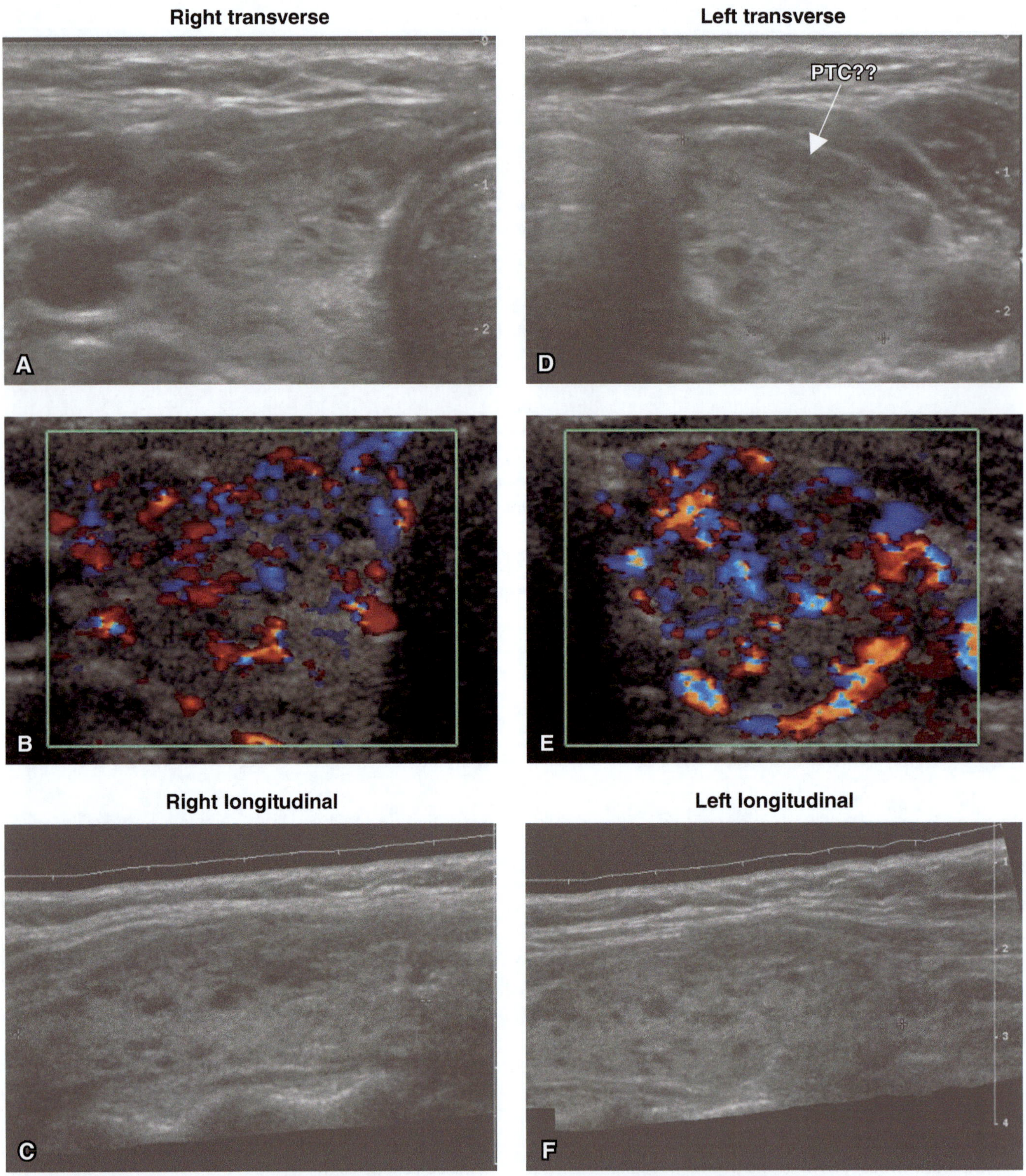

Figure 11-17. Ultrasound of thyroiditis in both lobes plus papillary thyroid carcinoma. **A**, Right lobe transverse. **B**, Color Doppler, right lobe transverse. **C**, Right lobe longitudinal. **D**, Left lobe transverse. **E**, Color Doppler, left lobe transverse. **F**, Left lobe longitudinal.

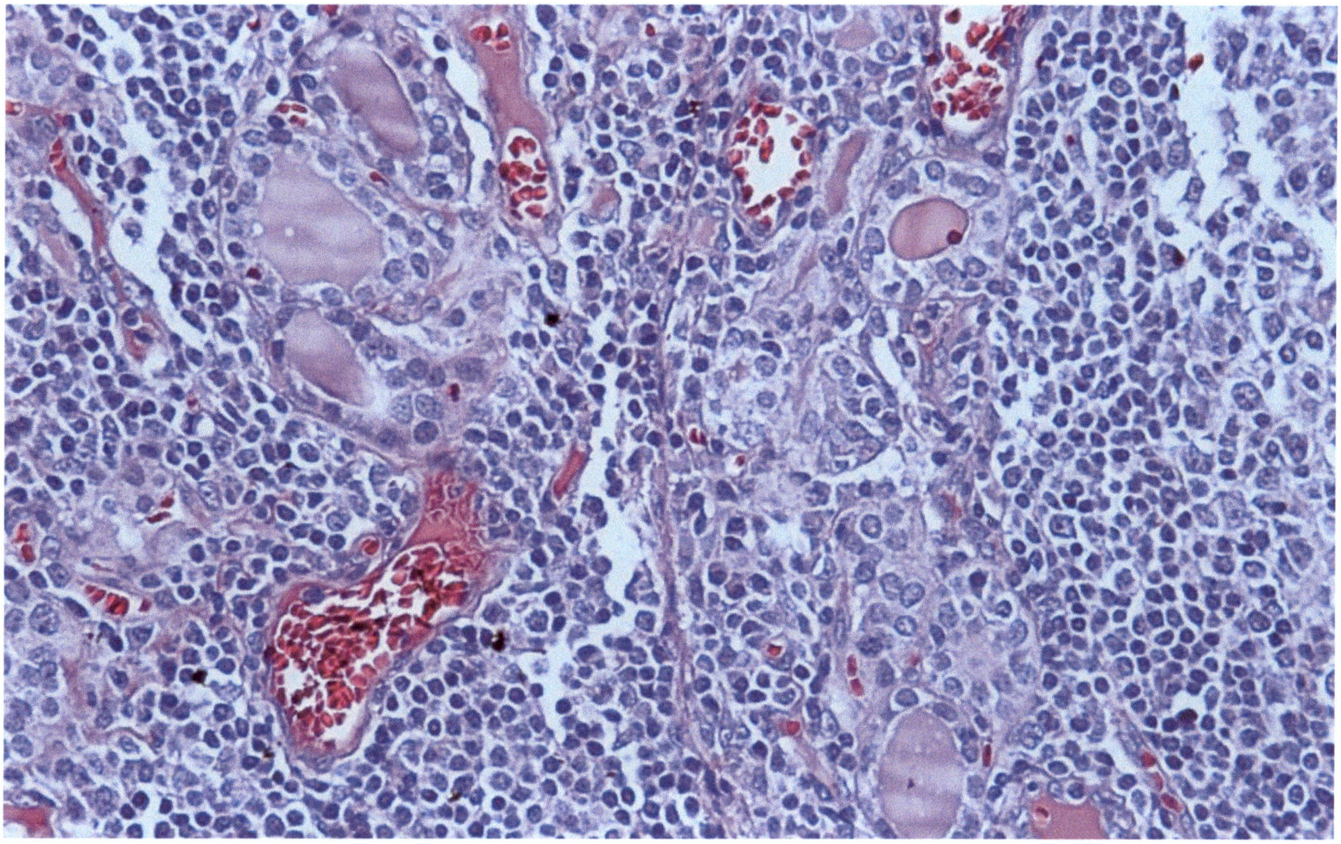

FIGURE 11-18. Histology: thyroiditis of Hashimoto's type.

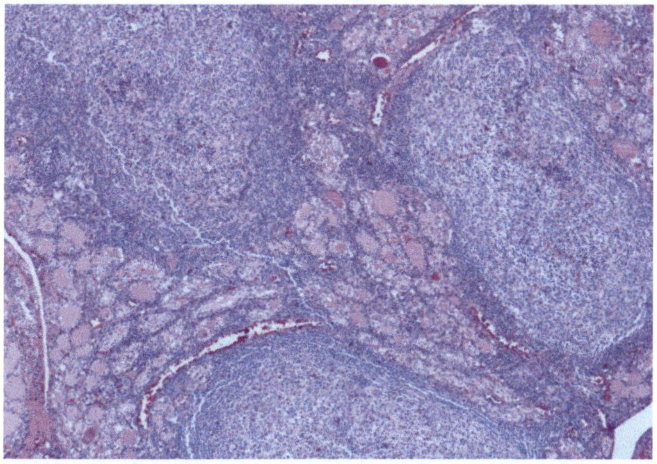

FIGURE 11-19. Histology: extensive thyroiditis.

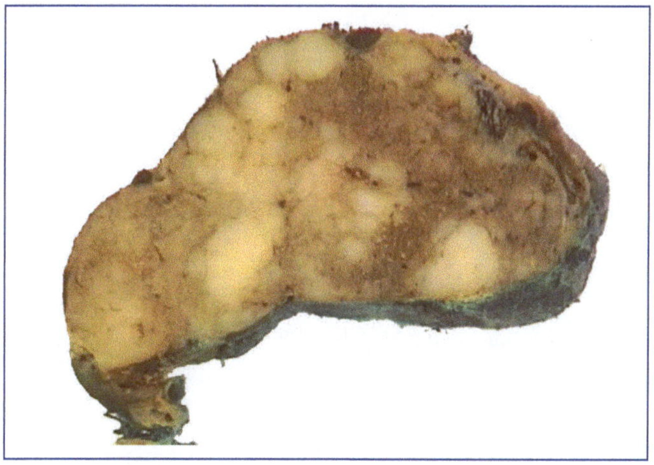

FIGURE 11-20. Gross section: diffusely dispersed, nonencapsulated nodules.

39-Year-old woman

- **Clinical history:** Cystic neck metastasis from papillary thyroid carcinoma (PTC) verified left side.
- **Ultrasound:** Thyroiditis. Also PTC?
- **Cytology:** Hashimoto's thyroiditis.
- **Thyroidectomy:** Three PTCs: 8, 2, and 1.2 mm + extensive Hashimoto's thyroiditis.

Features

Slightly hypoechoic with innumerable small hypoechoic nodules
Whole gland affected
One larger hypoechoic area anteriorly in left lobe
Moderate vascularity

Thyroiditis Both Lobes

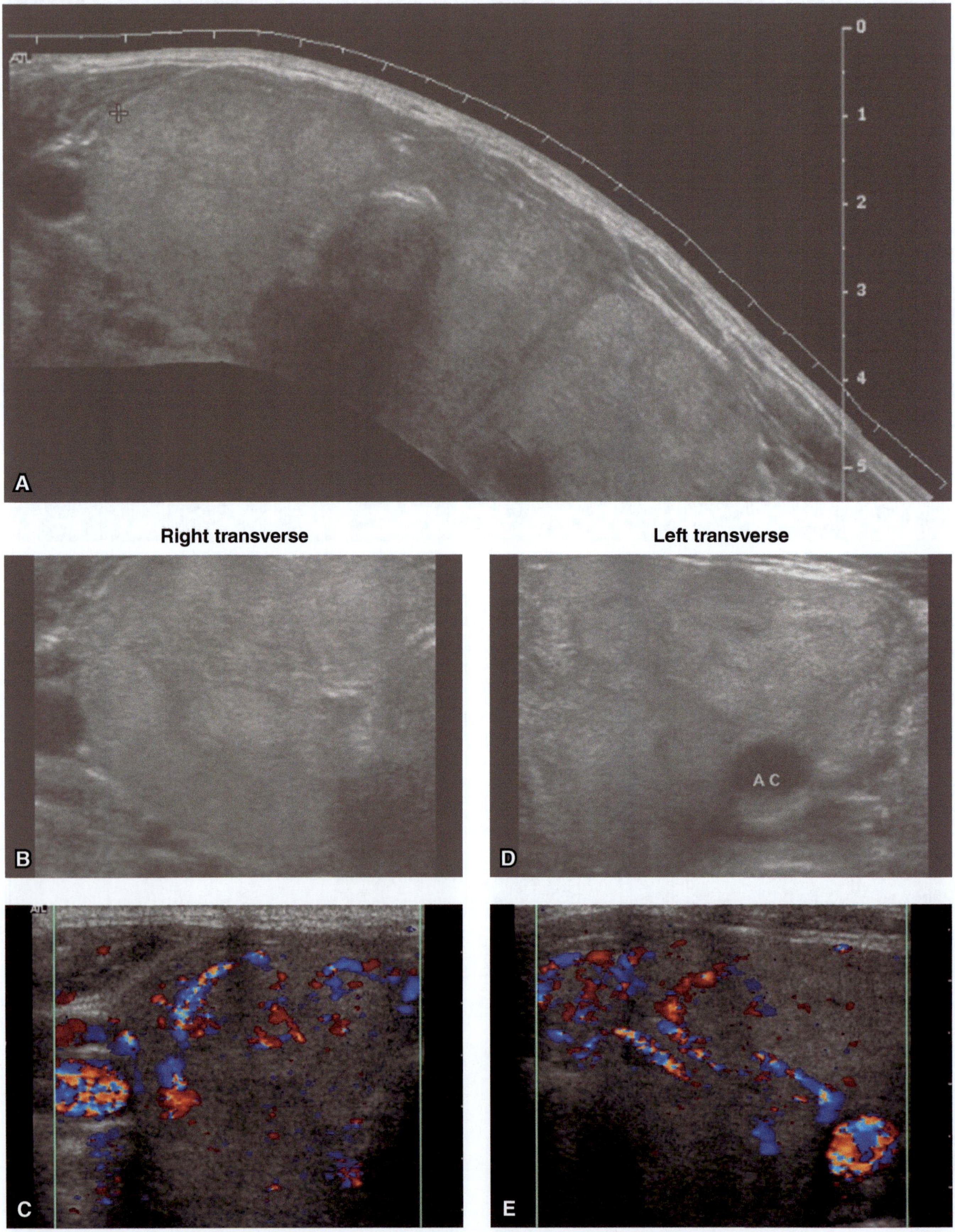

FIGURE 11-21. Ultrasound of thyroiditis in both lobes. **A**, Both lobes. **B**, Right lobe transverse. **C**, Color Doppler, right lobe transverse. **D**, Left lobe transverse. **E**, Color Doppler, left lobe transverse.

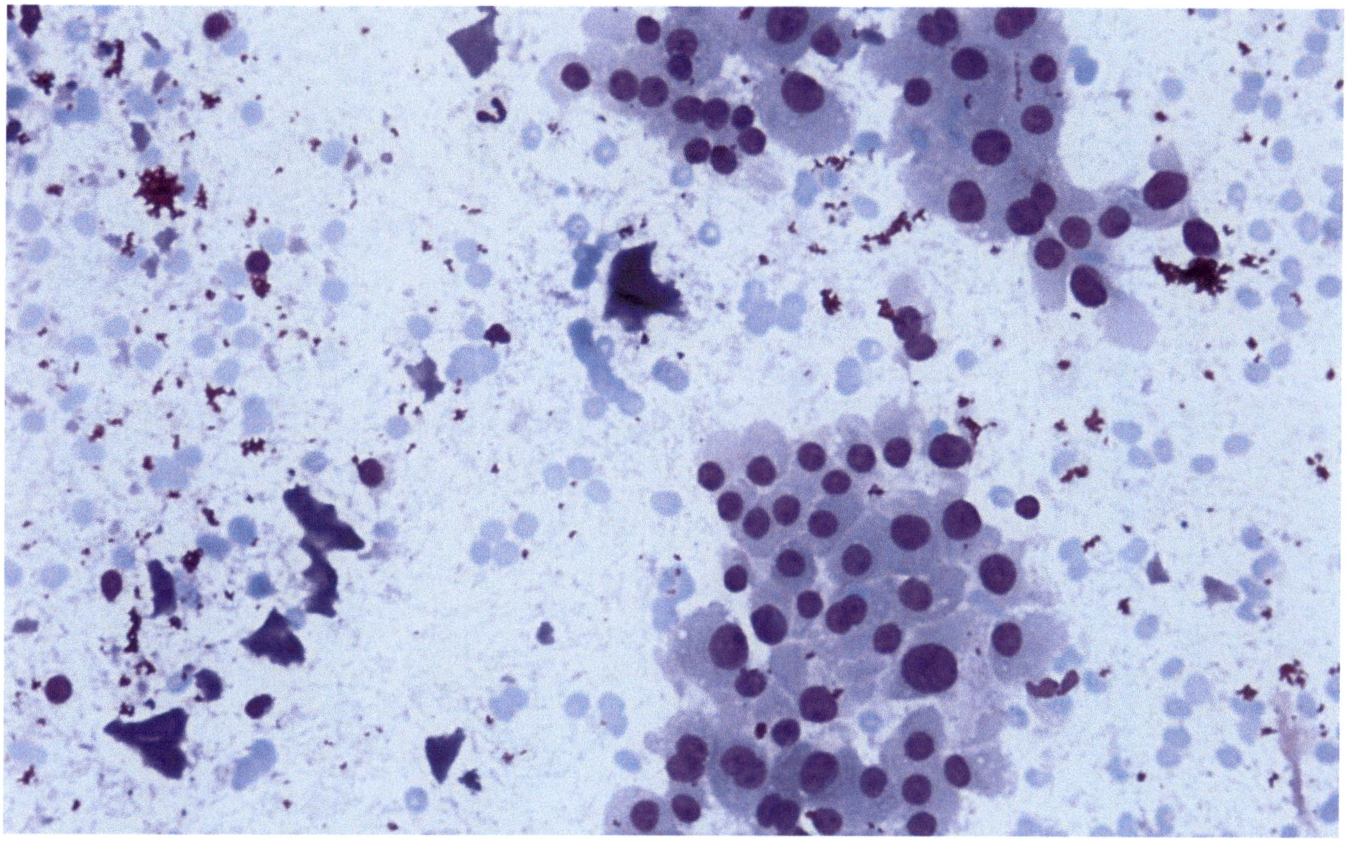

FIGURE 11-22. Cytology: dominated by metaplastic follicular cells. Few lymphoid cells.

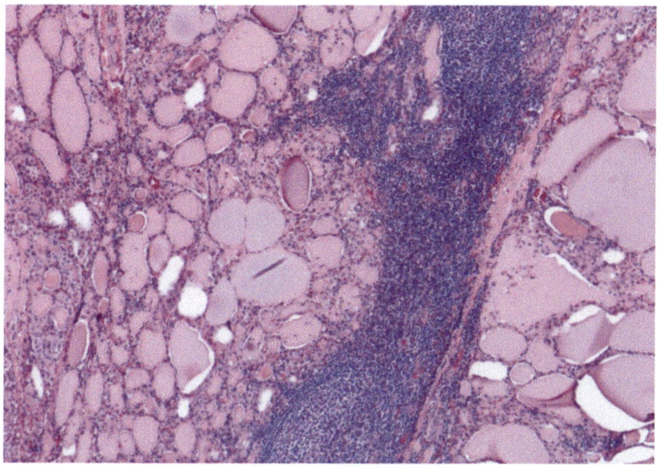

FIGURE 11-23. Histology: lymphocytic thyroiditis.

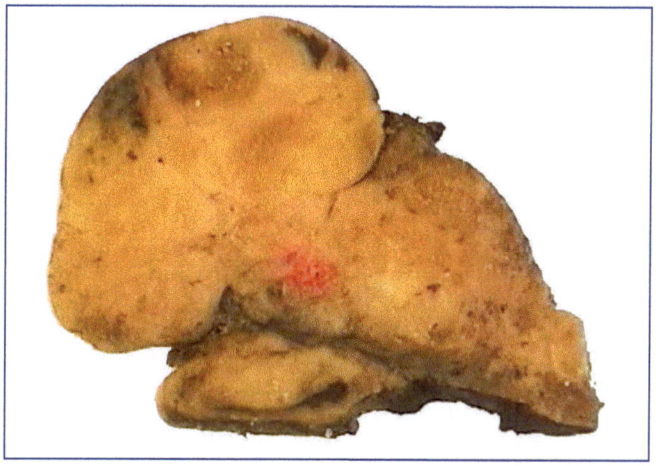

FIGURE 11-24. Gross section: diffusely enlarged lobe.

59-Year-old woman

- **Clinical history:** Not known.
- **Ultrasound:** Diffuse goiter.
- **Cytology:** Follicular cells with oncocytic features. Neoplasia?
- **Thyroidectomy:** Hashimoto's thyroiditis.

Features

Isoechoic
Homogeneous echo pattern
Whole gland affected
Scant vascularity

12 Metastases

Metastases in the thyroid gland are rare and the ultrasound appearance depends on the primary tumor. They are most commonly seen in patients with renal cell carcinomas, breast carcinomas, and malignant melanomas [6,7]. In renal cell carcinoma a metastasis may be the first sign of the disease, but when metastases from the other malignancies are found, the diagnosis of the primary tumor will usually already be known.

Cytologic Morphology

The possibility of metastasis must always be considered when the morphology demonstrates atypical cells of a type not usually found in the thyroid or thyroid-derived lesions. The differentiation of metastasis from lung carcinoma may be very difficult, both morphologically and with the use of immunohistochemistry (lung carcinoma and thyroid carcinoma are often positive for thyroid transcription factor-1 [TTF-1]). Clinical information is of crucial importance.

When it comes to metastasis from a renal cell tumor, the clear cells of this tumor may be indistinguishable from a follicular carcinoma of thyroid origin with clear cell metaplasia. Immunocytochemistry of unstained smears for the markers of renal cell carcinoma (RCC), TTF-1, and thyroglobulin may be of some help.

As Melan A and HMB45 may be helpful when there is a suspicion of metastasis from malignant melanoma, likewise estrogen, progesterone, and AP15 may be helpful when the morphology indicates the possibility of metastasis from breast carcinoma.

Metastasis Left Lobe (Leiomyosarcoma)

Transverse

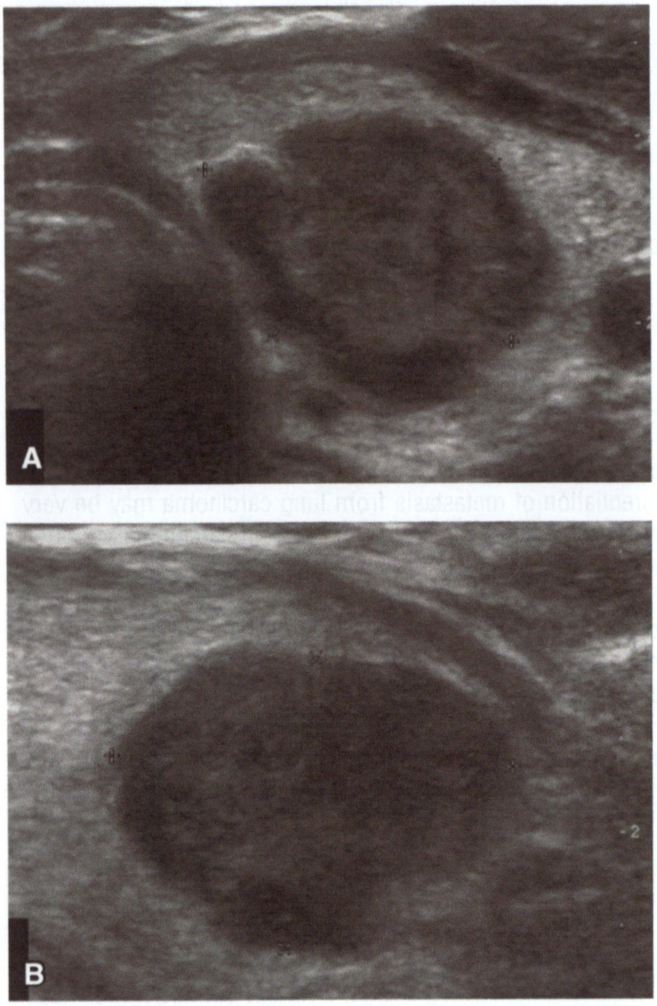

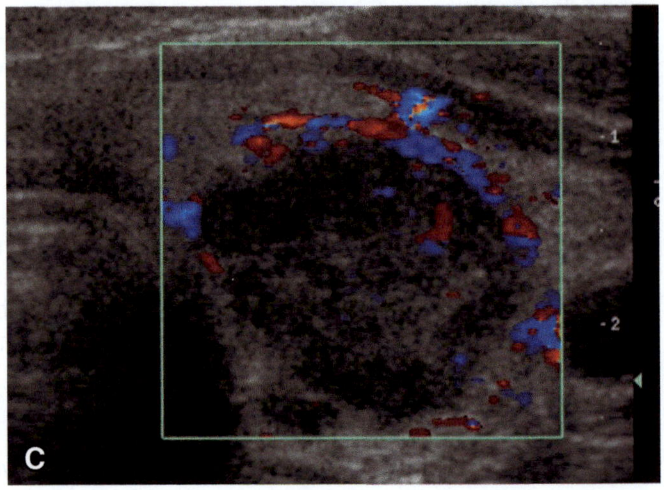

Figure 12-1. Ultrasound of metastasis in the left lobe (leiomyosarcoma). **A** and **B**, Transverse. **C**, Color Doppler.

44-Year-old woman

- **Clinical history:** Leiomyosarcoma with metastasis. CT showed incidentaloma in left thyroid lobe.
- **Ultrasound:** Malignant tumor in left lobe. Primary? Metastasis?
- **Cytology:** Metastasis from leiomyosarcoma.

Features

Strongly hypoechoic
Inhomogeneous echo pattern
Blurred margins
Some microcalcifications
Scant peripheral vascularity

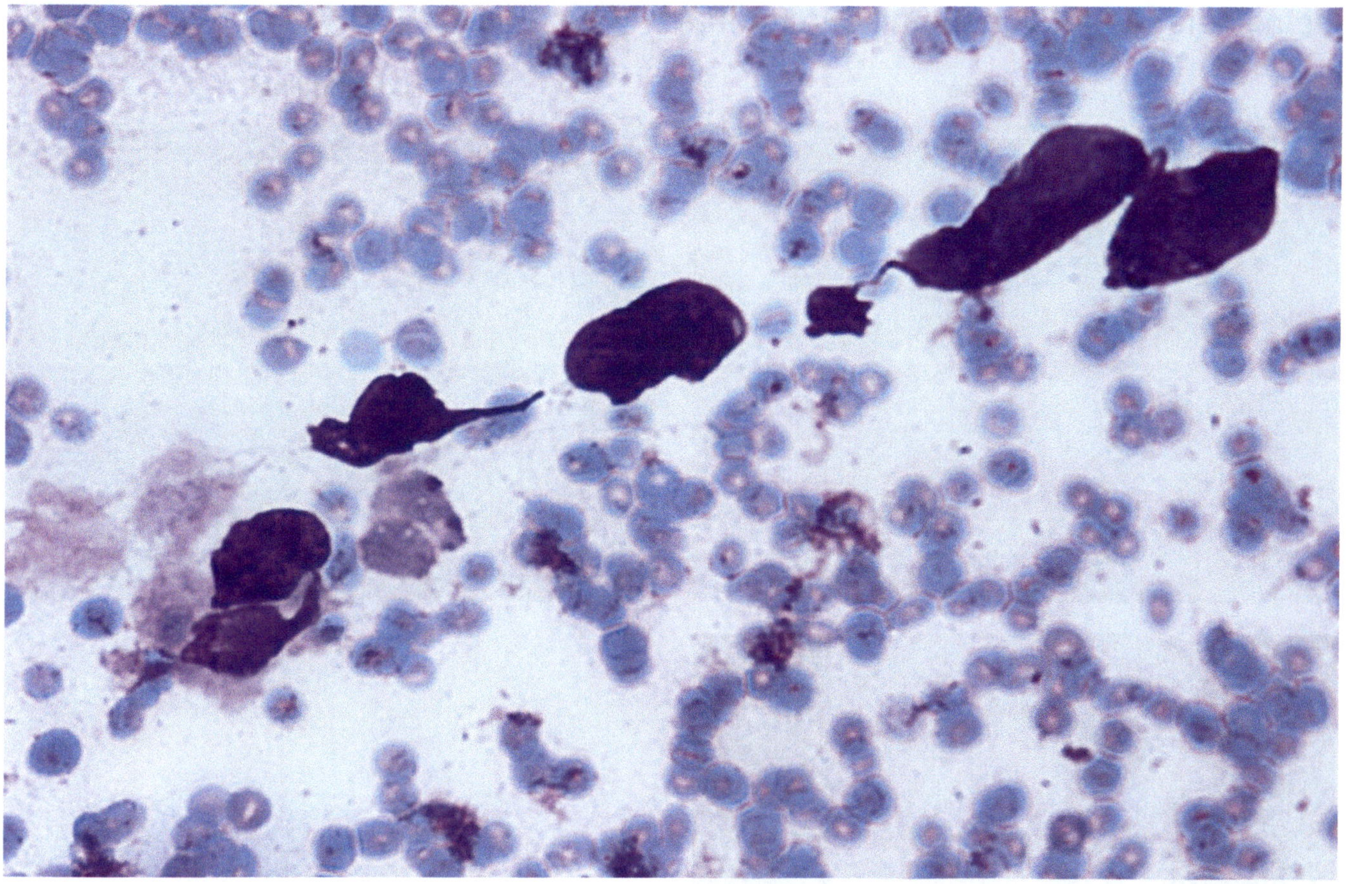

Figure 12-2. Cytology: high-grade malignant cells.

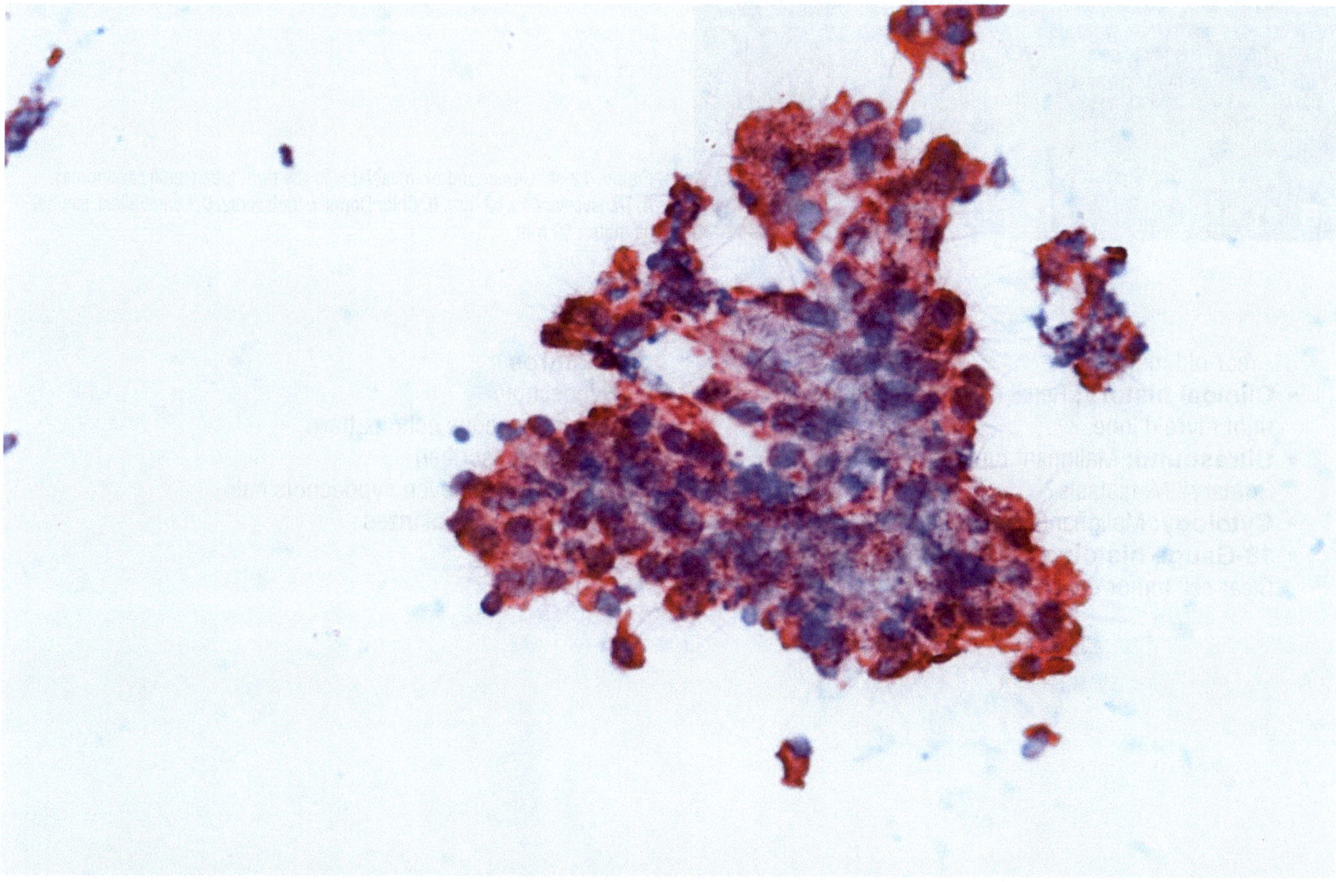

Figure 12-3. Cytology: malignant cells positive for desmin, consistent with metastasis from leiomyosarcoma.

Metastasis Right Lobe (Renal Carcinoma)

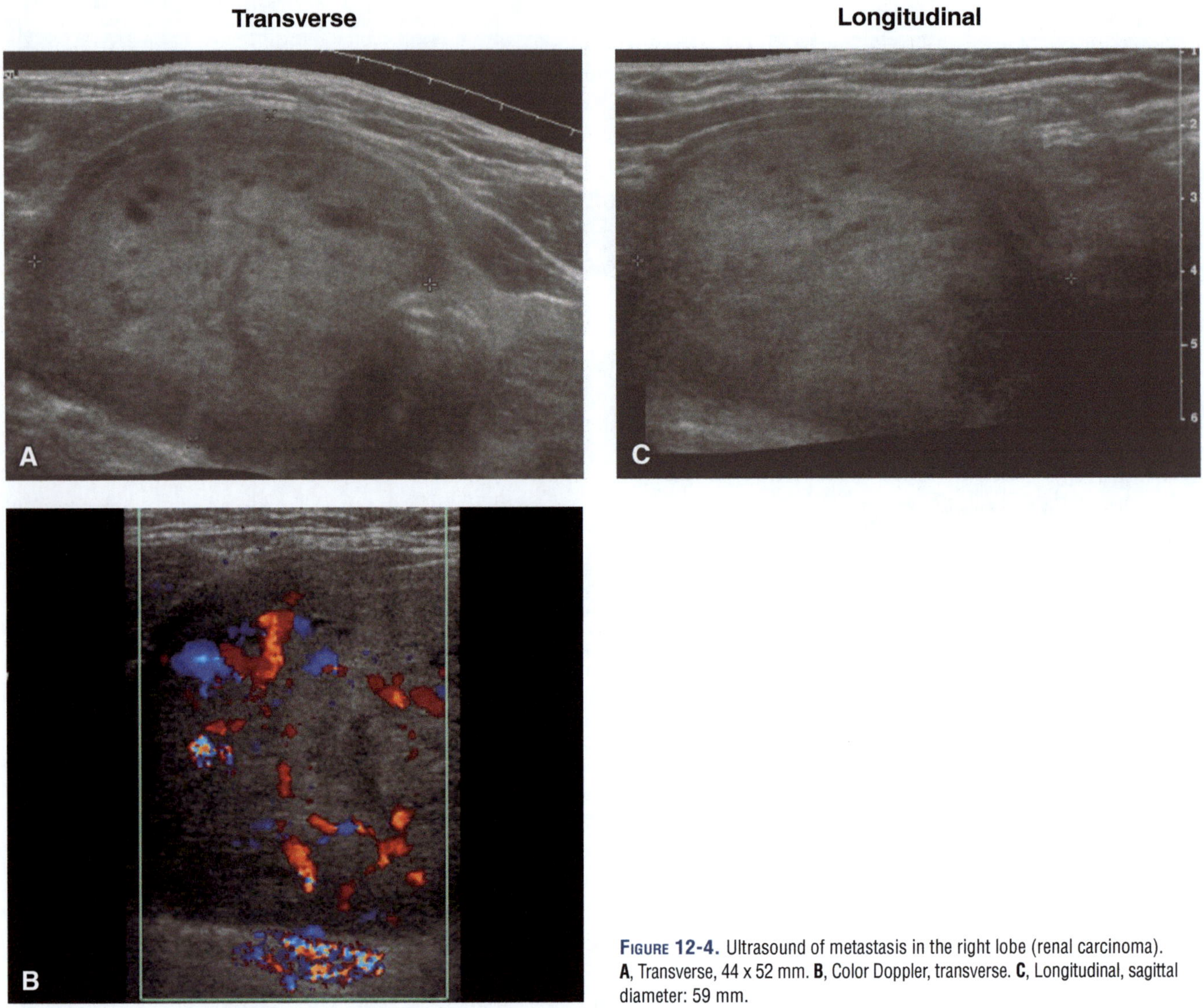

Figure 12-4. Ultrasound of metastasis in the right lobe (renal carcinoma). **A**, Transverse, 44 x 52 mm. **B**, Color Doppler, transverse. **C**, Longitudinal, sagittal diameter: 59 mm.

61-Year-old man

- **Clinical history:** Renal carcinoma. Tumor in right thyroid lobe.
- **Ultrasound:** Malignant tumor in right lobe. Primary? Metastasis?
- **Cytology:** Malignant clear cells.
- **18-Gauge histologic needle biopsy:** Clear cell tumor consistent with renal carcinoma.

Features

Hypoechoic
Inhomogeneous echo pattern
Well circumscribed
Partial thick, uneven hypoechoic halo
Moderately vascularized

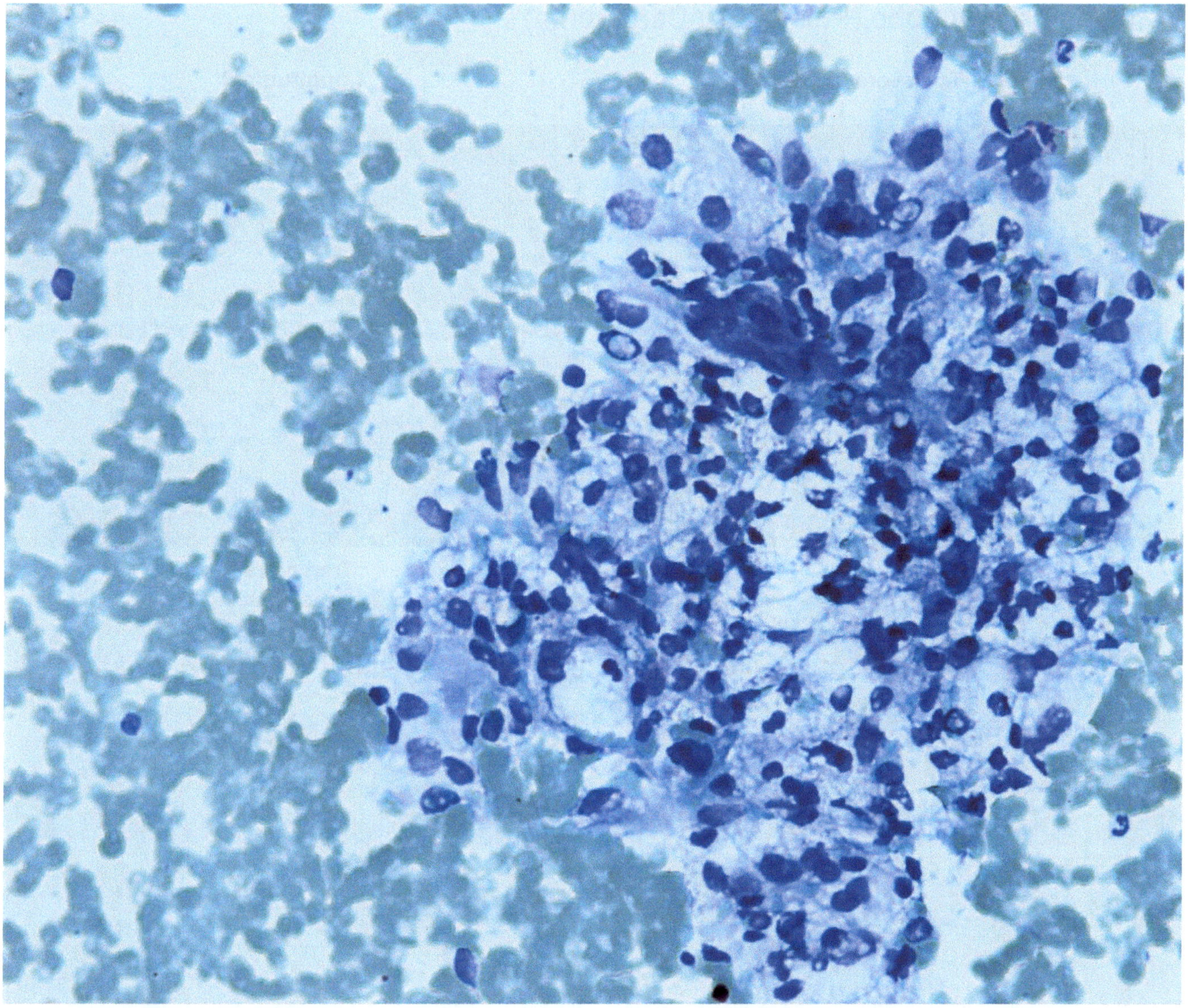

Figure 12-5. Cytology: malignant clear cells.

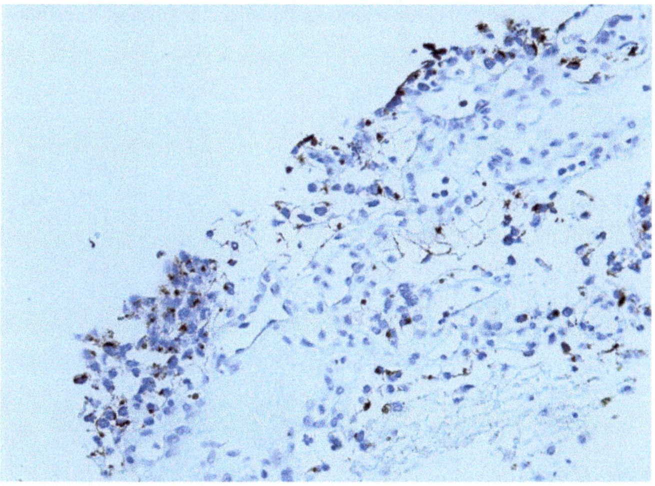

Figure 12-6. Immunohistochemistry: malignant cells positive for renal cell carcinoma marker (RCC).

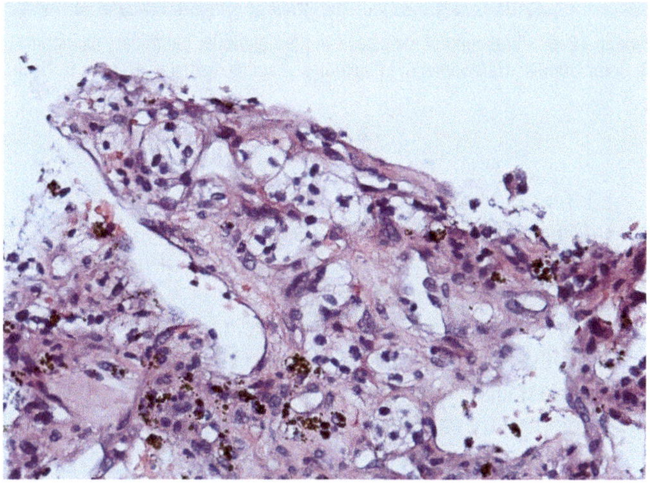

Figure 12-7. Histologic needle biopsy: metastasis from clear cell carcinoma.

Metastasis Right Lobe (Pulmonary Carcinoma)

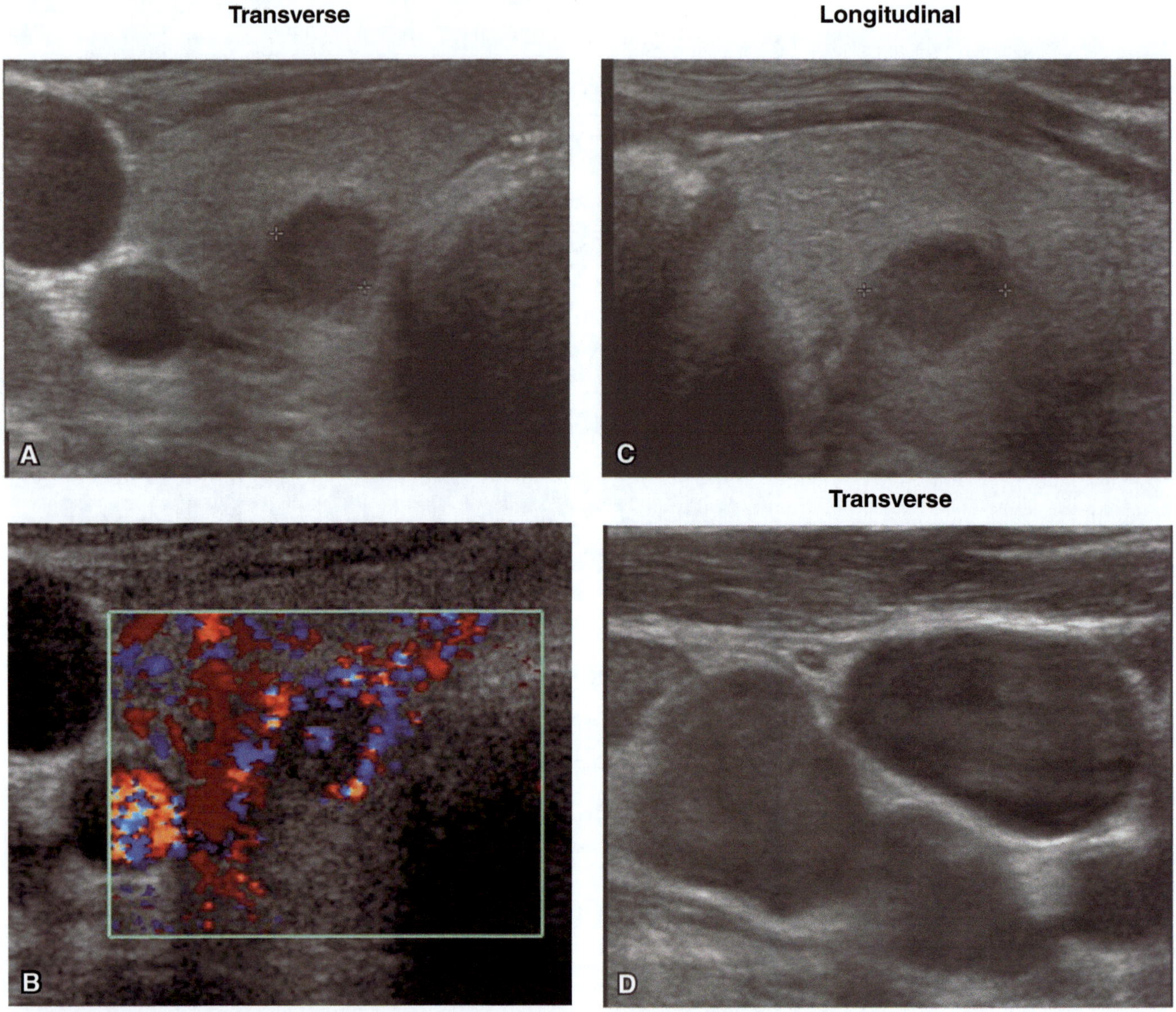

Figure 12-8. Ultrasound of metastasis in the right lobe (pulmonary carcinoma). **A**, Transverse diameter: 7 mm. **B**, Color Doppler, transverse. **C**, Longitudinal, sagittal diameter: 10 mm. **D**, Neck, transverse, metastases.

50-Year-old man

- **Clinical history:** Enlarged neck lymph nodes.
- **Ultrasound:** Lymph node metastases. Probably metastasis in right thyroid lobe.
- **Cytology:** Metastasis from carcinoma.
- **18-Gauge histologic needle biopsy:** Metastasis from mucinous adenocarcinoma (pulmonary carcinoma).

Features of thyroid tumor

Strongly hypoechoic
Homogeneous echo pattern
Well circumscribed
Scantly vascularized

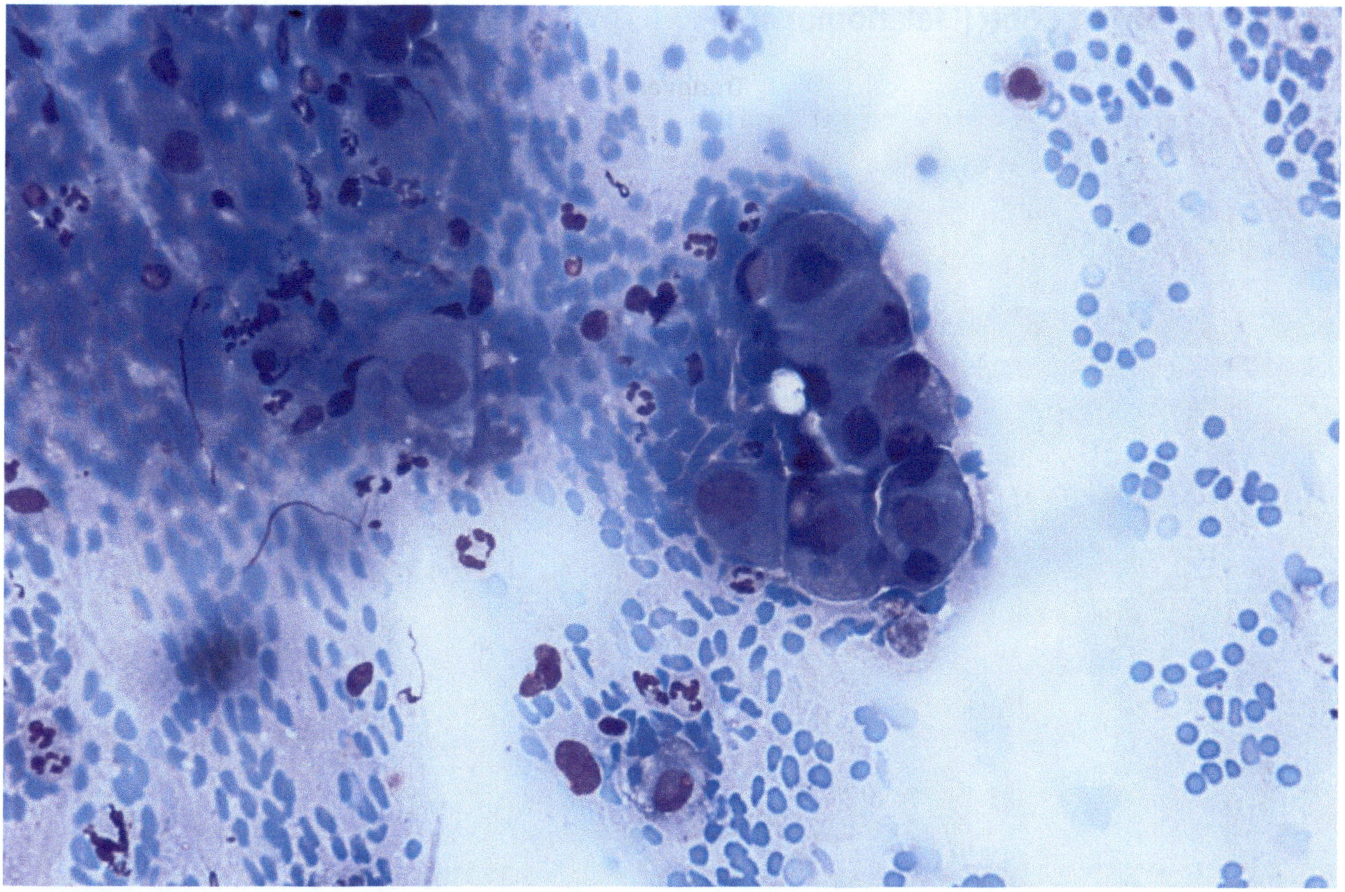

Figure 12-9. Cytology: carcinoma cells, metastasis from mucinous adenocarcinoma.

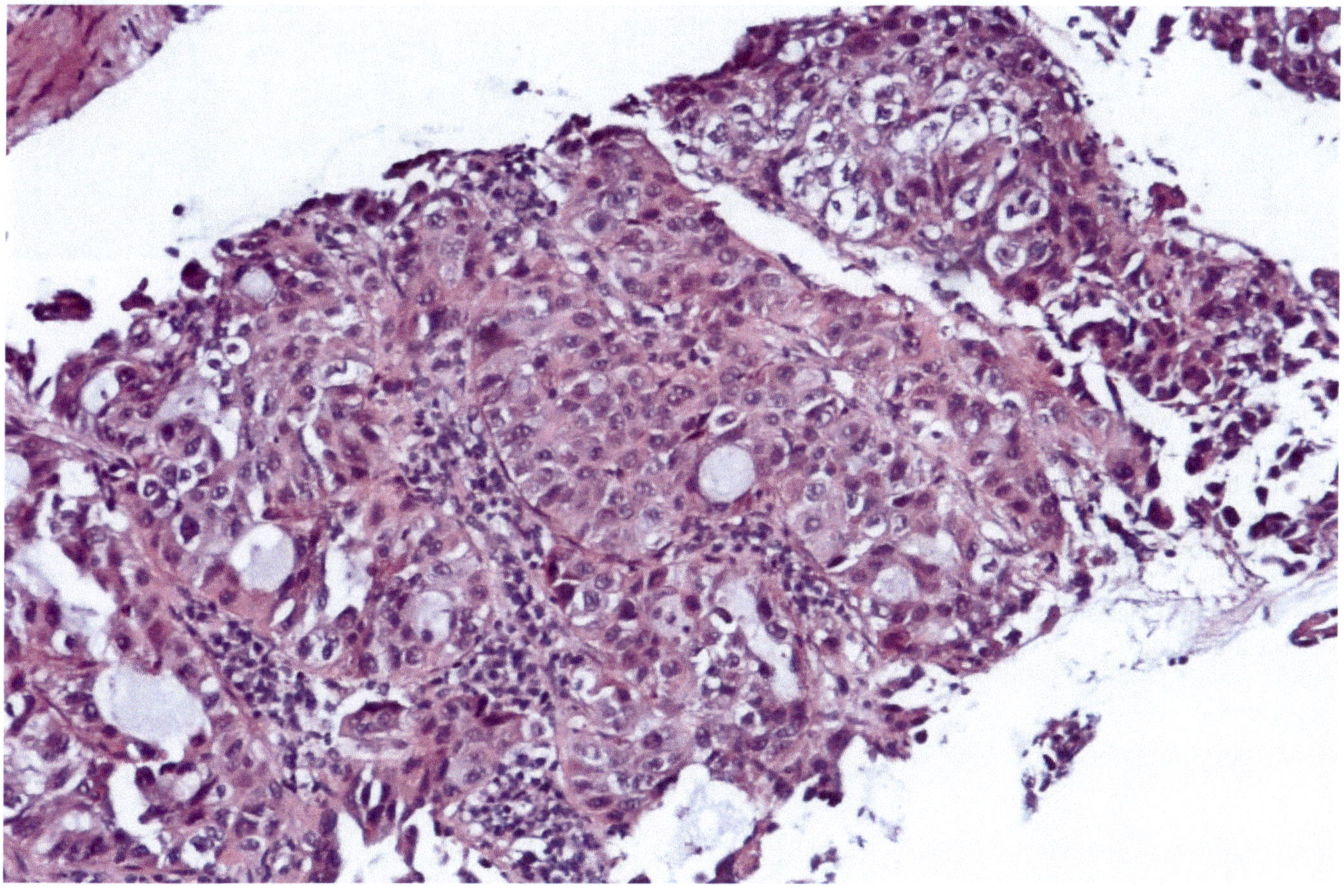

Figure 12-10. Histologic needle biopsy: metastasis from mucinous adenocarcinoma, poorly differentiated.

Metastasis Right Lobe (Melanoma)

Transverse

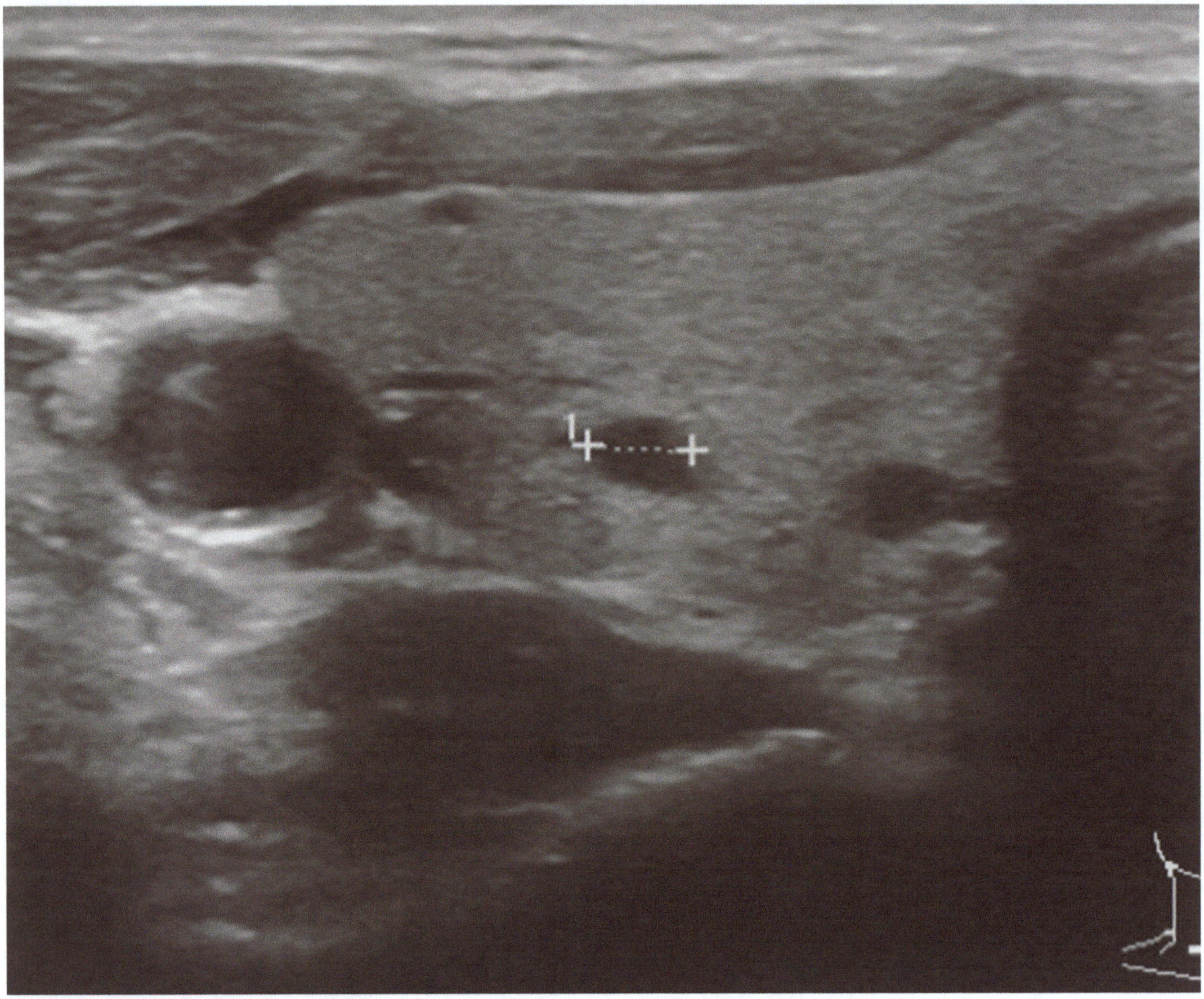

FIGURE 12-11. Ultrasound of metastasis from melanoma in the right lobe. Transverse diameter: 3 mm.

54-Year-old woman

- **Clinical history:** Surgery for skin melanoma on the back 12 years ago. April 2008 surgery for neck metastasis on right side. Controlled.
- **Ultrasound:** Two suspicious, 3 mm lesions in right thyroid lobe.
- **Cytology:** Metastasis from on the melanoma in central lesion.

Features of central lesion

Strongly hypoechoic/anechoic
Echo enhancement behind lesion
Sharply circumscribed

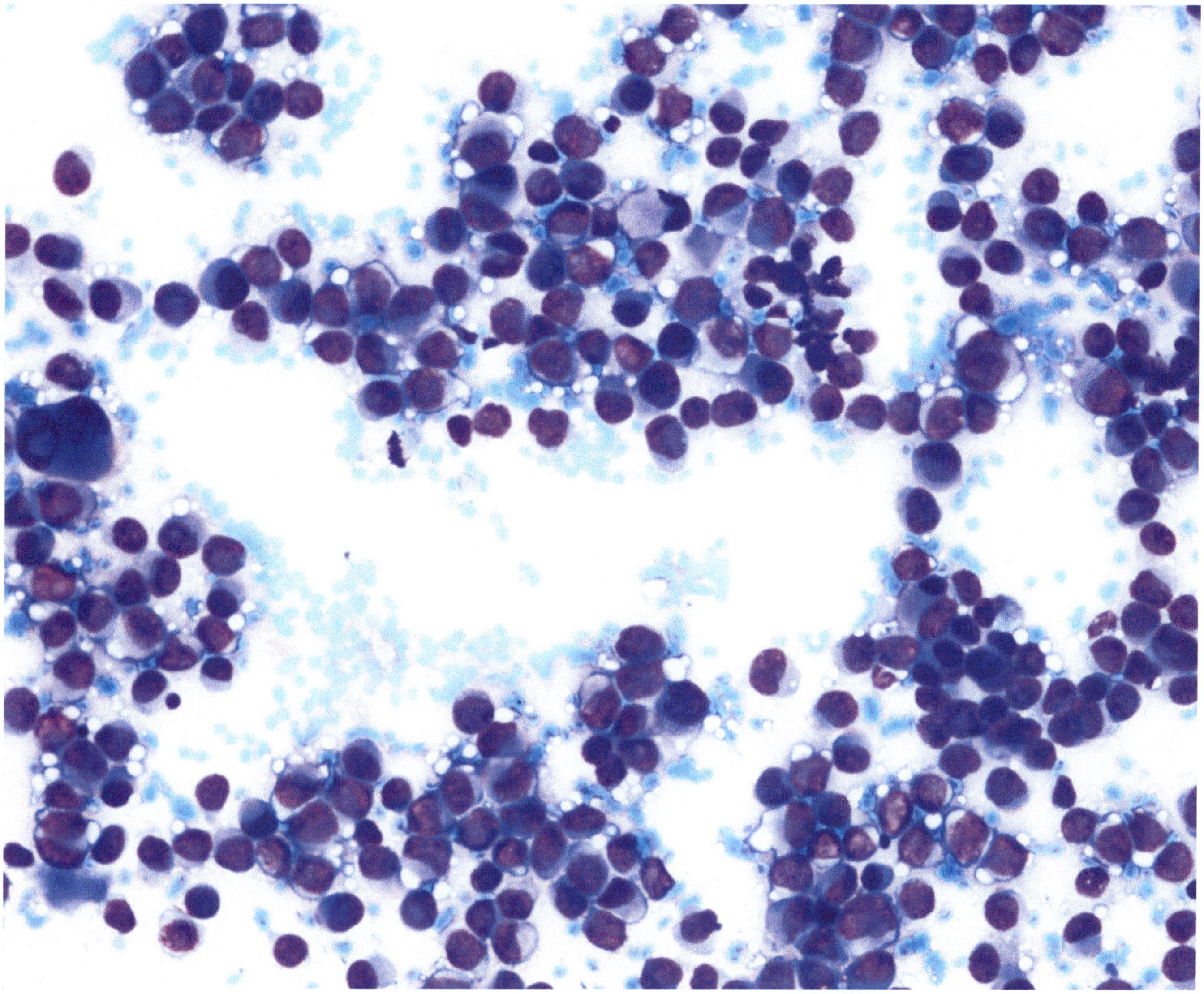

Figure 12-12. Cytology: metastasis from malignant melanoma. Dispersed malignant cells.

13 Regional Lymph Node Metastases

Regional lymph node metastases are a common finding in papillary and medullary carcinomas, but they are very rare in follicular carcinoma because this tumor usually spreads hematogenically. Lymph node affection is often seen in thyroid lymphomas, and reactive lymph nodes are found in thyroiditis. Reactive lymph nodes are usually enlarged, but metastatic infiltration does not necessarily cause enlargement. Thus, lymph node size is not a reliable criterion in the differential diagnosis [6,23].

Most normal neck lymph nodes are flat or oval shaped like an almond or a grape. Malignant lymph nodes usually have a more round shape, or they may show eccentric cortical hypertrophy due to focal infiltration [23,24]. Metastases, however, are also found in normally shaped lymph nodes. The echo pattern of these normal lymph nodes consists of a moderately hypoechoic cortex and a hyperechoic medulla and hilum. Low-velocity color Doppler demonstrates scant vascularity in the hilum and medulla.

Lymph nodes with metastastic infiltration from papillary thyroid carcinoma may have normal size and shape, but most often they will be enlarged with a more round shape. They may be partially or completely cystic [4,6,24], but both cystic and solid metastases can be found at the same time. The solid metastases often have a grayish heterogeneous echo pattern in the whole lymph node, or they may show thickened hypoechoic cortex with compressed or lost echogenic medulla and hilum like other lymph node metastases. The lymph node capsule is most often sharply defined, but infiltration through the capsule causes blurred margins.

The most striking features indicating metastatic lymph node infiltration from papillary thyroid carcinoma (PTC) are increased blood flow in pathologic vessels in the cortex, microcalcifications, cystic degeneration, and heterogeneous echo pattern [6]. Sometimes a pathologic vascularity is virtually the only sign of metastasis. Microcalcifications are often found in both papillary and medullary carcinoma, but the calcifications from medullary carcinoma may be more coarse, like in the primary tumor [6].

The location of neck metastases in this atlas refers to the map made by the American Joint Committee on Cancer having segments from 1-7, see page 4.

Features

Microcalcifications
Pathologic vascularity
Cystic
Heterogeneous echo pattern

Cytologic Morphology

Until a few years ago, the most frequent difficulties when examining smears from neck lymph nodes were deciding the etiology of a cystic specimen and clarifying whether the material could originate from a cystic lymph node metastasis from PTC. This was because many of these cystic specimens did not demonstrate atypical epithelium, or epithelium at all. With the aid of thyroglobulin measurement in wash-out specimens, most of these metastases were easily and reliably confirmed. Non-cystic metastases from well-differentiated PTC are usually no challenge for the experienced cytopathologist. Metastases from malignancies originating in other organs can, however, sometimes be difficult to classify. The finding of atypical epithelium with no characteristic features for PTC, especially when a thyroid tumor is not found on ultrasound examination, should make the cytopathologist analyze the specimen more thoroughly and ask for additional material for further and extended investigation. Metastases from well-differentiated PTC may demonstrate a picture almost devoid of cytologic atypia, misleading the cytopathologist to think that it represents an aberrant/ectopic thyroid gland. In these cases the information from the radiologist concerning the exact location of the lesion will be of crucial importance, as well as the information concerning lesions located within the thyroid gland.

Lymph Node Metastases from Papillary Thyroid Carcinoma: Left Levels III and IV

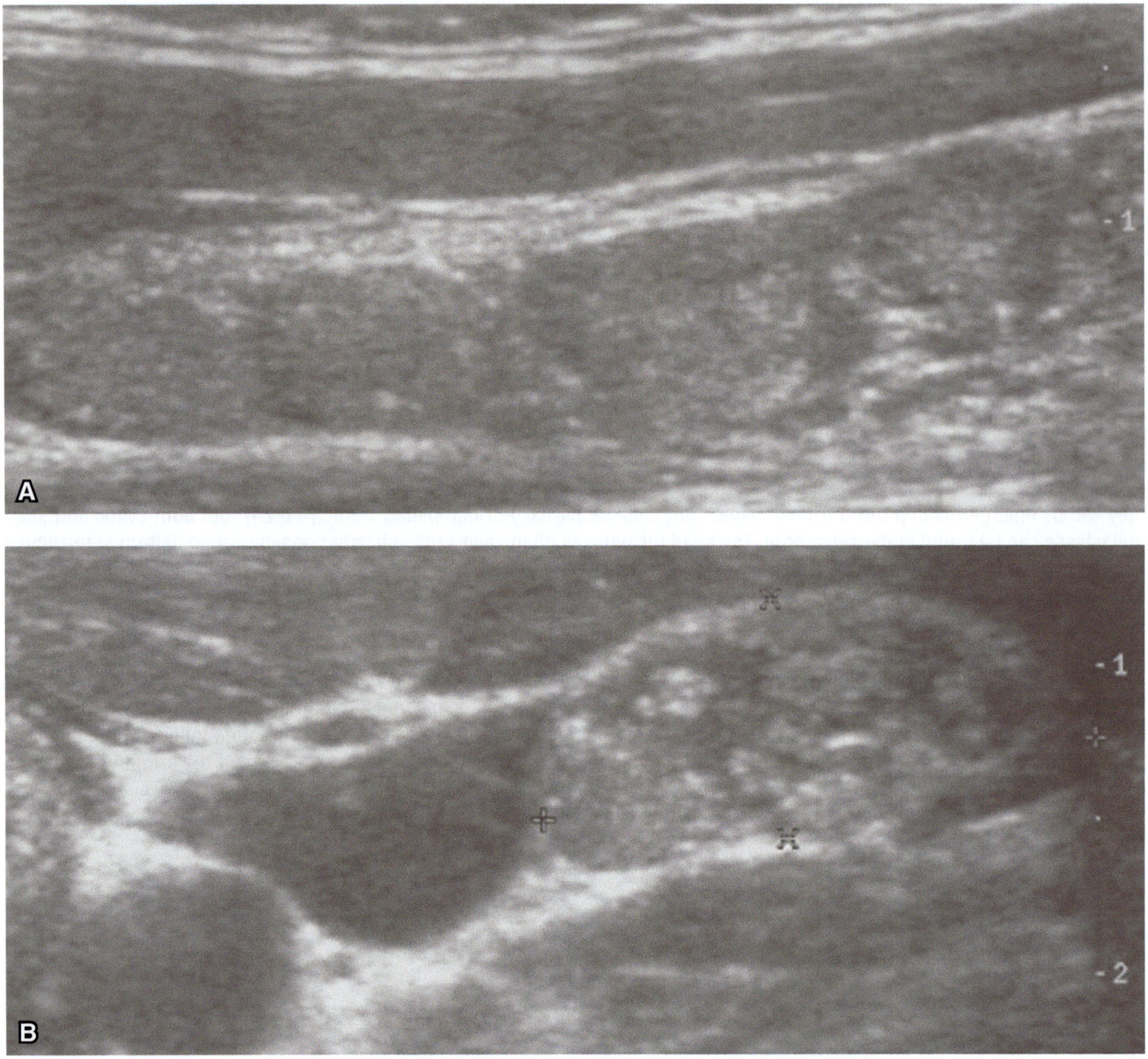

Figure 13-1. Ultrasound of lymph node metastases from papillary thyroid carcinoma: left levels III and IV. **A**, Longitudinal transverse diameter: 13 mm. **B**, Transverse, 8 x 18 mm.

Features

Chain of enlarged pathologic lymph nodes
Pathologic shape
Heterogeneous, light grayish echo pattern
Microcalcifications
Quite sharply defined capsules

Lymph Node Metastasis from Papillary Thyroid Carcinoma: Right Level IV

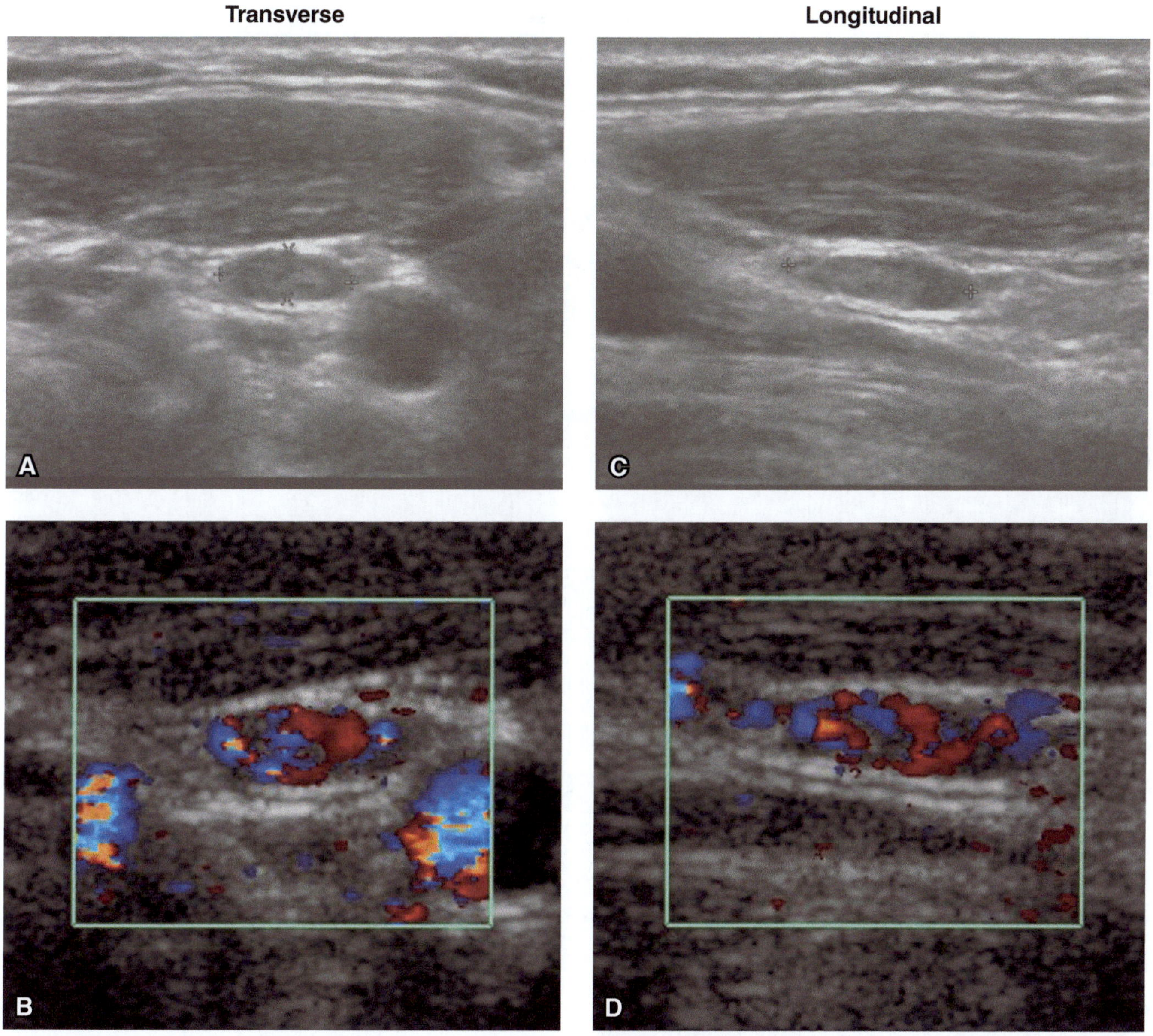

FIGURE 13-2. Ultrasound of lymph node metastasis from papillary thyroid carcinoma: right level IV. **A**, Transverse, 3 x 7 mm. **B**, Color Doppler, transverse. **C**, Longitudinal, sagittal diameter: 10 mm. **D**, Color Doppler, longitudinal.

Features

Normal shape
Normal size
Somewhat heterogeneous echo pattern
Typical malignant hypervascularity
Sharply defined capsule

Transverse

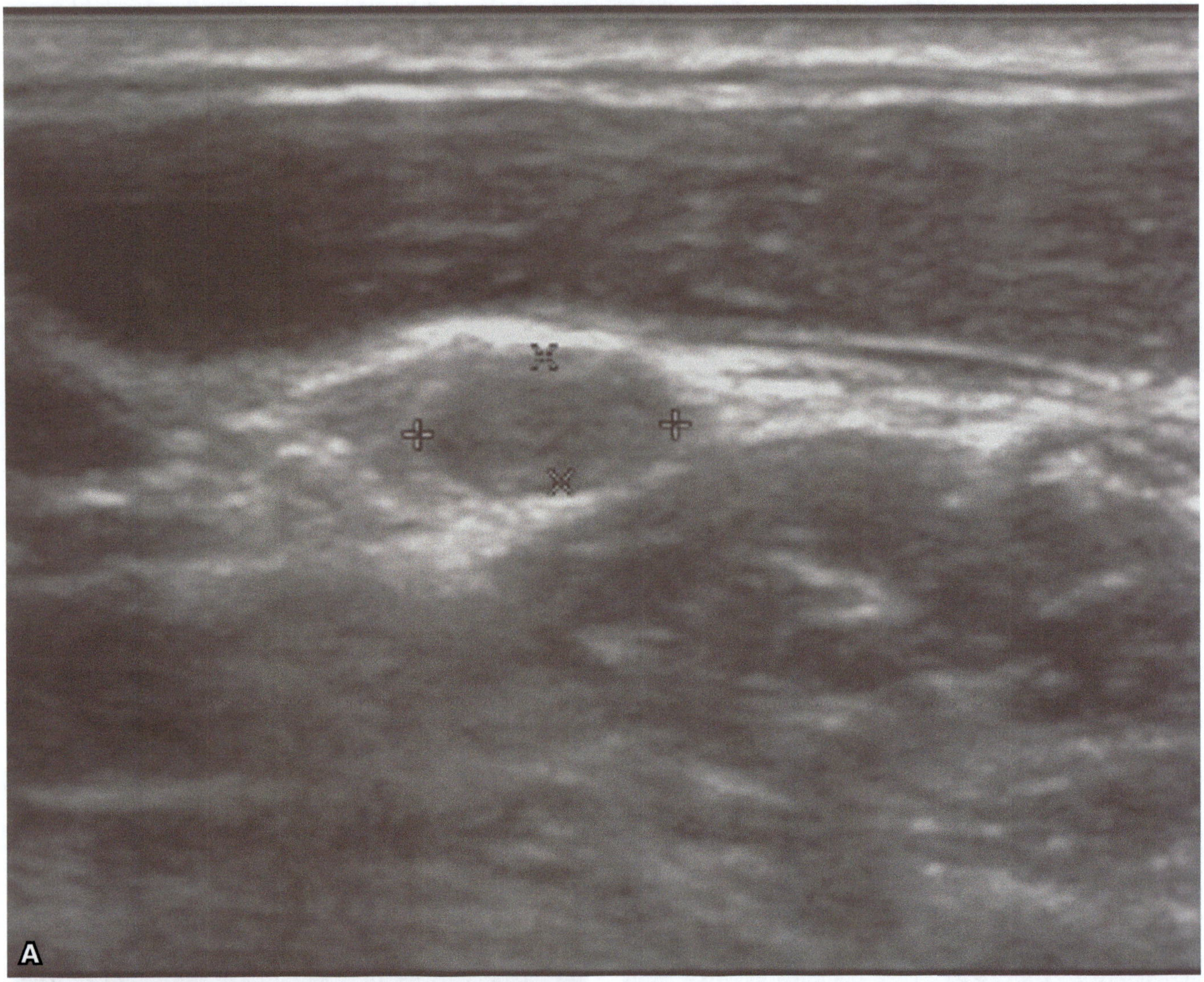

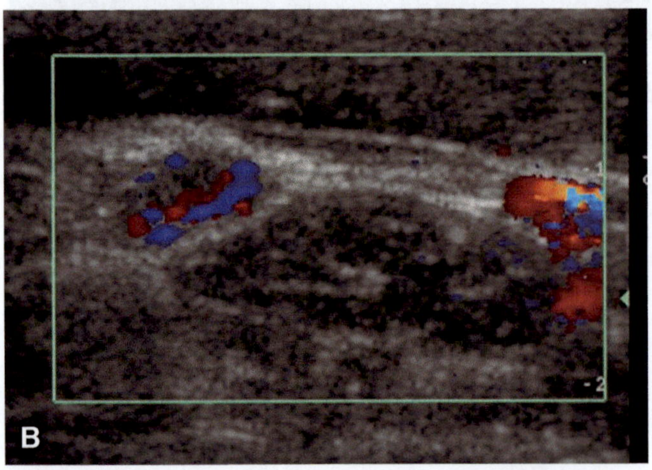

Features

Normal shape
Normal size
Heterogeneous echo pattern
Typical malignant hypervascularity
Sharply defined capsule

Figure 13-3. Ultrasound of lymph node metastasis from papillary thyroid carcinoma: right side level VI. **A**, Transverse, 3 x 6 mm. **B**, Color Doppler, transverse.

Lymph Node Metastasis from Papillary Thyroid Carcinoma: Right Level III

Transverse

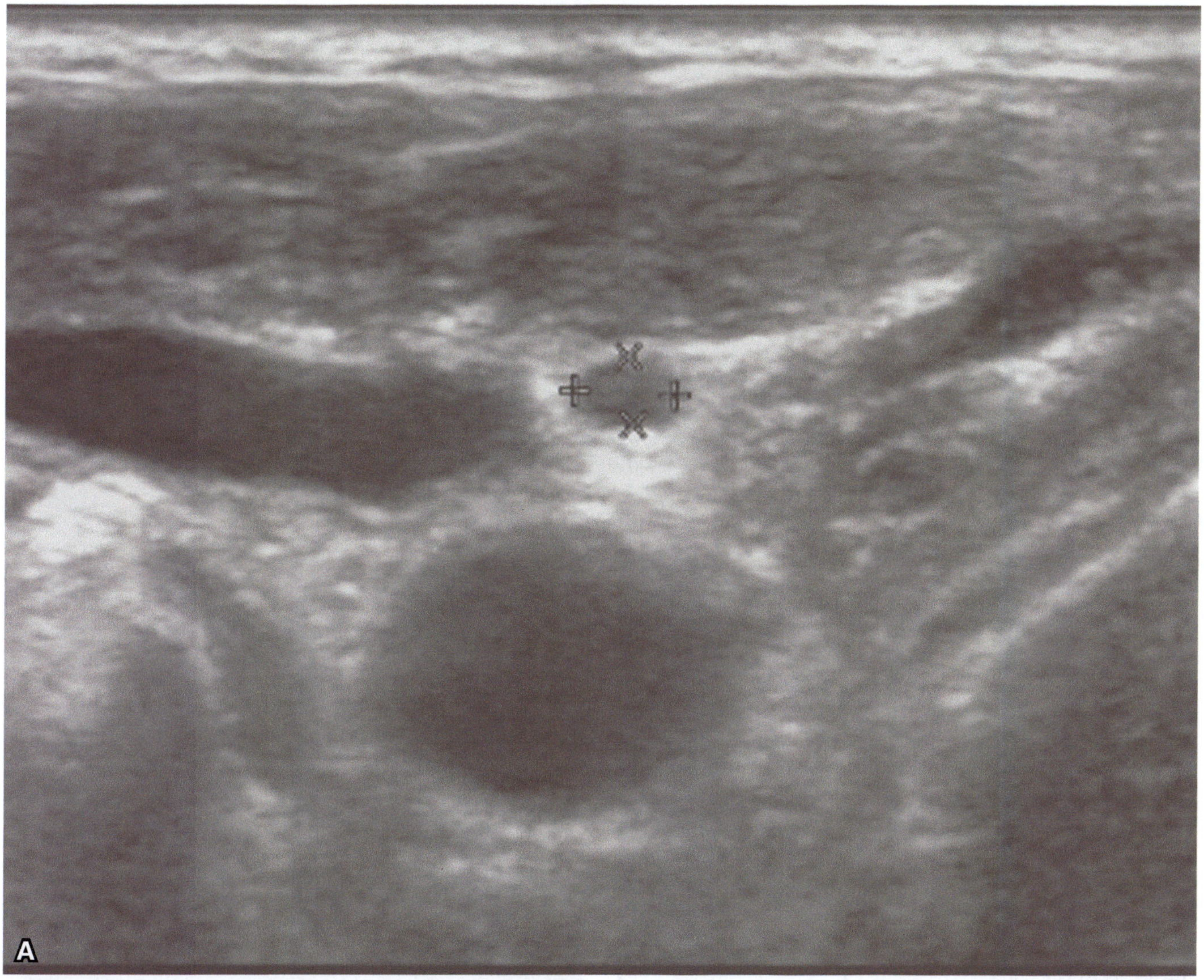

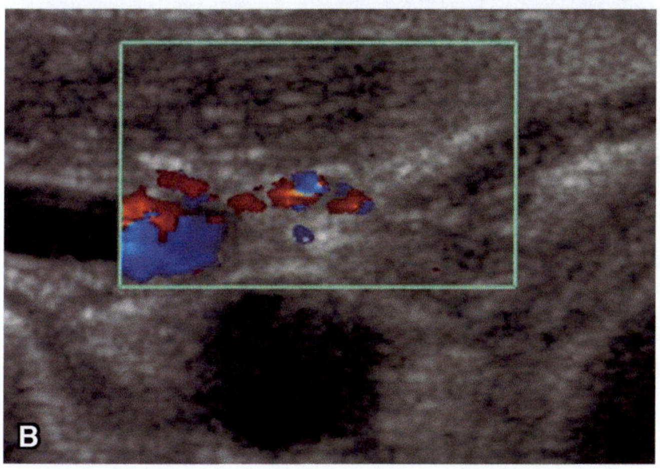

Features

Round shape
Hypoechoic without hyperechoic hilum
Hypervascularity
Sharply defined capsule

Figure 13-4. Ultrasound of lymph node metastasis from papillary thyroid carcinoma: right level III. **A**, Transverse, 1.7 x 2.5 mm. **B**, Color Doppler, transverse.

Longitudinal

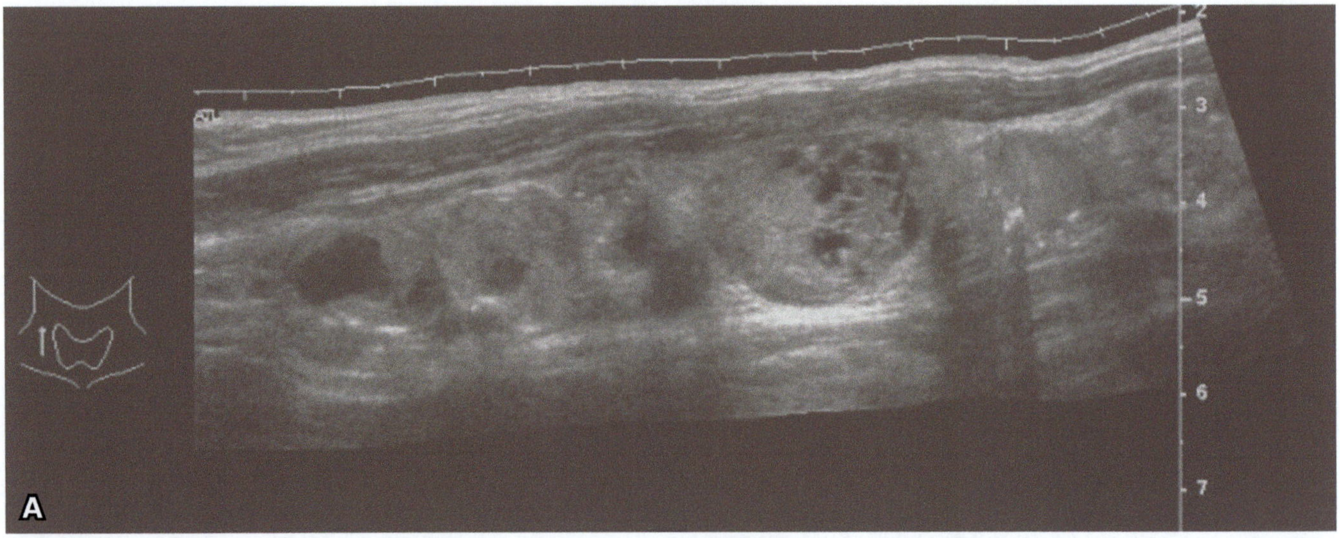

Transverse

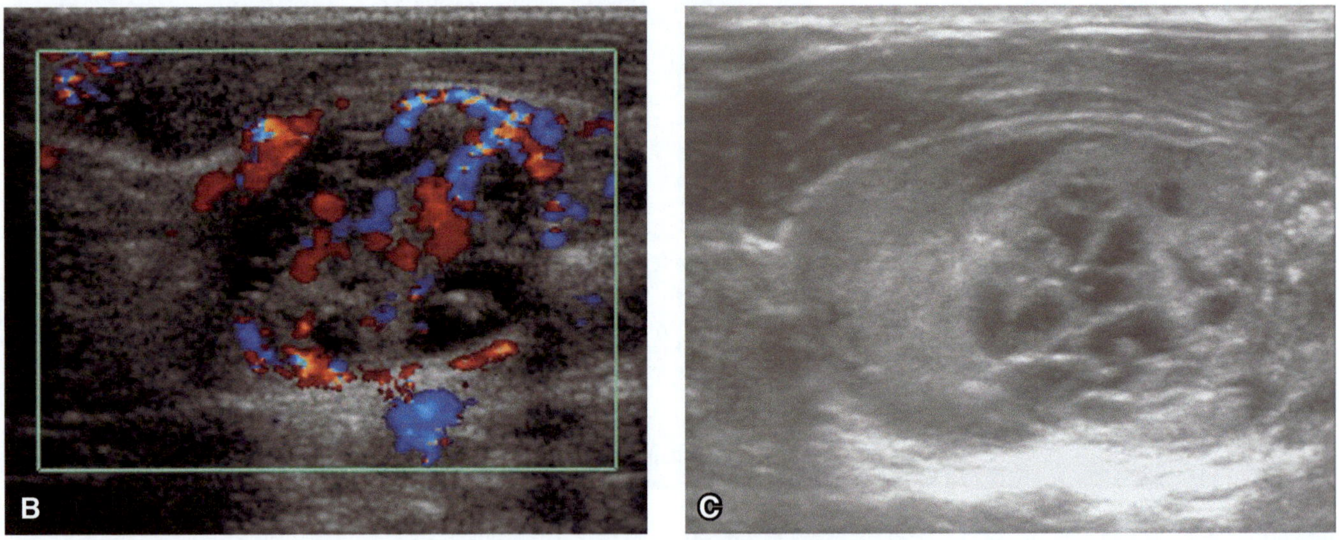

Figure 13-5. Ultrasound of lymph node metastases from papillary thyroid carcinoma: right levels III and IV. **A**, Longitudinal, **B**, Color Doppler, transverse. **C**, Transverse.

Features

Chain of partially cystic lymph nodes
Heterogeneous, grayish echo pattern
Microcalcifications
Typical malignant, peripheral vascularity
Quite sharply defined capsules

Lymph Node Metastasis from Papillary Thyroid Carcinoma: Right Level IV

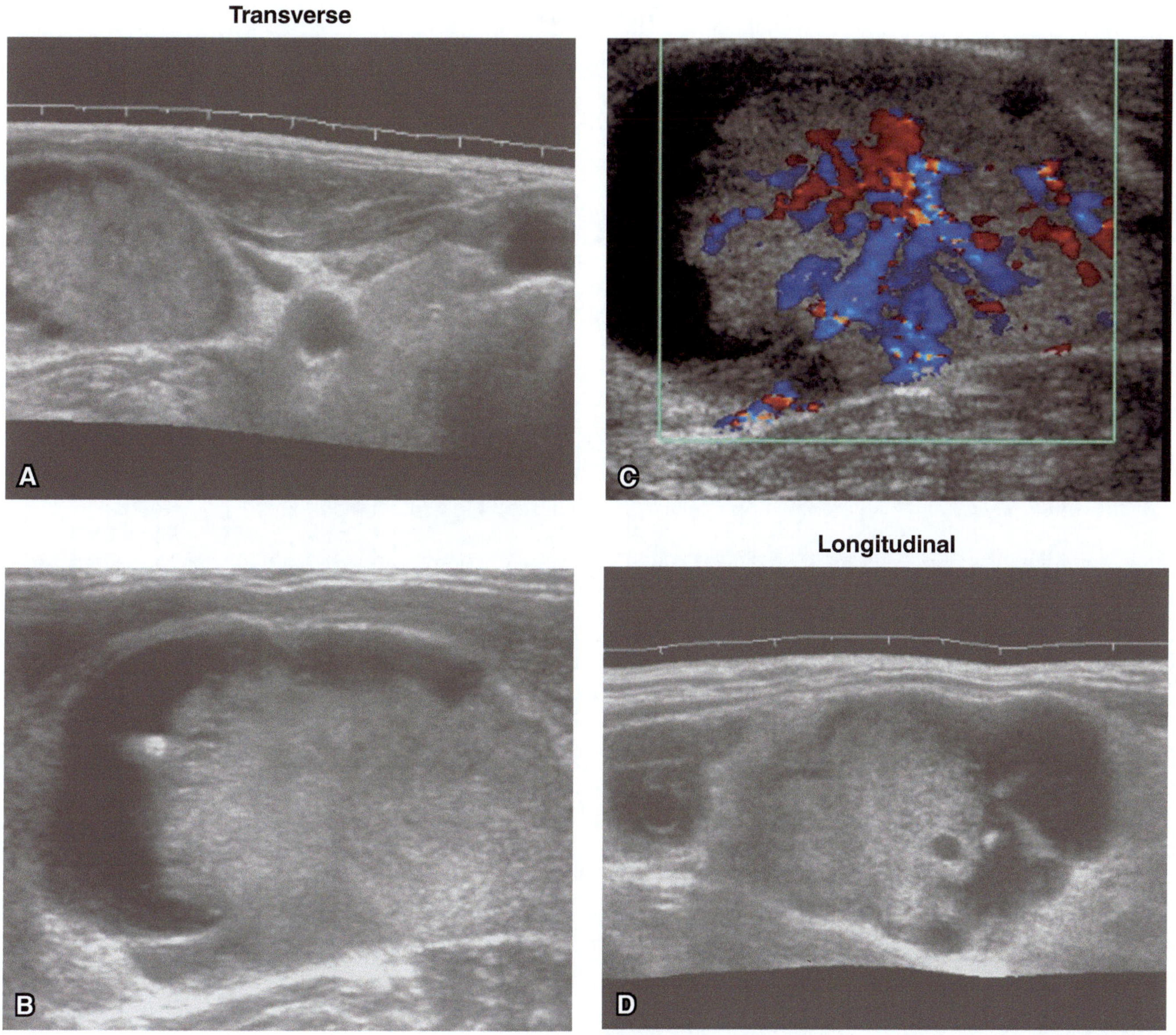

Figure 13-6. Ultrasound of lymph node metastasis from papillary thyroid carcinoma: right level IV. **A**, Transverse diameter: 35 mm. **B**, Transverse. **C**, Color Doppler, transverse. **D**, Longitudinal.

Features
Enlarged
Partially cystic
Hypervascular
Sharply defined capsule

Lymph Node Metastasis from Papillary Thyroid Carcinoma: Left Level III

Transverse

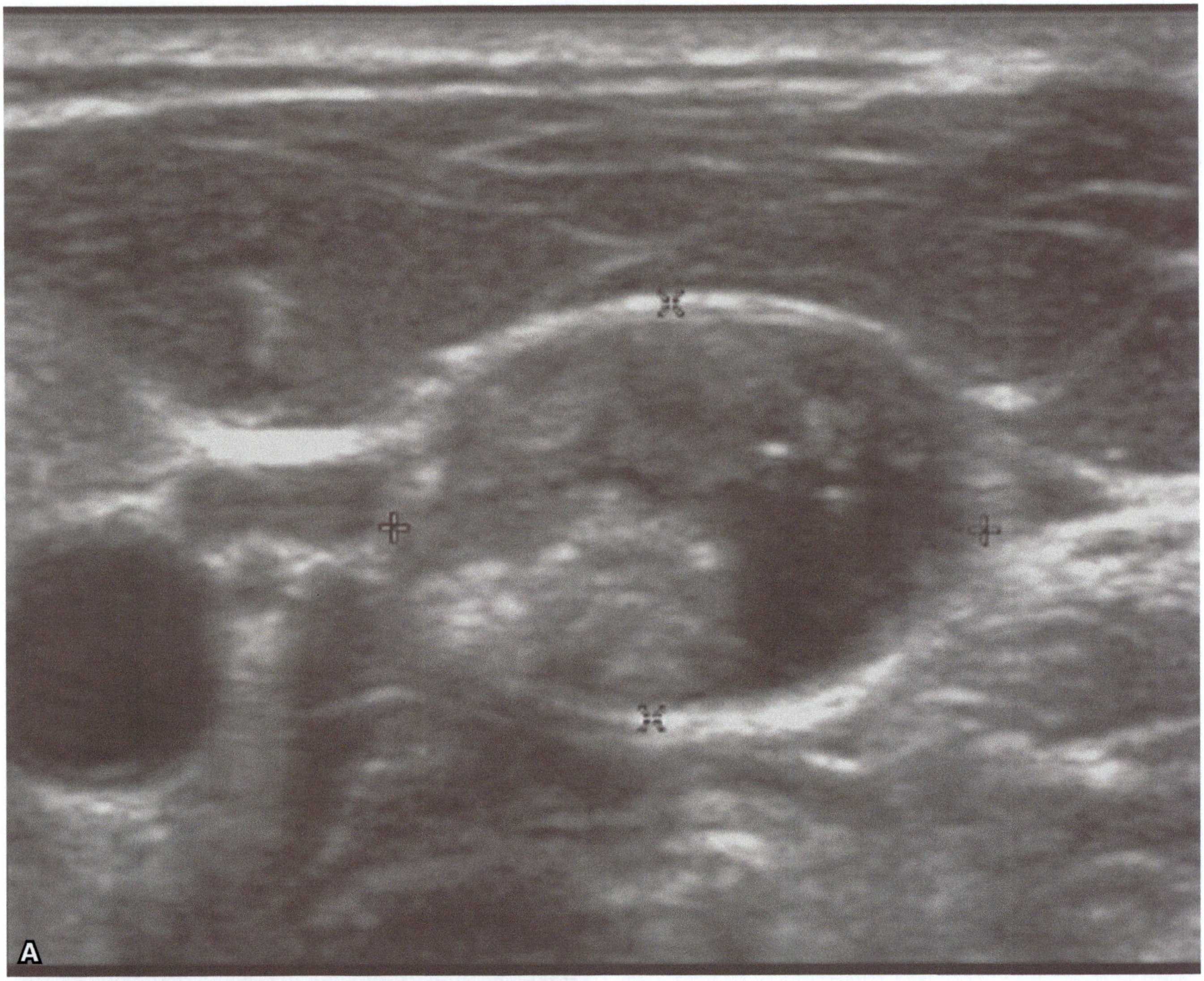

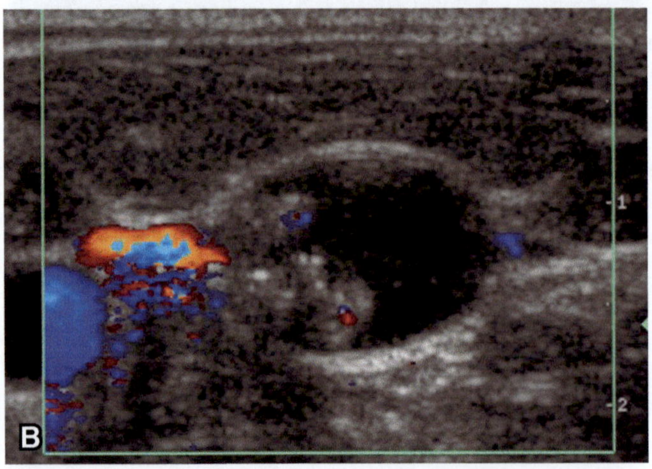

Figure 13-7. Ultrasound of lymph node metastasis from papillary thyroid carcinoma: left level III. **A**, Transverse, 11 x 15 mm. **B**, Color Doppler, transverse.

Features

Enlarged
Mostly cystic
Heterogeneous echo pattern in solid tissue
Microcalcifications
Almost avascular
Sharply defined capsule

Transverse

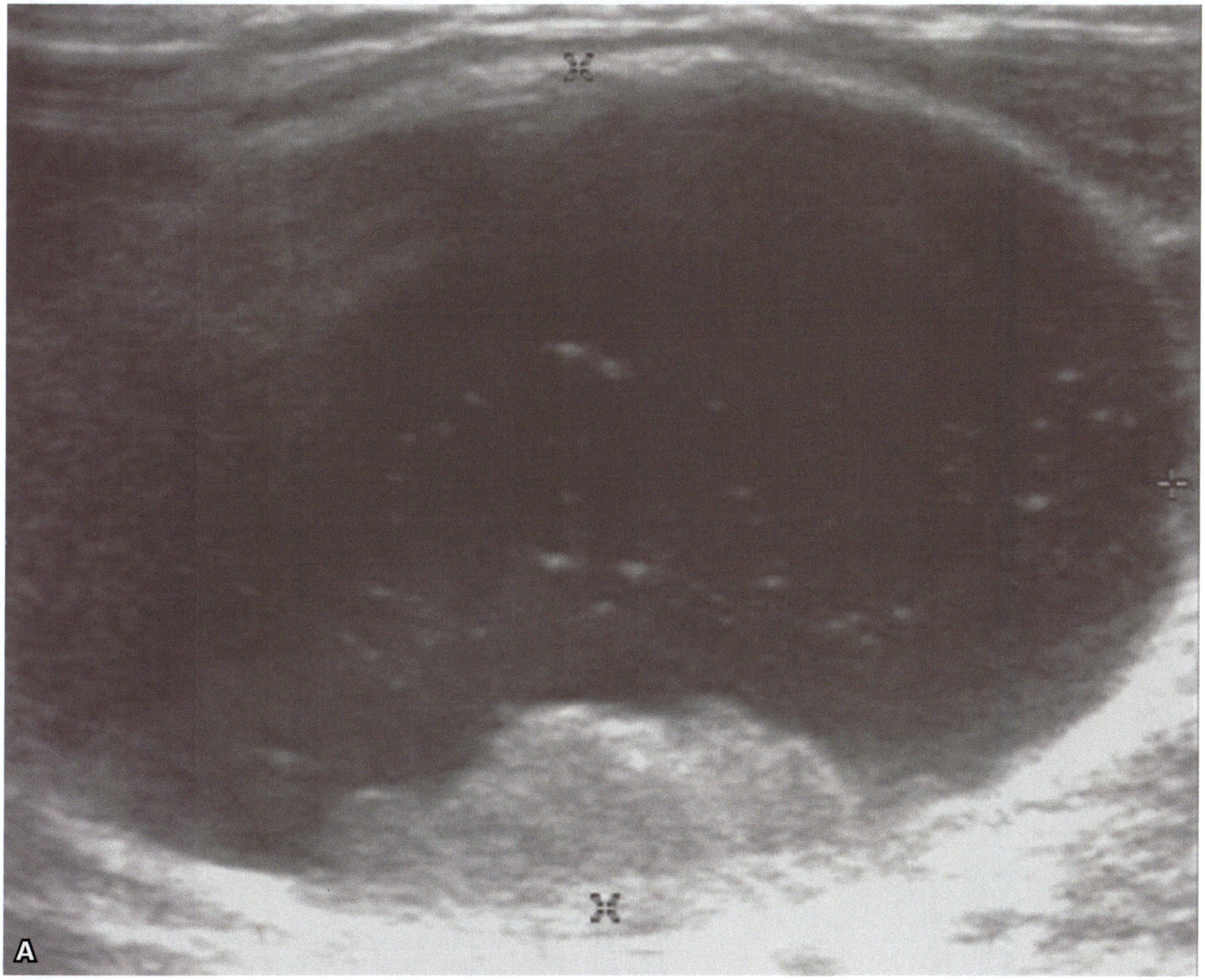

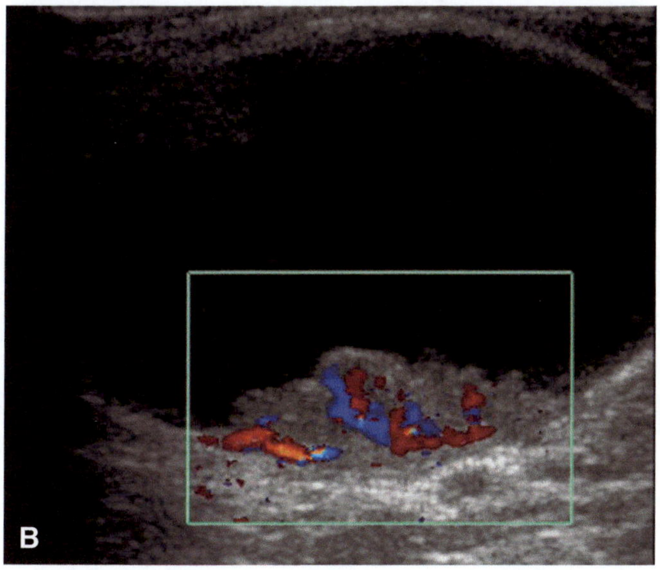

Features
Enlarged
Mostly cystic
Homogeneous echo pattern in solid tissue
Pathologic vascularity
Sharply defined capsule

Figure 13-8. Ultrasound of lymph node metastasis from papillary thyroid carcinoma: right level IV. **A**, Transverse, 26 x 37 mm. **B**, Color Doppler, transverse.

Lymph Node Metastasis from Follicular Variant of Papillary Thyroid Carcinoma: Right Level IV

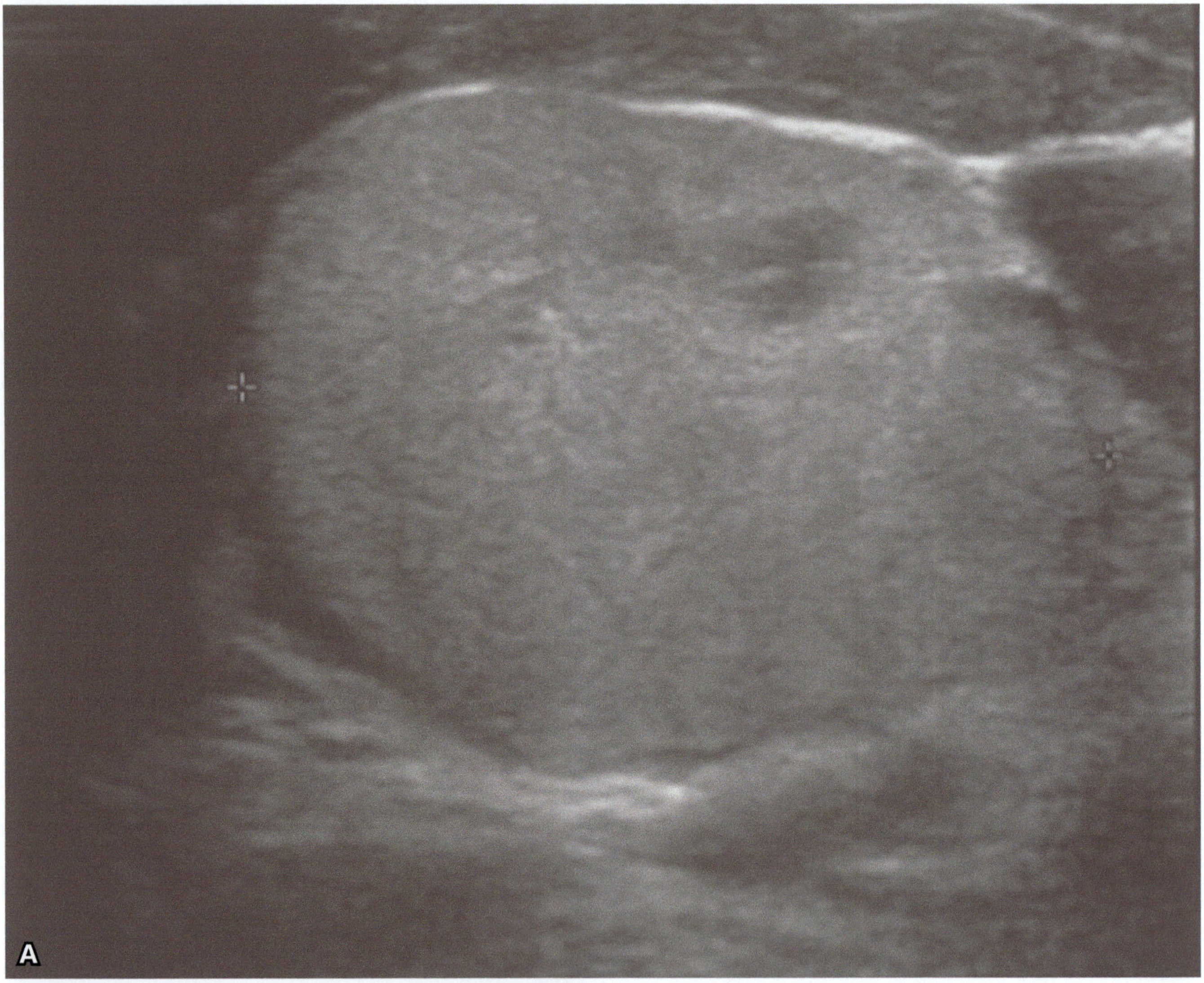

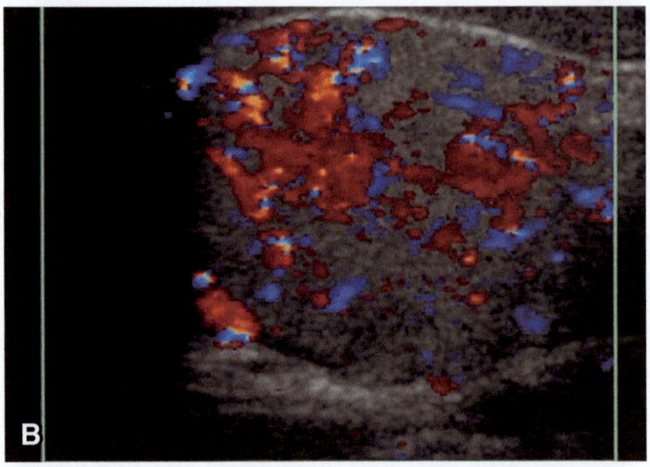

Features
Enlarged
Hyperechoic homogeneous echo pattern
Hypervascular
Sharply defined capsule

Figure 13-9. Ultrasound of lymph node metastasis from follicular variant of papillary thyroid carcinoma: right level IV. **A**, Transverse diameter: 27 mm. **B**, Color Doppler, transverse.

Transverse

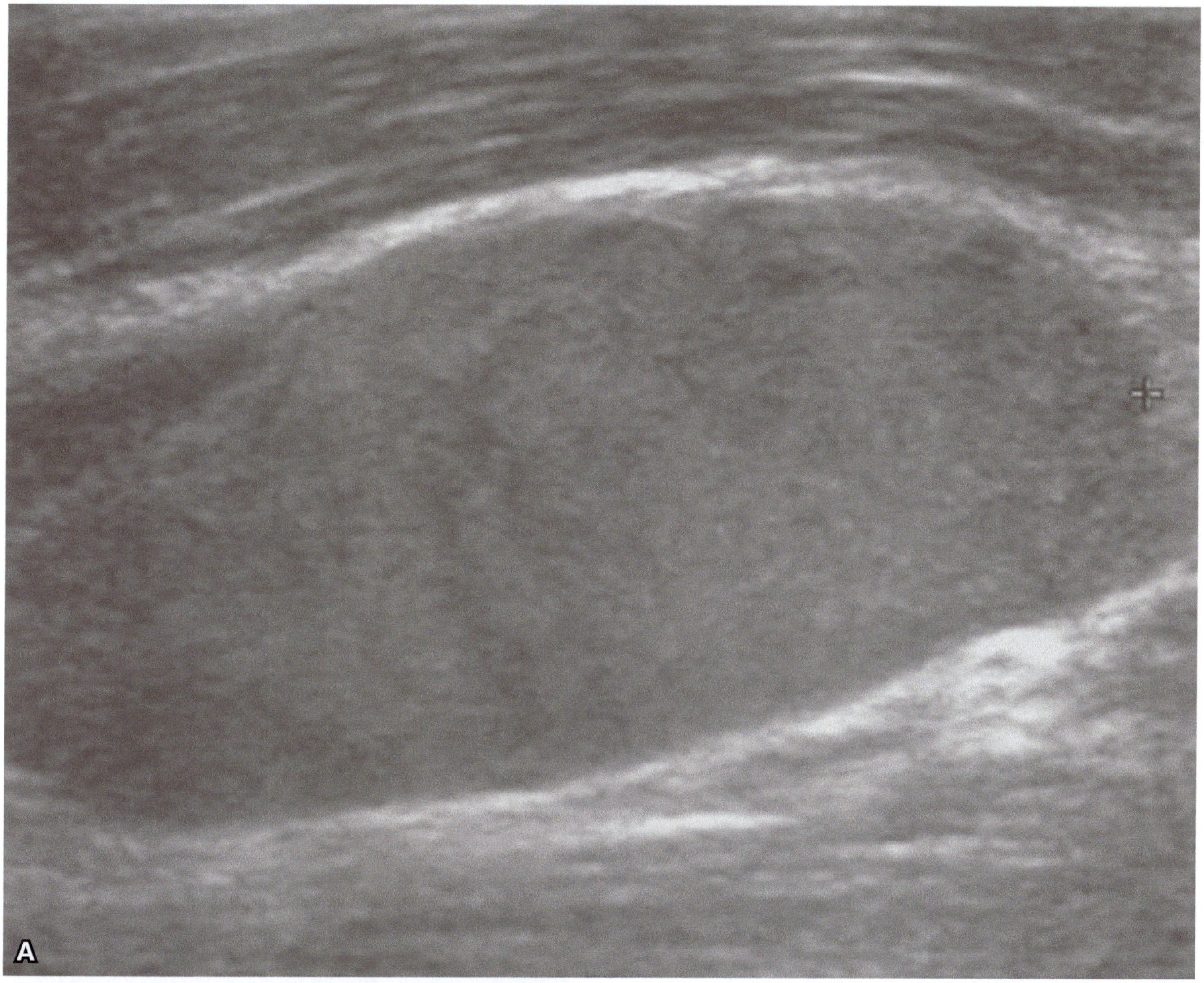

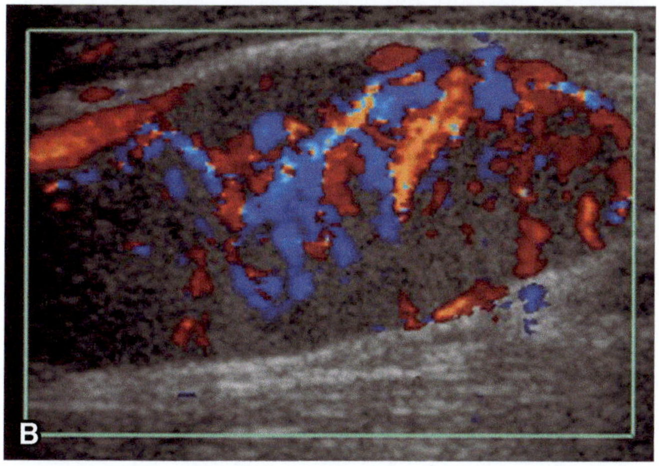

Features
Enlarged
Heterogeneous, dark grayish echo pattern
Typical malignant hypervascularity
Sharply defined capsule

Figure 13-10. Ultrasound of lymph node metastasis from medullary thyroid carcinoma: right level III. **A**, Transverse, sagittal diameter: 37 mm. **B**, Color Doppler, transverse.

Lymph Node Metastasis from Medullary Thyroid Carcinoma: Left Level IV

Longitudinal

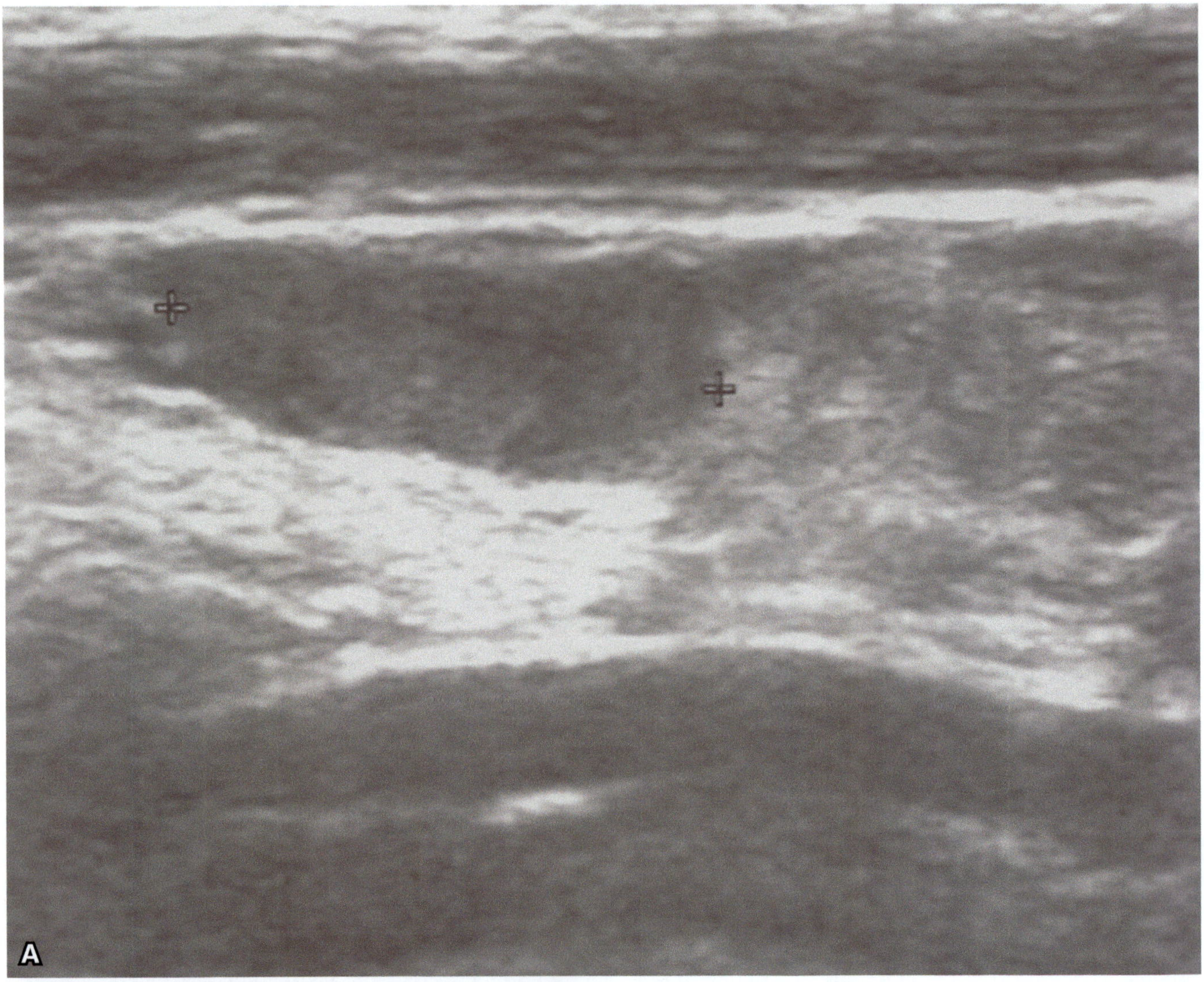

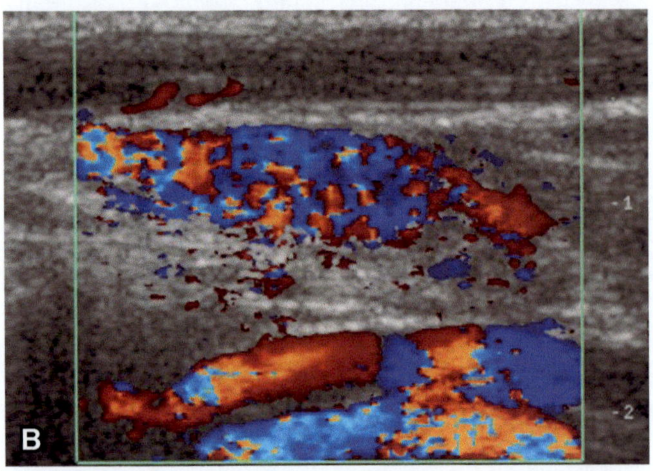

FIGURE 13-11. Ultrasound of lymph node metastasis from medullary thyroid carcinoma: left level IV. **A**, Longitudinal, sagittal diameter: 13 mm. **B**, Color Doppler, longitudinal.

Features

Abnormal shape
Heterogeneous, grayish echo pattern
Malignant hypervascularity
Sharply defined capsule

Lymph Node Metastasis from Medullary Thyroid Carcinoma: Right Level IV

Transverse

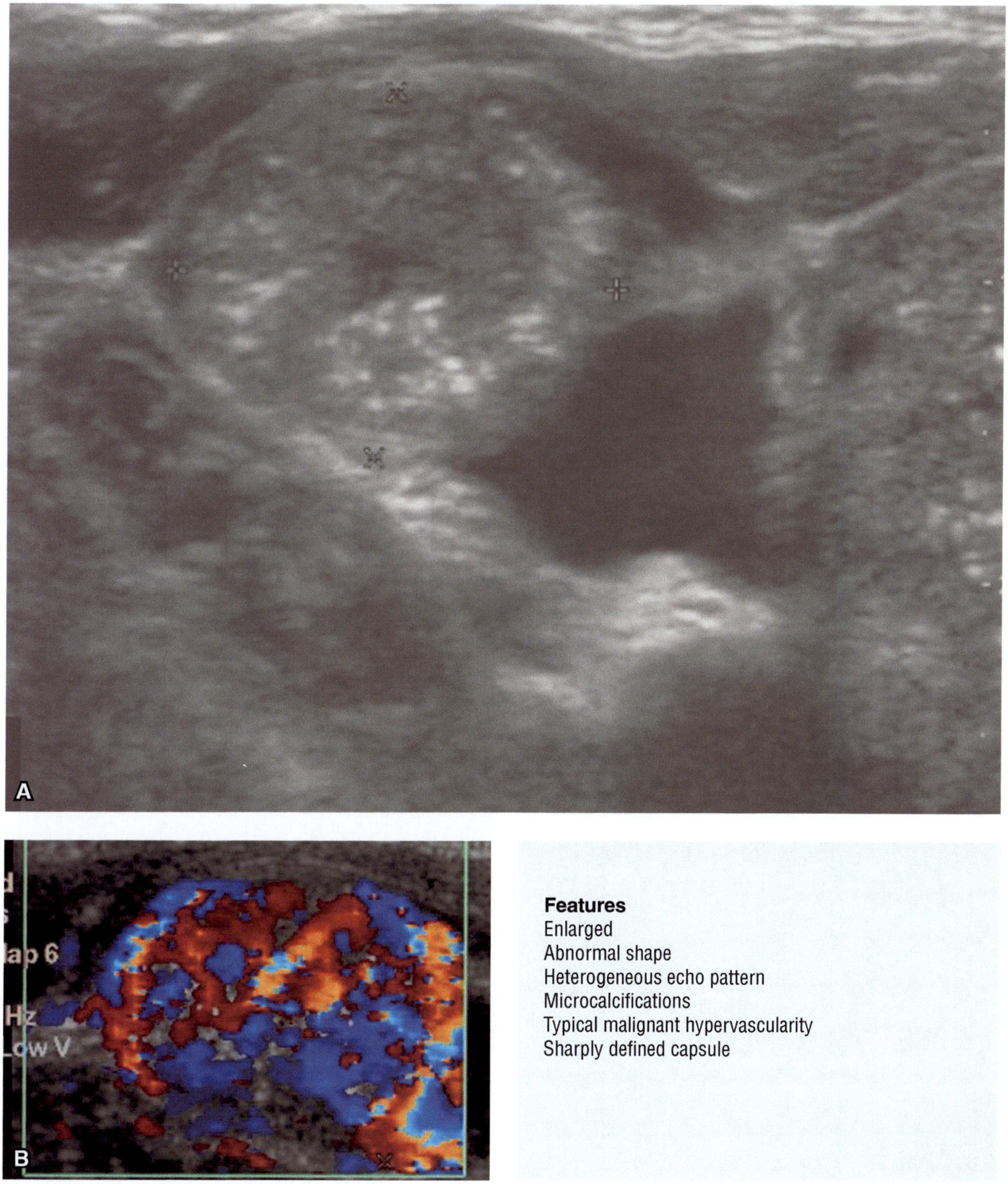

Features
Enlarged
Abnormal shape
Heterogeneous echo pattern
Microcalcifications
Typical malignant hypervascularity
Sharply defined capsule

Figure 13-12. Ultrasound of lymph node metastasis from medullary thyroid carcinoma: right level IV. **A**, Transverse, 12 x 15 mm. **B**, Color Doppler, transverse.

Transverse

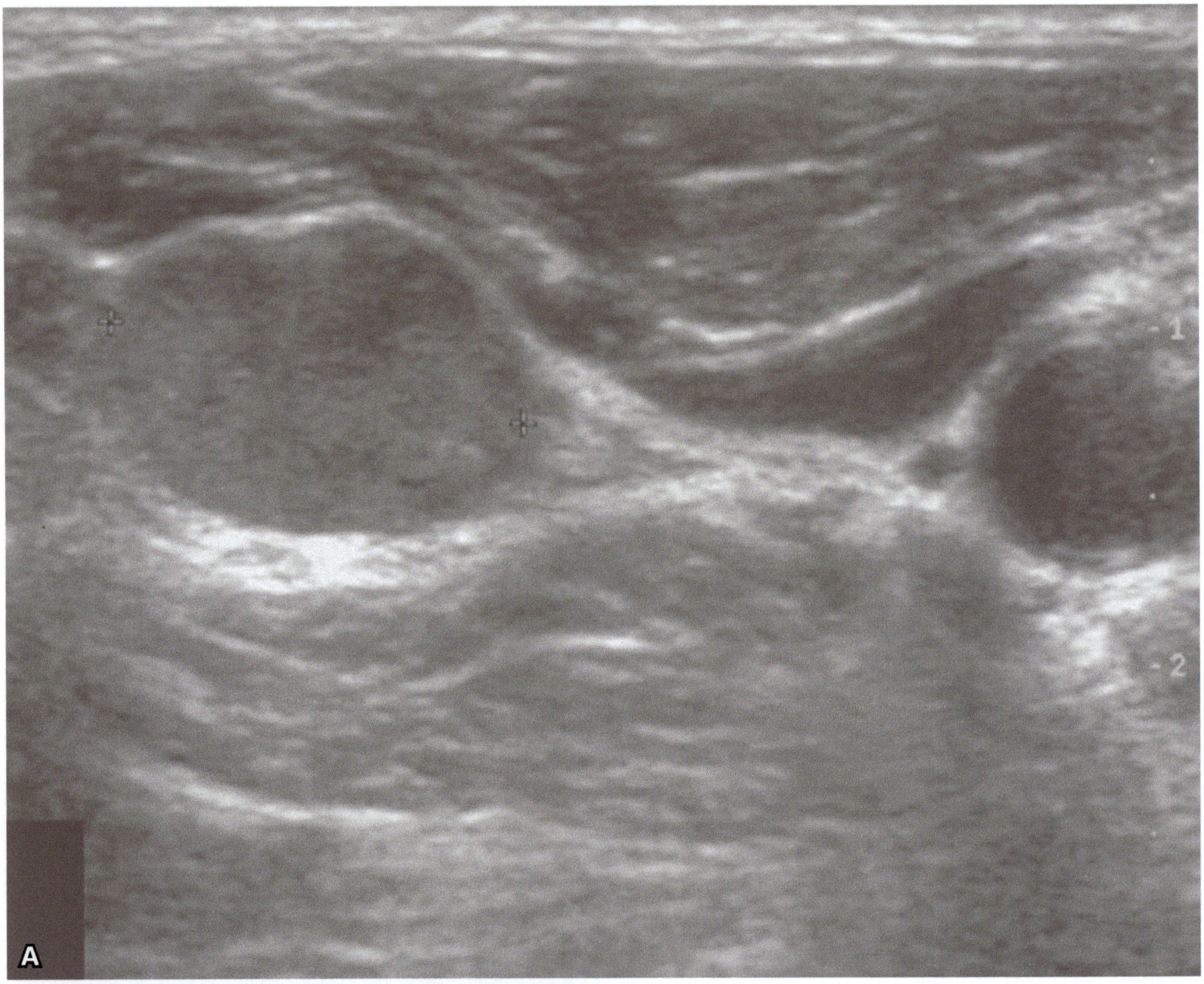

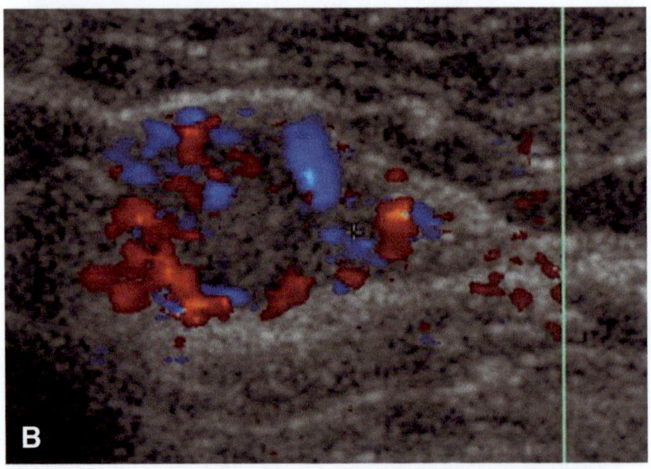

Features
Pathologic shape
Heterogeneous, dark grayish echo pattern
Typical malignant peripheral vascularity
Sharply defined capsule

Figure 13-13. Ultrasound of lymph node metastasis from anaplastic carcinoma: right level IV. **A**, Transverse diameter: 13 mm. **B**, Color Doppler, transverse.

References

1. Manangement guidelines for patients with thyroid nodules and differentiated thyroid carcinoma. The American Thyroid Association Guidelines Taskforce. *Thyroid* 2006, 16:1–33.
2. European consensus for the management of patients with differentiated thyroid carcinoma of the follicular epithelium. *Eur J* of *Endocrinol* 2006, 154:787–803.
3. Nasjonale retningslinjer for diagnostikk, behandling og oppfølging av differensiert carcinoma thyroideae. http://www.kreftforeningen.no/vp/multimedia/archive/00003/Retningslinjer_differ_3352a.pdf.
4. Baskin HJ, Duick DS, Levine RA: *Thyroid Ultrasound and Ultrasound-Guided FNA*, edn 2. Springer; New York: 2008.
5. Blank W, Braun B: Sonography of the thyroid – part 1. *Eur J Ultrasound* 2007, 6:555–568.
6. Solbiati L, Charboneau JW, Osti V, *et al.* The thyroid gland. In *Diagnostic Ultrasound*, edn 3. Edited by Rumack CM, Wilson SR, Charboneau JW and Johnson JA. Philadelphia: Mosby; 2005.
7. Wong KT, Ahuja AT. Ultrasound of thyroid carcinoma. *Carcinoma Imaging* 2005, 5:167–176.
8. Moon WJ, Jung SL, Lee JH, *et al.*: Benign and malignant nodules: US differentiation - multicenter retrospective study. *Radiology* 2008, 247:762–770.
9. Frates MC, Benson CB, Charboneau JW, *et al.*: Management of thyroid nodules detected at US: Society of Radiolgists in Ultrasound Consensus Conference Statement. *Radiology* 2005, 237:794–800.
10. Reading CC, Charboneau JW, Hay ID, Sebo TJ: Sonography of thyroid nodules: a "classic pattern" diagnostic approach. *Ultrasound* 2005, 21:157–165.
11. Kakkos SK, Scopa CD, Chalmoukis AK, *et al.*: Relative risk of carcinoma in sonographically detected thyroid nodules with calcifications. *J Clin Ultrasound* 2000, 28:347–352.
12. Takashima S, Fukuda H, Nomura N, *et al.*: Thyroid nodules: re-evaluation with ultrasound. *J Clin Ultrasound* 1995, 23:179–184.
13. Kim MJ, Kim EK, Kwak JY, *et al.*: Differentiation of thyroid nodules with macrocalcifications. *J Ultrasound Med* 2008, 27:1179–1184.
14. Roti E, Uberti EC, Bondanelli M, Braverman LE: Thyroid papillary carcinoma: a descriptive and meta-analysis study. *Eur J Endocrinol* 2008, 159:659–673.
15. Rago T, Vitti P, Chiovato L, *et al.*: Role of conventional ultrasonography and color flow-Doppler sonography in predicting malignancy in "cold" thyroid nodules. *Eur J Endocrinol* 1998, 138:41–46.
16. Frates MC, Benson CB, Doubilet PM, *et al.* Can color doppler sonography aid in the prediction of malignancy of thyroid nodules? *J Ultrasound Med* 2003, 22:127–131.
17. Salajegheh A, Petcu EB, Smith RA, Lam AKY: Follicular variant of papillary thyroid carcinoma: a diagnostic challenge for clinicians and cytopathologists. *Postgrad Med J* 2008, 84:78–82.
18. Chan BK, Desser TS, McDougall IR, *et al.*: Common and uncommon sonographic features of papillary thyroid carcinoma. *J Ultrasound Med* 2003, 22:1083–1090.
19. Leboulleux S, Baudin E, Travagli JP, Schlumberger M: Medullary thyroid carcinoma. *Clin Endocrinol* 2004, 61:299–310.
20. Takashima S, Morimoto S, Ikezoe J, *et al.*: Primary thyroid lymphoma: comparison of CT and US assessment. *Radiology* 1989, 171:439–443.
21. Chaganti S, Gurunathan RK, McNaboe EJ: Solitary extramedullary plasmacytoma of thyroid. A case report and review of literature. *The Internet Journal of Head and Neck Surgery.* http://www.ispub.com/ostia/index.php?xmlFilePath=journals/ijhns/vol2n1/thyroid.xml
22. Langer JE, Khan A, Nisebaum HL, *et al.*: Sonographic appearance of focal thyroiditis. *Am J Roentgenol* 2001, 176:751–754.
23. Ahuja A, Ying M: Sonography of neck lymph nodes. Part II: abnormal lymph nodes. *Clin Radiol* 2003, 58:359–366.
24. Wunderbaldinger P, Harisinghani MG, Hahn PF, *et al.*: Cystic lymph node metastases in papillary thyroid carcinoma. *Am J Roentgenol* 2002, 178:693–697.

Suggested Further Reading in Pathology

Zubair W, Baloch ZW, *et al.* Diagnostic terminology and morphologic criteria for cytologic diagnosis of thyroid lesions: a synopsis of the National Cancer Institute Thyroid Fine-Needle Aspiration State of the Science Conference. *Diagn Cytopathol* 2008, 36:425–437.

DeLellis RA, Lloyd RV, Heitz PU, Eng C, eds. WHO histological classification of thyroid and parathyroid tumours.

World Health Organization classification of tumours. In *Pathology and Genetics of Tumours of Endocrine Organs.* Lyon: IARC Press; 2004.

Orell SR, Philips J: *The Thyroid. Fine-Needle Biopsy and Cytological Diagnosis of Thyroid Lesions.* Basel: Karger AG; 1997.

Clark DP, Faquin C: *Thyroid Cytopathology.* New York, Springer: 2005.

DeMay RM: *The Art and Science of Cytopathology.* Chicago: ASCP Press; 1996.

Index

A

B

C

D

E

F

G

H

I

L

M

N

O

P

R

S

T

U

V

MIX
Papier aus verantwortungsvollen Quellen
Paper from responsible sources
FSC® C105338

If you have any concerns about our products,
you can contact us on
ProductSafety@springernature.com

In case Publisher is established outside the EU,
the EU authorized representative is:
Springer Nature Customer Service Center GmbH
Europaplatz 3, 69115 Heidelberg, Germany

Printed by Libri Plureos GmbH
in Hamburg, Germany